Core Curriculum for
Neonatal Intensive Care Nursing

Core Curriculum for Neonatal Intensive Care Nursing

Edited by

Patricia Beachy, RN, MS
Perinatal Program Coordinator
University Hospital
University of Colorado Health Sciences Center
Denver, Colorado

Jane Deacon, RNC, MS, NNP
Neonatal Nurse Practitioner
The Children's Hospital
Denver, Colorado

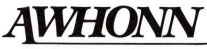

*Association of Women's Health,
Obstetric, and Neonatal Nurses*
——————— *(formerly naacog)*

W. B. SAUNDERS COMPANY
A Division of Harcourt Brace & Company
Philadelphia London Toronto Montreal Sydney Tokyo

W. B. SAUNDERS COMPANY
A Division of
Harcourt Brace & Company

The Curtis Center
Independence Square West
Philadelphia, PA 19106

Library of Congress Cataloging-in-Publication Data

Core curriculum for neonatal intensive care nursing / edited by
  Patricia Beachy, Jane Deacon.
       p.   cm.
    ISBN 0-7216-3121-5
    1. Neonatal intensive care.   I. Beachy, Patricia.
  II. Deacon, Jane.
    [DNLM: 1. Curriculum—outlines.   2. Education, Nursing—outlines.
  3. Intensive Care, Neonatal—methods—outlines.   WY 18 C7967]
  RJ253.5.C67   1992
  618.92'01—dc20

  DNLM/DLC   91-37727

Dedicated to:

Dave, Jamie, Kristy, and Becky
whose patience, understanding, encouragement, and support
have never wavered

Bruce, Jill, and Mark
for their patience and understanding
during the many hours spent working on this text

Contributors

Patricia Beachy, RN, MS • Perinatal Program Coordinator, University Hospital, University of Colorado Health Sciences Center; Clinical Faculty, School of Nursing, University of Colorado Health Sciences Center, Denver, Colorado • *Gastrointestinal Disorders*

Janice Bernhardt, RN, MS • Perinatal Clinical Specialist, Ramsey, New Jersey • *Renal/ Genitourinary Disorders*

Mary Ann Best, RN, PhD • Assistant Professor, The University of Texas School of Nursing at Galveston, Galveston, Texas • *The Family in Crisis*

Candice Cook Bowman, RN, MS • Lecturer, School of Nursing, University of Canberra, Australian Capital Territory, Australia • *The Teenage Family*

Margaret Brennan-Behm, RNC, MS • Adjunct Faculty, The University of Illinois at Chicago, Chicago, Illinois; Neonatal Clinical Nurse Specialist, Lutheran General Children's Medical Center, Park Ridge, Illinois • *Neonatal Nutrition*

Anne B. Broussard, RNC, MSN, ACCE • Assistant Professor and Coordinator of Maternal-Child Nursing, Department of Baccalaureate Nursing, College of Nursing, University of Southwestern Louisiana, Lafayette, Louisiana • *Antepartum-Intrapartum Complications*

Mary K. Buser, RNC, MS, NNP • Clinical Faculty, School of Nursing, University of Colorado Health Sciences Center; Nursing Director, Children's Emergency Transport Service and Department of Neonatal Nurse Practitioners, The Children's Hospital, Denver, Colorado • *Neonatal Transport*

Wendy Griffith Cornell, RNC, MS • Instructor, School of Nursing, University of Rochester; Interim Clinical Chief of Pediatric Nursing, University of Rochester Medical Center, Rochester, New York • *Research*

Pamela Creger, RN, BSN • Divisional Nursing Director, Maternal-Child Health, Medical Center Hospital, Odessa, Texas • *Developmental Support in the NICU*

Margaret Crockett, RNC, MSN, NNP • Neonatal Clinical Nurse Specialist, Sutter Memorial Hospital, Sacramento, California • *Cardiovascular Disorders*

Cindy Davis, RNC, MSN, NNP • Neonatal Nurse Practitioner, Presbyterian Hospital, Albuquerque, New Mexico • *Common Technical Procedures*

Jane Deacon, RNC, MS, NNP • Clinical Faculty, University of Colorado Health Sciences Center, School of Nursing; National Faculty, NAACOG NICU Review Course; Neonatal

Nurse Practitioner, The Children's Hospital, Denver, Colorado • *Radiological Evaluation of the Newborn*

Elizabeth A. Estrada, RNC, MS • Neonatal Clinical Nurse Specialist, Children's National Medical Center, Washington, DC • *Neonatal Nutrition*

Diane Gilchriest, RN, MS • Maternal-Child Instructor, Crouse-Irving Memorial Hospital School of Nursing, Syracuse, New York • *Quality Assurance*

Mary Anne Givhan, RNC, BSN, NNP • Charge Nurse—NICU, University of South Alabama Children's and Women's Hospital, Mobile, Alabama • *Respiratory Distress*

Sharon M. Glass, RNC, BSN, NNP • National Faculty, NAACOG NICU Review Course; Neonatal Nurse Practitioner, The Children's Hospital, Denver, Colorado • *Hematological Disorders; Neonatal Pain Management* (Appendix C)

Peggy Cohen Gordin, RNC, MS • Neonatal Clinical Nurse Specialist, Children's Hospital of Philadelphia, Philadelphia, Pennsylvania • *High-Frequency Ventilation*

Harriet A. Harrell, RNC, BSN, NNP • National Faculty, NAACOG NICU Review Course, National Faculty, AAP/AHA Neonatal Resuscitation Program; Assistant Director of Neonatal Nurse Practitioners and Outreach Education Coordinator, Section of Neonatology, Department of Pediatrics, Arizona Health Sciences Center, University of Arizona, Tucson, Arizona • *Neonatal Delivery Room Resuscitation*

Lynn Hornick, RN, BSN • Nurse Specialist, Prenatal Diagnosis and Genetics, University Hospital, University of Colorado Health Sciences Center, Denver, Colorado • *Fetal Anomalies: Diagnosis and Management*

Joanne Riley Kilb, RN, MS, NNP • Neonatal Nurse Practitioner at the Carolinas Medical Center, Charlotte, North Carolina • *Assisted Ventilation*

Stephen Kilb, RN, BSN, NNP • Neonatal Nurse Practitioner at the Carolinas Medical Center, Charlotte, North Carolina • *Assisted Ventilation*

Robin Kriedeman, RNC, BSN, NNP • St. John's Northeast Hospital—Neonatal Nurse Practitioner, Minneapolis, Minnesota • *Apnea of the Newborn*

Sharon L. Kuhrt, RNC, BSN • Clinical Supervisor, Central Maine Medical Center, Alfred, Maine • *Fetal Anomalies: Diagnosis and Management*

Nanette Landry, RN, MS, CNM • Certified Nurse Midwife, University Hospital, University of Colorado Health Sciences Center, Denver, Colorado • *Uncomplicated Antepartum, Intrapartum, and Post-partum Care*

Roger G. Martin, RN, MS, NNP • Adjunct Faculty, South Dakota State University, College of Nursing, Neonatal Nurse Practitioner/Clinical Nurse Specialist, Sioux Valley Hospital, Sioux Falls, South Dakota • *Pharmacology in Neonatal Care*

Mary McCulloch, RNC, MS, NNP • Clinical Director, Neonatal Nurse Practitioner Program, College of Nursing, University of Utah; Neonatal Nurse Practitioner, University of Utah Hospital, Salt Lake City, Utah • *Neurological Disorders*

Jan Nugent, RNC, MSN • Medical Student, Louisiana State University School of Medicine, New Orleans, Louisiana • *Extracorporeal Membrane Oxygenation (ECMO) in the Neonate*

Josanne M. Paxton, RN, MSN, NNP • Adjunct Clinical Assistant Professor of Nursing, The

University of Arizona; Certified Neonatal Nurse Practitioner, The University of Arizona, Arizona Health Sciences Center, Tucson, Arizona • *Neonatal Infections*

Joy Hinson Penticuff, RN, PhD, FAAN • Associate Professor, School of Nursing, The University of Texas at Austin, Austin, Texas • *Ethical Issues*

Janet Pinelli, RN, MSN • Associate Professor, School of Nursing, McMaster University; Clinical Nurse Specialist/Neonatal Practitioner, Chedoke-McMaster Hospitals, Hamilton, Ontario, Canada • *Case Studies*

Donna J. Rodden, RN, BSN • Senior Professional Research Assistant, Neonatal Clinical Research Center, University of Colorado Health Sciences Center, Denver, Colorado • *Surfactant Replacement Therapy*

Bonny Sham, RN, MN • Head Nurse ICNN/Newborn Nursery, Valley Presbyterian Hospital, Van Nuys, California • *Perinatal Substance Abuse*

Carla R. Shapiro, RN, MN • Clinical Nurse Specialist, Maternal/Child Nursing, St. Boniface General Hospital, Winnipeg, Manitoba, Canada • *Ophthalmologic Disorders*

Leann Sterk, RN, BS, NNP • Neonatal Nurse Practitioner, Rapid City Regional Hospital, Rapid City, South Dakota • *Neonatal Orthopedic Conditions*

Laura Campbell Stokowski, RNC, MS • Staff Nurse, 130th Station Hospital, Heidelberg, Germany • *Metabolic Disorders; Endocrine Disorders*

Linda Henry Therrien, RN, MS • Director of Community Health Programs, The Children's Hospital, Denver, Colorado • *Discharge Planning for the High-Risk Neonate*

M. Terese Verklan, RNC, MSN • Doctoral Candidate, University of Pennsylvania, School of Nursing, Philadelphia, Pennsylvania • *Legal Issues in the NICU*

Catherine L. Witt, RNC, MS, NNP • Neonatal Nurse Practitioner, Presbyterian/St. Lukes Medical Center, Denver, Colorado • *Neonatal Dermatology*

Patti Witt, RNC, BSN, NNP • Faculty Member at the Minnesota Association of Public Teaching Hospitals; Coordinator of the Neonatal Nurse Practitioners, Hennepin County Medical Center, Minneapolis, Minnesota • *Physical Assessment of the Newborn*

Christine Zabloudil, RN, BSN, NNP • Staff Nurse, Valley Medical Center, Renton, Washington • *Adaptation to Extrauterine Life*

Preface

Providing neonatal intensive care is a multi-faceted, constantly evolving area of health care. Those involved in the nursing care of high-risk newborns and their families are constantly faced with the task of integrating the best of themselves, their knowledge of pathophysiology and physical processes, their understanding of family dynamics, and, sometimes, their very personal struggles with the ethics involved in caring for the high-risk newborn, into the role of the neonatal nurse. This role is frequently to ''bring together'' all of these pieces to provide comprehensive, clinically excellent, and compassionate care to sick newborns and their families.

Core Curriculum for Neonatal Intensive Care Nursing is intended to meet the needs of neonatal nurses at all levels of their careers as they strive for ever-increasing clinical excellence. Divided into sections and designed in outline format, it provides easy reference for the most current information on problems affecting infants in the NICU. Neonatal nurses are confronted daily by the medical problems of neonates and must have an in-depth understanding of the pathophysiology of these problems to assess the infants' responses to medical treatment and to provide families with the information they need to understand the medical care of their infants. Accordingly, physiological problems of the sick newborn are the major focus of this book. To make this text comprehensive, we included information on families, ethics, legal aspects of care, and quality assurance issues. Our intent is to provide information on the entire spectrum of neonatal nursing.

This text is the collaborative effort of many contributing authors representing various regions of the United States, Canada, and Australia. The goal is to provide a comprehensive guide for the management and care of sick newborns that is universal in nature and not guided by regional differences.

Our hope is that this book will be taken to work and used as a reference guide. The format and soft cover were designed specifically to make this a user-friendly manual of neonatal care. We hope it is marked in, that notes are written in the margins, and that in a few years it will become an even richer manual of neonatal information, which the neonatal nurse can use to enhance the practice of neonatal care.

PATRICIA BEACHY
JANE DEACON

Acknowledgments

The authors would like to express their thanks to the chapter contributors and reviewers for their excellent work. Reviewers included Grace T. Clancy, RNC, MS, Boston, Massachusetts; Kit Sharon Devine, RNC, MSN, LaGrange, Kentucky; Sheila Ecklund, RNC, MSN, Lincoln, Nebraska; Lynn E. Lynam, RNC, MS, NNP, Newark, Delaware; Donna Middaugh, RN, MSN, CCRN, Little Rock, Arkansas; Christine O. Newman, MS, RNC, Detroit, Michigan; Katherine L. Peters, RN, BScN, MN, PhC, Seattle, Washington; Mary E. Polleys, RNC, MS, NNP, Salt Lake City, Utah; Maribeth Stein, RN, MN, Seattle, Washington; Diane Strandlund, RNC, CCRN, BAN, Burnsville, Minnesota; Peter Tallerico, RNC, CCRN, MSN, Columbia, Missouri; and Cheryl M. Ward-Simons, RN, MA, Middletown, New York.

Also, thanks are expressed to the Departments of Nursing at The Children's Hospital and University Hospital in Denver for supplying the resources and allowing us the time to complete this text.

Lastly, heartfelt thanks to our colleagues in the NICU and Perinatal Units who helped us with their encouragement and review of much of this text.

PATRICIA BEACHY
JANE DEACON

Contents

SECTION

I OBSTETRICAL CARE AND THE INFANT IN TRANSITION   1

CHAPTER

1 Uncomplicated Antepartum, Intrapartum, and Post-partum Care • 3
Nanette Landry

Terminology • 3
Normal Physiological Changes of Systems • 4
Endocrine and Metabolic Changes • 6
Antepartum Care • 6
Assessment of Gestational Age • 7
Antepartum Visits • 8
Antepartum Fetal Surveillance • 9
Normal Labor • 10
Intrapartum Labor Management • 10
Puerperium: Fourth Trimester • 11

CHAPTER

2 Antepartum-Intrapartum Complications • 14
Anne B. Broussard

Anatomy and Physiology • 14
Conditions Related to Antepartum • 17
Conditions Related to Intrapartum Period • 20
Obstetrical Analgesia and Anesthesia • 28
Operative Delivery • 31

CHAPTER

3 Adaptation to Extrauterine Life • 35
Christine Zabloudil

Anatomy and Physiology • 35
Routine Care Considerations • 40

CHAPTER

4 Physical Assessment of the Newborn • 57
Patti Witt

Perinatal History Review • 57
Assessment of Gestational Age • 58
Physical Examination Overview • 65
Physical Assessment • 65

CHAPTER
5   Neonatal Delivery Room Resuscitation • 76
Harriet A. Harrell

Introduction • 76
Anatomy and Physiology • 77
Risk Factors • 78
Anticipation of and Preparation for Resuscitation • 79
Equipment for Neonatal Resuscitation • 80
Decision Making Process • 81
Neonatal Resuscitation: ABCs • 81
Unusual Situations • 87
Complications of Resuscitation • 89
Post-Resuscitation Care • 89

SECTION
**II   NEONATAL CARDIOPULMONARY DISORDERS AND
MANAGEMENT   93**

CHAPTER
6   Respiratory Distress • 95
Mary Anne Givhan

Lung Development • 95
Physiology of Respiration • 97
Respiratory Disorders • 98
Bronchopulmonary Dysplasia (BPD) • 111
Chronic Lung Disease in Premature Infants • 116
Air Leaks • 117
Pulmonary Hypoplasia • 119
Pulmonary Hemorrhage • 119
Non-Respiratory Causes of Respiratory Distress • 120

CHAPTER
7   Apnea of the Newborn • 125
Robin Kriedeman

Definitions of Apnea • 125
Types of Apnea • 126
Pathogenesis of Apnea in the Premature Infant • 127
Causes of Apnea • 128
Evaluation of Apnea • 129
Management Techniques • 131
Home Monitoring • 133

CHAPTER
8   Surfactant Replacement Therapy • 136
Donna J. Rodden

Historical Overview of Surfactant • 137
The Pulmonary Surfactant System • 137
Functional Characteristics of Surfactant • 137
Types of Replacement Surfactants • 138
Clinical Use of Surfactants • 138
Conclusion • 145

CHAPTER
9   Assisted Ventilation • 148
Joanne R. Kilb
Stephen Kilb

Physiology • 149

Treatment Modalities • 152
Monitoring During Therapy • 154
Medications Used During Ventilation Therapy • 156
Nursing Care • 161
Weaning from the Ventilator • 163
Blood Gas Interpretation • 164

CHAPTER
10 **High-Frequency Ventilation** • 170
Peggy Cohen Gordin

Physiology of High-Frequency Ventilation • 170
Types of HFV and Terminology • 172
Indications for Use of HFV • 172
High-Frequency Oscillatory Ventilation: Clinical Application • 172
High-Frequency Jet Ventilation: Clinical Application • 173
Summary of Research and Outcome Data • 175

CHAPTER
11 **Extracorporeal Membrane Oxygenation (ECMO) in the Neonate** • 177
Jan Nugent

ECMO: A Historical Perspective • 177
Criteria for Use of ECMO • 178
Venoarterial (VA) Perfusion • 178
Circuit Components • 179
Blood Gas Monitoring Device • 181
Physiology of Extracorporeal Circulation • 182
Care of the Infant • 182
Parental Support • 188
Follow-up and Outcome • 188

SECTION
III **NEONATAL PATHOPHYSIOLOGY: MANAGEMENT AND
TREATMENT OF COMMON DISORDERS** **191**

CHAPTER
12 **Cardiovascular Disorders** • 193
Margaret Crockett

Cardiovascular Embryology and Anatomy • 194
Congenital Heart Disease (CHD) • 199
Approach to Diagnosis of Cardiac Disease • 200
Congenital Heart Lesions: Acyanotic • 207
Congenital Heart Lesions: Cyanotic • 216
Congestive Heart Failure • 224
Shock • 227

CHAPTER
13 **Gastrointestinal Disorders** • 233
Patricia Beachy

Gastrointestinal Embryonic Development • 233
Functions of the Gastrointestinal Tract • 234
Disorders of the Gastrointestinal Tract: Abdominal Wall Defects • 234
Care of the Neonate with an Abdominal Wall Defect (Omphalocele and
Gastroschisis) • 235
Prune-belly Syndrome • 236
Disorders of the Gastrointestinal Tract: Intestinal Obstruction • 237
Hyperbilirubinemia • 245
Hydrops Fetalis • 251

CHAPTER
14   Neonatal Nutrition • 254
Elizabeth A. Estrada
Margaret Brennan-Behm

Anatomy and Physiology of the Pre-term Infant's GI Tract • 255
Standards for Adequate Growth • 256
Nutritional Requirements and Feeding for Full-Term Infants • 256
Nutritional Requirements for Pre-term Infants • 257
Parenteral Nutrition • 264
Enteral Feedings: Human Milk and Commercial Formulas • 269
Enteral Feeding Methods • 271
Nutritional Assessment • 275
Nursing Interventions to Facilitate Tolerance of Enteral Feedings • 276

CHAPTER
15   Metabolic Disorders • 281
Laura Campbell Stokowski

Glucose Metabolism and Disorders • 282
Fluid Balance and Disorders • 286
Electrolyte Balance and Disorders • 290
Acid-Base Balance • 296
Inborn Errors of Metabolism • 298
Specific Disorders of Metabolism • 300

CHAPTER
16   Endocrine Disorders • 306
Laura Campbell Stokowski

The Endocrine System • 306
Thyroid Gland Disorders • 307
Adrenal Gland Disorders • 311
Disorders of Sexual Development • 314

CHAPTER
17   Hematological Disorders • 322
Sharon M. Glass

Development of Blood Cells • 322
Coagulation • 327
Anemia • 328
Hemorrhagic Disease of the Newborn • 333
Disseminated Intravascular Coagulation (DIC) • 334
Thrombocytopenia • 336
Polycythemia • 338
Blood Products • 339
Transfusion Therapies • 340
Complete Blood Count (CBC) Evaluation • 341

CHAPTER
18   Neonatal Infections • 345
Josanne M. Paxton

Immunology • 346
Transmission of Bacterial Organisms • 348
Clinical Assessment • 348
Clinical Manifestations • 348
Hematological Evaluation • 349
Diagnostic Evaluation • 352
Bacterial Infection • 353

Specific Bacterial Pathogens • 354
Intervention • 356
Fungal Infections • 357
Viral Infections • 358
Other Infections • 361
Infection Control • 362

CHAPTER
19   **Renal/Genitourinary Disorders** • 365
Janice Bernhardt

Embryology • 365
Gross Renal Anatomy • 366
Microscopic Renal Anatomy • 366
Renal Hemodynamics • 367
Renal Physiology • 368
Acute Renal Failure • 369
Hypertension • 373
Potter's Syndrome • 375
Infantile Polycystic Kidney Disease • 376
Multicystic Dysplastic Kidney Disease • 378
Hydronephrosis • 379
Renal Vein Thrombosis • 381
Urinary Tract Infections • 382
Patent Urachus • 383
Hypospadias • 384
Exstrophy of the Bladder • 385
Inguinal Hernia • 387
Undescended Testicles (Cryptorchidism) • 388
Circumcision • 389

CHAPTER
20   **Neurological Disorders** • 394
Mary McCulloch

Anatomy of the Neurological System • 394
Physiology of the Neurological System • 397
Neurological Assessment • 398
Neurological Disorders • 399
Craniosynostosis • 405
Birth Injuries • 407
Intracranial Hemorrhages • 410
Seizures • 414
Hypoxic-Ischemic Encephalopathy (HIE) • 417
Periventricular Leukomalacia (PVL) • 419
Meningitis • 420

CHAPTER
21   **Developmental Support in the NICU** • 426
Pamela Creger

Concepts of Developmental Care • 426
Behavioral Organization • 427
Neuromotor Development • 430
Positioning Techniques: Therapeutic Handling • 430
Assessment of Feeding Abilities • 433
Auditory Assessment and Follow-Up of Infant at Risk for
Impairment • 437
Fostering Parent-Infant Interaction • 440
The Developmental Care Plan • 441

CHAPTER
22 **Fetal Anomalies: Diagnosis and Management** • 443
Sharon Kuhrt
Lynn Hornick

Basic Genetics • 443
Chromosomal Defects • 445
Prenatal Diagnosis • 446
Newborn Care Management • 451
Evaluation of the Malformed Infant • 451
Beckwith-Wiedemann Syndrome • 452
Cleft Lip and Palate • 453
Cornelia de Lange Syndrome • 454
Craniosynostosis • 455
Crouzon Syndrome • 456
Trisomies • 456
Turner's Syndrome • 459
Vater Association • 459

CHAPTER
23 **Neonatal Orthopedic Conditions** • 462
Leann Sterk

Skeletal System • 462
Muscular System • 463
Clinical Assessment • 463
Pathological Conditions • 464
Neck Abnormalities • 465
Lower Extremities • 466

CHAPTER
24 **Neonatal Dermatology** • 471
Catherine L. Witt

Anatomy and Physiology • 471
Care of the Newborn's Skin • 473
Assessment of the Newborn's Skin • 474
Common Skin Lesions • 474

CHAPTER
25 **Ophthalmologic Disorders** • 485
Carla Shapiro

Anatomy of the Eye • 485
Patient Assessment • 487
Pathological Conditions and Management • 488
Congenital Infections • 495

CHAPTER
26 **Pharmacology in Neonatal Care** • 501
Roger G. Martin

Principles of Pharmacology • 502
Drug Categories • 511
Specific Nursing Implications for Drug Administration in the
Neonate • 517

SECTION

IV   SOCIAL TRENDS AND FAMILY CARE   **521**

CHAPTER
27   Perinatal Substance Abuse • 523
     Bonny Sham

Cocaine • 523
How Cocaine Works • 524
Cocaine in Pregnancy • 524
Methamphetamine • 525
Fetal Alcohol Syndrome • 526
Heroin and Methadone • 528
Neonatal Abstinence Syndrome • 529
Marijuana Smoking • 530
Cigarette Smoking • 531
Problems Associated with Maternal Drug Use • 531
Management Recommendations • 532
Nursing Intervention • 533
Breast-feeding and the Drug-dependent Woman • 534
Ethical Considerations • 534

CHAPTER
28   The Family in Crisis • 537
     Mary Ann Best

Crisis and the Birth of the Less-Than-Perfect Infant • 538
Identification of the Family in Crisis • 538
Grief and Loss • 540
Interventions for Facilitating Grief • 541
Interventions for Parents Experiencing a Perinatal Loss • 541
Interventions for Parents with a Pre-term or Malformed Infant • 541
Family-Infant Bonding • 542
Interventions to Encourage Family-Infant Bonding • 543
Evaluation of Parent-Infant Bonding • 544
Summary of Parental Needs to Be Met by NICU Staff • 545

CHAPTER
29   The Teenage Family • 548
     Candice Cook Bowman

The Teenage Parent in the NICU: Multiple Crises Needing Resolution • 549
Crisis Origins • 550
Personal Crisis Manifestations • 556
Crisis Resolution • 558
Aids to a Positive Resolution • 560
Summary • 562

CHAPTER
30   Discharge Planning for the High-Risk Neonate • 565
     Linda Henry Therrien

Goals and Objectives of Discharge Planning • 565
Challenges that Influence the Value of Discharge Planning • 566
Criteria for Consideration of Discharge Planning • 566
The Discharge Planning Process: The Nurse's Role • 566

SECTION

V   CLINICAL PRACTICE   571

CHAPTER
31   Neonatal Transport • 573
Mary K. Buser

Historical Aspects • 573
Philosophy of Neonatal Transport • 574
Selection of Transport Vehicles • 575
Transport Personnel • 576
Transport Equipment • 577
The Neonatal Transport Process • 579
Documentation • 581
Transport Environment • 581
Legal/Ethical Considerations • 582
Quality Assurance/Quality Control • 582

CHAPTER
32   Case Studies • 586
Janet Pinelli

CHAPTER
33   Radiological Evaluation of the Newborn • 612
Jane Deacon

Basic Concepts • 612
Terminology • 613
X-Ray Views Commonly Used in the Newborn • 613
Radiographical Densities • 614
Approach to Interpreting an X-Ray • 614
The Respiratory System • 616
Thoracic Surgical Problems • 622
Cardiovascular System • 624
Gastrointestinal System • 627
Skeletal System • 634
Indwelling Lines and Tubes • 635

CHAPTER
34   Common Technical Procedures • 638
Cindy Davis

Capillary Blood Sampling • 639
Venipuncture • 640
Radial Artery Puncture • 640
Peripheral Intravenous Line Placement • 641
Thoracentesis • 643
Endotracheal Intubation • 644
Umbilical Artery Catheterization • 646

SECTION

VI   CURRENT ISSUES AND TRENDS IN NEONATAL CARE   651

CHAPTER
35   Research • 653
Wendy Cornell

Basic Principles of Research • 653
Identifying Research Questions • 655
Steps in the Research Process • 656

The Role of Research in Neonatal Nursing • 660
Interdisciplinary Research: Implications for Nursing • 661

CHAPTER
36 **Ethical Issues** • 665
Joy Hinson Penticuff

Definitions • 665
Principles of Ethics • 666
Ethical Decision Making • 666
Creation of Ethical Dilemmas in High-Risk Neonatal Nursing • 668
Resources for Resolving Ethical Dilemmas • 670

CHAPTER
37 **Legal Issues in the NICU** • 673
M. Terese Verklan

Standard of Care • 673
Liability • 674
Documentation • 676
Informed Consent • 678
Scope of Practice • 679
Malpractice • 680

CHAPTER
38 **Quality Assurance** • 684
Diane Gilchriest

Quality Assurance • 684
Assessment • 685
Evaluation • 686

APPENDIX
A **Newborn Metric Conversion Tables** 691

APPENDIX
B **Recommended Schedule for Hepatitis B Vaccine** 694

APPENDIX
C **Neonatal Pain Management** 695
Sharon M. Glass

APPENDIX
D **Apgar Score** 698

INDEX 699

OBSTETRICAL CARE AND THE INFANT IN TRANSITION

Nanette Landry

Uncomplicated Antepartum, Intrapartum, and Post-partum Care*

Objectives

1. Define term, pre-term, and post-term pregnancy.

2. Define Näegele's rule for estimated date of confinement (EDC).

3. Identify normal physiological changes of each system in pregnancy.

4. Identify three methods of antepartum fetal surveillance.

5. Define the normal stages of labor.

6. Contrast low-risk intrapartum fetal monitoring management vs. high-risk fetal monitoring management.

7. Identify normal post-partum assessments and management.

Antepartum, intrapartum, and post-partum care is not usually thought of as within the practice parameters of the neonatal nurse. Yet, an understanding of the normal processes of pregnancy provides a framework to begin to understand factors that affect the developing fetus and the high-risk neonate. This chapter discusses uncomplicated antepartum, intrapartum, and immediate post-partum nursing care. In addition, an overview of the normal physiologic changes that can be expected in a healthy mother is included.

Terminology

A. **Pregnancy's length of gestation** is defined as 280 days. This corresponds to 40 post-menstrual weeks or 10 lunar months.

B. **Gestation is divided into 3 trimesters.**

1. First trimester: 0–12 weeks.
2. Second trimester: 13–27 weeks.
3. Third trimester: 28–40 weeks.

---

*The author wishes to thank Dr. Alan M. Rapaport for his help in reviewing this chapter.

C. **Term pregnancy.** Term pregnancy is defined as 38–42 weeks; pre-term is defined as <37 weeks; and post-term as >42 weeks.

Normal Physiological Changes of Systems

Pregnancy affects all body systems. Some of the normal physiological changes of systems include the following:

A. **Alimentary tract.**
1. There will be an increase in appetite up to 300 kcal/day. The recommended calorie intake for the average woman in pregnancy is 2200 kcal/day. Pregnant teenagers need an additional 100–200 kcal/day.
2. Approximately 70% of pregnancies are affected by morning sickness from the 4th through the 16th week.
3. The stomach loses tone and has delayed emptying time.
4. Gastroesophageal junction also relaxes and, in combination with increased intra-abdominal pressure, leads to reflux and resulting heartburn.
5. The small bowel has reduced motility, and, in the colon, constipation is a problem due to mechanical obstruction from the uterus, reduced motility, and increased water absorption.
6. The gallbladder empties much more slowly in the second and third trimesters with high residuals, increasing the chance of gallstone formation.
7. The liver remains unchanged in pregnancy as far as size and hepatic blood flow are concerned; however, some laboratory values mimic liver disease, such as reduced serum albumin, elevated alkaline phosphatase, and elevated serum cholesterol. Serum levels of bilirubin, aspartate aminotransferase (AST), alanine aminotransferase (ALT), and prothrombin time are unchanged in normal pregnancy.

B. **Respiratory system.**
1. Hypersecretion of mucus from the nasopharynx leads to nasal stuffiness and epistaxis during pregnancy.
2. The chest wall profile changes, resulting in an expansion of the circumference and increase in the subcostal margin angle. This results in the diaphragm being elevated by 4 cm in the third trimester.
3. Up to 60–70% of all pregnant women experience dyspnea with increased tidal volume and reduced P_{ACO_2} levels.

C. **Skin.**
1. Due to elevated levels of estrogen, spider angiomata (vascular, red elevations with tiny vessels branching out from a central body) and palmar erythema (diffuse or blotchy spots on palms) are frequently seen on the neck, face, throat, and arms.
2. Striae gravidarum, or "stretch marks," occur as a result of a genetic predisposition to stretching of the skin or connective tissue.
3. There is increased pigmentation due to increased levels of estrogen, progesterone, and melanocyte-stimulating hormone. This is most marked on the nipples, areola, perineum, and midline lower abdomen (commonly called the linea nigra).
4. There is also sun-sensitive hyperpigmentation of the face called chloasma or melasma, also referred to as the "mask of pregnancy." This results in a dark, blotchy appearance of the face, forehead, and upper lip.
5. During gestation, a greater percentage of the hair remains in the anagen or growth phase, decreasing normal hair loss. Hair loss commonly occurs between 2 and 4 months post-delivery due to an increase in the telogen or resting phase of hair growth. The hair will return to a normal growth phase by 6 months to 1 year.

D. **Urinary system.**
1. The kidneys enlarge and the ureters dilate. The consequences of these changes are as follows:
   a. An increase in asymptomatic bacteriuria. This can lead to cystitis and pyelonephritis.
   b. Difficulty in diagnosing obstruction on x-ray and interference with studies of glomerular filtration, renal blood flow, and tubular function.
2. The glomerular filtration rate (GFR) increases in pregnancy by 50%. This leads to:
   a. An increase in creatinine clearance and a decrease in nitrogen levels.
   b. Increased filtration of sodium with increased reabsorption of sodium by renal tubules to balance the loss.
   c. A lower threshold at which glucose will be excreted by the kidneys. This leads to:
      (1) Inability to utilize urine glucose measurements in management of pregnant women with diabetes mellitus.
      (2) Increase in susceptibility to urinary tract infections (UTIs).

E. **Cardiovascular system.**
1. Cardiac output increases 30–50% in pregnancy.
2. The maternal heart rate increases during pregnancy by 15–20 beats above non-pregnant rates by the third trimester.
3. Blood pressure remains normal at the pre-pregnancy level in the first trimester and drops during the second trimester at approximately 24 weeks' gestation by 5–10 mm Hg systolic and 10–15 mm Hg diastolic. It returns to normal pre-pregnancy levels during the end of pregnancy.
4. In late pregnancy, there can be pressure obstruction of the inferior vena cava in the supine position. This causes a 25% fall in cardiac output and is called *supine hypotension.*
5. Edema in the legs is common due to an increase in venous pressure in the legs and obstruction of the lymphatic flow.

F. **Breasts.**
1. Early changes in the breasts include tingling, heaviness, tenderness, and enlargement; these begin to occur by 4 weeks' gestation. These symptoms usually subside at the end of the first trimester.
2. The areolae enlarge and darken.
3. Montgomery's glands appear on the areolae. These are secretory glands.
4. Colostrum may be expressed in late pregnancy.

G. **Skeletal changes.**
1. Compensating for the anteriorly positioned growing uterus, the lower back curves. This lordosis shifts the center of gravity back over the lower extremities and causes low back pain, a common complaint in pregnancy.
2. Joints loosen during pregnancy, secondary to the hormone relaxin.
3. These changes and an unsteady gait lead to falls, a common occurrence in pregnancy.

H. **Hematologic changes.**
1. Plasma volume is increased by 50% at term.
2. The white blood cell (WBC) count rises progressively during pregnancy and labor and then returns to normal pre-pregnancy levels.
3. The red blood count (RBC) rises by 18–30% throughout pregnancy, and the plasma volume increases by 50%, reaching its peak at 30–34 weeks. This change in the ratio of RBCs to plasma causes a drop in hematocrit (Hct), resulting in "physiologic anemia of pregnancy." The plasma volume increase levels off as the Hct begins to rise, resulting in a more normal ratio of RBCs to plasma and a rise in Hct near term.

4. Platelet count decreases during pregnancy but remains within the normal range.
5. Pregnancy has been called a "hypercoagulable state." Fibrinogen is increased and Factors VII through X increase. Bleeding and clotting times remain normal. There is an increase in the incidence of thromboembolism during pregnancy that is greatest during the post-partum period.

Endocrine and Metabolic Changes

A. **Thyroid.** The thyroid enlarges during pregnancy; however, there is little transplacental transfer of the hormones triiodothyronine (T_3) and thyroxine (T_4).

B. **Peripheral resistance to insulin.** This is referred to as the "diabetogenic effect of pregnancy." The hormones responsible for this effect are human placental lactogen (HPL), progesterone, and estrogen.

C. **Basal metabolic rate.** The basal metabolic rate is increased by 25%.

D. **Carbohydrate metabolism.** This is significantly altered by HPL. The effects are in direct proportion to placental mass.

E. **Glucose.** Glucose is actively transported to the fetus; however, insulin and glycogen do not cross the placenta.

Antepartum Care

A. **Initial antepartum visit.**
1. A thorough past obstetrical history should be obtained to include the following:
   a. Gravidity—number of pregnancies; Parity—number of births.
      (1) When one is describing a patient's obstetrical history, this is often written in the form $G_3P_2A_,L_2$, where G is gravity, P is parity, A is the number of abortions, and L is the number of living children at this time.
      (2) Parity may be subdivided into term (T) and preterm (P).
      (3) Abortions include all pregnancies terminated prior to 24 weeks. This includes spontaneous and elective abortions as well as ectopic pregnancies.
   b. Weeks of gestation achieved with each pregnancy.
   c. Hours of labor.
   d. Type of delivery (i.e., vaginal or operative).
   e. Size of babies at birth.
   f. Any complications.
2. Medical history of the patient and immediate family should be obtained to include the following:
   a. Complete medical history.
   b. Infection history.
      (1) Hepatitis.
      (2) HIV (Human immunodeficiency virus).
      (3) Herpes.
      (4) Rubella.
      (5) Varicella.
      (6) Sexually transmitted diseases (STDs).
   c. Risk assessment to include the following:
      (1) Drug or alcohol use.
      (2) Smoking.
      (3) Age.
      (4) Educational level.
      (5) History of emotional problems.
      (6) Support systems.
      (7) Attitude toward pregnancy.

3. Obtain a genetic background to identify factors that may lead you to screen for Down syndrome, open neural tube defects in the immediate family, or any other possible genetic defects.
4. Obtain current history of the pregnancy.
5. Perform a complete physical examination, including a complete pelvic examination.

B. **Initial lab work.**
1. Blood type and Rh.
2. Antibody screen.
3. Hematocrit/hemoglobin.
4. Pap smear.
5. Rubella titer.
6. Serology.
7. Urinalysis for protein, glucose, and evidence of infections.
8. HBsAg (hepatitis B surface antigen).
9. HIV (human immunodeficiency virus), *Chlamydia*, and gonorrhea culture (depending on history and population).
10. Sickle cell screen, Tay-Sachs screen for appropriate population.

C. **Routine and diagnostic lab work and procedures.**
1. 8–18 weeks: ultrasound may be indicated to establish accurate dates or to detect genetic abnormalities.
2. CVS (chorionic villus sampling) at 9–11 weeks for chromosomal evaluation.
3. 14–18 weeks: offer maternal serum alpha-fetoprotein (MSAFP) measurement to screen for open neural tube defects and other potential problems with the pregnancy.
4. 15–20 weeks: amniocentesis for genetic evaluation and measurement of alpha-fetoprotein. Other studies as suggested by the genetic history may be performed.
5. 24–28 weeks: a glucose screen for gestational diabetes is performed. A 50 g glucose load is given, and a plasma glucose concentration is determined 1 hour later. A level above 140 mg/dl is abnormal.
   a. A glucose tolerance test is performed on all patients with an abnormal screen. This includes a fasting plasma glucose concentration as well as hourly values for 3 hours after a 100 g glucose load. The diagnosis of gestational diabetes is made if two values are elevated. (Plasma values: fasting, 105 mg/dl; 1 hour, 190 mg/dl; 2 hours, 165 mg/dl; 3 hours, 145 mg/dl.)
6. 28 weeks: repeat antibody titer on Rh-negative mothers; administer Rh immune globulin 300 μg/M if no anti-D antibody detected.
7. Early third trimester: repeat hemoglobin/hematocrit (Hgb/Hct) determinations to recheck for anemia.
8. 36–40 weeks.
   a. Ultrasound may be indicated for serial growth evaluation, amniotic fluid volume testing, or placental assessment.
   b. If patient is at risk, repeat Hct/Hgb. Serology and cultures for gonorrhea and *Chlamydia* may be necessary. Some physicians will routinely culture for group B beta-hemolytic streptococci at this time.

Assessment of Gestational Age

A. **Last menstrual period (LMP).** Pregnancy may be detected by 5–6 weeks after the LMP. Estimating gestational age by counting from the LMP is a reliable method.
1. A history should include the following:
   a. Length of periods.
   b. Heaviness of flow.

c. Past menstrual history.
d. Oral contraceptive use.
2. Näegele's rule determines the estimated date of confinement (EDC) or due date using the following formula: EDC = LMP − 3 months + 7 days.

B. Pelvic examination and fundal height.
1. Size of the uterus on an early examination (before 12–14 weeks) is quite accurate if the mother is of normal height and not grossly obese. Fundal height measurements in centimeters from 16 to 35 weeks approximate gestational age within 3 weeks. The uterus is generally at the umbilicus at 20 weeks.
2. Quickening: the first feelings of fetal movement.
   a. Primigravida: 18–20 weeks.
   b. Multigravida: 16–18 weeks.

C. Fetal heart tones (FHT). Fetal heart tones can be detected by an electronic Doppler device as early as 9 weeks and commonly by 12 weeks. They may be auscultated with a fetoscope by 19–20 weeks.

D. Sonography.
1. Ultrasound is most accurate in the first trimester (6–14 weeks), with crown-rump measurement accurately reflecting gestational age plus or minus 3 days.
2. Fetal heart motion can be detected by real-time ultrasound as early as 6 weeks' gestation by vaginal sonography.
3. Biparietal diameter (BPD) is the most frequently used method to establish gestational age; it is most accurate before 26 weeks.
4. Abdominal circumference (AC) can be used to assess gestational age and intrauterine growth retardation (IUGR). Combining BPD and AC can give an accurate estimate of fetal weight within 10%.
5. Fetal femur length (FL) may also be used to determine gestational age. Fetal weight within 7–10% can be determined by combining AC and FL.

E. Laboratory assessments. Laboratory assessments (for documenting fetal lung maturity) include the following:
1. Lecithin/sphingomyelin (L/S) ratio: L/S ratios greater than 2:1 occur when fetal lung surfactant is present in amniotic fluid (approximately 35 weeks). A level greater than or equal to 2:1 suggests that the baby will not need respiratory support after birth.
2. Phosphatidylglycerol (PG); PG is also present in amniotic fluid at around 35 weeks and increases rapidly at 37 weeks. PG is a component of surfactant and is a more reliable test of lung maturity in diabetic mothers than the L/S ratio. PG is reported as present or not present.
3. Fluorescence polarization NBD-PC (FPOL) is another test for lung maturity in the newborn that is growing in popularity. It is less expensive, is easier to perform, and has fewer false-negative results than L/S or PG. FPOL is reported as follows: <260: mature lungs; 261–289: 20% risk of respiratory distress in the newborn; >290: 80% risk of respiratory distress in the newborn.

Antepartum Visits

A. Frequency.
1. In general, OB visits are recommended every 4 weeks until 28 weeks; then every 2 weeks until 36 weeks; then weekly. Additional visits may be necessary around 18–20 weeks to establish heart tones with a fetoscope and quickening, or if the pregnancy shows any signs of complications.

B. Routine assessments. Routine assessments, as appropriate, including the following:
1. Psychosocial assessments.
2. Weight.
3. Blood pressure.

4. Urine for glucose and protein.
5. Gestational age in weeks.
6. Fundal height in centimeters.
7. Presence of edema.
8. Fetal heart tones (FHT).
9. Fetal movement (after 20 weeks).
10. Fetal presentation.
11. Vaginal bleeding.
12. Prematurity signs and symptoms:
    a. Increased discharge/mucus show.
    b. Contractions, abdominal cramping, intestinal cramping.
    c. Dysuria/frequency/costovertebral angle tenderness.
    d. Increased pelvic pressure.
13. Pregnancy-induced hypertension (PIH) signs and symptoms:
    a. BP, proteinuria, edema.
    b. Epigastric pain.
    c. Nausea/vomiting.
    d. Hyper-reflexia.
    e. Clonus.
    f. Visual disturbances.
    g. Headaches.

Antepartum Fetal Surveillance

A. **Non-stress test (NST).** This is the most widely used screening method for fetal well-being.
1. It is indicated for patients at risk for placental insufficiency and may be started as early as 30–32 weeks' gestation. Conditions that are of concern include the following:
    a. Post dates.
    b. Diabetes mellitus.
    c. Hypertension.
    d. Previous stillbirths.
    e. IUGR.
    f. Decreased fetal movements.
    g. Rh disease.
2. Testing is repeated one to two times weekly. With a reactive test, the perinatal death rate is approximately 5 in 1000.
3. A reactive NST is two to three fetal heart rate accelerations of 15 beats' amplitude over 15 seconds during a 20 minute period; a non-reactive test is no fetal movements after 40 minutes associated with fetal heart rate (FHR) or no FHR accelerations associated with fetal movements.
4. Whereas a reactive NST is reassuring, a non-reactive test is an indication for further studies.

B. **Contraction stress test (CST).** This was the first test of fetal well-being. It evaluates the reserve function of the placenta. Indications are the same as for the NST; it is most often used following a non-reactive NST.
1. CST can be achieved by the following:
    a. Spontaneous contraction test: three spontaneous contractions in a 10 minute period.
    b. Nipple stimulation test: naturally induced oxytocin by stimulation of nipples (endogenous).
    c. Oxytocin challenge test (OCT): artificially induced oxytocin by intravenous administration (exogenous).
2. The CST requires three contractions of moderate intensity lasting 40–60 seconds in a 10 minute period. This stimulates a labor pattern and allows the fetus

to be stressed as in normal labor. The CST looks for decelerations or decreases in the FHR in relation to the onset of uterine contractions.
3. A positive CST is defined as late decelerations of the FHR that are present with the majority (>50%) of contractions in a 10 minute window. Delivery should be considered with a positive CST. Results may also be termed suspicious, hyperstimulation, equivocal, or unsatisfactory. These cases require retesting in the next 24 hours for adequate interpretation of fetal well-being.
4. Frequency of CSTs is usually weekly, but can be performed more frequently, as the fetus' condition warrants.

C. Biophysical profile (BPP).
1. The BPP uses real-time ultrasound to evaluate five parameters, each receiving either 0 or 2 points; maximum score is 10 points.
   a. Fetal breathing movements.
   b. Gross body movements.
   c. Fetal tone.
   d. Quantitative amniotic fluid volume.
   e. Non-stress test (NST).
2. Management is based on the assigned score:
   a. 8–10 points: normal; weekly tests are indicated.
   b. 6 points: requires repeat test in 4–6 hours or delivery if oligohydramnios is present.
   c. 4 points: suspect chronic asphyxia. Delivery will be determined based on gestational age and lung maturity.
   d. 2 points or less: strongly suspect chronic asphyxia, requires delivery regardless of gestational age.

Normal Labor

A. Phases of labor. According to Friedman, there are three phases of labor:
1. Latent phase: onset of labor to change in slope of dilatation.
2. Active: approximately 3 cm to complete dilatation.
3. Descent: coincides with 2nd stage.

B. Seven cardinal movements. These are the movements of the head and fetus enroute to delivery.
1. Engagement: the head enters the pelvis.
2. Descent: the head descends into the pelvis, past the pelvic brim.
3. Flexion: with flexion of the head, the narrowest diameter of the head is presented to the pelvis.
4. Internal rotation: the head enters the pelvis transversely, then rotates to an anterior-posterior position.
5. Extension: the flexed head extends to be delivered.
6. External rotation: the head rotates back to the transverse position.
7. Expulsion: the body is expelled.

Intrapartum Labor Management

A. Assessments. Review the prenatal records and obtain a current history, including the following:
1. Vital signs.
2. Contraction pattern, intensity.
3. Membrane status—intact, ruptured, leaking.
4. Fetal heart tones.
5. Vaginal examination (if no bleeding or spontaneous rupture of membranes) to assess:
   a. Dilatation of the cervix.

    b. Effacement or thinning of the cervix.

    c. Station or position of the presenting part in the pelvis.

      (1) 0 station represents when the head enters the pelvis. As descent occurs, station is expressed as +1, +2, +3 and is measured in centimeters.

    d. Presenting part.

    e. Position: the position of the head relative to the pelvis—i.e., anterior, posterior, or transverse.

Based on the available data, the patient should be identified as being at low or high risk.

B. **Management of low-risk patient.** A patient determined to be at low risk during labor does not require continuous electronic fetal monitoring. According to the ACOG Technical Bulletin Number 132 (1989), auscultation should be performed at least every 15 minutes following a contraction for 30 seconds. In the second stage of labor, auscultation should be performed every 5 minutes. If electronic monitoring is used, the patient should be evaluated at the same intervals. Any detectable deceleration of the FHR should alert the nurse to apply the electronic fetal monitor to determine if the fetal heart rate is reassuring.

1. Auscultation. A non-reassuring fetal heart rate detected by auscultation for which electronic fetal monitoring should be performed is indicated by the following:

    a. A baseline rate (average rate between contractions) of less than 100 beats/minute.

    b. A rate of less than 100 beats/minute 30 seconds after a contraction.

    c. Unexplained baseline tachycardia of more than 160 beats/minute, especially with at-risk patients in whom the tachycardia persists through three or more contractions (10–15 minutes) despite corrective measures.

2. Electronic fetal monitoring. This allows systematic evaluation of the fetal heart rate and labor. The contractions should be evaluated for polysystole (more than five contractions in 10 minutes), prolonged contractions lasting more than 90 seconds, and tetanic contractions. These conditions may cause increased stress for the fetus or mother. The fetal baseline heart rate should be observed for variability, periodic changes, and trends over time.

3. Fetal heart rate patterns that have been reported to be associated with increased incidence of fetal compromise are as follows:

    a. Severe bradycardia, a rate less than 80 beats/minute for over 3 minutes.

    b. Repetitive late decelerations, a symmetrical fall in the fetal heart rate, beginning at or after the peak of the uterine contraction and returning to baseline only after the contraction has ended.

    c. Undulating baseline, a pattern of rapid change between tachycardia (rates over 160) and bradycardia (rates less than 100).

    d. Any nonreassuring pattern associated with explained poor or absent baseline variability. This would appear as a flat or nearly flat baseline.

Puerperium: Fourth Trimester

The period of time following delivery through the sixth week.

A. **Uterine involution.** Involution begins immediately following delivery; the fundus is at the level of the umbilicus.

B. **Placental site regeneration.** Takes approximately 6 weeks after delivery.

C. **Lochia.** Post-delivery uterine discharge, changes as follows:

1. Lochia rubra: dark red or reddish brown; 3–4 days
2. Lochia serosa: pink or brown; 4–10 days.
3. Lochia alba: yellow to white; approximately 10 days after delivery to 4–6 weeks after delivery.

D. **Breasts.** The breasts should be soft until the third or fourth post-partum day, when engorgement occurs. This resolves spontaneously within 24–36 hours. In non–breast-feeding mothers, lactation ceases within a week.

E. **Immunizations.**
1. Rubella vaccination should be administered in the immediate post-partum period to all women who are not immune.
2. Rh (D) immune globulin (300 μg IM) is administered to the mother within 72 hours of delivery to prevent sensitization from fetal-maternal transfusion of Rh-positive fetal RBCs.

STUDY QUESTIONS

1. A baby delivered at 35 weeks is classified:
   a. post-term.
   b. pre-term.
   c. term.

2. A woman's LMP is September 4th. By Näegele's rule, her calculated EDC would be:
   a. June 4.
   b. June 11.
   c. July 11.

3. In pregnancy, plasma volume increases by:
   a. 25%.
   b. 35%.
   c. 50%.

4. In routine antepartum visits, three assessments routinely performed include:
   a. Blood pressure, weight, and urine for glucose and protein.
   b. Fundal height, fetal heart rate, maternal heart rate.
   c. Hct/Hgb, blood pressure, fetal heart rate.

5. Fetal heart tones (FHTs) can be detected by an unamplified fetoscope by:
   a. 10–12 weeks.
   b. 19–20 weeks.
   c. 24 weeks.

6. The screening method commonly used initially for determining fetal well-being is:
   a. Biophysical profile (BPP).
   b. Contraction stress test (CST).
   c. Non-stress test (NST).

7. Post-delivery uterine discharge at 7 days that is light pink to brown is referred to as:
   a. Lochia alba.
   b. Lochia rubra.
   c. Lochia serosa.

Answers to Study Questions

1. b	4. a	6. c
2. b	5. b	7. c
3. c		

BIBLIOGRAPHY

American College of Obstetricians and Gynecologists (ACOG): Technical Bulletin Number 79, Prevention of Rho(D) Isoimmunization. Washington, DC, 1984.

American College of Obstetricians and Gynecologists (ACOG): Technical Bulletin Number 89, Gonorrhea and Chlamydia Infections. Washington, DC, 1985.

American College of Obstetricians and Gynecologists (ACOG): Technical Bulletin Number 90, Management of Isoimmunization in Pregnancy. Washington, DC, 1986.

American College of Obstetricians and Gynecologists (ACOG): Technical Bulletin Number 99, Prenatal Detection of Neural Tube Defects. Washington, DC, 1987.

American College of Obstetricians and Gynecologists (ACOG): Technical Bulletin Number 108, Antenatal Diagnosis of Genetic Disorders. Washington, DC, 1987.

American College of Obstetricians and Gynecologists (ACOG): Technical Bulletin Number 110, Induction and Augmentation of Labor. Washington, DC, 1987.

American College of Obstetricians and Gynecologists (ACOG): Technical Bulletin Number 116, Ultrasound in Pregnancy. Washington, DC, 1988.

American College of Obstetricians and Gynecologists (ACOG): Technical Bulletin Number 122, Perinatal Herpes Simplex Virus. Washington, DC, 1988.

American College of Obstetricians and Gynecologists (ACOG): Technical Bulletin Number 130, Diagnosis and Management of Post Term Pregnancy. Washington, DC, 1989.

American College of Obstetricians and Gynecologists (ACOG): Technical Bulletin Number 132, Intrapartum Fetal Heart Rate Monitoring. Washington, DC, 1989.

Bobak, I.M., and Jensen, M.D.: Essentials of Maternity Nursing: The Nurse and the Childbearing Family, 2nd ed. St. Louis, C.V. Mosby Co.

Caring for Our Future: The Content of Prenatal Care. A Report of the Public Health Service Expert Panel on the Content of Prenatal Care. Washington, DC, 1989.

Cunningham, F.G., MacDonald, P.C., and Gant, N.F.: Williams Obstetrics, 18th ed. Norwalk, CT: Appleton and Lange, 1989.

Friedman, E.A.: Graphic appraisal of labor: A study of 500 primigravidas. Bull. Sloan. Hosp. Women 1:42, 1955.

Gabbe, S.G., Neibyl, J.R., and Simpson, J.L.: Obstetrics: Normal and Problem Pregnancies. New York, Churchill Livingstone, 1986.

Kilpatrick, S.J., and Laros, R.K.: Characteristics of normal labor. Obstet. Gynecol., 74(1), 1989.

Manning, F.A.: Assessment of fetal condition & risk: Analysis of single and combined biophysical variable monitoring. Semin. Perinatol. 9:168, 1985.

Olds, S.B., London, M.L., and Ladewig, P.A.: Maternal-Newborn Nursing: A Family-Centered Approach, 2nd ed. Menlo Park, CA, Addison-Wesley Publishing Co., 1984.

Pritchard, J.A., MacDonald, P.C., and Gant, N.F.: Williams Obstetrics, 17th ed. Norwalk, CT, Appleton-Century-Crofts, 1985.

Schifrin, B.S., and Cohen, W.R.: Clinical commentary: Labor's dysfunctional lexicon. Obstet. Gynecol., 74(1):121–124, 1989.

Sterat, G.M.: Obstetrics, 2nd ed. Oxford, Blackwell Scientific Publications, 1986.

Tait, J., Foerdr, C., Ashwood, E., and Benedett, T.: Improved fluorescence polarization assay for use in evaluating fetal lung maturity. I. Development of the assay procedure. Clin. Chem., 33:554, 1987.

Vestal, K.W., and McKenzie, C.A.M.: High Risk Perinatal Nursing: The American Association of Critical-Care Nurses. Philadelphia: W.B. Saunders Co., 1983.

CHAPTER 2

Anne B. Broussard

Antepartum-Intrapartum Complications

Objectives

1. List maternal risk factors that may exist prior to pregnancy.

2. Discuss the effects of pregnancy-induced hypertension and diabetes on the maternal-placental-fetal complex.

3. Categorize intrapartum conditions that may result in complications for the newborn.

4. Assess the fetus/newborn for effects of tocolytic drugs.

5. Describe the effect on the fetus/newborn of these intrapartum crises: abruptio placentae, placenta previa, cord prolapse, and shoulder dystocia.

6. List neonatal complications associated with breech delivery.

7. Examine the effect of obstetrical analgesia/anesthesia and operative delivery on the newborn.

An understanding of maternal complications enhances the ability of the nurse to anticipate and recognize neonatal complications and to intervene appropriately. The purpose of this chapter is to provide a comprehensive view of possible neonatal complications secondary to maternal risk factors. These risk factors may exist prior to the pregnancy or develop during the antepartum and intrapartum periods (Table 2–1).

Anatomy and Physiology

A. **The fetus.** The fetus is a part of the maternal-placental-fetal complex.

B. **Conditions and substances that affect the pregnant woman.** These have the potential to affect placental functions of respiration, nutrition, excretion, and hormone production. Decreased placental function can in turn adversely affect the fetus.

C. **The placenta.** In addition, the old concept of the placenta as a barrier to noxious substances has long been superseded by the concept of the placenta as a sieve that permits transport of desirable *and* undesirable substances to the fetus.

Table 2-1
GUIDE FOR PERINATAL ASSESSMENT OF THE NEWBORN: IDENTIFICATION OF RISK FACTORS BY MATERNAL COMPONENTS

General Information	Risk		Risk		Risk
Age: <18 or >40	2				
Marital status		**Maternal medical/ surgical problems**		**Duration of labor**	
Single, separated, divorced, widowed	2	Diabetes	3	1st stage >16 hours	2
		Heart disease	2	2nd stage >2 hours	3
Socioeconomic level		Chronic hypertension	2	2nd stage <10 minutes	3
Low	2	Thyroid disease	2	Total >20 hours	2
Low-middle	1	Other endocrine disorders	2	<3 hours	2
Ethnic-cultural group: minority	2	Anemia		**Identified-intrapartal problems**	
Educational level: 10th grade	1	Iron deficiency	2	CPD	2
Hereditary disorder: genetic	3	Sickle cell	3	Pre-eclampsia	2
Familial health history		Other	3	Eclampsia	3
Diabetes	2	Pulmonary disease	2	Rx MgSO$_4$ >25 g	3
Chronic hypertension	1	Chronic renal disease	2	Meconium staining	3
Prepregnancy weight: <100 or >200 lb	2	Neurologic disease	2	Placenta previa	3
History of infertility		PID	2	Abruptio placentae	3
Para 0, >35 years	2	Pelvic surgery	2	Cord compression	2
Problem conceiving	1	Habits/present pregnancy		Prolapsed cord	3
Pregnancy interval >4 years	1	Heavy smoker: ≥20/day	2	Uterine inertia	3
Rx for infertility	2	Alcohol use or abuse	3	Uterine tetany	3
				Multiple birth	3
				Maternal fever ≥100°F	3
Obstetrical History				**Fetal heart monitoring**	
Gravida: ≥6	2			Base line FHR <100 or >160	3
Parity: ≥5	2	**Drug abuse**	3		
Abortions		**Complications**		Bradycardia >30 minutes	3
≥1 (≤20 weeks)	3	Pre-eclampsia	2	Tachycardia ≥30 minutes	3
Gravida <1 + para	3	Eclampsia	3	Poor beat-to-beat variability	3
Stillbirths: ≥1 (≥37 weeks)	3	Hyperemesis gravidarum	3	Increasing number of variables	3
Prematurity: <37 weeks	3	Early bleeding ≤20 weeks	2	Late decelerations	3
SGA		Late bleeding >20 weeks	3	**Analgesia**	
<37 weeks	3	Bleeding with pain	3	Total Demerol >200 mg	3
37-41 weeks	2	Hydramnios	2	Demerol >25 mg IV within 1/2 hour of delivery	3
≥42 weeks	2	Oligohydramnios	3		
LGA		Rubella infection (8-12 weeks)	3	Demerol >25 mg IM within 1 hour of delivery	3
<37 weeks	3	Sexually transmitted disease	3		
37-41 weeks	2	Other infections	2	**Course of delivery**	
≥42 weeks	2	Maternal FUO	2	**Presentation**	
Neonatal death: ≤4 weeks	3	Rh sensitization	3	**Breech**	3

Continued

Table 2–1
GUIDE FOR PERINATAL ASSESSMENT OF THE NEWBORN: IDENTIFICATION OF RISK FACTORS BY MATERNAL COMPONENTS (*Continued*)

General Information	Risk		Risk		Risk
History of congenital anomalies	2	Antepartal diagnostic tests		Transverse lie	3
History of neonatal asphyxia	2	Estriol level: no rise >36 weeks	3	Position: vertex other than OA	2
Prevous prenatal history		Ultrasonography; growth retardation >2 weeks	3	Forceps	
Pre-eclampsia	2			Outlet	1
Eclampsia	3	Amniocentesis		Low	2
PROM	2	L/S ratio <2:1	3	Mid or >	3
Ectopic pregnancy	2	Bilirubin present	3	Vacuum extraction	2
Placenta previa	2	Meconium present	3	Identified problems	
Abruptio placentae	2	Other evidence of immaturity	3	Shoulder dystocia	3
CPD	2	NST: nonreactive	3	Nuchal cord ×1	1
Uterine dystocia	3	OCT: positive	3	≥×2	3
Cesarean section	2	Duration of pregnancy		Short cord	2
Induction	1	<37 weeks	3	Cesarean section	
Rh sensitization	3	>42 weeks	2	Repeat	2
ABO incompatibility	2			Emergency	3
Present Pregnancy		**Present Pregnancy**		Episiotomy: none, with laceration	1
Antepartal Course		**Intrapartal Course**		Anesthesia	
General prenatal information		Onset of labor		General	3
Prenatal care: little or none	3	Early labor: <37 weeks	3	Spinal 15 minutes before delivery	2
Weight gain: ≤15 lb or ≥35 lb	2	PROM	3	Maternal bonding	
Medications other than dietary supplement	3	Induction	2	No bonding	2
		Cesarean section	2	Inappropriate affect	2

Risk significance: 3 = high risk; 2 = moderate risk; 1 = slight risk.
Modified from Brodish, M.: Perinatal assessment. J. Obstet. Gynecol. Neonatal Nursing, *10*:42, 1981.

D. **Placental transport mechanisms.** These mechanisms, including passive and facilitated diffusion, are affected by a number of factors (Martin and Gingerich, 1976):
1. Placental area.
    a. The placenta normally increases in size as the pregnancy advances in order to supply the increased growth needs of the fetus.
    b. A placenta that is not keeping pace with fetal growth or that has decreased functional area as a result of infarct or separation does not allow optimum transport of materials between fetus and mother.
    c. The outcome of decreased functional placental area can include decrease in fetal growth, fetal distress, and even fetal death.
2. Concentration gradient.
    a. Passive and facilitated diffusion of unbound substances dissolved in maternal and fetal plasma occurs in the direction of lesser concentration.
    b. The greater the concentration gradient, the faster the rate of diffusion will occur.
    c. Concentration gradients are maintained when dissolved substances are removed from plasma via metabolism, cellular uptake, or excretion. For exam-

ple, the excretion of CO_2 from the maternal lungs maintains the concentration gradient for CO_2, permitting fetal plasma CO_2 to cross from fetal plasma to maternal plasma. Inefficient maternal excretion of CO_2 may lead to maternal respiratory acidosis and fetal acidosis.

3. Diffusing distance.
   a. The greater the distance between maternal and fetal blood in the placenta, the slower the diffusion rate of substances will be.
   b. Any edema that develops in the placental villi increases the distance between the fetal capillaries within the villi and the maternal arterial blood in the intervillous spaces, thus slowing the diffusion rate of substances between the maternal and fetal circulations.
   c. Edema of villi may occur in:
      (1) Maternal diabetes.
      (2) Transplacental infections.
      (3) Erythroblastosis fetalis.
4. Uteroplacental blood flow.
   a. 85–90% of uterine blood flow reaches the placenta.
   b. Decreased blood flow to the uterus or within the intervillous spaces will decrease the transport of substances to and from the fetus.
   c. Causes of decreased uteroplacental blood flow include:
      (1) Maternal vasoconstriction in hypertension, cocaine abuse, diabetic vasculopathy, and smoking.
      (2) Decreased maternal cardiac output in supine hypotension.
      (3) Decreased maternal blood flow in intervillous spaces due to edema of placental villi.
      (4) Hypertonic uterine contractions.
      (5) Severe maternal physical stress.

Conditions Related to Antepartum

PREGNANCY-INDUCED HYPERTENSION (PIH)

PIH, which includes pre-eclampsia and eclampsia, is a major cause of perinatal morbidity and mortality in the U.S. In addition, it is the third leading cause of maternal death in this country. The main pathophysiologic events in PIH are vasospasm, hematologic changes, deposition of fibrin and fibrinogen in vessels, hypovolemia secondary to fluid shifts, and increased CNS irritability.

A. Incidence. 5–7% of all pregnancies (May and Mahlmeister, 1990).

B. Etiology/predisposing factors.
1. The exact etiology has not been determined.
2. Associated with primigravidas, younger and older women, family history of PIH, multiple gestation, hydatidiform mole, malnutrition and low weight gains in pregnancy, diabetes, lack of a second trimester decrease in mean arterial pressure (Remich and Youngkin, 1989), multigravidas with changed paternity for subsequent pregnancies, and previous use of barrier contraceptives (Klon-off-Cohen et al., 1989).

C. Clinical presentation.
1. Evaluated BPs after the 20th week of pregnancy: either BPs of 140/90 or above, or a rise of 30 mm Hg/systolic and/or 15 mm Hg/diastolic or more over the early pregnancy baseline.
2. Proteinuria due to decreased renal perfusion resulting in development of glomerular capillary endotheliosis.
3. Edema due to sodium retention and decreased plasma colloid osmotic pressure.
4. Other signs and symptoms: headache, hyper-reflexia with clonus, visual and retinal changes, irritability, nausea and vomiting, epigastric pain, dyspnea, and oliguria.

D. Potential complications.
1. Maternal.
   a. Eclampsia (grand mal seizure).
   b. Cardiopulmonary failure; peripartum cardiomyopathy (Schmidt et al., 1989).
   c. Hepatic rupture.
   d. Cerebrovascular accident.
   e. Renal cortical necrosis.
   f. Disseminated intravascular coagulation (DIC).
   g. HELLP syndrome (*h*emolysis, *e*levated *l*iver function tests, and *l*ow *p*latelet count).
   h. Retinal detachment.
2. Placental/fetal.
   a. Premature placental aging, placental infarction, and decrease in amniotic fluid.
   b. Abruptio placentae.
   c. Intrauterine growth retardation (IUGR) secondary to decreased placental blood flow.
   d. Fetal distress.
   e. Pre-term delivery.

E. Assessment and management.
1. Severe pre-eclampsia.
   a. Hospitalization, with complete bedrest in left lateral recumbent position.
   b. Limitation of stimuli such as noise and visitors.
   c. Seizure precautions.
   d. Frequent assessments of the cardiopulmonary, neurologic, hepatic, renal, and hematopoietic systems for signs and symptoms of progression.
   e. High-protein diet (1.5 g/kg/day) with moderate sodium intake (Olds et al., 1988).
   f. Supportive care, including teaching and emotional support of the woman and her family.
   g. Lab work: complete blood count (CBC), liver enzymes, blood urea nitrogen (BUN), uric acid, serum creatinine, and 24-hour urine protein.
   h. Placental-fetal function tests: fetal movement, ultrasound to determine fetal age and detect IUGR, serial non-stress tests and/or contraction stress test to detect uteroplacental insufficiency, and amniocentesis for lecithin/sphingomyelin (L/S) ratio or fluorescence polarization (FPOL) to determine fetal lung maturity.
   i. Drugs.
      (1) Use of magnesium sulfate ($MgSO_4$) IV as a CNS depressant to prevent convulsions. $MgSO_4$ is usually given IV. Monitor fetus for changes in short-term variability.
      (2) Sedation with phenobarbital. Non-stress test may be non-reactive as a result of sedation. Monitor fetus for loss of short-term variability.
      (3) Apresoline (hydralazine) for antihypertensive effect. Monitor fetus for signs of hypoxia (tachycardia, bradycardia, late decelerations), which can occur with a sudden decrease in maternal BP.
   j. Monitor fetus for late decelerations caused by decreased uterine perfusion.
   k. Delivery by induction or cesarean if fetus is mature or if worsening maternal condition warrants.
2. Eclampsia.
   a. Immediate notification of physician.
   b. Safety measures for woman during and after convulsion.
   c. Support breathing with airway management, O_2, and suctioning.
   d. Monitor fetus for bradycardia.
   e. Continuous maternal assessment.
   f. $MgSO_4$ IV push and Apresoline.
   g. Delivery by induction or cesarean when woman and fetus recover.

3. Assess newborn for:
   a. IUGR.
   b. Pre-term gestational age.
   c. Hypoxia and acidosis.
   d. Signs of hypomagnesemia when mother is a young primipara who developed eclampsia (Bliss-Holtz, 1983).
   e. Specific drug effects on the newborn:
      (1) Signs of hypermagnesemia, including weakness, lethargy, hypotonia, flaccidity, respiratory depression, poor suck, decrease in GI motility, hypotension, urinary retention, and increase in atrioventricular and ventricular conduction when maternal administration of high doses of $MgSO_4$ occurs near the time of delivery.
      (2) Hypothermia with maternal administration of Valium.
      (3) Poor suck, decrease in responsiveness, and respiratory depression with maternal administration of phenobarbital.
      (4) Thrombocytopenia with maternal administration of Apresoline.

DIABETES MELLITUS

The insulin-dependent diabetic woman who becomes pregnant and the pregnant woman who develops gestational diabetes are at risk during the antepartum period because of altered carbohydrate metabolism. The fetus/newborn is therefore also at risk. Strict control of maternal blood glucose and anticipatory management of the newborn are important elements of perinatal care.

A. **Incidence.** 2–3% of all pregnancies. Of these women, 90% are gestational diabetics (Gabbe, 1984). When undiagnosed, gestational diabetes doubles the perinatal mortality rate (Herbert et al., 1986).

B. **Etiology/predisposing factors in gestational diabetes.**
1. In the second half of pregnancy, secretion of estrogen, progesterone, and human placental lactogen increases cellular resistance to insulin. The pancreas of the woman who is predisposed to diabetes cannot meet the increased demand for insulin, and hyperglycemia results.
2. Associated with obesity; family history of diabetes; age over 40; multiparity; and a previous history of a large for gestational age (LGA) newborn, hydramnios, congenital anomaly, or stillbirth.

C. **Clinical presentation in gestational diabetes.**
1. Cardinal signs of polyuria, polydipsia, polyphagia, and weight loss.
2. Abnormally high glucose levels on glucose tolerance tests.

D. **Potential complications.**
1. Maternal.
   a. Hypoglycemic reactions in the first trimester.
   b. Ketoacidosis in the second and third trimesters.
   c. Progression of vasculopathy, nephropathy, and retinopathy with pre-existing diabetes.
   d. Hydramnios.
   e. PIH.
   f. Anemia.
   g. Infections such as monilial vaginitis and urinary tract infections (UTIs).
2. Fetal/newborn.
   a. Pre-term birth.
   b. Macrosomia (greater than 4000 g) with possible traumatic vaginal delivery. IUGR in advanced maternal diabetes (White's classifications D, F, R, and H).
   c. Fetal demise.
   d. Respiratory distress syndrome
   e. Hypoglycemia, hypocalcemia, and hypomagnesemia.
   f. Polycythemia, hyperviscosity, and hyperbilirubinemia.

g. Cardiomyopathy with congestive heart failure.

h. Congenital malformation as a consequence of poorly controlled pre-existing diabetes: renal and CNS anomalies, caudal regression syndrome, facial clefts, patent ductus arteriosus, transposition of the great vessels, ventricular septal defect, and small left colon syndrome.

E. Assessment and management.

1. In pre-existing diabetes:
   a. Pre-conception counseling with optimal control of blood glucose levels and use of insulin if necessary (oral hypoglycemic agents are considered teratogenic).
   b. Home blood glucose monitoring, diet, and insulin (Lente or NPH, and regular in divided doses) prescribed to maintain rigid control of blood glucose, which is associated with decreased risk of macrosomia, perinatal morality, and congenital malformations.
   c. Weekly prenatal visits after 28 weeks, with fetal assessment via non-stress test, contraction stress test, and fetal activity determination.
   d. Baseline ultrasound at 20–26 weeks, repeated every 4–6 weeks.
   e. Delivery at 38 weeks if phosphatidylglycerol present in amniotic fluid and L/S ratio or FPOL indicates the lungs of the fetus are mature. Insulin IV drip prior to induction of labor to control glucose levels at 60–90 mg/dl.
   f. Delivery prior to 38 weeks if maternal or fetal complications develop. Immediate delivery by cesarean if fetal distress occurs.

2. In gestational diabetes:
   a. Many authorities recommend that all pregnant women be screened for gestational diabetes via a one hour 50 g glucose screening test, followed by a three hour 100 g glucose tolerance test if the results are positive (O'Brien and Gilson, 1987; O'Sullivan et al., 1973; Scupholme and Kamons, 1988).
   b. 15–20% of gestational diabetics have significant hyperglycemia requiring the management described above (Herbert et al., 1986).
   c. 2000–2500 calorie diet with no simple carbohydrates.
   d. Assessment of glucose levels every 2 weeks.
   e. Fetal assessment via estriols and non-stress tests performed twice a week, beginning at 32 weeks. Delivery by induction is delayed until 40 weeks if possible.

3. In newborn:
   a. Assess for gestational age and size (LGA or IUGR).
   b. Assess for:
      (1) Respiratory distress.
      (2) Hypoglycemia, hypocalcemia, and hypomagnesemia.
      (3) Polycythemia and hyperviscosity.
      (4) Complications resulting from decreased blood flow, RBC hemolysis, and thrombosis.
      (5) Congenital malformations.
      (6) Birth injuries: fractured clavicles, intracranial bleeding, facial nerve paralysis, brachial palsy, and skull fractures.

Conditions Related to Intrapartum Period

PRE-TERM LABOR

Pre-term labor is defined as labor occurring prior to the 37th week of pregnancy. If pre-term labor is recognized in time, measures can be taken to stop the contractions. The prognosis for the fetus improves with each week of pregnancy gained.

A. Incidence. Occurs in about 7% of all pregnancies in the U.S. (May and Mahlmeister, 1990).

B. **Etiology/predisposing factors.**

1. The exact cause is unknown.
2. A number of socioeconomic, medical, obstetrical, and lifestyle factors have been associated with an increased incidence of pre-term labor.
3. Risk scoring systems (Table 2–2) have been designed to screen women during pregnancy.

C. **Clinical presentation.**

1. Painless or painful uterine contractions.
2. Low, dull, intermittent or constant backache.
3. Intermittent or constant menstrual-like cramping.
4. Intermittent pelvic pressure that may extend along the inner thigh.
5. Abdominal cramps that may be accompanied by diarrhea.
6. Increased vaginal discharge, which may be mucousy, watery, or slightly bloody in character.
7. Spontaneous and premature rupture of membranes.
8. A generalized feeling that something is wrong.
9. Progressive cervical effacement and dilatation unless intervention occurs.

D. **Potential complications.**

1. Maternal.
   a. No particular physical complications other than adverse reactions to tocolytic agents.
   b. Emotional stress and financial problems may occur.
2. Fetal/newborn.
   a. Pre-term birth with an increase in neonatal mortality and morbidity.
   b. Adverse reactions to tocolytic agents.

E. **Assessment and management.**

1. Screening of pregnant women at the first and subsequent prenatal visits for pre-term labor risk factors. Presence of one or more major factors or two or more minor factors on the risk scoring system in Table 2–2 would indicate that a woman is at high risk for pre-term labor.
2. Teaching *all* pregnant women the symptoms of pre-term labor and the actions to take if they occur (lie down on the left side and drink several glasses of fluid; report to physician or midwife if contractions are still occurring after one hour).
3. Helping high-risk women modify their risk factors and take measures to prevent pre-term labor—e.g., stop smoking, improve nutrition and hydration,

Table 2–2
MAJOR AND MINOR RISK FACTORS OF THE MODIFIED SCORING SYSTEM FOR SPONTANEOUS PRE-TERM LABOR

Major Factors*	Minor Factors†
Multiple gestation	Febrile illness during pregnancy
Prevous pre-term delivery	Bleeding after 12 weeks
Previous pre-term labor, term delivery	History of pyelonephritis
Abdominal surgery during pregnancy	Cigarette smoking (>10 per day)
Diethylstilbestrol exposure	One second-trimester abortion
Hydramnios	More than two first-trimester abortions
Uterine anomaly	
History of cone biopsy	
Uterine irritability (admission to rule out preterm labor)	
More than one second-trimester abortion	
Cervical dilation (>1 cm) at 32 weeks	
Cervical effacement (<1 cm length) at 32 weeks	

*Presence of one or more indicates high risk.
†Presence of two or more indicates high risk.
From Holbrook, R. et al.: Evaluation of a risk-scoring system for prediction of pre-term labor. Am. J. Perinatol., *6*:62, 1989.

treat infections, decrease work hours and stress, increase bedrest, and avoid nipple preparation that initiates signs of preterm labor.

4. Gently examine the cervix of high-risk women at weekly or bi-weekly prenatal visits to detect changes that are indicative of impending pre-term labor (Catalano et al., 1989).

5. For high-risk women, use of a home contraction monitoring system with telephone counseling from a nurse to increase early diagnosis of pre-term labor and provide psychosocial support (Gill and Katz, 1986; Newman et al., 1986).

6. Treatment of episodes of pre-term labor with hospitalization, hydration with IV fluid, bedrest in left lateral position, and sedation.

7. When appropriate and not contraindicated, use of drug therapy:
   a. Ritodrine (Yutopar) given IV drip and by mouth, inhibits uterine contractility. Potential fetal/neonatal side effects include tachycardia and hypoglycemia (Fitzgerald, 1983).
   b. MgSO$_4$ given IV drip for uterine relaxation. Monitor fetus for loss of cardiac variability and neonate for respiratory depression.
   c. Terbutaline (Brethine) can be given IV drip, subcutaneously, or by mouth. For long-term use at home, women can be taught to give themselves terbutaline in programmed continuous and bolus doses via a miniature subcutaneous automatic infusion pump, in conjunction with a home contraction monitoring system (Lam, 1989).

8. If the above measures are not successful and the cervix continues to efface and dilate, the following measures are important:
   a. No rupture of membranes is performed, in order to allow the amniotic fluid to cushion the fetal skull.
   b. The head is delivered in a slow, controlled fashion.
   c. Cesarean delivery is often suggested for the fetus presenting breech, due to the risk of cord prolapse and the potential risk of difficult delivery of the head.

ABRUPTIO PLACENTAE

In abruptio placentae, the placenta separates suddenly and prematurely from the uterine wall during pregnancy or labor. It is a common cause of bleeding in the second half of pregnancy.

A. **Incidence.** 1 in 100–250 deliveries (Moore, 1983; Hayashi and Castillo, 1986).

B. **Etiology/predisposing factors.**

1. The etiology is not really established, but there is a high correlation with hypertensive disorders during pregnancy and with high multiparity.

2. Other factors that are considered predisposing include short umbilical cord, maternal abdominal trauma, uterine leiomyomas or anomalies, polyhydramnios and multiple pregnancy, supine hypotension, history of previous abruption, maternal cigarette smoking and poor weight gain, and cocaine use.

C. **Clinical presentation.**

1. Types.
   a. Marginal.
   b. Central.
   c. Complete.

2. Maternal signs and symptoms.
   a. Sharp, continuous abdominal pain.
   b. Board-like and tender abdomen.
   c. Dark or bright red vaginal bleeding (unless the bleeding is concealed behind the placenta) ranging from spotting to frank hemorrhage.
   d. Amniotic fluid that is port-wine colored (Hayashi and Castillo, 1986).
   e. Enlargement of the uterus as blood accumulates.

3. Fetal signs.
   a. Weak or absent fetal heart tones.
   b. Tachycardia.
   c. Late decelerations.
   d. Decreased fetal heart rate variability.

D. Potential complications.
1. Maternal.
   a. Anemia.
   b. Hypovolemic shock, sometimes resulting in anterior pituitary necrosis (Sheehan's syndrome) (Oxorn, 1986).
   c. Couvelaire uterus (blood forced between the muscle fibers of the uterus).
   d. Disseminated intravascular coagulation (DIC).
   e. Kidney necrosis leading to renal shutdown.
   f. Death.
2. Fetal/newborn.
   a. Neonatal anemia.
   b. Hypoxia and asphyxia.
   c. Death.

E. Assessment and management.
1. If bleeding is not severe.
   a. Bedrest in left lateral position, close assessment of abdomen for rigidity and pain, and close assessment of vaginal bleeding.
   b. Monitoring of maternal vital signs and fetal heart for rate, decelerations, and variability.
   c. Ultrasound to locate placenta and determine degree of placental separation.
   d. IV with large-gauge intracatheter.
   e. Urine for drug screening may be requested.
2. If bleeding is severe or becomes severe.
   a. Preparation for cesarean delivery.
      (1) Inform and support parents and ensure that "surgical consent" is obtained.
      (2) Order lab tests (CBC, type and crossmatch blood, coagulation studies)
      (3) Prep abdomen and insert urinary catheter.
      (4) Notify NICU and pediatrician.

PLACENTA PREVIA

Placenta previa is a placenta that is implanted near the cervix (marginal) or in varying degrees over the cervix (partial or total). Cervical dilatation at or near term is accompanied by bleeding from the placenta. Placenta previa is a common cause of bleeding in the second half of pregnancy.

A. Incidence. 1 in 200 pregnancies (Oxorn, 1986).

B. Etiology/predisposing factors.
1. The precise etiology is unknown, but placenta previa occurs most frequently in multiparas and older women.
2. Other associated and predisposing factors include previous placenta previa, past history of low-segment cesarean delivery, history of myomectomy or post-partum endometritis, and increased placental size.

C. Clinical presentation.
1. Bright red, painless vaginal bleeding. Although first bleeding episode may be slight in amount, more blood is usually lost in subsequent episodes.
2. Uterine contractions in 10% of cases, but otherwise uterus is soft and non-tender (Hayashi and Castillo, 1986).

3. Found on routine ultrasound in 10% of cases (Hayashi and Castillo, 1986).
4. Presenting part of fetus is unengaged. Fetus may lie transversely or breech.

D. **Potential complications.**
1. Maternal.
   a. Anemia.
   b. Hypovolemic shock.
   c. Endometritis.
   d. Decreased contractile strength of the lower uterine segment can lead to postpartum hemorrhage and need for hysterectomy.
2. Fetal/newborn.
   a. Hypoxia and asphyxia.
   b. Developmental anomalies.
   c. IUGR.
   d. Fetal hemorrhage and death.
   e. Prematurity.

E. **Assessment and management.**
1. Marginal placenta previa and low-lying placenta with minimal bleeding is managed conservatively:
   a. Ultrasound to confirm diagnosis (95% accuracy) and to rule out IUGR.
   b. Bedrest with no vaginal examinations.
   c. Avoidance of intercourse and orgasm, which can cause uterine contractions. Resumption of intercourse only if placenta subsequently "migrates" away from the cervix (Osofsky and Drukker, 1986).
   d. Weekly non-stress test or contraction stress test.
   e. If the fetus is mature, the physician may choose to perform a vaginal examination under a double set-up (preparation for an immediate cesarean delivery), although the use of ultrasound has generally obviated the use of the double set-up. Vaginal delivery can be accomplished if bleeding is minimal.
2. Partial or total placenta previa or greater amounts of bleeding are handled as above, except that vaginal delivery may not be possible. In addition:
   a. Frequent assessment of vaginal bleeding, with pad counts and/or weighing of pads.
   b. Frequent assessment of maternal vital signs and fetal heart tones, and palpation of abdomen.
   c. Semi-Fowler's position to allow fetus to compress placenta.
   d. Lab work: CBC, type and crossmatch for blood.
   e. With significant bleeding, IV with large-gauge intracatheter for blood administration.
   f. Method of delivery:
      (1) Vaginal delivery only if less than 30% of placenta overlies cervix and bleeding remains minimal. Artificial rupture of membranes may be performed to allow presenting part of fetus to compress placental site.
      (2) If a greater degree of placenta previa is present or if bleeding is significant, cesarean delivery is performed.

UMBILICAL CORD PROLAPSE

Umbilical cord prolapse is an event that is life-threatening to the fetus and requires immediate and effective management by the nurse. It occurs when the cord falls below the presenting part or is compressed between the presenting part and the pelvis or cervix.

A. **Incidence.** Estimated to be between 0.25 and 0.6% (1 in 400 to 1 in 166 deliveries) (McKenzie, 1983; Oxorn, 1986).

B. **Etiology/predisposing factors.**
1. The fetal presenting part does not fill the pelvic inlet well, and the cord slips past it, often when the membranes rupture.

2. Predisposing factors include malposition (transverse lie and breech presentation), pre-term or small for gestational age (SGA) fetus, multiple pregnancy, polyhydramnios, long cord, cephalopelvic disproportion that prevents fetal engagement, placenta previa, and lack of engagement prior to the onset of labor (as is common with multiparas).

C. Clinical presentation.
1. Cord is protruding from vagina or is palpable on vaginal examination.
2. In an occult prolapse, cord is not visible or palpable but is located between the presenting part and the pelvis or cervix.
3. Station of presenting part is 0 to −4 cm, and membranes are often ruptured.
4. Fetal heart rate accelerates to 180–200, then decreases rapidly if adequate treatment is not given. With occult prolapse, variable fetal decelerations may precede these changes.

D. Potential complications.
1. Maternal.
   a. Trauma to the birth canal from rapid forceps delivery.
   b. General anesthesia resulting in uterine atony with subsequent post-partal bleeding.
   c. Blood loss from cesarean delivery.
2. Fetal/neonatal.
   a. Perinatal mortality of 35%, with mortality increasing as increased time elapses between cord prolapse and delivery (Oxorn, 1986).
   b. Fetal anoxia leading to long-range neurologic complications.
   c. Neonatal infection.

E. Assessment and management.
1. Assessments on admission to labor and delivery.
   a. Presenting part and its station.
   b. Dilatation of cervix.
   c. Status of membranes.
   d. Estimated fetal weight and fetal heart rate.
   e. Review of prenatal record for evidence for polyhydramnios or placenta previa.
2. Ambulation during labor and artificial rupture of membranes may be contraindicated in certain situations—e.g., in the presence of polyhydramnios and lack of engagement of presenting part.
3. Assessments to make with artificial or spontaneous rupture of membranes.
   a. Monitor fetal heart for rate and variable decelerations.
   b. Perform vaginal examination to detect prolapse.
4. If prolapse has occurred:
   a. Keep examining hand in vagina to push presenting part away from cord until delivery of fetus.
   b. Have assistant help woman into knee-chest or Trendelenburg position, with hips elevated and head down.
   c. Have O_2 administered to woman.
   d. Monitor fetal heart rate continuously and palpate cord for continued pulsation.
   e. Tocolytic agents may be used.
   f. For immediate delivery, internal podalic version may be used to turn fetus to a breech position if woman is fully dilated; emergency cesarean delivery may be preferable, especially if woman is not fully dilated and fetal heart rate is affected.
   g. Continuous emotional support of parents.

SHOULDER DYSTOCIA

Shoulder dystocia is defined as an inability of the physician or midwife to deliver the shoulders of the infant by the usual maneuvers after the delivery of the head.

A. **Incidence.** 0.15–0.2% overall, but increased incidence in babies over 4000 g (Oxorn, 1986).

B. **Etiology/predisposing factors.**
1. The fetal shoulders are too broad to be delivered between the symphysis pubis and the sacrum.
2. Predisposing factors include maternal obesity, excessive weight gain, oversized infants, history of large siblings, maternal diabetes, and contracted pelvic outlet.

C. **Clinical presentation.**
1. History of large babies or high estimated fetal weight.
2. Second stage longer than 2 hours, with slow descent of head.
3. After delivery of the head, the head recoils against the perineum and restitution does not occur ("turtling"). The usual traction from below with fundal pressure is not successful in delivering the baby.

D. **Complications.**
1. Maternal.
   a. Vaginal or perineal lacerations.
   b. Ruptured uterus.
   c. Hemorrhage.
2. Fetal/neonatal.
   a. Birth injuries such as brachial palsy and fractured clavicles.
   b. Anoxia, brain damage, and late neuropsychiatric abnormalities (McCall, 1982).
   c. Intrapartum or neonatal death.

E. **Assessment and management.**
1. Anticipate shoulder dystocia if descent of the head is slow and estimated weight is large.
2. If shoulder dystocia occurs, physician or midwife will:
   a. Clear infant's airway.
   b. Perform large mediolateral episiotomy.
   c. Consider anesthesia to relax woman's perineal muscles.
   d. Perform one or several maneuvers to expedite delivery:
      (1) Manually rotate shoulders from the anteroposterior to the oblique diameter in the pelvis and have suprapubic pressure exerted to deliver anterior shoulder.
      (2) Extract posterior shoulder and arm.
      (3) Utilize "Screw Principle of Woods," in which abdominal pressure is exerted along with rotation of the posterior shoulder to anterior for delivery under the pubic bone, with the maneuver repeated for the other shoulder (Oxorn, 1986).
      (4) Utilize knee-chest position (McRoberts maneuver) (May and Mahlmeister, 1990) or turn woman on all fours to widen the pelvic outlet.
      (5) Fracture the clavicle in order to collapse the diameter of the shoulders.

BREECH DELIVERY

A. **Incidence.** 3.7% of all pregnancies after 37 weeks (Hill, 1990). Incidence increases in multiple gestation and in pre-term birth (Oxorn, 1986; May and Mahlmeister, 1990).

B. **Etiology/predisposing factors.**
1. Maternal.
   a. High multiparity with uterine relaxation.
   b. Polyhydramnios with free movement of fetus.
   c. Oligohydramnios with resultant lack of ability of fetus to move from breech position common in second trimester.

    d. Uterine anomalies and leiomyomas.
    e. Contracted pelvis.
  2. Placental/fetal.
    a. Placenta previa.
    b. Multiple gestation.
    c. Hydrocephalus or anencephalus or other fetal anomalies.
    d. Fetal demise.
    e. Large fetus or pre-term fetus.

C. Clinical presentation.
  1. Woman feels fetus kicking in lower abdomen.
  2. Fetal heart sounds are heard loudest above umbilicus.
  3. Use of Leopold's maneuvers indicates head is in fundal area and breech is in pelvis.
  4. On bimanual examination, it is found that the presenting part is soft, no fontanelles are felt, and the genitalia may be identified.

D. Complications.
  1. Maternal.
    a. Lacerations of the birth canal may occur if the delivery is rapid and forceful.
    b. Usual maternal morbidity of 25–40% if cesarean delivery is performed.
  2. Fetal/neonatal complications resulting from vaginal delivery.
    a. Prolapsed cord.
    b. Asphyxia from too slow delivery of fetal head or from compression of umbilical cord between pelvis and head during delivery.
    c. Aspiration of amniotic fluid with potential for meconium aspiration syndrome.
    d. Vertebral injury, subdural hemorrhage, and skull fracture.
    e. Central nervous system abnormalities such as cerebral palsy, mental retardation, and hemiplegia.
    f. Mortality rate with vaginal delivery is three times the rate of cephalic presentations (Oxorn, 1986).

E. Assessment and management.
  1. If the presentation is discovered to be breech in the last few weeks of pregnancy, the physician may attempt external cephalic version with use of a uterine relaxant, and vaginal delivery if the fetus remains in a cephalic presentation (Van Veelen et al., 1990).
  2. Another procedure that may help the fetus turn from breech to cephalic presentation is postural exercise in which the woman assumes either the knee-chest or an elevated-hips posture several times a day until the fetus turns (Young and Mahan, 1989).
  3. Assessments on admission to labor and delivery.
    a. Perform Leopold's maneuvers and vaginal examination to determine presentation.
    b. Report breech presentation immediately to physician or midwife.
  4. Ultrasound may be ordered to confirm breech presentation, determine degree of flexion of the fetal head, evaluate size of fetal head, estimate fetal weight, diagnose fetal anomalies, and locate placenta.
  5. A trial of labor for vaginal delivery may be attempted.
    a. The fetus is at term, a frank breech (buttocks only presenting), with head flexed and pelvis adequate.
    b. The estimated fetal weight must be between 2500 and 3800 grams (Oxorn, 1986), and no other indications for cesarean delivery must exist.
    c. The nurse should perform, at the time of rupture of the membranes, a vaginal examination to check for prolapsed cord and should monitor the fetal heart tones closely.
    d. Meconium in the amniotic fluid is not necessarily a sign of fetal hypoxia when the fetus is breech. However, meconium aspiration at the time of delivery may be a serious complication.

6. With vaginal delivery, the woman will probably receive a large episiotomy, and Piper's forceps may be used to deliver the baby's head. The nurse may be asked to perform suprapubic pressure to keep the baby's head flexed while certain maneuvers are performed during the delivery.
7. Many physicians will perform cesarean delivery when the fetus is breech in these situations: primigravida, small pelvis, premature rupture of membranes, large fetus, hyperextension of head, footling breech, and pre-term fetus.
8. A manual breech extraction with the woman under deep anesthesia may be performed if fetal distress occurs and cesarean delivery cannot be performed immediately.
9. Assessment of the neonate may reveal:
   a. Edema of the external genitalia.
   b. A continuation of the frank breech position for a while after the birth.
   c. Congenital hip dislocation, which is increased in incidence with breech presentation.

Obstetrical Analgesia and Anesthesia

Up to 10% of maternal deaths in the U.S. are related to anesthesia (Gillespie, 1983). Though many of these deaths result from poor technique or overdosage, most anesthesiologists and obstetricians would agree that there is no method of obstetric pain relief that is completely safe for all women. In addition, side effects or adverse reactions in the woman affect the fetus to some degree.

OBSTETRICAL ANALGESIA

Obstetrical analgesia is given by either the IM or the IV route, and in as small a dose as possible. Analgesics are given when the women has reached 4 or 5 cm of dilatation, but not in the last hour or two before delivery. The most commonly used analgesic is the narcotic meperidine (Demerol); butorphanol (Stadol) and nalbuphine (Nubain) are also commonly used.

A. Potential complications.
1. Maternal.
   a. Respiratory depression.
   b. Nausea and vomiting.
   c. Slowing of labor if given in the latent phase.
   d. Orthostatic hypotension.
   e. Drowsiness and dizziness.
2. Fetal/newborn.
   a. Decreased fetal activity and short-term variability, and late decelerations if mother experiences hypotension.
   b. Neonatal respiratory depression.
   c. Decreased Apgar scores.
   d. Respiratory acidosis.
   e. Neurobehavioral abnormalities.
   f. Hypotonia.
   g. Lethargy.
   h. Thermoregulation problems.

B. Assessment and management.
1. Do not administer analgesics too early or too late in labor.
2. Administer IV analgesics slowly; give during a uterine contraction to minimize amount of drug fetus receives.
3. Observe woman for side effects and monitor fetus continuously with electronic fetal monitor or periodic auscultation.
4. With maternal hypotension, turn woman on her left side, increase infusion of IV fluids, and closely monitor fetal heart tones as well as woman's BP.

5. Have naloxone (Narcan), oxygen, and ventilatory equipment available for use with newborn if respiratory depression occurs.
6. Document use of analgesic, and communicate this information to nursery nurse.
7. In nursery, observe newborn for side effects of maternal analgesia.

OBSTETRICAL ANESTHESIA

Several types of anesthesia are used with women in labor and delivery. General anesthesia is used only for emergency cesarean deliveries and complicated vaginal deliveries when it is not possible to have immediate and effective regional anesthesia. Regional anesthesia includes continuous lumbar epidural, saddle block, and pudendal block.

A. **Potential complications with general anesthesia.**
1. Maternal.
   a. Vomiting and aspiration of gastric contents with chemical pneumonitis as a consequence.
   b. Respiratory depression.
   c. Cardiac irritability and arrest.
   d. Hypotension or hypertension.
   e. Tachycardia.
   f. Laryngospasm.
   g. Post-partum uterine atony.
2. Fetal/newborn.
   a. Decreased fetal cardiac variability and movements.
   b. Fetal depression in proportion to the amount of anesthesia.
   c. Neonatal respiratory depression.
   d. Hyperbilirubinemia.
   e. Hypotonicity.

B. **Assessment and management with general anesthesia.**
1. Keep the woman NPO in labor if there is any possibility that she will receive general anesthesia.
2. Note the time of her last meal.
3. Physician may order 30 ml of clear antacid to be administered prior to general anesthesia to increase the pH of the stomach contents in case of aspiration.
4. Endotracheal tube and cricoid pressure are techniques used by the anesthesiologist to prevent aspiration.
5. Place wedge under right hip to cause displacement of uterus from aorta and vena cava and to prevent supine hypotensive syndrome during surgery.
6. Monitor woman's cardiorespiratory status during and after surgery, and uterine bleeding afterward.
7. Monitor fetus during surgery and newborn after surgery for complications.

C. **Potential complications with regional anesthetics.**
1. Maternal.
   a. With spinal and epidural anesthesia:
      (1) 25–70% incidence of hypotension (Gibbs, 1986).
      (2) Allergic reaction.
      (3) Toxic reaction from overdose or intravascular injection.
      (4) Respiratory paralysis from inadvertent high spinal administration.
      (5) Post-spinal headaches.
      (6) Anesthetic failure.
      (7) Urinary retention during labor and post-partum.
      (8) Slowing of labor with need to use oxytocin and forceps if given too early.
   b. With epidural anesthesia:
      (1) Shearing off of epidural catheter.
      (2) Trauma to spinal cord or nerve roots.
      (3) Anterior spinal artery syndrome.

(4) Epidural hematoma with permanent nerve damage (Nicholson and Ridolfo, 1989).
  c. With pudendal block.
    (1) Sciatic nerve trauma.
    (2) Perforated rectum.
    (3) Broad ligament hematoma (Olds, 1988).
2. Fetal/newborn.
  a. Toxic reaction from overdose or intravascular injection.
  b. Fetal compromise with prolonged maternal hypotension, as evidenced by late decelerations and decrease in short-term variability.

D. **Assessment and management with regional anesthetics.**
1. Note history of allergies to local anesthetics.
2. Pre-hydrate with 500–1000 ml IV fluid prior to spinals and epidurals to minimize hypotensive effects from sympathetic blockade.
3. Position and reassure woman during administration of anesthetic. Position woman on alternate sides after epidural or spinal to prevent supine hypotension.
4. Monitor woman's BP after spinal or epidural, and fetal heart after any type of regional anesthetic.
5. Monitor bladder distention, and catheterize if necessary.
6. Monitor for and help manage complications.
  a. Hypotension
    (1) Signs and symptoms.
      (a) Drop in BP.
      (b) Dizziness or affected vision.
    (2) Management.
      (a) Increase IV fluids.
      (b) Elevate legs and lower head.
      (c) Displace uterus from aorta and vena cava.
      (d) Administer oxygen and IV ephedrine.
      (e) Monitor fetus for hypoxia and fetus/newborn for side effects of ephedrine (tachycardia, jitteriness, and increased muscular activity) (Ostheimer and Warren, 1984).
  b. High spinal
    (1) Signs and symptoms.
      (a) Rising level of anesthesia.
      (b) Difficulty in breathing.
    (2) Management.
      (a) Maintain airway and ventilation
      (b) Reassure woman.
      (c) Monitor fetal heart tones.
  c. Toxic reaction.
    (1) Signs and symptoms.
      (a) Metallic taste.
      (b) Ringing in ears.
      (c) Slurring of speech.
      (d) Numbness of tongue and mouth.
      (e) Convulsions.
      (f) Cardiovascular and respiratory depression.
    (2) Management.
      (a) Cardiorespiratory support.
      (b) Drugs to control convulsions.
      (c) Monitor newborn for seizures, bradycardia, apnea, hypotonia.
  d. Allergic reaction.
    (1) Signs and symptoms.
      (a) Bronchospasm.

(b) Laryngeal edema.

(c) Urticaria.

(2) Management: IV antihistamine.

Operative Delivery

A. **Incidence.** Cesarean delivery has risen from 4.5% in 1965 to 24.7% in 1988 (Myers and Gleicher, 1991).

B. **Indications.**

1. Maternal.
   a. Cephalopelvic disproportion.
   b. Failure to progress in labor.
   c. Previous cesarean delivery, unless low transverse uterine incision used.
   d. Pregnancy-induced hypertension.
   e. Cardiac disease.
   f. Diabetes.
   g. Premature rupture of membranes with failed induction.
   h. Active herpes.
2. Placental.
   a. Abruptio placentae.
   b. Placenta previa.
   c. Placental insufficiency.
3. Fetal.
   a. Distress.
   b. Breech or other malpresentation.
   c. Multiple gestation.
   d. Pre-term.

C. **Potential complications.**

1. Maternal.
   a. Infection.
   b. Anemia.
   c. Hemorrhage.
   d. Morbidity and mortality from anesthesia.
   e. Inadvertent operative injuries.
   f. Pulmonary embolus.
   g. Thrombophlebitis.
2. Fetal/newborn.
   a. Asphyxia.
   b. Pre-term birth.
   c. Respiratory distress due to retained fluid in the lungs.
   d. Anemia from blood loss from incision of placenta and lack of full placental transfusion.

D. **Assessment and management.**

1. Perform usual interventions to prepare woman for operative delivery.
2. Notify infant's physician per policy.
3. Give antacid if ordered.
4. Insert indwelling urinary catheter.
5. Arrange for support person to be with woman for delivery.
6. Remove fetal scalp electrode prior to surgery.
7. Place wedge under woman's right hip to displace uterus to left to avoid supine hypotension and fetal hypoxia.
8. Suction newborn well and observe closely for cardiorespiratory and thermoregulatory status.

STUDY QUESTIONS

1. A maternal risk factor that exists prior to pregnancy is:
   a. Age 32 and no previous pregnancy.
   b. Previous treatment for infertility.
   c. Twelfth grade education.

2. Potential effects of pregnancy-induced hypertension on the maternal-placental-fetal complex include:
   a. Fetal hyperproteinemia, maternal hyporeflexia, and polyuria.
   b. Maternal hyperglycemia, placenta previa, and respiratory distress in the newborn.
   c. Maternal seizures, abruptio placentae, and fetal distress during labor.

3. Potential effects of diabetes on the maternal-placental-fetal complex include:
   a. Fetal diabetes.
   b. Maternal nephropathy.
   c. Neonatal hypermagnesemia.

4. An intrapartum condition that may result in complications for the newborn is:
   a. Baseline fetal heart rate of 118 beats per minute.
   b. Demerol 25 mg given IV 3 hours before delivery.
   c. First stage of labor lasting 17 hours.

5. Effects of ritodrine (Yutopar) on the newborn include:
   a. Bradycardia and hyperglycemia.
   b. Bradycardia and hypoglycemia.
   c. Tachycardia and hypoglycemia.

6. Potential effects on the fetus/newborn that are common to abruptio placentae, placenta previa, prolapsed cord, and shoulder dystocia are:
   a. Anoxia and death.
   b. Birth injuries and variable decelerations.
   c. Infection and prematurity.

7. Which of the following is the best indication that a serious complication may have occurred for a woman in labor with a breech presentation?
   a. An ultrasound reveals poor flexion of the fetal head.
   b. Presence of meconium in the amniotic fluid is noted.
   c. She states she feels something in her vagina.

8. A laboring woman has received two doses of Demerol IV. When the nurse notes late decelerations on the monitor, her first actions are to turn the woman on her side and increase the IV fluid infusion rate. Her next action should be to:
   a. Call the physician.
   b. Check the woman's blood pressure.
   c. Document this on the chart at the desk.

9. After a cesarean delivery, it would be particularly important to assess the newborn's:
   a. Hips.
   b. Liver.
   c. Lungs.

Answers to Study Questions

1. b	4. c	7. c
2. c	5. c	8. b
3. b	6. a	9. c

REFERENCES

Bliss-Holtz, J.: Renal and metabolic crises. *In* Vestal, K., and McKenzie, C. (eds.): AACN High Risk Perinatal Nursing. Philadelphia, W.B. Saunders Co., 1983, pp. 429–451.

Brodish, M.: Perinatal assessment. J. Obstet. Gynecol. Neonatal Nursing, 10:42–46, 1981.

Catalano, P., Ashikaga, T., and Mann, L.: Cervical change and uterine activity as predictors of preterm delivery. Am. J. Perinatol., 6(2):185–190, 1989.

Fitzgerald, G.: Preterm labor. Part 2: Management. NAACOG Update Series, Lesson 3, Volume 1. Princeton, Continuing Professional Education Center, Inc., 1983.

Gabbe, S.: Diabetes mellitus in pregnancy. *In* Stern, L.: Drug Use in Pregnancy. Boston, ADIS Health Sciences Press, 1984, pp. 177–189.

Gibbs, C.: Anesthesia in pregnancy. *In* Knuppel, R., and Drukker, J. (eds.): High-Risk Pregnancy: A Team Approach. Philadelphia, W.B. Saunders Co., 1986, pp. 277–289.

Gill, P., and Katz, M.: Early detection of preterm labor: Ambulatory home monitoring of uterine activity. J. Obstet. Gynecol. Neonatal Nursing, *15*:439–442, 1986.

Gillespie, S.: Intrapartum crises. *In* Vestal, K., and McKenzie, C. (eds.): AACN High Risk Perinatal Nursing. Philadelphia, W.B. Saunders Co., 1983, pp. 191–257.

Hayashi, R., and Castillo, M.: Bleeding in pregnancy. *In* Knuppel, R., and Drukker, J. (eds.): High Risk Pregnancy: A Team Approach. Philadelphia, W.B. Saunders Co., 1986, pp. 419–439.

Herbert, W., Kaufman, M., and Cefalo, R.: Nutrition in pregnancy. In Knuppel, R., and Drukker, J. (eds.): High Risk Pregnancy: A Team Approach. Philadelphia, W.B. Saunders Co., 1986, pp. 125–147.

Hill, L.: Prevalence of breech presentation by gestational age. Am. J. Perinatol. *7*:92–93, 1990.

Holbrook, R., Laros, R., and Creasy, R.: Evaluation of a risk-scoring system for prediction of preterm labor. Am. J. Perinatol. *6*:62–68, 1989.

Klonoff-Cohen, H., Savitz, D., Cefalo, R., and McCann, M.: An epidemiologic study of contraception and preeclampsia. JAMA, *262*:3143–3147, 1989.

Lam, F.: Miniature pump infusion of terbutaline—an option in preterm labor. Contemp. OB/GYN, *33*(1):52–70, 1989.

Martin, V., and Gingerich, B.: Uteroplacental physiology. J. Obstet. Gynecol. Neonatal Nursing, *5*:16s–25s, 1976.

May, K., and Mahlmeister, L.: Comprehensive Maternity Nursing. Philadelphia, J.B. Lippincott, 1990.

McCall, J.: Shoulder dystocia: A study of after effects. Am. J. Obstet. Gynecol., *83*:1486–1489, 1982.

McKenzie, C.: Prolapse of cord. *In* Vestal, K., and McKenzie, C. (eds.): AACN High Risk Perinatal Nursing. Philadelphia, W.B. Saunders Co., 1983, pp. 205–208.

Moore, E.: Antepartal crises. *In* Vestal, K., and McKenzie, C. (eds.): AACN High Risk Perinatal Nursing. Philadelphia, W.B. Saunders Co., 1983, p. 153–190.

Myers, S., and Gleicher, N.: A successful program to reduce cesarean section rates: friendly persuasion. Quality Rev. Bull. (QRB), *17*:162–166, 1991.

Newman, R., Gill, P., Wittreich, P., and Katz, M.: Maternal perception of prelabor uterine activity. Obstet. Gynecol. *68*:765–769, 1986.

Nicholson, C., and Ridolfo, E.: Avoiding the pitfalls of epidural anesthesia in obstetrics. J. Am. Assn. Nurse Anesthetists, *57*:220–230, 1989.

O'Brien, M., and Gilson, G.: Detection and management of gestational diabetes in an out-of-hospital birth center. J. Nurse-Midwifery, *32*(2):79–84, 1987.

Olds, S., London, M., and Ladewig, P.: Maternal-Newborn Nursing: A Family-Centered Approach. New York, Addison-Wesley Publishing Co. 1988.

Osofsky, J., and Drukker, J.: Sexual intimacy in pregnancy. *In* Knuppel, R., and Drukker, J. (eds.): High Risk Pregnancy: A Team Approach. Philadelphia: W.B. Saunders Co., 1986, pp. 187–199.

Ostheimer, G., and Warren T.: *In* Stern, L. (ed.): Drug Use in Pregnancy. Boston, ADIS Health Sciences Press, 1984, pp. 225–269.

O'Sullivan, J., Mahan, C., Charles, D., and Dandrow R.: Screening criteria for high-risk gestational diabetic patients. Am. J. Obstet. Gynecol., *116*: 895, 1973.

Oxorn, J.: Human Labor and Birth, 5th ed. Norwalk, CT, Appleton-Century-Crofts, 1986.

Remich, M., and Youngkin, E.: Factors associated with pregnancy-induced hypertension. Nurse Pract., *14*:20–24, 1989.

Schmidt, J., Boilander, M., and Abbott, S.: Peripartum cardiomyopathy. J. Obstet. Gynecol. Neonatal Nursing, *18*:465–472, 1989.

Scupholme, A., and Kamons, A.: Validating change in risk criteria for a birth center: Gestational diabetes. J. Nurse-Midwifery, *33*(3):129–133, 1988.

Van Veelen, A., Van Cappellen, A., Flu, P., et al.: Effect of external cephalic version in late pregnancy on presentation at delivery: A randomized control trial. Obstet. Gynecol. Survey, *45*, 243–244, 1990.

Young, D., and Mahan, C.: Unnecessary Caesareans: Ways to Avoid Them. Minneapolis, The International Childbirth Education Association, Inc., 1989.

BIBLIOGRAPHY

Brengman, S., and Burns, M.: Hypertensive crisis in L & D. Am. J. Nursing, *88*:325–328, 1988.

Engel, N.: Insulin therapy in pregnancy. MCN, Am. J. Maternal/Child Nursing, *14*:19, 1989.

Fedorkow, D., Stewart, T., and Parboosingh, J.: Fetal heart rate changes associated with general anesthesia. Am. J. Perinatol., *6*:287–288, 1989.

Fitzgerald, G.: Preterm labor. Part 2: Management. NAACOG Update Series, Lesson 3, Volume 1. Princeton, Continuing Professional Education Center, Inc., 1983.

Johnson, F.: Assessment and education to prevent preterm labor. MCN, Am. J. Maternal/Child Nursing, *14*:157–160, 1989.

Klaus, M., and Fanaroff, A. (eds.): Care of the High-Risk Neonate, 3rd ed. Philadelphia, W.B. Saunders Co., 1986.

Knuppel, R., and Drukker, J. (eds.): High Risk Pregnancy: A Team Approach. Philadelphia, W.B. Saunders Co., 1986.

Robertson, C.: When your pregnant patient has diabetes. *RN*, *50*(11), 18–22, 1987.

Shannon, D.: HELLP syndrome: A severe consequence of pregnancy-induced hypertension. J. Obstet. Gynecol. Neonatal Nursing, *16*:395–402, 1987.

Spencer, R., Nichols, L., Lipkin, G., et al., Clinical Pharmacology and Nursing Management, 3rd ed. Philadelphia, J.B. Lippincott, 1989.

Stern, L. (ed.): Drug Use in Pregnancy. Boston, ADIS Health Sciences Press, 1984.

Vestal, K., and McKenzie, C. (eds.): AACN High Risk Perinatal Nursing. Philadelphia, W.B. Saunders Co., 1983.

Zimmer, E., Divon, M., and Vadasz, A.: Influence of meperidine on fetal movements and heart rate beat-to-beat variability in the active phase of labor. Am. J. Perinatol., *5*:197–200, 1988.

Christine Zabloudil

Adaptation to Extrauterine Life

Objectives

1. Identify primary features of fetal circulation.

2. Identify physiological changes that occur at birth in the newborn's transition to extrauterine homeostasis.

3. Identify routine care considerations for a newborn with an abnormal assessment at 1–2 hours of age.

4. Identify signs/symptoms of common problems in the transition period.

5. Define the methods and intervention times for parental teaching.

The transition period is defined as from the moment of birth to 6 hours of age, but, more than a period of time, it is a process of physiological change in the newborn that begins in utero as the child prepares for transition from intrauterine placental support to extrauterine self-maintenance. The fetus prepares for transition over the course of gestation in such ways as storing glycogen, producing catecholamines, and depositing brown fat. The newborn's ability to accomplish transition to extrauterine life will depend on the gestational age and on the quality of placental support during gestation.

As the newborn adapts over the course of the first hours of life, the level of nursing intervention will vary with the baby's needs. The need for intervention will then determine the level of care required at the end of the transition period.

Anatomy and Physiology

CHARACTERISTICS OF PLACENTAL/FETAL CIRCULATION

A. **Placenta.**
1. Blood oxygenation and elimination of waste products of metabolism; O_2 and CO_2 transfer across the placenta is by simple diffusion.
2. High rate of metabolism; utilizes 1/3 of all the oxygen and glucose supplied to it by the maternal circulation for its own metabolic needs.
3. Low-resistance circuit; receives approximately 50% of fetal cardiac output.

4. Uterine venous blood as it enters the intervillous space has a P_{CO_2} of 38 mm Hg, a P_{O_2} of 40–50 mm Hg, and a pH of 7.36.

B. **Fetal shunts/blood flow** (Fig. 3–1) (Moore, 1988).
   1. Umbilical vein (P_{O_2} = 30 mm Hg) carries oxygenated blood from the placenta to the fetus.
   2. Ductus venosus: 1/2 of the umbilical venous blood bypasses the liver through the ductus venosus to the inferior vena cava; the other half passes through the liver and enters the inferior vena cava via the hepatic veins. This mixing of blood slightly lowers the P_{O_2}.
   3. Inferior vena caval blood (P_{O_2} = 25–28 mm Hg) is largely deflected across the right atrium through the foramen ovale into the left atrium.
   4. Left atrium: receives the blood from the right atrium and mixes it with a small amount of blood returning from the lungs via the pulmonary veins.
   5. Left ventricular blood (P_{O_2} = 25–28 mm Hg) is virtually all from the inferior vena cava by way of the right atrium–foramen ovale–left atrium pathway. Left ventricular blood is pumped out through the aorta to the brain from the upper part of the aortic arch. Approximately 2/3 of the blood from the ascending aorta flows into the brain and upper extremities.
   6. Superior vena cava receives unoxygenated blood returning from the brain and upper extremities. Ninety-seven per cent enters the right atrium and flows to the right ventricle; only 3% goes to the left atrium via the foramen ovale.
   7. Right atrium: some mixing occurs here between the unoxygenated superior vena caval blood and the oxygenated inferior vena caval blood not shunted directly into the left atrium via the foramen ovale.
   8. Right ventricle: the dominant ventricle (P_{O_2} = 19–22 mm Hg), ejecting about 2/3 of the total cardiac output. Most of the blood is directed away from the lungs through the ductus arteriosus to the descending aorta and subsequently to the placenta through the umbilical arteries.
   9. Ductus arteriosus: equal in size to the aorta; connects the pulmonary artery to the descending aorta. The blood flows right to left (pulmonary artery to aorta) across the ductus arteriosus because of high pulmonary vascular resistance and low placental resistance.
   10. Low pulmonary blood flow (only 8–10% of right ventricular output) results from high pulmonary vascular resistance.
   11. Descending aorta supplies kidneys and intestines, divides into two arteries, and returns blood to the placenta for oxygenation.

FETAL LUNG CHARACTERISTICS

A. **Decreased blood flow.** Due in part to the compression of the pulmonary capillaries by the fetal lung fluid.

B. **Pulmonary arteries.** The small pulmonary arteries of the fetus have a thick muscular medial layer; they are very reactive and are actively constricted by the low P_{O_2} levels normally present during fetal life.

C. **Lung fluid secretion.** Decreased secretion of lung fluid toward term.

D. **Fetal breathing.** In utero fetal breathing movements have been detected as early as 11 weeks' gestation.

E. **Surfactant.** Surfactant is secreted into the amniotic fluid by the fetal lung prior to 20 weeks' gestation. The absolute quantity of surfactant increases throughout the gestation in both lung and amniotic fluid.

FETAL METABOLISM AND HEMATOLOGY

A. **Glucose.** Fetal blood glucose concentrations are 70–80% of maternal blood glucose concentrations. Glucose is exchanged via the placenta by facilitated diffusion.

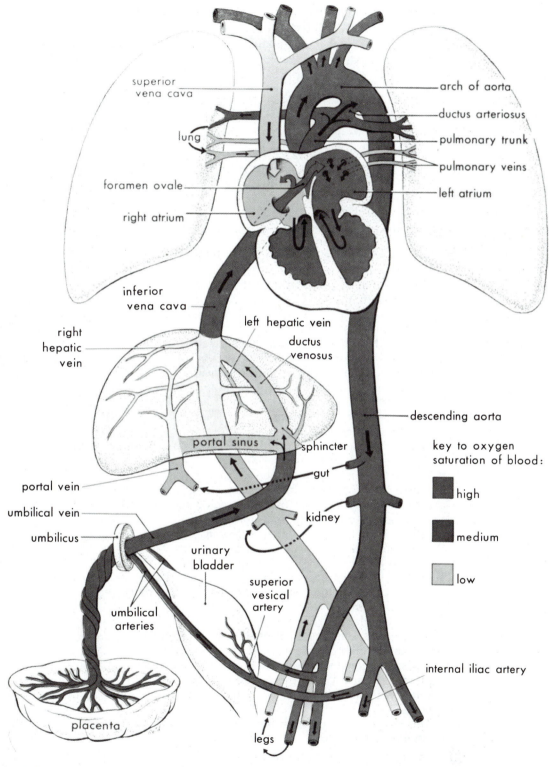

Figure 3–1
A simplified scheme of the fetal circulation. The shaded areas indicate the oxygen saturation of the blood, and the arrows show the course of the fetal circulation. The organs are not drawn to scale. (From Moore, K.L.: *The Developing Human—Clinically Oriented Embryology*, 4th ed. Philadelphia, W.B. Saunders Co., 1988.)

B. **Glycogen.** Large glycogen stores (2–10 times that of an adult) provide large energy reserves to sustain the newborn through the transition period.

C. **Hemoglobin.** Fetal hemoglobin has an increased affinity for oxygen. Fetal hemoglobin is progressively replaced by adult hemoglobin from about 32–36 weeks' gestation on and is approximately 80% of total hemoglobin at term.

LABOR

A. **Placenta.** There is cessation of maternal placental perfusion with uterine contractions.

B. **Stress hormones.** High concentrations of stress hormones (predominantly norepinephrine) are released secondary to a direct effect of the resultant hypoxia on the adrenal medulla.

CARDIOPULMONARY ADAPTATION AT BIRTH

A. **Cardiovascular** (Fig. 3–2) (Moore, 1988).
1. The umbilical cord is clamped.
   a. The placenta is separated from the circulation, and the umbilical arteries and veins constrict.
   b. As the low-resistance placental circuit is removed, there is a resultant increase in systemic blood pressure; the systemic vascular resistance then exceeds the pulmonary vascular resistance.
2. The three major fetal shunts (ductus venosus, foramen ovale, and ductus arteriosus) functionally close during transition.
   a. Ductus arteriosus: the lungs now provide more efficient oxygenation of the blood, and the arterial tension rises. This rise in the Po_2 is the most potent stimulus to constriction of the ductus arteriosus. Circulating prostaglandins also contribute to ductal closure.
   b. Foramen ovale: the fall in pulmonary vascular resistance results in a drop in right ventricular and right atrial pressure, and the increased systemic vascular resistance results in an increase in left atrial and left ventricular pressures, causing the foramen ovale to close.
      (1) The foramen ovale becomes sealed by the deposit of fibrin and cell products during the first month of life.
      (2) Until the foramen ovale is anatomically sealed, anything that produces a significant increase in right atrial pressure can re-open the foramen ovale and allow a right-to-left shunt.
   c. Ductus venosus: absent umbilical venous return leads to closure of the ductus venosus. Functionally closes within 2–3 days; becomes the ligamentum venosum.
3. Postnatal circulation.
   a. Systemic venous blood enters the right atrium from the superior vena cava and the inferior vena cava.
   b. Poorly oxygenated blood enters the right ventricle and passes through the pulmonary artery into the pulmonary circulation for oxygenation.
   c. The oxygenated blood returns to the left atrium through the pulmonary veins.
   d. This blood passes through the left ventricle and into the aorta to supply the systemic circulation.

B. **Pulmonary adaptation at birth.**
1. Stimuli for initiating respiration: the mild hypercapnia, hypoxia, and acidosis that result from normal labor; due partially to the intermittent cessation of maternal-placental perfusion with contractions. The decreased pH stimulates the respiratory center directly; the low Po_2 and high Pco_2 stimulate the respiratory center via central and peripheral chemoreceptors. Other stimuli include cold, light, noise, and touch.

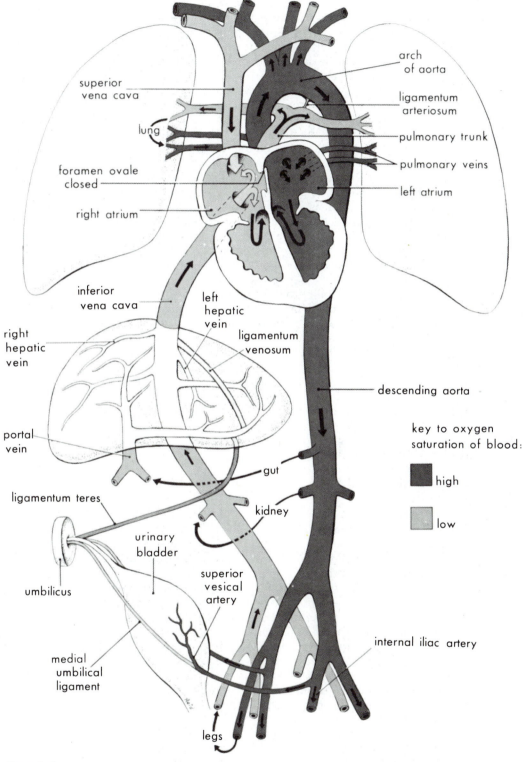

Figure 3-2
A simplified representation of the circulation after birth. The adult derivatives of the fetal vessels and structures that become non-functional at birth are also shown. The arrows indicate the course of the neonatal circulation. The organs are not drawn to scale. (From Moore, K.L.: *The Developing Human—Clinically Oriented Embryology*, ed. 4. Philadelphia, W.B. Saunders, Co., 1988.)

2. With the first breath, air enters the lungs.
   a. Transpulmonary pressure drives fluid into the interstitium; it is then absorbed through the lymphatic and pulmonary circulation.
   b. The pulmonary vessels respond to the increase in Po_2 with vasodilation. Pulmonary vascular resistance progressively decreases until adult levels are reached at 2–3 weeks of age.
3. After the thoracic squeeze (during vaginal delivery this empties the lungs of approximately 1/3 of the fetal lung fluid), the subsequent recoil of the chest wall causes inspiration of air and expansion of the lungs. Negative intrathoracic pressures generated with the first breath may be as high as 40–80 cm H_2O due to the mechanical advantage created by the high resting level of the diaphragm in the non-aerated lung.
4. Respiratory augmentation: Head's paradoxical reflex is a vagally mediated hyperinflation triggered by distention of stretch receptors in the large airways.
5. The work of inspiration is mainly (80%) devoted to overcoming the surface tension of the walls of the terminal lung units at the gas-tissue interface. On expiration, the ability to retain air depends on surfactant.
   a. Surfactant is a complete lipoprotein produced by type II alveolar pneumocytes; surfactant release increases in response to increased catecholamines at birth.
   b. Surfactant has the ability to lower surface tension at an air-liquid interface.
   c. As surfactant lowers surface tension in the alveolus at end-expiration, it stabilizes the alveoli and prevents collapse.
6. There is an increased functional residual capacity with each breath; thus less inspiratory pressure is required for subsequent breaths.
7. Lung compliance improves in the hours following delivery secondary to circulating catecholamines. The increased levels of catecholamines (especially epinephrine) also clear the lungs by decreasing secretion of lung fluids and increasing their absorption through the lymphatic system.

Routine Care Considerations

DELIVERY/RESUSCITATION

Nursery*

A. Assessment/observation.
1. Measurements will include head circumference, length, and weight.
2. Vital signs on admission will include heart rate, respiratory rate, axillary temperature, and blood pressure.
3. Gestational age assessment: graph the weight, head circumference, and length against the assessed gestational age and record. (Refer to Chapter 4.)
4. During the first hours of life, newborns follow a sequence of clinical behavior as summarized in Figure 3–3 (Desmond et al., 1966). The time sequence of changes is altered in infants with low Apgar scores, immaturity, maternal medications, and intrinsic disease. (See Appendix D.)
5. A head-to-toe physical examination is performed. (Refer to Chapter 4.) The following findings seen during transition are within normal limits as the infant progresses through the physiological changes described under cardiopulmonary adaptation.
   a. Skin
      (1) Acrocyanosis; vasoconstricted peripheral vessels resulting in a mottled appearance; decreased peripheral pulses initially. (These findings are a sequela of catecholamine release, mild acidosis, and cold stress).
      (2) Petechiae of the face and facial bruising may be seen in the infant born

---

*Refer to Chapter 5 for management of the infant in the delivery room.

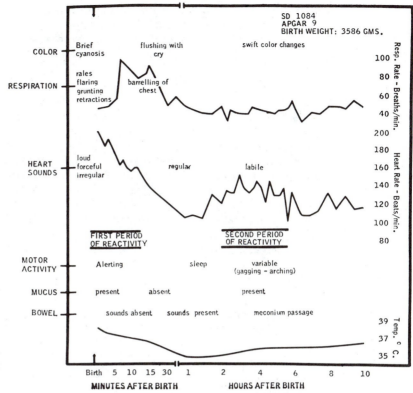

Figure 3-3
A summary of the physical findings noted during the first 10 hours of extrauterine life in a representative high-Apgar-score infant delivered under spinal anesthesia without prior pre-medication. (From Desmond, M.M., Rudolph, A.J., and Phitaksphraiwan, P.: The transitional care nursery: A mechanism for preventive medicine in the newborn. Pediatr. Clin. North Am., *13*:651–668, 1966.)

vertex after a rapid second stage or after a tight nuchal cord. (With severe facial bruising, central color may be assessed by looking at the mucous membranes in the mouth.)
  b. Head.
    (1) The newborn head is large relative to the body; during vaginal delivery, considerable molding of the skull bones may take place to facilitate passage through the birth canal. Molding resolves over the first hours and days.
    (2) Caput succedaneum may be present. (See Birth Trauma Chapter.)
  c. Respirations/breath sounds.
    (1) Initially, coarse rales and moist tubular breath sounds are present until clearing of lung fluid is complete.
    (2) Prolonged expiratory phase.
    (3) Respiratory rate 30–60/minute
    (4) Grunting and retracting (intercostal, substernal) may be present during the first hours of life as lung fluid is cleared.
  d. Heart sounds.
    (1) Loud second heart sound during first 2 hours; splitting of the second heart sound is usually detectable at 2–4 hours of age and increases during the next 12 hours (pulmonic ahead of aortic component).
    (2) Murmur: soft, grade II/VI systolic murmur may be present; represents a left-to-right shunt across the ductus arteriosus prior to its closure.
  e. Heart.
    (1) Normal rate 120–160 beats/minute; increased initially, with mean peak of 180 beats/minute, then decreased or irregular.
    (2) See Heart Sounds.
  f. Intestines.
    (1) Reduced blood flow initially.

(2) As the bowel begins to fill with air, normal motility and bowel sounds are present within 15 minutes.

g. Falling body temperature: mean low temperature is 35.6°C; lowest temperature is reached at a mean age of 75 minutes after delivery (Desmond et al., 1966).

h. Extremities: findings may include deformities secondary to intrauterine position.

B. **Neutral thermal environment (NTE).** (The admission assessment/observation should be done in a neutral thermal environment, such as a radiant warmer or incubator.) Defined as the ambient air temperature at which oxygen consumption for heat production is minimal with body temperature in normal range (Merenstein and Gardner, 1989) (axillary = 36.5–37°C; skin = 36.0–36.5°C); dependent on weight, gestational age, and chronological age (Table 3–1). Temperatures outside the NTE may result in development of either hypothermia or hyperthermia, which have serious metabolic consequences.

1. Heat production.

a. Heat is generated through oxidation of glucose and free fatty acids.

Table 3–1
NEUTRAL THERMAL ENVIRONMENTAL TEMPERATURES

Age and Weight	Range of Temperature (°C)	Age and Weight	Range of Temperature (°C)
0–6 hours		**72–96 hours**	
Under 1200 g	34.0–35.4	Under 1200 g	34.0–35.0
1200–1500 g	33.9–34.4	1200–1500 g	33.0–34.0
1501–2500 g	32.8–33.8	1501–2500 g	31.1–33.2
Over 2500 g (and >36 weeks)	32.0–33.8	Over 2500 g (and >36 weeks)	29.8–32.8
6–12 hours		**4–12 days**	
Under 1200 g	34.0–35.4	Under 1500 g	33.0–34.0
1200–1500 g	33.5–34.4	1501–2500 g	31.0–33.2
1501–2500 g	32.2–33.8	Over 2500 g (and >36 weeks)	
Over 2500 g (and >36 weeks)	31.4–33.8	4–5 days	29.5–32.6
12–24 hours		5–6 days	29.4–32.3
Under 1200 g	34.0–35.4	6–8 days	29.0–32.2
1200–1500 g	33.3–34.3	8–10 days	29.0–31.8
1501–2500 g	31.8–33.8	10–12 days	29.0–31.4
Over 2500 (and >36 weeks)	31.0–33.7	**12–14 days**	
24–36 hours		Under 1500 g	32.6–34.0
Under 1200 g	34.0–35.0	1501–2500 g	31.0–33.2
1200–1500 g	33.1–34.2	Over 2500 g (and >36 weeks)	29.0–30.8
1501–2500 g	31.6–33.6	**2–3 weeks**	
Over 2500 (and >36 weeks)	30.7–33.5	Under 1500 g	32.2–34.0
36–48 hours		1501–2500 g	30.5–33.0
Under 1200 g	34.0–35.0	**3–4 weeks**	
1200–1500 g	33.0–34.1	Under 1500 g	31.6–33.6
1501–2500 g	31.4–33.5	1501–2500 g	30.0–32.7
Over 2500 (and >36 weeks)	30.5–33.3	**4–5 weeks**	
48–72 hours		Under 1500 g	31.2–33.0
Under 1200 g	34.0–35.0	1501–2500 g	29.5–32.2
1200–1500 g	33.0–34.0	**5–6 weeks**	
1501–2500 g	31.2–33.4	Under 1500 g	30.6–32.3
Over 2500 (and >36 weeks)	30.1–33.2	1501–2500 g	29.0–31.8

Adapted from Scopes, J., and Ahmed, I.: Arch. Dis. Child. *41*:417, 1966. For his table, Scopes had the walls of the incubator 1° to 2° warmer than the ambient air temperatures.

Generally speaking, the smaller infants in each weight group will require a temperature in the higher portion of the temperature range. Within each time range, the younger the infant, the higher the temperature required.

From Klaus, M., Fanaroff, A., and Martin, R.: *In* Klaus, M., and Fanaroff, A.: Care of the High-Risk Neonates, 3rd ed. Philadelphia, W.B. Saunders Co., 1986, pp. 96–112.

    b. Much of the heat production takes place in brown fat (unique to the newborn) that is present around the blood vessels and muscles in the neck with extensions under the clavicles and into the axillae and accompanying the great vessels entering the thoracic inlet. Also envelops the kidneys and adrenal glands.

2. Heat loss: newborns have an increased body surface area in relation to body mass; as a result, there is an increased rate of heat loss.
    a. Routes of heat loss.
       (1) Evaporation: heat is lost from the skin and respiratory tract as moisture is evaporated (e.g., immediately after delivery when the skin is wet with amniotic fluid).
       (2) Radiation: heat is lost to cool surfaces close to the infant such as cold walls or windows; is independent of ambient temperature.
       (3) Conduction: heat is lost to cool surfaces during direct contact with the infant such as x-ray plates, scales, or a cold mattress.
       (4) Convection: heat is lost to cool air moving past the infant (i.e., drafts or cold oxygen). The amount of heat lost through this route is dependent on the temperature gradient between the infant and air, the amount of body surface exposed to the air, and the speed of the air movement.

3. Pathophysiology of cold stress and hypothermia.
    a. Cold stress: an infant responds to cold stimulus with increased oxygen consumption, glucose utilization, and acid production; these physiologic responses can be present even when core body temperature is normal.
    b. Sequence of physiological responses to cold stimulus at receptors (nerve endings in the skin, especially of the face).
       (1) Release of norepinephrine; stimulates lipolysis in brown fat; the byproducts of the lipolysis, fatty acids and glycerol, are used as fuel by the liver and muscles.
       (2) Peripheral vasoconstriction to conserve core temperature.
       (3) Chemical thermogenesis: lipolysis and fatty acid oxidation in brown fat produce heat that is released to the perfusing blood.
       (4) In the production of heat through chemical thermogenesis, there is an increased oxygen consumption leading eventually to hypoxia and impaired cellular function.
          (a) Anaerobic metabolism ensues with the production of lactic acids and a metabolic acidosis.
          (b) Metabolic acidosis leads to decreased surfactant release and to pulmonary vasoconstriction.
          (c) These result in reduced ventilation and perfusion of the lungs and persistence of the hypoxia.
          (d) With anaerobic metabolism, there is a marked increase in the consumption of glucose and breakdown of glycogen stores, leading eventually to hypoglycemia.
    c. Hypothermia: core temperature drops (less than 36.5°C) only when the infant's physiological efforts to produce heat have failed.
    d. Severe cold stress can present with moderate to severe respiratory distress, shock, disseminated intravascular coagulation and pulmonary hemorrhage.
    e. Signs and symptoms of cold stress and hypothermia.
       (1) Apnea.
       (2) Bradycardia.
       (3) Tachypnea.
       (4) Poor perfusion.
       (5) Acrocyanosis.
       (6) Oxygen requirement.
       (7) Seizures.
       (8) Acidosis.
       (9) Dusky color with crying.
      (10) Feeding intolerance.

      (11) Lethargy.

      (12) Irritability.

      (13) Jitteriness.

      (14) Hypoglycemia.

      (15) Cyanosis.

  f. Infants most susceptible to cold stress and hypothermia.

      (1) Already stressed infants with severe birth asphyxia, hypoglycemia, respiratory distress, or sepsis.

      (2) Infants with poor glucose stores, decreased amounts of subcutaneous tissue, and little or no brown fat stores—i.e., prematures and infants who are small for gestational age.

  g. Consequences of thermal instability.

      (1) Acute.

        (a) Hypoglycemia; hypoxia; metabolic acidosis due to the metabolism of brown fat, release of fatty acids, and anaerobic metabolism.

        (b) Pulmonary vasoconstriction due to metabolic acidosis.

        (c) Increased respiratory distress due to hypoxia and acidosis.

      (2) Chronic.

        (a) Impaired weight gain due to consumption of calories for heat production.

        (b) If the degree and duration of cold exposure exceed the infant's ability to compensate, a gradual fall in core temperature will occur, accompanied by respiratory failure, heart failure, depletion of energy resources, and eventually death.

4. Temperature care considerations in the nursery.

  a. Monitor temperature.

      (1) Check axillary temperature every 30 minutes to 1 hour during transition when the child is under a radiant warmer. Avoid hyperthermia (skin temperature greater than 37°C or axillary temperature greater than 37.5°C). *Note:* Monitoring the axillary temperature allows time for successful intervention before a fall in core temperature indicates failure of the body's compensatory heat regulation mechanisms.

      (2) First bath should be delayed until body temperature has stabilized at 36.5–37°C. Check temperature 30 minutes after the bath and 1 hour after transfer to open crib.

      (3) Check temperature at least every 4 hours until infant is stable, then every 8 hours until discharge.

      (4) Record the environmental temperature (incubator or warmer) with temperature checks of the infant in order to monitor infant's environmental temperature requirements. *Note:* These requirements can be checked against the normal ranges of neutral thermal environmental temperature needs as a tool in evaluating an infant.

C. Transition nursery: medications, teaching, feeding.

1. Eye care: given OU before 1 hour of age.

  a. Recommendation: 1% silver nitrate solution or an ophthalmic ointment containing 0.5% erythromycin or 1% tetracycline for prophylaxis of ophthalmia neonatorum due to *Neisseria gonorrhoeae*. Prophylaxis for *Chlamydia trachomatis* requires erythromycin or tetracycline (AAP, ACOG, 1988).

  b. Instill into conjunctival sac within 1 hour of birth; medication should not be flushed from the eye following application. A new tube should be used for each infant. Prophylaxis should be administered to infants born by cesarean section as well as those delivered vaginally.

  c. Side effects include sensitivity reaction. Chemical conjunctivitis can be observed following silver nitrate instillation.

2. Vitamin K (AquaMEPHYTON): given IM or PO within 4 hours of age.

  a. Recommendation: IM (single dose) 0.5 mg if infant is less than 1.5 kg in weight; 1 mg IM if infant is greater than 1.5 kg in weight (AAP, ACOG,

1988). *Note:* Vitamin K may be given PO in 1 mg dose; PO vitamin K is used extensively in Canada and England (Birbeck, 1988) but is not yet recommended by the American Academy of Pediatrics.

b. Maternal dietary inadequacy of vitamin K, hepatic immaturity, reduced liver stores and absence of intestinal flora predispose the child to neonatal deficiency of vitamin K; gut bacteria are a substantial source of vitamin K.

Vitamin K is needed to promote the hepatic biosynthesis of vitamin K–dependent clotting factors, including prothrombin (Factor II), proconvertin (Factor VII), plasma thromboplastin component (Factor IX), and Stuart factor (Factor X). Deficiency results in hemorrhagic disease of the newborn (HDN).

   (1) Classic HDN—Occurs from 1–7 days of life. The infant is normal at birth but develops cutaneous or GI bleeding. Other sites of bleeding include nasal bleeding or bleeding after circumcision. Can be prevented with vitamin K prophylaxis.

   (2) Early HDN—Occurs with maternal exposure to drugs that may affect coagulation, including warfarin, anticonvulsants, and antituberculosis drugs. Severe or life-threatening hemorrhage may occur during delivery or in the 1st day of life. Intracranial hemorrhage is a common complication. Early HDN is the only type that cannot be prevented by vitamin K prophylaxis.

   (3) Late HDN—May occur between 1 and 3 months of life. Acute intracranial hemorrhage is the most common initial finding and is often fatal or neurologically devastating. Other findings include GI or mucous membrane bleeding. Can be prevented by vitamin K prophylaxis.

3. Hepatitis vaccine/hepatitis B immune globulin.

   a. Infants born to mothers positive for hepatitis B surface antigen have a 70–90% chance of acquiring perinatal hepatitis B virus infection, and 85–90% of infected infants will become chronic hepatitis B virus carriers.

   b. Treatment recommendations.

      (1) Child is bathed as soon as temperature is stable.

      (2) Hepatitis vaccine (Heptavax or Recombivax) 0.5 ml IM and hepatitis B immune globulin (contains high-titer antibodies to hepatitis B virus) 0.5 ml IM are given within 12 hours of age; may be given concurrently at different sites; 85–95% effective in preventing the development of the hepatitis B virus carrier state (CDC, 1988).

      (3) Continue the vaccine series. The second dose is given at 1 month of age, and the third dose is given at 6 months of age.

   c. The Centers for Disease Control has recommended that hepatitis B vaccine be administered to all infants, including those born to hepatitis B surface antigen, (HBsAg)–negative mothers. See Appendix B for recommended doses and administration schedule of hepatitis B vaccine.

4. Glucose needs/first feeding.

   a. The stress of delivery causes increased conversion of fats and glycogen to glucose for the increase energy needs of temperature maintenance, skeletal muscles, and breathing/crying. Breakdown products of this conversion are glucose, free fatty acids, and glycerol.

   b. Hepatic glycogen is mobilized immediately after birth in response to the increased catecholamines to provide a continuing source of glucose to the brain in the absence of placental supply; in a healthy, full-term infant, up to 90% of the hepatic glycogen stores may be consumed by 3 hours of life.

   c. Blood glucose concentration at birth is 70–80% of the maternal level. Glucose level then falls over 1–2 hours, stabilizes at a minimum of 35–40 mg/dl, and rises by 6 hours to 45–60 mg/dl in healthy, nonstressed infants.

   d. A screening blood glucose determination by Chemstrip bG or Dextrostix (done on capillary whole blood) should be performed on infants with the following risk factors at 30 minutes to 1 hour of age. A STAT serum glucose determination is recommended if the screening glucose level is less than 25 mg/dl. (See Initial Stabilization of the Sick Newborn.) *Note:* The whole blood glucose concentration is usually 10–15% lower than the corresponding serum glucose level.

(1) Asphyxia, cold stress, increased work of breathing, and sepsis lead to an increased metabolic response and increased utilization of glucose.

(2) Premature and small for gestational age infants have reduced stores of glucose.

(3) Infants of diabetic or gestational diabetic mothers and large for gestational age infants present with hyperinsulinemia resulting in rapid removal of glucose from the circulation.

(4) Any symptomatic infant: one with jitteriness, hypothermia, apnea. (See Common Problems and Clinical Presentation: Metabolic.) *Note:* Capillary samples from a unwarmed heel may lead to a falsely low glucose value due to stasis of blood and ongoing transfer of glucose to the cells.

e. Feeding: Early frequent feedings ad lib demand; not to exceed 5 hours between feedings (maximum of 3 hours between feedings for infants weighing less than 2.5 kg). Allow the infant to begin feeding when he is demanding nutrition and evaluation is within normal limits; nursing or bottle feeding can be used (type of formula is per family's or physician's choice).

(1) Evaluation prior to feeding.

    (a) Physical examination: normal bowel tones, abdomen soft and nontender. Normal suck, swallowing mucus without excessive accumulation in oropharynx. No emesis; patent anus; patent nares. Respiratory rate less than 70/minute, and pattern of breathing is normal. (Passage of orogastric tube is often done prior to feeding to check for patency.)

    (b) Contraindications to bottle feeding or nursing. (Consider gavage feeding based on infant's condition.)

        i. Choanal atresia.

        ii. Respiratory rate greater than 70/minute without other signs of respiratory distress.

        iii. Weak suck.

        iv. Absent coordination of suck/swallow.

    (c) Contraindications to enteral feedings.

        i. Cyanosis.

        ii. Severe birth asphyxia.

        iii. Shock.

        iv. Increased work of breathing and oxygen requirement.

        v. Suspicion of GI obstruction.

(2) Sterile water "test" feeding: it is difficult to evaluate an infant's ability to suck/swallow with sterile water because most infants do not like the taste and on occasion will refuse to suck or swallow; therefore, it is advisable to forego "sips of water" in favor of a thorough evaluation prior to feeding.

(3) Five per cent dextrose in water (D5W) is not indicated as a "test" feeding, as studies show D5W is as irritating to lungs following aspiration as formula (Olson, 1970). Not indicated after feeding unless:

    (a) Ordered by a physician.

    (b) Requested by mother (e.g., at one night feeding in the nursery or if infant doesn't settle down after effective nursing). Mother may be planning to introduce bottle feedings to complement nursing.

(4) Guidelines for feeding in transition nursery for decreased glucose screen.

    (a) May nurse or bottle feed if glucose screen 30–40 mg/dl and there are no contraindications. Check Chemstrip/Dextrostix 1 hour after feeding.

    (b) Give formula if glucose screen is less than 30 mg/dl (See Initial Stabilization of the Sick Newborn) and there are no contraindications to oral feedings. Check Chemstrip/Dextrostix 1 hour after feeding.

      (c) See Initial Stabilization of the Sick Newborn for management of infants with low glucose screen who must be NPO.

  f. Ongoing teaching in the transition nursery.

    (1) Talk with family about the infant's ability to see and hear with a preference for black/white contrast initially and the sound of a high-pitched voice.

    (2) Demonstrate/point out infant's response to stimuli (tactile, visual, auditory): self-consolability, body movements, gaze, head turning.

    (3) Discuss physical findings.

      (a) Transient: acrocyanosis, birth trauma, positional deformities.

      (b) Permanent: congenital anomalies, birthmarks.

    (4) If infant is stable, may be returned to the family by 1–2 hours of age to visit, breast-feed, be given first bottle feeding. Provide an open crib, warm blankets, and a warm hat.

  g. Transfer out of transition nursery when the following are stable:

    (1) Temperature.

    (2) Glucose screen.

    (3) Respiratory rate and color. (Infants requiring further intervention will need to be transferred to an intensive care setting.)

RECOGNITION OF THE SICK NEWBORN

Review Perinatal History

A. **Ultrasound/biophysical profile:** estimated date of confinement, evidence of congenital anomalies such as bowel obstruction or enlarged heart, twins, breech position, pre-term.

B. **Medications or history of substance abuse:** $MgSO_4$, terbutaline; history of cocaine or alcohol use.

C. **Maternal illnesses:** pregnancy-induced hypertension, diabetes, herpes, hepatitis B surface antigen positive.

D. **Perinatal fetal distress/delivery complications:** abnormal fetal heart rate pattern, meconium staining of the amniotic fluid, rapid delivery, difficult delivery.

E. **Cesarean section and indications:** breech presentation, fetal distress, placenta previa, cephalopelvic disproportion, failure to progress in labor.

PHYSICAL ASSESSMENT, INCLUDING GESTATIONAL AGE ASSESSMENT AND VITAL SIGNS

A. **Skin.**
1. Cyanotic.
2. Pale.
3. Mottled.
4. Cool to touch.
5. Poor perfusion.

B. **Respiratory system.**
1. Poor color.
2. Tachypnea.
3. Decreased air entry.
4. Increased work of breathing: grunting, flaring, retracting.
5. Apnea.
6. Unequal breath sounds.
7. Oxygen requirement.

C. **Cardiovascular system.**
1. Abnormal heart sounds/murmurs.
2. Weak, absent, or unequal pulses.
3. Hepatosplenomegaly.

D. Central nervous system.
1. Hyper- or hypotonic.
2. Jitteriness/tremors.
3. Lethargy.
4. Bulging fontanel.
5. Seizures.
6. Irritability.

E. Morphology.
1. Congenital anomalies.
2. Severe birth trauma.
3. Absent or decreased limb movement.
4. Asymmetry.

DIAGNOSTIC TOOLS/STUDIES

A. Pulse oximetry (peripheral monitoring of oxygen saturation).
1. The oxygen saturation (So_2) of blood is that percentage of the total hemoglobin concentration that is chemically combined with oxygen.
2. A baseline Po_2 value needs to be obtained to correlate the existing Po_2 to the pulse oximetry reading (Hay, 1987).

B. Arterial blood gas: if persistent oxygen requirement, decreased saturations in room air or cyanosis is present.

C. Chest x-ray: AP and lateral views if respiratory distress is present.

D. Transillumination using a high-intensity light: if suspicion of pneumothorax is present.

E. Chemstrip/Dextrostix as a glucose screen or serum glucose: indicated by history or assessment. (See Glucose Needs; Routine Care Considerations.)

F. Hematocrit.
1. History of blood loss.
2. Plethoric or pale infant.
3. Twins (to rule out twin-to-twin transfusion).
4. Heelstick (capillary) samples tend to have higher results of approximately 10%.
5. Highest hematocrit is at 2–4 hours of age, then progressively falls due to beginning of RBC breakdown and cessation of erythropoiesis in response to comparatively oxygen-enriched environment.

G. Complete blood count with differential.

H. Blood culture.

I. Urine sample for:
1. Urinalysis.
2. Urine culture.
3. Drugs of abuse screen.
4. Latex agglutination test for group B streptococcal antigen.

J. Lumbar puncture.
1. Protein/glucose.
2. Cell count/Gram's stain.
3. Culture.

K. Ultrasound.
1. Cranial.
2. Abdominal.

L. Echocardiogram/electrocardiogram.

M. Passage of orogastric tube.
1. To check patency of esophagus in infants with excessive pooling of mucus in oropharynx.

2. To decompress a distended abdomen.
3. If history of excessive amniotic fluid or pre-natal ultrasound positive for bowel obstruction.

COMMON PROBLEMS AND CLINICAL PRESENTATION

A. **Birth trauma.** (Refer to Chapter 20.)

  Birth asphyxia.
1. Defined as that state in which pulmonary or placental gas exchange ceases.
2. Fetal distress is indicated by abnormal fetal heart rate pattern, meconium staining of the amniotic fluid, scalp pH less than 7.25, Apgar scores less than 5 at 1 minute of age and less than 7 at 5 minutes of age. (See Appendix D.)
3. Pathophysiological sequelae include:
   a. Decreasing Po_2: the tissue hypoxia that ensues leads to anaerobic metabolism with release of lactic acid into the circulation.
   b. Respiratory acidosis from elevated levels of carbon dioxide.
   c. Metabolic acidosis.
      (1) Results in high pulmonary vascular resistance.
      (2) Leads to decreased surfactant release.
   d. Hypoxic-ischemic damage to less vital organs such as kidney and gut following redistribution of blood to vital organs.
   e. Eventually severe hypoxia, acidosis, and hypoglycemia cause reduced myocardial function with decreased blood flow to vital organs (Phibbs, 1987).
4. All newborns have some degree of respiratory acidosis and hypoxia during labor and vaginal delivery; a healthy, full-term infant has increased tolerance and reserves. The asphyxiated newborn has more prolonged hypoxia and respiratory acidosis and may have additional metabolic acidosis, hypothermia, and hypoglycemia.
5. Clinical findings.
   a. Mild to moderate perinatal asphyxia.
      (1) Extended awake, alert state (45 minutes to 1 hour).
      (2) Dilated pupils.
      (3) Normal muscle tone.
      (4) Active suck.
      (5) Regular or slightly increased respiratory rate.
      (6) Normal or slightly increased heart rate.
   b. Moderate to severe perinatal asphyxia.
      (1) Hypothermia.
      (2) Hypoglycemia.
      (3) Pupils constricted.
      (4) Respiratory distress including grunting, flaring, retracting, tachypnea, and an oxygen requirement.
      (5) Seizures (subtle and multifocal clonic; 12–24 hours of age).
      (6) Acute tubular necrosis following reduced blood flow to the kidneys.
      (7) Hypotonia initially; lethargy.
      (8) Bradycardia.
   c. Severe perinatal asphyxia: requires constant monitoring in a Level II (intermediate care) or Level III (intensive care) nursery.
      (1) Pale; poor perfusion.
      (2) Cerebral edema.
      (3) Seizures.
      (4) Apnea.
      (5) Intracerebral hemorrhage.

C. **Pulmonary.**
1. Pneumothorax (2% of all births)/pneumomediastinum.
   a. Tachypnea, unequal breath sounds, shift of heart tones, distant heart tones.
   b. Transillumination of chest is positive for free air.

2. Retained lung fluid, respiratory distress syndrome (RDS) (secondary to prematurity or birth asphyxia), pneumonia.
   a. Decreased air entry with RDS/pneumonia.
   b. Increased work of breathing: grunting, flaring, retracting.
   c. Tachypnea, apnea.
   d. Decreased saturations (So_2), cyanosis, continued oxygen requirement.
3. Aspiration syndromes (meconium, blood).
   a. Coarse rales.
   b. Tachypnea.
   c. Barrel chest.
4. Upper airway obstruction (e.g., choanal atresia or micrognathia).
5. Extrapulmonary (e.g., phrenic nerve injury with resultant diaphragm paralysis or eventration of the diaphragm).

D. **Cardiovascular.**
1. Congenital heart disease.
   a. Acyanotic lesions.
      (1) Patent ductus arteriosus with a left-to-right shunt.
      (2) Ventricular septal defect.
      (3) Atrial septal defect.
      (4) Endocardial cushion defect.
   b. Obstructive lesions.
      (1) Aortic stenosis.
      (2) Coarctation of the aorta.
      (3) Pulmonary stenosis/atresia.
   c. Admixture lesions.
      (1) Right-to-left shunt with normal or increased pulmonary blood flow.
         (a) Complete transposition of the great vessels.
         (b) Truncus arteriosus.
      (2) Anomalous venous connection of the pulmonary veins.
      (3) Left-to-right shunt with decreased pulmonary blood flow.
         (a) Tetralogy of Fallot.
         (b) Tricuspid atresia.
2. Persistent fetal shunts.
   a. Patent ductus arteriosus with right-to-left shunt.
   b. Persistent pulmonary hypertension.
3. Clinical findings.
   a. Cyanosis with or without increased work of breathing, decreased oxygen saturations. *Note:* Absence of any signs of abnormal respiratory function in the presence of cyanosis suggests congenital heart disease.
   b. Unequal or absent pulses, bounding pulses, decreased blood pressure in the lower extremities, decreased perfusion.
   c. Increased precordial activity, shift of point of maximal intensity of heart tones, murmur.
   d. Congestive heart failure: tachypnea, moist breath sounds, tachycardia, peripheral edema, cardiomegaly.

E. **Hemodynamics.**
1. Acute hypovolemic shock.
   a. Internal hemorrhage resulting from birth trauma, intracranial hemorrhage.
   b. External hemorrhage resulting from placenta previa or abruption, cord accident, fetal-maternal or twin-to-twin transfusion.
   c. Respiratory distress, pale, poor perfusion, hypotension, weak or absent pulses.
2. Polycythemia.
   a. Plethoric, cyanotic, or excessively flushed with crying.
   b. Hypoglycemia.
   c. CNS symptoms including jitteriness, hypotonia, lethargy.
3. Anemia.
   a. Acute or chronic blood loss.

b. Hemolysis from sepsis or ABO incompatibility.

c. Reduced red blood cell production: severe asphyxia, sepsis, aplastic anemia.

d. Pale, murmur, tachypnea, normotensive, signs of congestive heart failure including hepatosplenomegaly.

F. Metabolic.

1. Hypoglycemia.
   a. Observed in large for gestational age infants, small for gestational age infants, and prematures.
   b. Clinical findings:
      (1) Poor perfusion.
      (2) Apnea/tachypnea.
      (3) Bradycardia.
      (4) Jitteriness/irritability.
      (5) Seizures.
      (6) Hypothermia.
      (7) Cyanosis.
      (8) Poor feeding.
2. Maternal medications/drugs of substance abuse.
   a. Magnesium sulfate: infants present with respiratory depression, decreased tone, decreased serum calcium.
   b. Tocolytics: infants may present with hypoglycemia.
   c. Narcotics: infants present with apnea, respiratory depression, periodic breathing.
   d. Cocaine: infants present with apnea, poor tone initially then irritability and agitation, tremors, feeding difficulties.
   e. Marijuana/methadone: infants present with hyperthermia, agitation, diarrhea.
   f. Alcohol: fetal alcohol syndrome with dysmorphic and behavioral abnormalities.

G. Sepsis.

1. A generalized bacterial or viral disease; acquired in utero or nosocomial.
2. Clinical findings.
   a. Hyperthermia or hypothermia.
   b. Tachypnea/apnea.
   c. Bradycardia.
   d. Cyanosis.
   e. Hypotension/shock.
   f. Disseminated intravascular coagulation.
   g. Hepatosplenomegaly.
   h. Poor feeding.
   i. Jaundice.
   j. Purpura.
   k. Hypoglycemia.
3. In utero viral infection may cause infant to be small for gestational age with microcephaly.

H. Congenital anomalies: frequently obvious on gross examination.

1. Diaphragmatic hernia.
   a. Present at birth with initial gasp then apnea or immediate onset of significant respiratory distress.
   b. Shift in heart tones, decreased or unequal breath sounds, bowel tones heard in chest, scaphoid abdomen.
2. Esophageal atresia with or without tracheal esophageal fistula.
   a. Excessive amniotic fluid.
   b. Increased pooling of secretions in oropharynx, respiratory distress, unable to pass an orogastric tube.
3. Abdominal wall defects—e.g. omphalocele/gastroschisis.
4. Limb anomalies: amniotic banding, talipes equinovarus, polydactyly, syndactyly.

5. Neural tube defects.
6. Intestinal obstruction.
7. Chromosomal abnormalities—e.g., trisomy 21 or trisomy 18.

INITIAL STABILIZATION OF THE SICK NEWBORN

A. **Observation.** Short-term observation in transition nursery to monitor infant's trend prior to transfer to NICU.
1. Infant may be capable of resolving the problem on his own if given time—e.g., correction of mild acidosis from asphyxia, clearing of lung fluid, stabilizing blood glucose, stabilizing blood pressure.
2. Monitor and record trends—i.e., improved respiratory rate toward normal, improved perfusion, follow glucose screens.

B. **Avoid excessive handling.**
1. Organize care and interventions to avoid frequent, unnecessary stimulation of an already stressed infant.
2. Use pulse oximeter and/or cardiorespiratory monitor to reduce hands-on vital signs.
3. Reduce background stimulation such as loud noises or bright lights.
4. Use non-nutritive sucking to lower activity levels and reduce energy needs.
   a. Infant may be more comfortable in a prone position.
   b. Crying can be stressful: similar to a Valsalva maneuver with prolonged exhalation, obstructed venous return, quick inspiratory gasp, right-to-left shunting at the foramen ovale.
   c. Crying depletes energy reserves and increases oxygen consumption.
5. Provide a neutral thermal environment. (See Point B. of Routine Care Considerations.)
   a. Observe for apnea and hypotension during warming.
   b. Avoid hyperthermia.
6. Supply glucose.
   a. Oral treatment of glucose 30–40 mg/dl: early frequent feedings by nipple, gavage, or nursing.
      (1) Give at least 1/2–1 ounce of formula by nipple or gavage. If infant is stable, may be allowed to nurse 5–10 minutes on each breast.
      (2) Begin maintenance formula at 50–70 kcal/kg/day or breast feed ad lib demand every 2–5 hours.
      (3) Check glucose 1 hour after feeding.
   b. Oral treatment of glucose less than 30 mg/dl. (STAT serum glucose if glucose screen is less than 30 mg/dl.)
      (1) Give at least 1/2–1 ounce of formula by nipple or gavage if there are no contraindications to oral feeds.
      (2) Consider giving a formula designed for premature infants.
         (a) These formulas provide carbohydrate in the form of glucose polymers that are easily absorbed (Menon and Sperling, 1988).
         (b) Fat is provided as medium chain triglycerides; medium chain fatty acids are absorbed in the stomach of the newborn.
         (c) Fatty acid oxidation and ketogenesis spare glucose for brain energy needs.
         (d) Free fatty acids and ketones promote glucose production by providing essential gluconeogenic cofactors.
         (e) Normal newborns respond to a protein meal by preferentially increasing glucagon, which elicits a glycemic response (Menon and Sperling, 1988).
      (3) Intravenous treatment of glucose less than 30 mg/dl. *Note:* Do not administer bolus of glucose IV greater than 25% dextrose in water because of reactive hypoglycemia and hypertonic solution. Always follow a glucose bolus with a continuous infusion of glucose.

(a) If infant is asymptomatic and unable to take oral feeds, give IV glucose at 4–5 mg/kg/minute.
(b) If infant is symptomatic and NPO, give IV glucose as a "mini-bolus" of 2 ml/kg of 10% dextrose in water and begin an intravenous infusion at 6–8 mg/kg/minute.
(c) Monitor therapy with frequent glucose checks and titrate infusion to meet infant's glucose needs.

7. Supply oxygen. Assess needs using a pulse oximeter or transcutaneous monitor, arterial blood gases, and close observation.
   a. Extended oxygen use in the transition nursery requires notification of the physician and transfer to a Level II or Level III setting.
   b. Provide warmed, humidified oxygen per oxyhood, continuous positive airway pressure (CPAP), or assisted ventilation based on the infant's needs. (Refer to Chapter 9.)
   c. Monitor oxygen provided with an oxygen analyzer. Record blowby oxygen as liters/minute and distance from infant's face.
8. Volume expanders, including blood, normal saline, 5% albumin.
   a. For hypotension and blood loss.
   b. Require IV placement and transfer to Level II nursery for continued management and observation, including cardiorespiratory monitor and frequent blood pressure checks to titrate therapy.
9. Naloxone hydrochloride (Narcan).
   a. Administered for apnea with history of narcotics given to mother just prior to delivery.
   b. Do not use Narcan with history of opioid-dependent mother; may precipitate acute withdrawal symptoms.
10. Antibiotics.
    a. As indicated by history, current status of the infant, and initial laboratory results.
    b. Administer via peripheral IV or heparin lock IV.

PARENT TEACHING

Before Delivery

A. **History.** Review the obstetrical history; anticipate the needs of the infant at delivery.

B. **Complications.** If there are expected complications (pre-term delivery, congenital anomalies) and time permits, discuss anticipated plan of care with the family.
1. Discuss plans for managing their infant, including plans for transfer to a Level II or Level III nursery and any special equipment that may be used (oxygen hood, incubator, ventilator, monitors).
2. Allow the parents to tour the NICU if possible.

C. **Parental support.** Encourage parents to express their feelings, fears, misgivings; involve support persons.

At Delivery

A. **Place infant on mother's abdomen** when possible with uncomplicated deliveries; use family's "birth plan' as much as possible.

B. **After delivery room assessment on warmer**, return infant to family if stable.

C. **Answer questions** regarding acrocyanosis, Apgar scores, morphologic findings.

D. **Allow time** to visit, breast-feed, see extended family.

During Transition

A. **"Introduce" the baby** to the family by noting unique features (dimples, long eyelashes, hair color).

B. **Encourage support person** to touch and talk to the infant.

C. **Discuss physical findings** such as caput succedaneum, positional deformities, birth marks.

D. **Discuss infant's sensory capabilities**, including seeing, hearing, smell.

E. **Listen to the parents:** allow them to express their reactions as they compare their "dream" baby with the real baby they now have (too tiny, not the right sex, deformed, premature).

F. **After completion of admission procedures**, the infant is returned to the family for feeding and visiting.

G. **Allow family to participate in the infant's care that they desire**—i.e., giving the first bath or first bottle feedings.

Post-partum Period (Early Discharge/Short Stay)

A. **Parental involvement.** Involve the parents in evaluation of their learning needs; begin teaching as soon as delivery occurs.

B. **Short hospital stays and family instruction.** With shorter hospital stays, there is less time available for teaching and an increased importance of teaching. This may be the only information many families receive on caring for a newborn.
1. Classes/videotaped lectures.
   a. CPR/safety.
   b. Breast-feeding.
   c. Childbirth preparation.
   d. Developmental milestones.
2. Follow-up with public health nurse visits to the home, phone calls from post-partum nurses.
3. Follow-up visit with primary care physicians.
4. Return for newborn screening if needed.

Transfer to Level II or III Setting

A. **Pre-natal teaching** if possible with visits to NICU.

B. **Information booklets** with location, phone numbers, visiting regulations, parent-to-parent groups, necessary support personnel.

C. **Bring mother to infant's bedside** if infant is unable to return to mother after delivery. Allow family to be near infant as much as possible and encourage them to see past the equipment to the infant and his special needs (gentle touch, stroking, soft voice, a familiar person).

D. **When infant is stable**, allow family to visit in the privacy of their post-partum room or a parent room if condition warrants—e.g., an infant with a heparin lock for antibiotics.

E. **Provide a picture of the infant for the family.** This is especially important if the transfer to a Level II or III nursery will be to another facility.

F. **Facilitate family keeping in contact with the transfer facility and be available to explain information given to the family.**

STUDY QUESTIONS

1. The fetal shunt connecting the pulmonary artery and the aorta is the:
   a. Ductus arteriosus.
   b. Ductus venosus.
   c. Foramen ovale.

2. The formen ovale and the ductus arteriosus allow blood to bypass:
   a. The fetal brain.
   b. The fetal liver.
   c. The fetal lungs.

3. A cause of fetal hypoxia during labor is:
   a. Cold stress.
   b. Hypoglycemia.
   c. Uterine contractions.

4. During transition, catecholamines cause which of these physiological events to occur:
   a. Closure of the ductus arteriosus.
   b. Increased absorption of lung fluid and release of surfactant.
   c. Reduced blood flow to the brain.

5. At 1 and 5 minutes of age, the following parameters are scored in the delivery room:
   a. Color, tone, heart rate, respiratory rate, and reflex irritability.
   b. Temperature and blood pressure.
   c. Weight, head circumference, and length.

6. Immediate transfer from the delivery room to the nursery would be indicated with the presence of:
   a. Acrocyanosis.
   b. Facial bruising.
   c. Grunting, flaring, and retracting.

7. Cold stress can lead to:
   a. Anemia.
   b. Hypertension.
   c. Increased oxygen consumption.

8. Transfer to a Level II or Level III nursery from the transition nursery would be indicated for an infant presenting with:
   a. Hypothermia after the first bath and poor breast-feeding.
   b. Polydactyly, talipes equinovarus, and an initial glucose screen of 35 mg/dl.
   c. Respiratory rate of 70 with grunting, retracting, and cyanosis in room air in the first hours of life.

9. The following clinical presentation is abnormal during the transition period:
   a. Cyanosis and weak pulses in the lower extremities.
   b. Facial bruising and petechiae following a rapid delivery.
   c. Pink in room air with moist rales and a respiratory rate of 68.

Answers to Study Questions

1. a	4. b	7. c
2. c	5. a	8. c
3. c	6. c	9. a

REFERENCES

American Academy of Pediatrics (AAP) and American College of Obstetricians and Gynecologists (ACOG): Guidelines for Perinatal Care, 3rd ed. AAP: Elk Grove Village, IL; ACOG: Washington, DC, 1992, pp. 118–120.

Birbeck, J.A.: Vitamin K prophylaxis in the newborn: A position statement of the Nutrition Committee of the Pediatric Society of New Zealand. N. Z. Med. J. 101:421–422, 1988.

Centers for Disease Control (CDC): Prevention of perinatal transmission of hepatitis B virus: Perinatal screening of all pregnant women for hepatitis B surface antigen. MMWR, 37:341–346, 1988.

Desmond, M.M., Rudolph, A.J., and Phitaksphraiwan, P.: The transitional care nursery: A mechanism for preventive medicine in the newborn. Pediatr. Clin. North Am., 13:651–668, 1966.

Hay, W.W., Jr.: Physiology of oxygenation and its relation to pulse oximetry in neonates. J. Perinatol., 7:309–319, 1987.

Menon, R.K., and Sperling, M.A.: Carbohydrate metabolism. Semin. Perinatol., 12:157–162, 1988.

Merenstein, G.B., and Gardner, S.L.: Heat balance. In Merenstein, G.B., and Gardner, S.L. (eds.): Handbook of Neonatal Intensive Care, 2nd ed. St. Louis, C.V. Mosby, 1989.

Moore, K.L.: The Developing Human: Clinically Oriented Embryology, 4th ed. Philadelphia, W.B. Saunders Co., 1988.

Olson, M.: The benign effects of rabbits' lungs of the aspiration of water compared with 5% glucose or milk. Pediatrics, 46:538–547, 1970.

Phibbs, R.H.: Delivery management of the newborn. *In* Avery, G. (ed.): Neonatology—Pathophysiology and Management of the Newborn, 3rd ed. Philadelphia, J.B. Lippincott Co., 1987, pp. 212–231.

BIBLIOGRAPHY

Askin, D.: Neonatal thermoregulation. NAACOG–OGN Nursing Practice Resource. Washington, DC, 1990.

Avery, G. (ed.): Neonatology—Pathophysiology and Management of the Newborn, 3rd ed. Philadelphia, J.B. Lippincott Co., 1987.

Banta, S.A.: Transition to extrauterine life. Neonatal Network, 3:35–39, 1985.

Birbeck, J.A.: Vitamin K prophylaxis in the newborn: A position statement of the Nutrition Committee of the Pediatric Society of New Zealand. N. Z. Med. J. 101:421–422, 1988.

Boddy, K., and Dawes, G.S. Fetal breathing. Br. Med. J., 31:3–7, 1975.

Dodman, N.: Newborn temperature control. Neonatal Network, 5:19–23, 1987.

Fanaroff, A.A., and Martin, R.J. (eds.): Neonatal–Perinatal Medicine; Diseases of the Fetus and Infant, 4th ed. St Louis, C.V. Mosby, 1987.

Gill, N.E., White, M.A., and Anderson, G.C.: Transitional newborn infants in a hospital nursery: From first oral cry to first sustained cry. Nurs. Res., 33:213–217, 1984.

Greer, F.R., Mummah-Schendel, L.L., Marshall, S., and Suttie, J.W.: Vitamin K_1 (phylloquinone) and vitamin K_2 (menaquinone) status in newborns during the first week of life. Pediatrics, 81:137–140, 1988.

Jansen, A.H., and Chernick, V.: Onset of breathing and control of respirations. Semin. Perinatol. 12:104–112, 1988.

Lagercrantz, H., and Slotkin, T.: The "stress" of being born. Sci. Am., 254:100–107, 1986.

Lane, P.A.: Vitamin K in infancy. J. Pediatr., 103(3):351–359, 1985.

Padbury, J.F., and Martinez, A.M.: Sympathoadrenal system activity at birth: Integration of postnatal adaption. Semin. Perinatol., 12:163–172, 1988.

Polk, D.H.: Thyroid hormone effects on neonatal thermogenesis. Semin. Perinatol., 12:151–156, 1988.

Rudolph, A.M.: High pulmonary vascular resistance after birth. 1. Pathophysiologic considerations and etiologic classification. Clin. Pediatr., 19:585–590, 1980.

Tsang, R.C., and Nichols, B.L. (eds.): Nutrition in Infancy. St. Louis, C.V. Mosby Co., 1988.

Patti Witt

Physical Assessment of the Newborn

Objectives

1. Describe methods of determining gestational age pre-natally and post-natally.

2. Discuss the classification of newborns by birthweight and gestational age and relate problems that can be anticipated.

3. Describe management of infants identified to be at risk.

4. Relate risk factors associated with discordant growth patterns.

5. Become familiar with morbidity and mortality statistics for the various classifications and risk groups.

6. Describe the systematic approach to conducting a physical examination on a newborn.

7. Identify and differentiate normal and abnormal findings of a newborn physical examination.

8. Recognize abnormalities that require immediate intervention.

Decreasing morbidity and mortality is a goal we strive for in neonatology. Early recognition of existing or potential problems is important to initiate appropriate treatment as soon as possible. Reliable tools are available for determining gestational age both pre-natally and post-natally. From this information, we can identify those who are at risk for a variety of problems. A comprehensive physical examination must also be performed on every newborn. Information collected can be reassuring to the newborn's family or can identify problems that must be treated. This chapter discusses determinants of gestational age, reviews infants identified to be at risk, and reviews the systematic approach to conducting a physical examination.

Perinatal History Review

An assessment of the newborn begins with a review of the perinatal history. Valuable information may reveal existing pathology and problems that may require immediate attention.

A. Pre-natal history.
1. Family history and pedigree.
2. Maternal past medical history.
3. Reproductive history.
   a. Number of pregnancies.
   b. Number of live births.
   c. Spontaneous/elective abortions.
   d. Neonatal deaths.
4. Pregnancy history.
   a. Prenatal care.
   b. Blood type and rhesus factor (Rh).
   c. Prenatal lab tests: Venereal Disease Research Laboratory (VDRL), rubella screen, antibody screen, hepatitis screen, human immunodeficiency virus (HIV) screen.
5. Last menstrual period (LMP) and estimated date of confinement (EDC).
6. Ultrasound examinations.
7. Drugs taken during pregnancy.
8. Weight gain, nutrition, and general health during pregnancy.

B. Labor and delivery history.
1. Onset of labor: spontaneous or induced.
2. Duration of stages of labor.
3. Presence of fetal distress.
4. Rupture of membranes.
   a. Artificial or spontaneous.
   b. Duration of rupture before delivery.
5. Amniotic fluid volume and appearance: clear or meconium stained.
6. Type of delivery: vaginal or cesarean section.
7. Indication for operative delivery.
8. Instrumentation: forceps or vacuum extraction.
9. Type of analgesia or anesthesia.

C. Resuscitation required.
1. Apgar scores.
2. Intervention and response.

Assessment of Gestational Age

A. Purpose of determining gestational age.
1. Assignment of a newborn classification.
   a. Term, pre-term, or post-term.
   b. Birthweight.
      (1) Appropriate for gestational age (AGA).
      (2) Small for gestational age (SGA).
      (3) Large for gestational age (LGA).
2. Determination of the neonatal mortality risk.
3. Identification of potential morbidities.

B. Obstetrical methods for determining gestational age.
1. LMP and menstrual history.
2. Pregnancy test.
3. Ultrasound evaluation of fetal growth.
4. Detection of fetal heart tones, fundal height, quickening.
5. Amniotic fluid studies.
   a. Creatinine level increases as fetus approaches term.
   b. Bilirubin concentration decreases as pregnancy approaches term.
   c. Lecithin/sphingomyelin ratio increase at 34–36 weeks' gestation except in infants of diabetic mothers.

C. Pediatric methods of determining gestational age.
1. Physical characteristics.
2. Neurologic examination.

D. Gestational age assessment tools.
1. Dubowitz (Dubowitz et al., 1970): assessment of 10 physical and 11 neurological criteria.
2. Ballard: a simplified scoring system based on the Dubowitz method using 6 neurologic and 6 physical criteria (Fig. 4–1).
   a. Unlike the Dubowitz examination, all elements of the Ballard method can be performed on very ill or fragile babies, therefore giving a more accurate estimate.
   b. Highest reliability when performed within 42 hours of birth.
   c. Accurate within 2 weeks of gestation (Ballard et al., 1979).

Neuromuscular Maturity

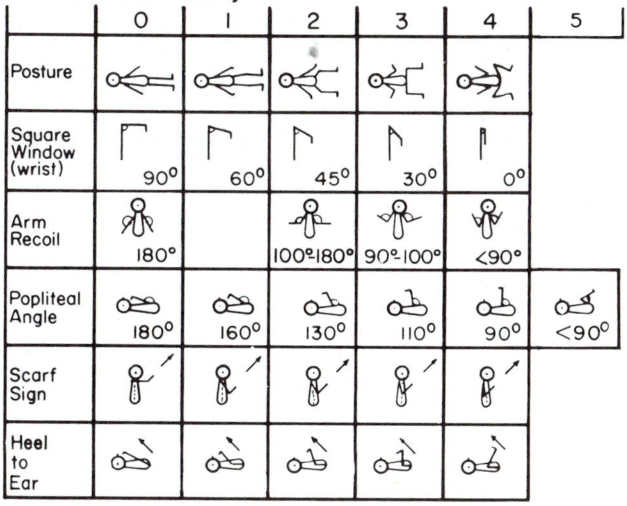

Physical Maturity

MATURITY RATING

Score	Wks.
5	26
10	28
15	30
20	32
25	34
30	36
35	38
40	40
45	42
50	44

Figure 4–1
Scoring system for simplified clinical assessment of maturation in newborn infants. (From Ballard, R.A., et al.: J. Pediatr., *95*:770, 1979.)

E. Assessment of individual physical signs.

1. Skin.
   a. The skin becomes less transparent, thicker, and tougher with increasing gestational age.
   b. By 36–37 weeks, the skin has lost its transparency and underlying vessels are no longer visible.
   c. As gestation progresses beyond 38 weeks, the subcutaneous tissue begins to decrease, causing wrinkling and desquamation.
2. Lanugo.
   a. Fine downy hair covering the body of the fetus from 20 to 28 weeks.
   b. At 28 weeks, it begins to disappear around the face and anterior trunk.
   c. At term, a few patches may be present over the shoulders.
3. Sole creases.
   a. First appear on the anterior portion of the foot and extend toward the heel as gestation progresses.
   b. An infant with intrauterine growth retardation and early loss of vernix may have more sole creases than expected.
   c. After 12 hours, sole creases are no longer a valid indicator of gestational age, due to drying of the skin.
4. Breast tissue and areola.
   a. The areola is raised by 34 weeks' gestation.
   b. A 1–2 mm nodule of breast tissue is palpable by about 36 weeks and grows to approximately 10 mm by 40 weeks' gestation (Black, 1978).
5. Ears.
   a. Incurving of the upper pinna usually begins by 34 weeks' gestation and by 40 weeks extends to the lobe.
   b. Before 34 weeks, the pinna has very little cartilage and will stay folded on itself.
   c. By 36 weeks, there is some cartilage and the pinna will spring back from folding.
6. Eyes.
   a. At 26–30 weeks' gestation, fused eyelids open.
   b. From 27 to 34 weeks' gestation, examination of the anterior vascular capsule of the lens is helpful in determining gestational age by examining the level of remaining embryonic vessels on the lens (Fig. 4–2).
7. Genitalia.
   a. Female.
      (1) Early in gestation, the clitoris is prominent with small, widely separated labia.
      (2) By 40 weeks, fat deposits have increased in size in the labia majora, so that the labia majora completely cover the labia minora.
   b. Male.
      (1) The testes begin to descend from the abdomen at 28 weeks.
      (2) At 37 weeks, the testes can be palpated high in the scrotum.
      (3) At 40 weeks, the testes are completely descended and the scrotum is covered with rugae.
      (4) As gestation progresses, the scrotum becomes more pendulous.
8. Hair.
   a. Appears on the head at 20 weeks.
   b. Eyelashes and eyebrows develop at 20–23 weeks' gestation.
   c. From 28 to 34–36 weeks, hair is fine and wooly and sticks together.
   d. At term, hair lies flat on the head and feels silky; single strands are identifiable.

F. Assessment of neurological signs.

1. Posture.
   a. Early in gestation, the infant's resting posture is hypotonic.
   b. At 30 weeks, there is often only slight flexion of the feet and knees.

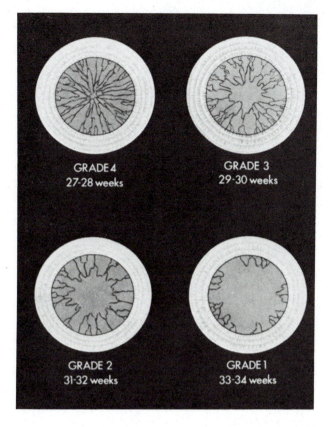

Figure 4-2
Grading system for assessment of gestational age by examination of the anterior vascular capsule of the lens. (From Hittner, H., et al.: J. Pediatr. *91*:455, 1977.)

GRADE 4
27-28 weeks

GRADE 3
29-30 weeks

GRADE 2
31-32 weeks

GRADE 1
33-34 weeks

    c. At 34 weeks, the thighs and hips are flexed (frog position) but usually the arms remain extended.

    d. By 35 weeks, beginning arm flexion can be observed.

    e. By 36–38 weeks, the resting posture of the healthy infant is of total flexion with prompt recoil of arms and legs.

2. Flexion angles and joint mobility.

    a. Flexion angle of the wrist decreases with increasing gestational age, denoting increasing joint mobility.

    b. The square window, a sign that describes flexion when the wrist is at a right angle to the forearm, shows little flexion until after 31 weeks. The flexion increases until term, when the angle disappears.

    c. Dorsiflexion is not noted until 34–35 weeks. This angle increases until it disappears at term.

    d. Popliteal angle is indirectly related to muscle tone in the lower extremities. The greater the gestational age, the smaller the angle.

    e. Reflexes that are the most helpful in determining gestational age are rooting and sucking movements, which occur at about 34 weeks.

G. **Classification of the newborn.**

1. Plot birthweight and gestational age on standard intrauterine growth charts (Fig. 4–3).

2. Clinical estimate of gestation is defined by weeks of gestation and is divided into several categories.

    a. Pre-term: through 37 weeks.

    b. Term: 38–41 completed weeks.

    c. Post-term: 42 weeks or greater.

3. Infants classified as small for gestational age (SGA) are those below the 10th percentile. Appropriate for gestational age (AGA) infants are those between the

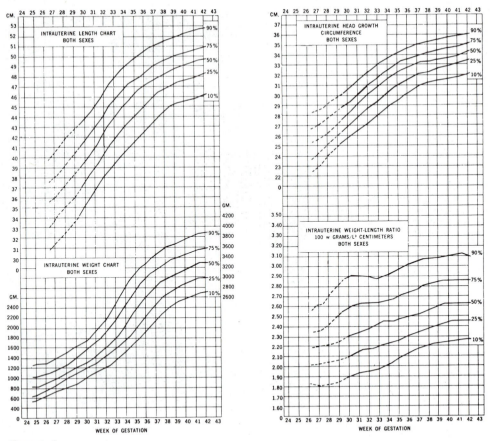

Figure 4-3
Colorado Intrauterine Growth Charts. (From Lubchenco, L.O., et al.: Pediatrics *37*:403, © 1966. Reproduced by permission of Pediatrics. Reprinted with permission of Ross Laboratories, Columbus, OH 43216, from CO Intrauterine Growth Charts. © 1966, Ross Laboratories.)

10th and 90th percentiles. Large for gestational age (LGA) infants are those above the 90th percentile.

4. Plot birthweight and gestational age on standard graphs to determine the neonatal mortality risk by birthweight and gestational age (Figs. 4–4 and 4–5).

5. Classification of the newborn assists in identification, observation, screening, and treatment of the most commonly occurring problems.

6. A problem list based on the morbidities should be formulated for each infant.

H. **Assessment of infants at risk.**

1. Infants determined to be pre-term, SGA, or LGA require specialized care due to an increased risk of respiratory disease, metabolic disorders (hypoglycemia/ polycythemia), and problems with thermoregulation.

2. Complications associated with SGA and LGA infants (Fig. 4–6).
   a. Large for gestational age infants (LGA).
      (1) Birth trauma.
         (a) May range from a large cephalohematoma to a depressed skull fracture.
         (b) Fractured clavicle.
         (c) Peripheral nerve injuries of the cervical or brachial plexus.
      (2) Infants of diabetic mothers may be large with an increased weight-over-length ratio. These infants have an increased incidence of respiratory distress, hypoglycemia, hypocalcemia, polycythemia, hyperbilirubinemia, and congenital anomalies (Goldkrand and Lin, 1987).

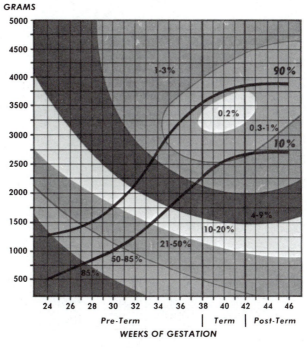

Figure 4–4
Neonatal mortality risk by birth weight and gestational age. (From Lubchenco, L.O., et al.: J. Pediatr. *81*:814, 1972. © 1982 Mead Johnson & Co.)

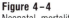

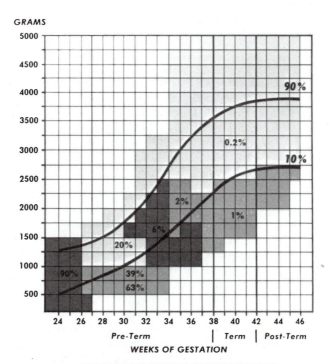

Figure 4–5
Neonatal mortality risk by birth weight and gestational age. (From Koops, B.L., et al.: J. Pediatr., *101*:969, 1982. © 1982 Mead Johnson & Co.)

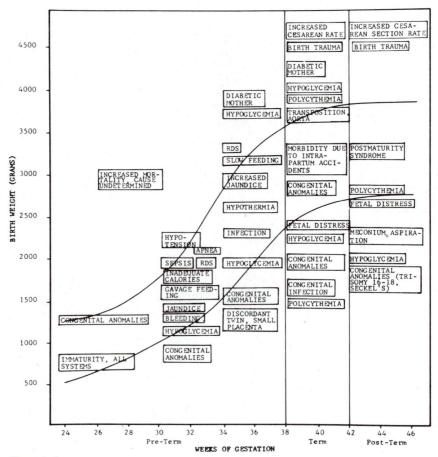

Figure 4–6
Specific neonatal morbidity by birthweight and gestational age. (From Lubchenco, L.O.: The High Risk Infant, Philadelphia, W.B. Saunders, Co., 1976.)

(3) Beckwith's syndrome is a syndrome characterized by LGA infants and consists of macroglossia, umbilical abnormalities (generally omphalocele) and hypoglycemia (Battaglia, 1973b).
(4) Asphyxia due to central nervous system trauma during the birth process.
(5) Hypoglycemia.
(6) Thermoregulation problems as a result of CNS trauma or infection.
b. Small for gestational age infants (SGA).
(1) Hypoglycemia occurs in almost two-thirds of SGA infants due to high metabolic rate and low glycogen stores (Battaglia, 1973a).
(2) Infants of diabetic mothers with advanced diabetes can also be SGA due to poor placental function.
(3) Increased incidence of fetal distress and asphyxia. SGA infants are at risk for aspiration of amniotic fluid frequently containing meconium. Complications of meconium aspiration include respiratory distress, pulmonary air leaks, and hypoxia.
(4) If intrauterine growth retardation is secondary to congenital infection, it may persist after birth.
(5) Chromosomal defects are commonly seen in SGA infants.
(6) Thermoregulation problems due to high demands for metabolic fuel. The SGA infant does not have adequate adipose tissue for insulation or stores of brown adipose tissue to maintain body temperature.

(7) Polycythemia (venous hematocrit greater than 65% during the first week of life) occurs from placental hypertransfusion or increased red blood cell production in utero due to endocrine, metabolic, or chromosomal disorders.

Physical Examination Overview

A. **A brief physical examination should be performed in the delivery room** to rule out obvious congenital anomalies, birth injuries, and cardiorespiratory distress. A more complete examination is performed in the nursery within 24 hours of birth.

B. **The infant must be kept warm during the examination**, either by a radiant warmer or by uncovering and examining only one body area at a time.

C. **The infant will generally be the most cooperative** during the examination, 1–2 hours after a feeding.

D. **A systematic, organized approach** to physical examination will ensure that no part is overlooked.

E. **Certain components of a physical examination may need to be modified** to match the infant's state.

F. **The physical examination should be documented** on the patient record.

G. **Abnormalities should be noted** and the infant's primary care provider notified.

Physical Assessment

A. Observation.
1. General condition.
   a. Size, contour, and general well-being.
   b. Posture.
      (1) Healthy term infants exhibit flexion of the extremities.
      (2) Breech infants exhibit extension of the legs and head, and frank breech infants have abduction and external rotation of the legs.
   c. Activity.
      (1) Motor activity consists of spontaneous activity of flexion and extension of arms and legs.
      (2) Lack of flexion is associated with hypotonia and may be seen in pre-term infants and as a result of CNS trauma.
      (3) Excessive flexion suggests hypertonicity and may be the result of CNS trauma.
      (4) Asymmetrical movements of arms, legs, or face may suggest birth injuries such as brachial plexus palsy, bone fractures, or congenital anomalies.
   d. Skin.
      (1) Observe for dry, peeling skin; rashes; pustules; petechiae; discolorations; pigmentation.
   e. State.
      (1) The infant should pass through all activity states from asleep to awake and crying during the examination.
      (2) The cry should be robust and vigorous in the term infant. Note high-pitched or hoarse cries.
   f. Respirations.
      (1) Respiratory rate and effort.
      (2) Nasal flaring.

      (3) Grunting, stridor.

      (4) Intercostal/substernal retractions.

  g. Morphology.

      (1) Obvious congenital defects.

      (2) Symmetry of like body parts.

      (3) Proportional body parts.

  h. Nutrition.

      (1) Well-nourished appearance.

      (2) Thin, lean, wasted appearance.

  i. Color.

      (1) The mucous membranes are the most reliable indicators of central color in all babies. Central cyanosis indicates low oxygen saturation in the blood, usually of a cardiac or respiratory origin.

      (2) Acrocyanosis suggests instability of the peripheral circulation and may be the result of cold, stress, shock, or polycythemia. May be a normal finding for 24 hours after birth.

      (3) Pallor at birth reflects poor perfusion and circulatory failure.

        (a) With bradycardia, pallor usually indicates anoxia.

        (b) With tachycardia, pallor usually indicates anemia.

      (4) Plethora: a beet-red color that may indicate polycythemia, which is confirmed by hemoglobin and hematocrit testing.

      (5) Jaundice appearing in the first 12 hours is abnormal and should be investigated.

B. Auscultation/palpation.

1. Auscultation is best accomplished on a quiet infant.

2. Warm hands, and stethoscope, and avoid overmanipulation of the infant to avoid disturbing the child, causing him to cry.

3. Heart.

  a. Heart rate counted for a full minute ranges from 110 to 160 beats/minute.

  b. Note rhythm and regularity at the apex.

  c. The point of maximal intensity (PMI) of the heart is normally lateral to the midclavicular line at the third to fourth interspace. Note the position.

  d. Precordial activity is associated with heart disease, fluid overload, and congestive heart failure. An active precordium can often be seen in premature infants with thin skin and little subcutaneous tissue.

  e. A heart rate less than 110 beats/minute is bradycardia, which may be associated with anoxia, cerebral defects, or increased intracranial pressure. In deep sleep, an infant may have a heart rate as low as 90. If it does not increase quickly to greater than 100 when the infant awakens, it may represent a congenital heart block.

  f. A heart rate greater than 160 beats/minute is tachycardia, which may be associated with respiratory problems, anemia, or congestive heart failure.

  g. Murmurs are heard frequently in the neonatal period. Most are systolic ejection murmurs that occur before the first heart sound and end at or before the second sound. Murmurs in the first 48 hours are often not pathological but should be followed.

  h. Continuous murmurs extend beyond the second heart sound into diastole.

  i. Note murmurs for loudness, quality, radiation, location, and timing.

  j. Transient murmurs occurring commonly at 4–8 hours of life are attributed to closing of the ductus arteriosus or to the change in pulmonary vascular resistance as the change from fetal to neonatal pulmonary pressure occurs.

  k. Note muffled or shifted heart sounds, which may indicate pneumothorax, pneumomediastinum, dextrocardia, or diaphragmatic hernia.

  l. Palpate pulses while the infant is quiet. Femoral pulses are normally palpable in all infants unless there is an obstruction to arterial flow or shock. Note volume and equality. Bounding pulses can be felt with a patent ductus arteriosus. Absent or decreased femoral pulses are associated with coarctation of the aorta. Blood pressures should be recorded at the time of admission to the nursery (Fig. 4–7). A differential in blood pressures greater than 20 mm Hg between upper and lower extremities may suggest an obstruction. Blood pressures in the lower extremities should be slightly higher than in the upper extremities.

4. Chest/lungs.
    a. Respirations should be easy and unlabored.
    b. Newborns are primarily nose breathers, and obstruction of the nares may lead to respiratory distress and cyanosis.
    c. The chest should be round, with the anteroposterior (AP) diameter equal bilaterally. An increased AP diameter may suggest pneumothorax or cardiomegaly.
    d. Inspect breasts and nipples for symmetry, size, number, and discharge.
        (1) Supernumerary nipples are small, raised pigmented areas found vertical to the main nipple line and require no treatment.
        (2) Enlarged breasts result from effects of maternal estrogen and are transient. A milk-like substance may occur uncommonly but is a normal finding. The enlargement lasts 1–2 weeks.
        (3) Widespread nipples: the distance between nipples is greater than 25% of the full chest circumference (Coen et al., 1988). May indicate congenital malformations such as Turner's syndrome.
    e. The respiratory rate and pattern should be noted. A normal respiratory rate is approximately 40–60/minute and can vary somewhat based on the activity of the infant.
    f. After birth, fine rales may be audible due to clearing of lung fluid.
    g. Bronchial breath sounds and air entry should be audible bilaterally and should be clear. Rales and rhonchi suggest respiratory disease.

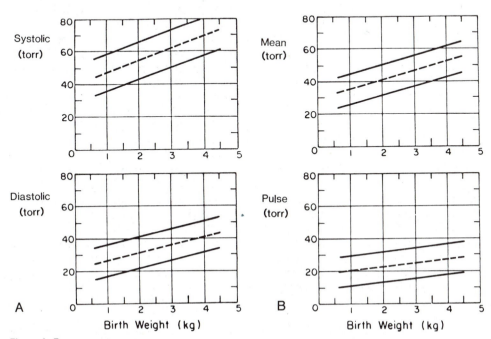

Figure 4–7
Blood pressure by birth weight. (From Versmold, H.T., Kitterman, J.A., Phibbs, R.H., et al.: Aortic blood pressure during the first 12 hours of life in infants with birth weight 610 to 4220 grams. Reproduced by permission of Pediatrics *67*(5):607, copyright 1981.) copyright © American Academy of Pediatrics, 1981.)

h. Retractions, tachypnea, and grunting are all symptoms of respiratory distress.
i. Asymmetrical breath sounds may indicate a tension pneumothorax or a diaphragmatic hernia.
j. The thoracic cage is small, and sound is easily transmitted throughout. Breath sounds are rarely entirely absent. Diminished breath sounds may suggest atelectasis, effusion, pneumothorax, or decreased respiratory effort.

5. Abdomen/trunk.
  a. The abdomen is slightly rounded, soft, and symmetrical.
  b. A concave abdomen may suggest diaphragmatic hernia, and a flabby abdomen may be associated with depressant effects of residual maternal medication or immaturity or the absence of muscles in the abdominal wall. Prune-belly syndrome exists when there are no muscles in the abdominal wall and is associated with other anomalies of the gastrointestinal and genitourinary tracts.
  c. Abdominal distention may be due to obstruction, infection, or enlargement of an abdominal organ.
  d. Observe for abdominal wall defects such as omphalocele, gastroschisis, or umbilical hernia.
  e. Palpate the abdomen gently for enlargement of organs or the presence of masses.
    (1) The liver edge is palpated 1–2 cm below the right costal margin in the midclavicular line.
      (a) Palpation is begun in the right lower quadrant and progresses upward so that a large liver edge will not be missed.
      (b) Hepatomegaly may be associated with congenital heart disease, infection, or hemolytic disease.
    (2) A palpable spleen tip more than 1 cm below the left costal margin is abnormal. A normal spleen is rarely palpable.
    (3) Kidneys are palpated by placing one hand under the flank and palpating from above with fingers from the other hand. A normal full-term kidney is 4.5–5.0 cm from pole to pole (Lawrence, 1984). Enlarged kidneys or absence of a palpable kidney suggests further evaluation.
    (4) Abnormal abdominal masses are most frequently of urinary tract origin.
    (5) The bladder can be palpated 1–4 cm above the symphysis.
  f. The umbilical cord should contain two arteries and one vein. A single artery may be associated with an increased incidence of congenital abnormalities, generally of the gastrointestinal and genitourinary systems.
    (1) The diameter of the cord varies, related to the quality of Wharton's jelly, and is an indicator of the nutritional status of the infant.
    (2) The cord begins to dry soon after birth and falls off 7–10 days after birth.
    (3) Redness, foul odor, or wetness of the cord may indicate omphalitis.
    (4) Herniation into the umbilical cord is a significant finding and needs immediate attention. The herniation may be small and present with just a large umbilical cord or may be an obvious omphalocele.
  g. Auscultate the abdomen for bowel sounds.
  h. Inspect the anal area for presence and patency of an anus. Patency can be determined by passage of meconium or passing a small rubber catheter 1–2 cm. Failure to pass meconium within 48 hours suggests obstruction. Passage of stool from any other orifice indicates a fistulous tract from the rectum.
  i. Inspect the infant's back while the child is in a prone position.
    (1) Observe for a flat, straight vertebral column.
    (2) Stroke one side of the vertebral column with your finger to check the incurving reflex. The infant should turn toward the stroked side.
    (3) Observe for curvature of the spine, pilonidal dimple or sinus, or open defects such as spina bifida or myelomeningocele.

C. **Genitalia.**
1. Male.
   a. The glans should be completely covered with foreskin in the non-circumcised infant.
   b. Hypospadias exists if the urethral opening is located on the ventral surface of the penis.
   c. Epispadias exists if the urethral opening is located on the dorsal surface.
   d. Any abnormality of the genitalia, including micropenis, epispadias, or hypospadia, is a contraindication to circumcision.
   e. Inspect the scrotum for size, rugation, and presence of testes. Testes may be palpable in the inguinal canal in a pre-term infant.
   f. A hydrocele is a collection of fluid in the scrotum that will light up when transilluminated. It is usually transient and may be either unilateral or bilateral. A mass that does not transilluminate may be a tumor or a torsion of the testes, which is a surgical emergency.
   g. Swelling and bruising of the scrotum may be evident in a breech delivery.
   h. If external genitalia are ambiguous, further evaluation is necessary.
2. Female.
   a. The labia majora covers the labia minora, clitoris, urethral opening, and external vaginal vault.
   b. In a preterm infant, the labia majora may not cover the labia minora and the clitoris will be prominent.
   c. An unusually large clitoris may indicate pseudohermaphroditism.
   d. A vaginal skin tag is a common finding and is hypertrophied vaginal tissue. It will regress over the first week of life.
   e. Palpate the labia majora for masses that may be hernias or ectopic gonads.
   f. Vaginal discharge is common in the first 48 hours of life.
   g. Ecchymosis and edema of the labia are common in breech deliveries.
   h. Observe for patency of the vaginal opening.
   i. If external genitalia are ambiguous, further evaluation is necessary.

D. **Body part examination.**
1. Head.
   a. The head is usually 2 cm larger in diameter than the newborn's chest.
   b. Note the size, shape, symmetry, and general appearance.
      (1) Microcephaly: small head size in proportion to body size.
      (2) Macrocephaly: large head size in proportion to body size. May be as a result of increased accumulation of cerebrospinal fluid within the ventricles of the brain (hydrocephalus).
      (3) The head of a newborn delivered vaginally from a vertex position will be molded to fit the configuration of the birth canal.
      (4) The head of a newborn delivered by cesarean section without labor is usually not molded.
      (5) The head of a newborn who was breech may be flat on top with the anterior-to-posterior measurement increased.
   c. Caput succedaneum: diffuse edema of the scalp resulting from compression of local blood vessels. The edema crosses suture lines and disappears in a few days.
   d. Cephalohematoma: subperiosteal hemorrhage (bleeding between scalp and bone) resulting from a traumatic delivery. Is limited to the surface of the bone and does not cross suture lines. Resolution may take up to several months.
   e. Sutures (Fig. 4–8).
      (1) Mobility of the sutures is checked by placing both thumbs on opposite sides of the suture and gently pushing in alternately while feeling for motion. The mobility of all sutures should be checked.

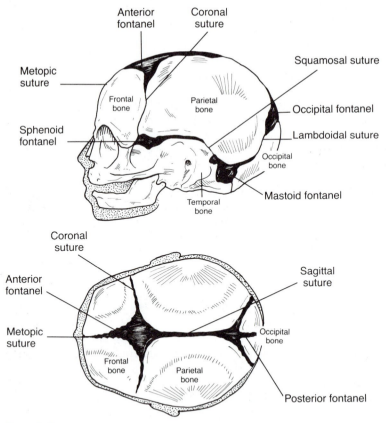

Figure 4–8
Two views of the skull showing fontanelles and sutures.

    (2) Craniosynostosis is the congenital ossification of cranial sutures that can lead to a restriction of brain growth.

    (3) Craniotabes is a soft ping-pong ball effect of the skull bones (usually parietal) that is benign and transient.

  f. Fontanelles.

    (1) The anterior fontanel is located at the junction of the sagittal and coronal sutures. It is diamond shaped and measures from 4 to 6 cm at the largest diameter and normally closes at 18 months.

    (2) The posterior fontanel is located at the junction of the lambdoidal and sagittal sutures. It is usually triangular shaped and barely admits a fingertip. It closes by 2 months of age.

    (3) A third fontanel may be located between the anterior and posterior fontanel and may vary in size. It may be associated with congenital anomalies.

    (4) Large fontanelles may be seen in hypothyroidism.

    (5) A bulging, full, or tense fontanel may be associated with intracranial pressure resulting from hydrocephalus, birth injury, bleeding, or infection.

    (6) A depressed fontanel is a late sign of dehydration.

  g. Scalp.

    (1) Observe for abrasions or lacerations that occasionally occur during delivery as a result of forceps, traumatic delivery, or internal monitor probe.

    (2) Observe for cutis aplasia, which is a localized congenital absence of skin. Lesions occur on the scalp and may be solitary or multiple and are

located just lateral to the midline. Associated abnormalities may be present.

(3) Observe hair pattern and quality and texture of hair. A number of syndromes exist that are characterized by the pattern of hair distribution.

2. Eyes.
   a. Eyes may be edematous for several days after birth due to the delivery process or chemical irritation following eye prophylaxis. Infectious conjunctivitis accompanied by purulent discharge is rarely seen on the first day of life.
   b. Subconjunctival hemorrhages occur frequently and result from pressure on the fetal head during delivery.
   c. The red reflex is normally present and represents an intact lens (may be pale in color in non-caucasian infants). Absence can indicate congenital cataracts. Cataracts may be the result of intrauterine viral infection or can be inherited as a dominant trait from an affected parent.
   d. Observe for pupil response to light and symmetry of eye movements. Pupils should be round and regular and react to light.
   e. Mongolian slanting and epicanthal folds may be indicative of trisomy 21 or may be a part of the fetal alcohol syndrome.
   f. Tears are not normally produced until 2 months of age.
   g. The iris is dark blue until 3–6 months of age, when eye color may change.

3. Ears.
   a. Inspect for maturity, symmetry, and size.
   b. Observe for unusual shape or abnormal position.
      (1) The helix of the ear normally attaches to the scalp at a point horizontal to the inner canthus of the eyes.
      (2) Low-set ears can be associated with various syndromes and chromosomal abnormalities.
   c. Observe for the presence of ear canals. Visualization of eardrums is not necessary unless indicated by the infant's history or other findings. If hearing loss is considered, a hearing examination should be conducted by an audiologist.
   d. Preauricular or auricular skin tags or pits are common and may be associated with renal problems or hearing loss or may be a normal variant.
   e. Malformed or malpositioned ears are often associated with renal, chromosomal, or congenital abnormalities.

4. Nose.
   a. Note the shape and size of the nose.
   b. Positional deformities may result from the birth process and most will resolve without treatment.
   c. Abnormal shape may be associated with congenital syndromes.
   d. Patency of the nostrils must be verified, since infants are obligate nose breathers. Hold a cold, flat, metal object under the nose and observe for fogging from the infant's exhalations.
   e. Obstruction may be caused by drugs, infections, tumors, or mucus.
   f. Choanal atresia is a membranous or bony obstruction in the nasal passage. It may be either unilateral or bilateral. Cyanosis, apnea, or noisy breathing may be evident in the infant with choanal atresia.

5. Mouth.
   a. The mouth should be symmetrical and positioned in the midline.
      (1) Microstomia: very small mouth. Can be associated with genetic syndromes such as trisomy 18.
      (2) Macrostomia: large mouth. May be associated with mucopolysaccharidoses.
   b. The hard and soft palates are examined to rule out cleft palate.
   c. Epstein's pearls are small, white keratin cysts found commonly on the hard and soft palate and gum margins.

d. The mucous membranes of the mouth and tongue should be pink in color. Cyanosis of the tongue and mucous membranes is indicative of a pathological condition.

e. Observe the lips for presence of a cleft lip, which can vary from a niche in the lip to a complete separation extending up onto the floor of the nose.

f. Natal teeth are not uncommon and are generally located on the lower gum. They are removed as soon as possible after birth to prevent the risk of aspiration.

g. Thrush or oral moniliasis is common in newborns. It is usually contracted from mothers with vaginal moniliasis at the time of delivery. The lacy white material is present on the surface of the oral mucous membranes and does not wipe away with a cotton-tipped swab.

h. Assess for root and gag reflexes (develop at 36 weeks' gestation) and suck and swallow reflexes (develop at 32–34 weeks' gestation).

i. A large tongue (macroglossia), cleft lip and palate, or a high, arched palate may be associated with other congenital anomalies such as Beckwith's syndrome, Pompe's disease (a type II glycogen storage disease), and hypothyroidism. A protruding tongue is often seen in trisomy 21.

j. Observe the jaw for size and relationship to the maxilla. Micrognathia (small jaw) may present a serious problem to the airway due to the tongue which is large for a small mandible. Frequently seen in Pierre Robin syndrome, Treacher Collins syndrome, and de Lange's syndrome (Jones, 1988).

6. Face.

a. Observe for symmetry and location of the eyes, nose, and mouth. The mouth can be divided into thirds, with one third encompassing the forehead, one third the eyes and nose, and one third of the mouth and chin.

b. Observe for symmetry of the face when the infant is crying. A facial palsy may result from a traumatic delivery.

c. Observe for wide-spaced eyes (hypertelorism); flat, broad nasal bridge; long philtrum; micrognathia; and size of the mouth. Facial characteristics may be familial or may be associated with chromosomal abnormalities.

7. Neck.

a. Palpate to rule out sternocleidomastoid hematoma and thyroid enlargement.

b. Webbing may be evident due to excessive skin along the posterolateral line.

c. A pouch of redundant skin located at the base of the neck posteriorly is seen in some syndromes (trisomy 21).

d. The most common neck mass is a cystic hygroma, which is a multiloculated cyst arising from lymphatic channels usually posterior to the sternocleidomastoid muscle and extending into the scapula and axillary and thoracic compartments. Most hygromas (65%) occur in the neck. The cysts invade and distort local anatomy. The airway can be distorted, and respiratory distress can be evident at birth.

e. Inspect the clavicles for fractures, which may occur during delivery. A palpable mass, crepitus, or tenderness is evident at the site. Arm movement may be limited on the affected side.

8. Extremities.

a. Examine extremities for malformations and trauma.

b. Length, contour, and symmetry of the extremities should be evaluated to rule out fractures resulting from a difficult delivery.

c. Full range of motion of each extremity should be evident.

d. Hands should be examined in detail.

(1) Simian crease: single palmar crease. Present in 40% of infants with trisomy 21.

(2) Polydactyly: extra digits of the hands or feet.

(3) Syndactyly: fusion of two digits into one structure.

(4) Shape and length of digits and fingernails should be noted.

e. Lower extremities.
   (1) Congenital hip dysplasia is ruled out by either Ortolani's maneuver or Barlow's test (Fig. 4–9).
   (2) Asymmetrical creases in the buttocks are suspicious of congenital hip dysplasia.
   (3) Feet may appear clubbed due to intrauterine positioning. A foot that can be put through full range of motion is clubbed due to intrauterine positioning.
   (4) Congenital equinovarus: a deformation of the ankle and forefoot adduction that will not return to midline with passive dorsiflexion.
9. Skin.
   a. The skin is soft, smooth, and opaque. Vernix covers the body of the fetus and decreases with increased gestational age. Discolored vernix occurs with postmaturity, hemolytic disease, and meconium staining.
   b. Skin in a post-term infant may be dry and peeling.
   c. Skin should be warm to the touch. Cold, clammy skin may indicate shock.
   d. Evaluate skin for signs of cyanosis and jaundice.
   e. Capillary refill should be evaluated by depressing the infant's skin over one or more areas. After blanching the skin, the time required to return to normal skin color is noted. A capillary filling time greater than 3–5 seconds is prolonged.
   f. Several lesions may be present as a result of the birth process.

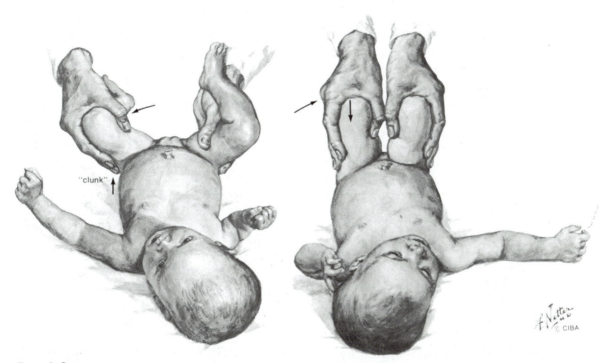

Figure 4–9
Recognition of congenital dislocation of the hip (CDH). *A* Ortolani (reduction) test. With baby relaxed and content on firm surface, the hips and knees are flexed to 90 degrees. Hips are examined one at a time. Examiner grasps baby's thigh with middle finger over greater trochanter, and lifts thigh to bring femoral head from its dislocated posterior position to opposite the acetabulum. Simultaneously, thigh is gently abducted, reducing femoral head into acetabulum. In positive finding, examiner senses reduction by palpable, nearly audible "clunk." *B,* Barlow (dislocation) test. Reverse of Ortolani test. If femoral head is in acetabulum at time of examination, the Barlow test is performed to discover any hip instability. Baby's thigh is grasped as above and adducted with gentle downward pressure. Dislocation is palpable as femoral head slips out of acetabulum. Diagnosis is confirmed with Ortolani test. (Copyright 1979 CIBA-GEIGY Corporation. Reproduced with permission from the CLINICAL SYMPOSIA by Frank H. Netter, M.D. All rights reserved.)

(1) Forceps marks: ecchymoses with rounded contours in the position the forceps were applied.
(2) Petechiae over the head and neck, typically from a nuchal cord.
(3) Abrasions or lacerations from scalp monitors, vacuum extractions, or scalpels.

g. Benign lesions.
(1) Ecchymoses: large areas of subcutaneous hemorrhage usually found over the presenting part in traumatic deliveries.
(2) Milia: white papules found over the forehead, cheeks, and chin that resolve spontaneously.
(3) Mongolian spots: macular lesions of gray-blue color usually located in the lumbosacral area. They occur in the majority of black, Latin American, Asian, and American Indian infants. They will fade over time.
(4) Vascular nevi: common cutaneous malformations that may occur anywhere on the body.
  (a) May present at birth or develop in early infancy.
  (b) Capillary hemangiomas: red or pink macular patches with diffuse borders that may be found over the forehead, nape of the neck, glabella, and eyelids. Frequently referred to as "storkbites." Resolve spontaneously.
  (c) Nevus flammeus (port-wine nevi): flat, sharply defined lesions. When present over the face, they may be associated with Sturge-Weber syndrome.
(5) Sucking blisters are single blister-like lesions on the forearm and hands in infants who have sucked on these areas in utero.
(6) Erythema toxicum (newborn rash: erythematous macules containing a central papule that may be yellow or white. The papules contain eosinophils and are sterile. The eruptions persist for a few days and then resolve spontaneously.

E. Neurological examination.
1. A neurological examination should be performed as part of the newborn examination. (Refer to chapter 20.)
2. Basic reflexes are presented in Figure 4–1.
3. The neurologic examination may not be valid in the first 24 hours of life, as the infant is recovering from the stress of delivery.

STUDY QUESTIONS

1. Which of the following statements is true?
   a. Acrocyanosis is cyanosis of the hands and feet and occasionally of the lips.
   b. Acrocyanosis indicates low O_2 saturation in the blood.
   c. Acrocyanosis is uncommon in the first 24 hours.

2. Which statement best defines a cephalohematoma?
   a. Diffuse edema of the scalp resulting from compression of local blood vessels.
   b. Subperiosteal hemorrhage resulting from a traumatic delivery.
   c. Temporary cone shaping of the skull resulting from the pressure of birth.

3. Which of the following statements is true?

   a. The skin is more transparent with decreasing gestational age.
   b. The areola is raised by 24 weeks' gestation.
   c. Lanugo is the fine downy hair covering the body of the fetus in abundance at 40 weeks' gestation.

4. Which of the following statements defines small for gestational age?
   a. Birth weight is less than 2500 g.
   b. Birth weight is one standard deviation below the mean for gestational age.
   c. Birth weight is two standard deviations below the mean or less than the 10th percentile for gestational age.

5. Which one of the following is abnormal in

the pre-term infant's physical examination and would require further follow-up?

a. Testes palpable in the inguinal canal.

b. The liver edge palpated 1.5 cm below the right costal margin.

c. Asymmetrical breath sounds.

Answers to Study Questions

1. a   3. a   5. c
2. b   4. c

REFERENCES

Ballard, R.A., et al.: A simplified score for assessment of fetal maturation of newly born infants. J. Pediatr., 95:769–774, 1979.

Battaglia, F.C.: The unique problems of small-for-dates babies. Contemp. OB/GYN, 1:35–38, 1973a.

Battaglia, F.C.: The large-for-gestational-age baby—an overlooked problem. Contemp. OB/GYN, 1:39–42, 1973b.

Black, M.: Assessment of weight and gestational age. Nurs. Clin. North Am., 13:13–22, 1978.

Coen, et al.: The detailed newborn examination. Patient Care, 22:93–102, 1988.

Dubowitz, L.M.S., et al.: Clinical assessment of gestational age in the newborn infant. J. Pediatr., 77:1–10,1970.

Goldkrand, J.W., and Lin, J.Y.: Large for gestational age: Dilemma of the infant of the diabetic mother. J. Perinatol., 7:282–287, 1987.

Jones, K.L.: Smith's Recognizable Patterns of Human Malformation, 4th ed. Philadelphia, W.B. Saunders Co., 1988, pp. 80, 196, 210.

Lawrence, R.A.: Physical examination. In Ziai, M., Clarke, T.A., and Merritt, T.A. (eds.): Assessment of the Newborn. Boston, Little, Brown, 1984, pp. 86–111.

BIBLIOGRAPHY

Barness, L.A.: Manual of Pediatric Physical Diagnosis, 4th ed. Chicago, Year Book Medical Publishers, 1979.

Battaglia, F.C.: Intrauterine growth retardation. Am. J. Obstet. Gynecol. 106:1103–1113, 1970.

Battaglia, F.C., and Lubchenco, L.O.: A practical classification of newborn infants by weight and gestational age. J. Pediatr., 71:159–163, 1967.

Behrman, R.E.: The field of neonatal-perinatal medicine and neonatal risk. In Fanaroff, A.A., and Martin, R.J. (eds.): Neonatal-Perinatal Medicine, 4th ed. St. Louis, C.V. Mosby, 1987, pp. 1–7.

Driscoll, J.M.: Physical examination. In Fanaroff, A.A., and Martin, R.J. (eds.): Neonatal-Perinatal Medicine, 4th ed. Philadelphia, J.B. Lippincott, 1987, pp. 343–348.

Hittner, et al.: Assessment of gestational age by examination of the anterior vascular capsule of the lens. J. Pediatr., 91:455–458, 1977.

Lubchenco, L.O.: Assessment of gestational age and development at birth. Pediatr. Clin. North Am., 17:125–145, 1970.

Lubchenco, L.O., and Koops, B.L.: Assessment of weight and gestational age. In Avery, G.B., (ed.): Neonatology, 3rd ed. Philadelphia, J.B. Lippincott, 1987, pp. 235–255.

Merenstein, G.B., and Gardner, S.L.: Handbook of Neonatal Intensive Care, 2nd ed. St. Louis, C.V. Mosby, 1989, pp. 58–100.

Resnick, M.B., et al.: Effect of birth weight, race, and sex on survival of low-birth-weight infants in neonatal intensive care. Am. J. Obstet. Gynecol. 161:184–187, 1989.

Sahu, S.: Birthweight, gestational age, and neonatal risks. Perinatol./Neonatol., 8:28–36, 1984.

Saigal, S., et al.: Decreased disability rate among 3-year-old survivors. J. Pediatr., 114:839–846, 1989.

Scanlon, J.W.: A System of Newborn Physical Examination. Baltimore: University Park Press, 1979.

Sweet, A.V.: Classification of the low-birth-weight infant. In Klaus, M.H., and Fanaroff, A.A. (eds.): Care of the High Risk Neonate, 3rd ed. Philadelphia, W.B. Saunders Co., 1986, pp. 69–95.

Walker, E.M., and Patel, N.B.: Mortality and morbidity in infants born between 20 and 28 weeks' gestation. Br. J. Obstet. Gynecol., 94:670–674, 1987.

Harriet A. Harrell

Neonatal Delivery Room Resuscitation

Objectives

1. Differentiate three anatomically unique features of the neonate that require special consideration during resuscitation.

2. Compare three physiological characteristics of the neonate that make neonatal resuscitation differ from adult resuscitation.

3. List three pre-partum, intrapartum, and post-partum factors that indicate the neonate may be at risk for asphyxia.

4. Assemble the equipment needed for neonatal resuscitation and discuss maintenance and use.

5. Explain the ABCs of neonatal resuscitation.

6. Discuss the appropriate application of the Apgar scoring system as it relates to neonatal resuscitation.

7. Describe three potential complications of neonatal resuscitation.

8. Construct a plan for post-resuscitation care, listing anticipated tests and nursing observations.

Resuscitation involves re-establishing heart and lung function after cardiac arrest or sudden death. Fortunately, neonates rarely have cardiac arrest. Neonates usually have respiratory insufficiency leading to respiratory arrest, and if there is no intervention cardiac arrest will ensue. The goal of resuscitation is to provide quick and efficient interventions to minimize the effects of hypoxia on the infant. This chapter provides comprehensive guidelines to delivery room resuscitation.

Definitions

Resuscitation: re-establish heart and lung function after cardiac arrest or sudden death (adult terminology).

- Neonates rarely have cardiac arrest.
- Neonates usually have respiratory insufficiency leading to respiratory arrest; if no intervention, this will lead to cardiac arrest.

• Rescue: save from current or impending danger. More appropriate for neonates when referring to delivery room interventions.

Anatomy and Physiology

A. **Physiological and anatomical characteristics.** Physiological and anatomical characteristics of the neonate make neonatal resuscitation different than adult resuscitation. In general, the need for cardiopulmonary resuscitation (CPR) in the neonate stems from respiratory compromise or failure rather than cardiac arrest. Intervention is often possible before the neonate is compromised to the point of cardiac failure.
1. Large head size to body size ratio.
    a. Problems:
        (1) Insensible water loss.
        (2) Heat loss: no insulating fat layer.
        (3) Decreased amount of hair.
2. Large surface area to body size ratio.
    a. Problems:
        (1) Insensible water loss.
        (2) Heat loss.
3. Decreased muscle mass.
    a. Problems:
        (1) Decreased ability to generate heat.
4. Decreased subcutaneous fat (premature, intrauterine growth retarded).
    a. Problems:
        (1) Decreased heat production (from brown fat metabolism).
        (2) Increased heat loss (from lack of insulation).
5. Immature systems:
    a. Central nervous system: inability to vasoconstrict (vasomotor instability).
    b. Neuromuscular system: inability to shiver.
    c. Liver: decreased ability to metabolize drugs.
    d. Renal: decreased ability to excrete drugs/fluids; low threshold for electrolyte losses.
    e. Gastrointestinal: air swallowing leading to gastric distention and respiratory compromise.
    f. Metabolism: glucose tolerance/intolerance.
    g. Lungs: decreased surface area for gas exchange.
    h. Immune: increased predisposition to infection.
6. Anteriorly situated glottis:
    a. Makes intubation difficult.
    b. Predisposes infant to airway compromise from positioning.
7. Short neck:
    a. Makes intubation difficult.
    b. Predisposes child to airway compromise from positioning.
8. Preferential nasal breather:
    a. Primary airway is nose; keep clear and patent.
    b. Check for anatomical patency.
9. Venous access (Fig. 5–1).
    a. Small veins: difficult to access.
    b. Difficult to restrain: access easily lost.
    c. Umbilical access.
        (1) Arterial.
        (2) Venous. *Remember:* Some medications can also be given via the endotracheal route while venous access is being established.
10. Small size/fragile skin and tissues: care must be taken to avoid undue roughness and trauma.

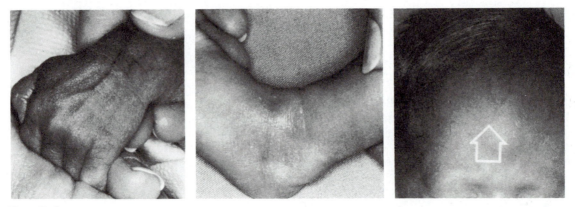

Figure 5-1
Preferred intravenous sites in the neonate for easy and rapid access. (Courtesy of Arizona Health Sciences Center.)

B. **Physiology of asphyxia.**
1. Perinatal asphyxia may be chronic, ongoing in utero for several days, or acute.
2. Decreased O_2 availability to tissues secondary to decreased placental blood flow or decreased O_2 content of maternal blood. Tissue hypoxia leads to acidosis and anaerobic metabolism, which lead to increased lactic acid production and further decrease of the pH. With placental circulatory compromise, PCO_2 increases as well as adding to the fetal acidosis. As acidosis worsens, availability of oxygen decreases and the need for glucose increases. Cardiac contractility may be affected by hypoxia, hypoglycemia, and acidosis (Wood, 1987).
3. Meconium in the amniotic fluid may indicate that the fetus has experienced a hypoxic event.
   a. Hypoxia secondary to decreased placental blood flow or maternal hypoxemia.
   b. Fetal tissue hypoxia affects the tone of the anal sphincter, which may relax, allowing passage of meconium into the amniotic sac.
   c. Fetal hypoxia causes gasping respirations in utero. Meconium may be taken into the upper airway. (*Remember:* Normal fetal respiratory efforts are minimal with the net flow of fluid through the lumen of the bronchial tree being outward. However, gasping respirations may allow meconium to enter even the distal airways.)
   d. At delivery, the mouth, nose, and posterior pharynx are suctioned thoroughly before the chest is delivered. Failure to do this may lead to aspiration of meconium into the lower airway when the neonate takes the first breath.
   e. Meconium in the airways may cause airway obstruction by:
      (1) Total blockage of an airway, leading to distal alveolar atelectasis.
      (2) Ball-valve effect: air enters on inspiration when the airway is dilated, allowing air to pass the obstruction. Air then gets trapped on expiration when the airway constricts. This leads to overdistention and alveolar rupture and can precipitate pulmonary air leaks (Avery, 1987). Thus, the typical x-ray findings of meconium aspiration reveal areas of atelectasis and air trapping, hyperinflation, and pulmonary air leads. (Refer to Chapter 33.)

Risk Factors

Warning signs that alert the perinatal team to the possibility of an adverse outcome and the need for anticipatory preparation of neonatal rescue or resuscitation.

A. Pre-partum (maternal). Conditions during pregnancy that predispose the mother and fetus to stress that can interfere with the fetus' successful transition to extrauterine existence.
1. Maternal age > 35 years old or < 15 years old.
2. Diabetes mellitus.
3. Hemorrhage or anemia.
4. Drug abuse.
5. No pre-natal care.
6. Poly- or oligohydramnios.
7. Cardiovascular disease.
8. Prolonged rupture of membranes.
9. Anatomical abnormalities of the uterus.
10. Rh or ABO incompatibilities.
11. Hypertension (toxemia, chronic).
12. Multiple gestation.
13. Previous pregnancy complication or fetal loss.
14. Chronic illness (renal, pulmonary, etc.) (Avery, 1987).

B. Intrapartum. Conditions that predispose the fetus to a difficult transition to extrauterine life or signs that the fetus is not tolerating the stresses of labor and that unsuccessful transition may ensue.
1. Abnormal fetal positioning or presentation—e.g., breech.
2. Cesarean section.
3. Fetal heart rate abnormalities.
4. Intrauterine growth retardation.
5. Intrapartum blood loss, mother or fetus.
6. Maternal sedation.
7. Maternal fever/infection.
8. Prolonged or difficult labor.
9. Prolonged rupture of membranes.
10. Prolapse of the umbilical cord (Avery, 1987).

C. Post-partum. Signs or conditions in the delivery room or transitional nursery that indicate that the baby is having difficulty making all the physiological changes needed for successful adaptation from intrauterine to extrauterine life.
1. Anomalous airway.
2. Cardiac arrhythmia—i.e., tachycardia or bradycardia.
3. Extreme color change.
4. Circulatory compromise.
5. Feeding intolerance.
6. Temperature instability.
7. Meconium staining.
8. Seizures.
9. Prematurity.
10. Postmaturity.
11. Respiratory distress/apnea.
12. Neurological depression (Avery, 1987).

Anticipation of and Preparation for Resuscitation

Institutional guidelines, protocols, policies, and procedures will dictate the method and frequency of equipment surveillance and staff certification. The Neonatal Resuscitation Program of the American Academy of Pediatrics/American Heart Association (AAP/AHA) is a national program designed for this purpose. All delivery rooms, emergency rooms, birthing centers, nurseries, and post-partum units must be fully equipped and staffed for neonatal resuscitation at all times. Although many resuscitative events are predictable and anticipated, there are unexpected events that must be handled as efficiently as anticipated ones.

A. General preparation.
1. Update all staff frequently.
2. Update and evaluate equipment needs frequently.
3. Periodic maintenance and evaluation of electrical equipment by Biomedical Engineering on a regularly scheduled basis.
4. Periodic maintenance and evaluation of all respiration equipment by Respiratory Therapy on a regularly scheduled basis.
5. Evaluate and replace supplies every shift (utilize equipment checklist).
6. Test alerting system for rapid, consistent response of personnel.

B. Delivery room preparation.
1. Identify high-risk situation.
2. Assemble equipment within easy reach and check functions.
3. Pre-heat warmer and blankets.
4. Review resuscitation protocol and familiarize self with drug doses, concentrations, routes, and side effects.
5. Designate resuscitation team captain and give assignments.
6. Reassure mother, significant others, and OB team that you are present and prepared. Explain that you will notify them of the neonate's well-being as soon as you can.
7. Remain calm and in control—remember you are prepared.

C. Personnel/roles.
1. Personnel designations for neonatal resuscitation is an institutional responsibility. Anyone working with neonates should be able to initiate rescue interventions while additional personnel are responding. In many institutions, a neonatal nurse practitioner is responsible for neonatal resuscitation; in others, an in-house medical staff member is responsible. It is important that each member of the resuscitation team know the scope and level of his or her responsibility.
2. Family support is important and is usually the responsibility of the OB nurse, since the pediatric personnel will be very busy. This function (family supporter) should not be assumed, it should be assigned in advance.

D. Non–delivery room preparation. As with delivery room resuscitation, being prepared for unforeseen events can facilitate success in a time of crisis. Unlike delivery room events, non–delivery room resuscitation is always unpredictable. Events precipitating respiratory or circulatory compromise include the following:
1. Apnea/periodic breathing.
2. Choking/aspiration.
3. Unwitnessed arrest.
4. Seizure.
5. Hypoxia or airway obstruction.

Equipment for Neonatal Resuscitation

Not every item on the equipment/supply list will be used, but it is important to have sufficient quantities to support a prolonged effort. New and revised products are available continually and should be critically evaluated before they are incorporated into existing stock. It is most important that staff be familiar with the equipment they will be using and practice with it frequently.

NEONATAL RESUSCITATION EQUIPMENT LIST

Light source
Heat source
Dry, warm, soft blankets

Treatment bed/table with removable or collapsible sides
Clock with second hand or timer
Wall suction
Oxygen: wall or cylinder (0–15 liter flow)
Air: wall or cylinder (0–15 liter flow)
Stethoscope: neonatal size
1/2 liter anesthesia bag with flow adjustment valve and manometer
1/2 liter self-inflating resuscitation bag with 100% O_2 adaptor
Premature size face masks
Newborn size face masks
Size 0 oral airways
Size 1 oral airways
Laryngoscope with Miller 0 and 1 curved and straight blades
Suction catheters (two each: 5 Fr, 8 Fr, and 10 Fr)
Sterile H_2O for suction
Sterile normal saline ampules for suction-lubrication
Bulb syringe
Cord clamp and sterile scissors
8 Fr feeding tube
Extra batteries and bulbs for laryngoscope
Non-cuffed endotracheal tubes (two each: 2.5, 3.0, 3.5, 4.0)
Stylets (2)
Liquid skin barrier
Adhesive tape 1″ and 1/2″
Alcohol swabs
Iodine swabs
1 cc, 3 cc, 10 cc, and 20 cc syringes

Heparinized blood gas syringes
25 g and 18 g needles
16 g intracath (over-the-needle intravascular catheter)
Umbilical catheters 3.5 Fr and 5.0 Fr
Three-way stopcock
Umbilical catheter tray
Meconium aspirator

Epinephrine 1:10,000 concentration
Normal saline IV solution
Ringer's lactate
5% albumin
Sodium bicarbonate 4.2%
Naloxone hydrochloride (Auvenshine and Enriquez, 1990)

Decision Making Process

For many years, delivery room resuscitation decisions were based on Apgar scores (see Appendix D). Current recommendations discourage use of the Apgar score for decision making in resuscitation. Components from the Apgar score are still used in the assessment and reassessment (i.e., heart rate, respirations, and color). Resuscitative interventions should never be delayed pending the 1 minute Apgar score. Currently, the action/evaluation/decision cycle is used (Fig. 5–2).

Neonatal Resuscitation: ABCs

The steps taken to rescue or resuscitate a neonate are best remembered using the familiar "ABCs" of resuscitation used in all AHA resuscitation programs.

The Action/Evaluation/Decision Cycle

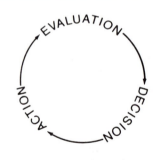

Figure 5-2
The circular process used during neonatal resuscitation to guide the events. (Reproduced with permission. © *Textbook of Neonatal Resuscitation*, 1987. Copyright American Heart Association.)

A. **ABCs defined.**
1. **A = Airway.**
   a. Establish and maintain an open airway.
   b. Position infant on back with neck slightly extended.
   c. Suction mouth, nose, and trachea as needed.
   d. Intubate the trachea if needed to maintain the airway or to remove meconium.
   e. Stabilize and secure endotracheal (ET) tube if needed.
2. **B = Breathing.**
   a. Evaluate respiratory effort and rate.
   b. Initiate breathing if infant is apneic by employing tactile stimulation.
   c. Begin bag and mask ventilation if needed.
   d. Initiate bag to tube ventilation if infant is intubated or if bag and mask are ineffective.
3. **C = Circulation.**
   a. Evaluate heart rate.
   b. Evaluate color and perfusion.
   c. Give chest compression by the thumb or two-finger method if needed.
4. **D = Drugs/medications.**
   a. Epinephrine: to stimulate heart by increasing rate and strength of contractions.
   b. Volume expander: to increase circulating blood volume when there are signs of hypovolemia, shock, or acute blood loss.
      (1) Whole blood.
      (2) 5% albumin.
      (3) Normal saline.
      (4) Ringer's lactate.
   c. Sodium bicarbonate: to correct metabolic acidosis.
   d. Naloxone: to reverse respiratory depression secondary to maternal narcotic administration.
5. **E = Environment.**
   a. Provide safety for patients and staff from sharp objects that may fall in the bed and from potentially infectious body secretions.
   b. Provide humidity if possible to prevent metabolic stress.
   c. Provide temperature control to prevent metabolic stress.
   d. Be gentle to prevent bruises and abrasions.

B. **Initial steps.** In most cases, the following steps (1–5) are all the intervention that will be necessary.

1. Prevent hypothermia, which may lead to increased metabolic requirement.
    a. Place and keep baby in pre-heated environment.
        (1) Warmed towels.
        (2) Heat lamps.
        (3) Radiant warmer.
        (4) Cover head.
        (5) Keep out of draft.
    b. Maintain dry, warm environment.
        (1) Dry thoroughly.
        (2) Remove wet linen immediately and replace with dry linen.
2. Open the airway.
    a. Position infant on back with neck slightly extended.
        (1) Do not hyperextend or underextend the neck.
        (2) A shoulder pad may help maintain the correct position.
        (3) Head may be turned to the side in this position without airway compromise (Fig. 5–3).
    b. Suction mouth and nares.
        (1) Use bulb syringe or wall suction (100 mm Hg).
        (2) Vigorous or prolonged deep suctioning can produce vagal-induced bradycardia and/or apnea.
        (3) If thick, particulate meconium is present or if any meconium is present

Positioning

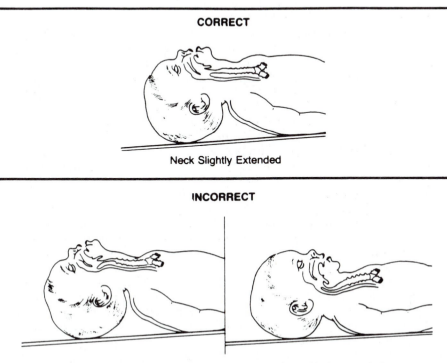

CORRECT

Neck Slightly Extended

INCORRECT

Neck Hyperextended   Neck Underextended

Figure 5–3
Positioning for neonatal resuscitation, appropriate for airway maintenance, bag and mask ventilation, and intubation. (Reproduced with permission. © *Textbook of Neonatal Resuscitation*, 1987. Copyright American Heart Association.)

and the baby is depressed, intubate and perform direct tracheal suction until clear.
  - (a) Clinical judgment must be used to decide if intubation is needed in a vigorous neonate with meconium.
  - (b) Clinical judgment must be used to decide how long to delay institution of positive-pressure ventilation in an asphyxiated neonate.
3. Stimulate respirations:
  - a. Slap the soles of the feet.
  - b. Rub the back.
  - c. Make two attempts. If respirations do not begin, move on to bag and mask ventilation (unless diaphragmatic hernia is suspected—then use bag to tube ventilation).
4. Evaluate:
  - a. Respiratory effort: rate, breath sounds, grunting, flaring, retracting.
  - b. Heart rate: count for 6 seconds and multiply by 10.
  - c. Color.
    - (1) Peripheral cyanosis is normal.
    - (2) Central cyanosis is abnormal.
5. Give blow-by oxygen if central cyanosis is present, heart rate is over 100, and respirations are adequate.
  - a. Use at least 80% oxygen.
  - b. Withdraw oxygen slowly if baby remains pink.

C. Positive-pressure ventilation.
1. Bag and mask ventilation.
  - a. Should be initiated for:
    - (1) Any apneic or gasping neonate.
    - (2) Any neonate whose ventilatory efforts are inadequate.
    - (3) Any neonate with a heart rate of less than 100 beats/minute.
  - b. Equipment.
    - (1) Self-inflating bags must have a reservoir tail to deliver 90–100% O_2.
    - (2) Anesthesia bags should have a pressure gauge and flow control valve.
    - (3) Should always be pre-set and tested before use.
    - (4) Mask of proper size should be used to obtain adequate seal.
    - (5) Should always be connected to 100% O_2 source at 5–10 liters of flow.
  - c. Procedure.
    - (1) Assemble, set, and test the equipment.
    - (2) Position the neonate as in "Initial Steps."
    - (3) Apply mask and ensure proper seal.
    - (4) Deliver 15–40 cm H_2O pressure at 40–60 breaths/minute for 15–30 seconds.
    - (5) Observe for easy rise and fall of chest.
    - (6) Pause to check 6 second heart rate and continue to ventilate until neonate begins spontaneous breathing and the heart rate is over 100.
    - (7) If bag and mask is ineffective or if the need for ventilation is prolonged, endotracheal intubation should be performed.
  - d. Exceptions.
    - (1) If the neonate has thick, particulate meconium present, intubate and perform tracheal suctioning before beginning bag and mask ventilation.
    - (2) If the neonate has, or is suspected of having, a diaphragmatic hernia, intubate, give bag to tube ventilation, and place orogastric tube for gastric decompression.
2. Bag to endotracheal tube ventilation.
  - a. Should be initiated:
    - (1) On any neonate who does not respond to bag and mask ventilation.
    - (2) When diaphragmatic hernia is suspected.
    - (3) When prolonged ventilation is required.
    - (4) When tracheal suctioning is required.

b. Equipment.
   (1) Laryngoscope, batteries, bulbs, size 0 and 1 blades (curved or straight).
   (2) Non-cuffed, non-tapered tubes in a variety of sizes, two each in sizes 2.5, 3.0, 3.5, and 4.0 with vocal cord maker.
   (3) Stylet.
   (4) Suction equipment with catheters in sizes 5 Fr, 8 Fr, and 10 Fr (two each).
   (5) Shoulder pad for positioning.
   (6) Adhesive tape/scissors.
   (7) 1/2 liter resuscitation bag, manometer, and masks.
   (8) Oxygen source, flowmeter, and tubing.
c. Procedure (see Chapter 34).
   (1) Intubate.
   (2) Confirm placement.
   (3) Secure tube.

D. Chest compressions.
1. Should be initiated when the heart rate is below 60 or between 60 and 80 and not increasing after 15–30 seconds of ventilation with 100% O_2.
2. Two methods:
   a. Thumb technique.
      (1) Both thumbs over the lower third of the sternum above the xiphoid.
      (2) The hands encircling the chest to provide support.
   b. Two-finger technique.
      (1) The tips of the middle and index finger of one hand over the lower third of the sternum.
      (2) The other hand under the infant's back to provide support.
3. Compressions should squeeze the heart between the spinal column and the sternum.
   a. Force of compression should be straight down to avoid rib or lung damage.
   b. Depress the sternum about 1.5–2.0 cm.
   c. Compress 2 times/second or 120 times/minute.
4. Compressions with ventilations.
   a. Difficult to coordinate ventilation and compressions at such rapid rates.
   b. Neonate should be ventilated with 100% O_2 at a rate of 60 breaths/minute. Optimally the neonate should be intubated. If not intubated, an orogastric tube should be placed to vent the stomach.

E. Chemical resuscitation. Most neonatal resuscitations do not require medications or volume expanders. An umbilical catheter will need to be placed to administer medications or volume expanders (see Chapter 34). Epinephrine and naloxone hydrochloride (Narcan) can be administered through an endotracheal tube.
1. Indications:
   a. Stimulate the heart.
   b. Increase tissue perfusion.
   c. Correct metabolic acidosis.
   d. When 100% O_2 with adequate ventilation and chest compressions do not revive the infant.
2. Drugs and solutions used (Table 5–1):
   a. Epinephrine: a cardiac stimulant. Increases the heart rate and strength of contractions. Causes peripheral vasoconstriction.
      (1) Indicated when:
         (a) Heart rate is below 80 after ventilation with 100% O_2, endotracheal tube, and chest compressions.
         (b) Heart rate is indetectable, while ventilations and compressions are being started.
      (2) Concentrations: 1 : 10,000 — neonatal strength.
      (3) Preparation: draw up 1 ml in a 1 ml syringe.
      (4) Dose: 0.1 to 0.3 ml/kg rapidly.

Table 5-1
DRUGS AND SOLUTIONS USED IN CHEMICAL RESUSCITATION

Drug or Volume Expander	Concentration to Administer	Preparation (based on recommended concentration)	Dosage	Route/Rate
Epinephrine	1:10,000	1 ml in a syringe Can dilute 1:1 with normal saline if giving IT	0.1-0.3 ml/kg	IV or intratracheal Give rapidly
Volume expanders	Whole blood 5% albumin/saline solution Normal saline Ringer's lactate	40 ml to be given by syringe or IV	10 ml/kg	IV Give over 5-10 minutes
Sodium bicarbonate	0.5 mEq/ml (4.2% solution)	20 ml in a syringe or 2 10 ml pre-filled syringes	2 mEq/kg	IV Give slowly over at least 2 minutes (1 mEq/kg/minute)
Naloxone hydrochloride	0.4 mg/ml or 1.0 mg/ml	1 ml in a syringe	0.1 mg/kg	IV, IM, SQ, or IT Give rapidly

Reproduced with permission. *Textbook of Neonatal Resuscitation*, 1990. © Copyright American Heart Association.

    (5) Route: IV, per endotracheal tube or per umbilical catheter (when given per endotracheal tube, the dose may be diluted in 0.1 ml of normal saline or followed with 0.1 to 0.2 ml of normal saline to facilitate delivery).

    (6) Response: should see effect within 30 seconds after administration. May be repeated every 5 minutes.

  b. Volume expanders: fluids that increase the neonate's blood volume to correct hypovolemia and thereby facilitate tissue perfusion.

    (1) Indicated when there is suspected or documented blood loss with signs of hypovolemia or shock.

      (a) Weak or absent peripheral pulses.

      (b) Low blood pressure.

      (c) Tachycardia.

      (d) Pale or mottled skin in spite of good oxygenation.

      (e) Unresponsiveness to initial attempts to resuscitate.

    (2) Solutions.

      (a) Whole blood.

      (b) 5% albumin/plasma substitute.

      (c) Lactated Ringer's solution.

      (d) Normal saline.

    (3) Preparation: draw up 40 ml.

    (4) Dose: 10 ml/kg over 5-10 minutes.

    (5) Route: IV or per umbilical catheter.

    (6) Response: should see an increase in blood pressure, improvement of perfusion of skin, and increase in the intensity of pulses. May be repeated if necessary.

  c. Sodium bicarbonate: a base buffer that will raise the pH of the blood.

    (1) Indicated when:

      (a) There is evidence of prolonged asphyxia.

      (b) Documented *metabolic* acidosis.

      (c) Adequate ventilation is ensured.

    (2) Concentration: 4.2% solution, 0.5 mEq/ml.

(3) Preparation: open a 10 ml pre-filled syringe.

(4) Dose: 2 mEq/kg slow IV push (do not exceed 1 mEq/kg/minute).

(5) Route: IV or per umbilical catheter.

(6) Response: should change pH and improve heart rate within 30 seconds.

d. Naloxone hydrochloride (Narcan): a short acting narcotic antagonist that displaces narcotics from receptor sites and reserves the physiologic depressant effects of the narcotic.

  (1) Indicated when:

    (a) There is severe respiratory depression in a neonate born to a mother who has recently been given a narcotic (usually within 4 hours).

    (b) There is a persistent apnea in a neonate who is being given assisted ventilation and there is any suspicion of maternal narcotics.

  (2) Concentration: 1.0 mg/ml or 0.4 mg/ml.

  (3) Preparation: draw up 1–2 cc in a syringe.

  (4) Dose: 0.1 mg/kg rapidly.

  (5) Route: may be given IV, per umbilical catheter, IM, or via the endotracheal tube.

  (6) Response:

    (a) Respiratory depression should abate within seconds to minutes after administration (depending on the route of administration). Duration of action is widely variable (1–4 hours). May be repeated several times if needed.

    (b) If given to a neonate of a narcotic-addicted mother, it may precipitate immediate and severe withdrawal, including seizures (Bloom and Cropley, 1990).

Unusual Situations

A. **Pulmonary hypoplasia.**

1. Definitions/characteristics.

  a. Associated with Potters syndrome, dysplastic renal conditions, chronic amniotic fluid loss, and diaphragmatic hernia.

  b. Underdeveloped lungs secondary to insufficient space within the thoracic cavity for normal development.

2. Acute clinical problems.

  a. Inability to ventilate adequately.

  b. Very high pressures required to expand small, stiff lungs.

  c. High risk for pulmonary air leak.

3. Management.

  a. Intubate to overcome upper airway resistance.

  b. Ventilate with 100% O_2 and as much pressure as necessary to expand the lungs.

  c. Transilluminate and auscultate chest frequently, looking for pulmonary air leaks.

  d. Place orogastric tube as soon as possible to prevent gastric and intestinal inflation, which could compromise the diaphragmatic excursions.

B. **Abdominal wall defects.**

1. Definition/characteristics.

  a. Gastroschisis: herniation of stomach, liver, and/or intestines through a defect next to the umbilical cord, usually to the right of the cord.

  b. Omphalocele: midline herniation of the bowel into the umbilical cord.

  c. Exstrophy of the bladder: externalization and aversion of the bladder, urethra, and/or ureteral orifices through a defect in the lower abdominal wall.

2. Acute clinical problems.

  a. Fluid and heat loss through exposed viscera (increases surface area).

  b. Potential for visceral damage from drying or trauma.

      c. Not associated with respiratory distress.

      d. Increased risk for infection.

  3. Management.

      a. Cover immediately with sterile plastic wrap and apply warm saline if necessary.

      b. Maintain infant in a moist, sterile, heated environment.

      c. Keep orogastric tube open to environment to prevent gastric and intestinal inflation, which would complicate repair.

      d. Maintain side lying position and provide support to exposed organs or sac.

C. Neural tube defects.

1. Definition/characteristics.

      a. Anencephaly: most severe form. Failure of neural tube closure with total brain involvement.

      b. Encephalocele: defect in closure of the neural tube at proximal end with outpouching of brain tissue through the skull.

      c. Myelomeningocele: defect in closure at the distal end with exposure of the neural tube at various levels of the spinal column.

2. Acute clinical problems.

      a. Question of viability of anencephalic infant.

      b. Heat and fluid losses through open defect.

      c. Increased risk of infection.

      d. Potential for damage of exposed nervous tissue secondary to trauma.

      e. Difficulty in handling baby due to exposed tissue on back.

3. Management.

      a. Cover defect with sterile, saline-soaked dressing sponges and a plastic barrier to prevent heat and fluid losses.

      b. Maintain baby in a neutral thermal environment.

      c. Keep child on side or abdomen.

      d. Infant may be ventilated on side if necessary.

      e. Manage all defects the same no matter how severe. Discuss viability issues *after* resuscitation and stabilization.

D. Choanal atresia.

1. Definitions/characteristics.

      a. Bony soft tissue obstruction of the posterior nares. May be bilateral or unilateral.

      b. Respiratory distress immediately after birth due to blockage of the primary airway, the nose.

2. Management:

      a. Stimulate the baby to cry, thereby using the secondary airway (mouth) for ventilation.

      b. Insert an oral airway.

      c. Give O_2 temporarily if needed.

      d. Suction secretions as needed.

E. Undiagnosed multiple gestation.

1. Definitions/characteristics.

      a. Unexpected twins, triplets, quadruplets, etc.

      b. Small size of neonates.

      c. Inadequate amount of supplies and equipment to manage multiple, prolonged resuscitative efforts.

      d. Immaturity of neonates.

2. Management:

      a. Always have extra equipment available.

      b. Always stock for twins and have back-up supplies close at hand when necessary.

      c. Have a system for secondary resuscitation teams who can be called upon when needed.

F. **Extremely low birthweight infant.**
1. Definitions/characteristics.
   a. Neonates less than 26 weeks' gestation and less than 600 g birthweight. Survival rates for these neonates range from 5% to 25% (Raju, 1986). Studies have shown the need for resuscitation within the first few days of life to be a poor prognostic indicator (Lantos et al., 1988).
   b. Very immature lungs.
   c. Very fragile skin.
   d. Very susceptible to system damage from resuscitative intervention.
   e. Very susceptible to infection and thermal instability.
2. Management:
   a. If at all possible, the family's physician, along with the neonatal team, should explore their feelings and wishes about resuscitation before the birth.
   b. Be as gentle as possible with the tiny baby.

Complications of Resuscitation

A. **Trauma.**
1. Skin: bruises and abrasions from chest compressions, handling, and tape application and removal.
2. Mucosa: laryngoscopy can cause trauma and bleeding to gums, lips, pharynx, and trachea.
3. Organ damage from chest compressions.

B. **Pulmonary air leaks.**
1. Pneumothorax.
2. Pneumomediastinum
3. Pneumopericardium.

C. **Dangers of umbilical vessel catheters.**
1. Vessel perforation.
2. Accidental blood loss.
3. Clots and emboli.
4. Organ and vessel endothelial damage from infusion of hypertonic solutions.
5. Organ ischemia from blockage of major vessels by the catheter tip.

D. **Intracranial hemorrhage.**
1. Subarachnoid.
2. Periventricular.
3. Intraventricular.

Post-Resuscitation Care

To evaluate for complications and help diagnose and treat underlying disease.

A. **Arterial blood gases (ABGs).**
1. To access oxygenation, ventilation, and acid-base balance:
   a. Check ABGs.
   b. Correlate with baby's clinical condition.
   c. Adjust baby's respiratory support as needed.

B. **Monitor glucose to ensure normoglycemia.**
1. Check Chemstrip/Dextrostix.
2. Treat hypoglycemia and adjust maintenance glucose.
3. Monitor Chemstrip/Dextrostix as ordered.

C. **Chest and abdominal x-rays.**
1. Looking for pneumothorax, pneumomediastinum, pneumopericardium, and pneumoperitoneum.

    a. Assess endotracheal tube position.

    b. Assess umbilical catheter position.

    c. Evaluate lung disease.

D. **Fluids/electrolytes.**

1. Calculate fluid volume received during resuscitation.
2. Determine ml/kg/day needed.
3. Adjust IV rate as needed.

E. **Monitor vital signs.**

1. Provide a neutral thermal environment to prevent the sequelae of hypothermia.
2. Perfusion.
3. Blood pressure.
4. Heart and respiratory rate.

F. **Screen for infection.**

1. Evaluate maternal history for risk factors.
2. Complete blood count, differential, platelet count.
3. Blood culture and sensitivity.
4. If high index of suspicion and neonate is stable, lumbar puncture.

G. **Support family.**

1. Report neonate's condition to mother and significant others.
2. Notify Social Service of new admission.

STUDY QUESTIONS

1. The neonate is predisposed to increased heat loss because anatomically he/she has:
   a. A large surface area to body size ratio.
   b. An immature liver.
   c. More brown fat than an adult.

2. The correct position to optimize airway patency and facilitate intubation in a neonate is:
   a. Prone with head turned to the side.
   b. Supine with slight neck extension.
   c. Supine with slight neck flexion.

3. Anaerobic metabolism in the neonate is a result of hypoxia and leads to:
   a. Decreased glucose utilization and alteration of cardiac function.
   b. Decreased insulin production and hemolysis.
   c. Increased lactic acid production and decreased pH.

4. Pre-partum risk factors that might alert the perinatal team to anticipate fetal/neonatal distress include:
   a. Breech presentation after 48 hours of labor with ruptured membranes.
   b. Non-compliance for pre-natal vitamin therapy in a 28 year old primiparous woman.
   c. Ten pre-natal visits in a 33 year old woman with gestational diabetes.

5. Preparation for resuscitation includes:
   a. Daily "mock-code" drills for the NICU staff.
   b. Monthly evaluation of all equipment and supplies.
   c. Yearly recertification of all staff members involved in neonatal resuscitation.

6. Decisions about which resuscitation measures to use are based on:
   a. Heart rate only.
   b. The 1 and 5 minute Apgar scores.
   c. The action/evaluation/decision cycle.

7. The ABCs of neonatal resuscitation are the same as the ABCs of adult resuscitation and stand for:
   a. A, assessment; B, bleeding; C, circulation.
   b. A, airway; B, breathing; C, calculation.
   c. A, airway; B, breathing; C, circulation.

8. The first pharmacological agent given in

the chemical resuscitation phase of neonatal resuscitation is:
a. Epinephrine: to correct acidosis.
b. Epinephrine: to stimulate the heart.
c. Sodium bicarbonate: to stimulate the heart.

9. A complication of resuscitation is:
a. Mucous membrane bleeding.
b. Thrombocytopenia.
c. Weight loss.

10. The goal of post-resuscitation care is to:
a. Collect data for resuscitation research.
b. Identify and treat underlying disease and complications.
c. Identify maternal risk factors.

Answers to Study Questions

1. a	5. c	8. b
2. b	6. c	9. a
3. c	7. c	10. b
4. a		

REFERENCES

Auvenshine, M.A., and Enriquez, M.G. (eds.): Comprehensive Maternity Nursing: Perinatal and Women's Health, 2nd ed. Boston, Jones and Bartlett, 1990.

Avery, G.B. (ed.): Neonatology: Pathophysiology and Management of the Newborn, 3rd ed. Philadelphia, J.B. Lippincott, 1987.

Bloom, R.S., and Cropley, C.: Textbook of Neonatal Resuscitation. Elk Grove Village, IL, American Heart Association and American Academy of Pediatrics, 1990.

Lantos, J.D., Miles, S.H. Silverstein, M.D., and Stocking, C.B.: Survival after cardiopulmonary resuscitation in babies of very low birth weight: Is CPR futile therapy? N. Engl. J. Med., *318*:91–95, 1988.

Raju, T.N.K.: An epidemiologic study of very and very, very low birth weight infants. Clin. Perinatol., *13*(2):233–250, 1986.

Wood, A.F.: Sequelae of perinatal asphyxia. Neonatal Network, *5*(5):21–23, 1987.

NEONATAL CARDIOPULMONARY DISORDERS AND MANAGEMENT

Mary Anne Givhan

Respiratory Distress

Objectives

1. Describe the anatomical and biochemical events associated with lung development.

2. Discuss the physiology of respiration.

3. Define common respiratory disorders found in the newborn.

4. Differentiate the common respiratory disorders found in the newborn.

5. Formulate plan of care for infants with respiratory disorders.

The most common group of life-threatening diseases in newborns are respiratory in origin. This is evidenced by the number of infants admitted to neonatal intensive care units (NICUs). The majority of cases are due to prematurity. Respiratory distress syndrome, retained lung fluid syndromes, aspiration syndromes, air leaks, and congenital pneumonia are commonly seen. These conditions account for approximately 90% of all respiratory distress in newborns.

Pulmonary disease is not the cause of all respiratory distress in newborn infants. Congenital malformations, metabolic abnormalities, central nervous system disorders, and congenital heart disease may also present with respiratory distress.

This chapter demonstrates the common respiratory problems found in the newborn and how to differentiate them. An understanding of the pathophysiology of these problems and the ability to make a specific diagnosis are important concepts to learn.

Lung Development

A. Anatomical events.
1. Embryonic development.
   a. *Embryonic period* (weeks 1–5). Lung bud appears and begins to divide; pulmonary vein develops and extends to join lung bud; trachea develops.
   b. *Pseudoglandular period* (weeks 5–17). Cartilage appears; main bronchi are formed; demarcation of major lobes occurs; formation of new bronchi com-

plete; capillary bed formed, connecting bronchial blood supply; no connection made with terminal air sacs.

c. *Canalicular period* (weeks 13–25). Appearance of glycogen-rich, cuboidal cells; inclusions for surface-active material storage are seen; capillaries invade terminal airway walls; type II alveolar epithelial cells appear. Airway changes from glandular to tubular and increases in length and diameter. Between weeks 24–26, alveolar sacs formed; air-blood surface area is limited for gas exchange; type II cells unable to release surfactant in sufficient quantity to maintain air breathing.

d. *Terminal sac period* (weeks 26–36). Capillary loops increase; type II cells cluster at alveolar ducts, become numerous, and mature; more budding occurs from alveolar ducts; lung size increases rapidly.

2. Biochemical events.
   a. Surface-active phospholipids.
      (1) Line terminal air spaces and maintain alveolar stability by reducing surface tension.
      (2) Surfactant is a surface-active agent composed of phospholipids (lecithin, sphingomyelin, cholesterol, phosphatidylinositol, phosphatidylcholine, and phosphatidylglycerol).
      (3) The changing pattern of phospholipids in amniotic fluid can be used to assess surfactant production and maturation of pathways.
         (a) Material from the fetal lung contributes to amniotic fluid.
         (b) Concentrations of various phospholipids can be measured and will assist in determining lung maturity.
      (4) Sphingomyelin concentration remains stable with a small peak at 28–30 weeks.
      (5) Lecithin and phosphatidylinositol concentrations remain low until 26–30 weeks, when an increase begins with peak occurring at 36 weeks.
      (6) Phosphatidylglycerol appears at 35–36 weeks and increases, and phosphatidylinositol level falls.
      (7) The lecithin to sphingomyelin ratio (L/S) has been used to assess fetal lung maturity.
         (a) Greater than 2:1 is considered mature.
         (b) An infant of a diabetic mother (IDM) may develop respiratory distress syndrome even with mature L/S ratio (presence of phosphatidylglycerol assures lung maturity).
         (c) Chronic fetal stress (e.g., maternal hypertension, retroplacental bleeding, maternal drug use, smoking) will tend to accelerate surfactant production, resulting in a mature L/S ratio in premature infants.
      (8) Use of phosphatidylinositol and phosphatidylglycerol concentrations is refining assessment of fetal lung maturity.

B. Role of steroids.

1. Glucocorticoids (e.g., betamethasone or dexamethasone) have been shown to affect lung maturation and present a strategy for preventing respiratory distress syndrome (RDS) (Gamsu et al., 1989; Papageorgiou et al., 1989; Block et al., 1977; Caspi et al., 1976; Liggins and Howie, 1972).
   a. Given concurrently with tocolytic agents (e.g., terbutaline, ritodrine) for premature labor. Generally not given if prolonged rupture of membranes (PROM) exists due to masking of infectious processes.
   b. Betamethasone is given intravenously in a 12 mg dose repeated at 12 or 24 hours; dexamethasone is given intravenously in a 4 mg dose every 8 hours for six doses (Lewis and Sammons, 1985).
2. Glucocorticoids have been effective for fetuses 27–34 weeks' gestation if given at least 48 hours before delivery and with delivery no longer than 7 days after treatment.
3. Infants exposed to chronic stress in utero are usually small for gestational age

(SGA) and have more mature lungs (they also have small thymuses and large adrenal glands, suggesting high glucocorticoid levels in utero).

Physiology of Respiration

A. In utero.
1. The alveoli contain fetal lung fluid and are open and stable at nearly normal lung volume. The lung fluid is produced by filtration of pulmonary capillary blood and secretions from alveolar cells.
2. Fetus spends almost 30% of time in a rapid, discoordinate form of "panting" (Patrick et al., 1978).
3. The fetus will inhale up to 600 ml of amniotic fluid a day by these breathing movements.
4. There is a high vascular pressure–low blood flow secondary to both passive and active pulmonary vascular resistance.
5. With the onset of respiration at birth, resistance reverses (pulmonary decreases, systemic increases).
   a. Success of reversal will determine adaptation to extrauterine life.
   b. Failure to decrease pulmonary vascular resistance and increase systemic vascular resistance will lead to a persistent pulmonary hypertension state.

B. First breath.
1. Vaginal birth compresses the thoracic cage from 30 to 160 cm H_2O pressure, resulting in ejection of tracheal fluid during passage through birth canal.
2. Recoil of chest wall pulls air into the upper airway, displacing fluid.
3. In larger airways, an air-liquid interface and surface retractive forces are established.
4. Aeration of the smaller airways will be easier if some fluid remains before the first active breaths are taken.
5. High distending pressures are needed for the first few lung breaths (up to 80 cm H_2O for first expansion if the lung is totally collapsed).
6. Pressures needed to maintain lung volume are quite low in normal lungs secondary to surfactant decreasing the surface tension of alveoli.

C. Stimulation to breathe.
1. Multiple factors.
   a. Cold.
   b. Light.
   c. Noise.
   d. Gravity.
   e. Handling.
   f. Asphyxia (hypercapnia, respiratory acidosis, and hypoxia) resulting from normal labor.
2. Normal birth produces gasping respirations (due to disruption of gas exchange through the placenta), improved oxygenation of the brain, and decreased tonic discharge of the expiratory neurons.
3. When the previous factors mentioned are combined, the rhythmicity of discharge in the respiratory centers is restored (Chernick, 1978).

D. Pulmonary adaptation: first active breath begins a chain of events.
1. Conversion of fetal to adult circulation.
2. Removal of lung liquid.
3. Lung volume and pulmonary function characteristics are established.
4. Establishment of lung retractive forces of surface tension with development of negative intrapleural and interstitial pressure as chest wall resists collapse.
5. Following onset of ventilation, there is an increase in blood and lymph flow through the lung.

E. Circulatory adaptation. (Refer to Chapter 3.)

Respiratory Disorders

RESPIRATORY DISTRESS SYNDROME (RDS)/HYALINE MEMBRANE DISEASE (HMD)

A. Definition.
1. Developmental disorder starting at or soon after birth occurring most frequently in infants with immature lungs.
2. Increasing respiratory difficulty in first 3–6 hours leading to hypoxia and hypoventilation.
3. Progressive atelectasis of prematurity.

B. Incidence.
1. Worldwide disorder.
2. Predominately seen in prematures but is more dependent on lung maturity than on gestational age.
3. 90% of infants at 26 weeks' gestation, 70% of infants at 30 weeks' gestation, 25% of infants at 34 weeks' gestation, and <1–2% of infants at term (Halliday et al., 1985).

C. Etiology.
1. Surfactant deficiency (see previous discussion).
2. Pulmonary hypoperfusion.
3. Anatomical immaturity (see previous discussion).
4. Precipitating factors associated with incidence of and/or severity of RDS.
   a. Prematurity, especially <35 weeks' gestation: the more premature, the more severe the disease.
   b. Cesarean section without labor.
   c. Infant of diabetic mother (IDM), especially if <38 weeks' gestation.
   d. Acute antepartum hemorrhage.
   e. Second twin.
      (1) May be due to greater risk of asphyxia.
      (2) First twin usually smaller, suggesting chronic stress leading to early lung maturation.
   f. Asphyxia at birth.
   g. RDS occurs at 2:1, males:females.
   h. RDS is more likely to occur in siblings of a low-birthweight (LBW) infant who had RDS.
   i. Decreased cord serum cortisol levels.
5. Unlikely factors for RDS development.
   a. Term birth.
   b. Intrauterine growth retardation (IUGR).
   c. Prolonged rupture of membranes (PROM).
   d. Chronic fetal stress.
      (1) Gradual placental insufficiency.
      (2) Maternal toxemia.
      (3) Smoking.
      (4) Retroplacental bleeding.
      (5) Maternal drug use.
      (6) Chronic maternal hypertension.

D. Pathophysiology.
1. Prerequisites for pulmonary adaptation.
   a. Adequate amounts of surface-active material to line air spaces (surfactant).
      (1) Must be regenerated at a rate equal to its utilization.
      (2) Must have intact and viable type II alveolar cells.
   b. Adequate surface area for gas exchange requires sufficient capillary bed in contact with an alveolar surface area covered with type I epithelial lining cells (cells adapted for gas diffusion).

2. Contributing factors.
   a. Pulmonary ischemia due to hypoperfusion.
   b. Lack of surfactant from several causes.
      (1) Extreme immaturity of cells lining alveoli.
      (2) Diminished production rate due to transient fetal stress or early neonatal stress.
      (3) Release mechanism for phospholipids within membrane of type II cells is impaired.
      (4) Cell death of those responsible for production.
   c. The very immature infant.
      (1) Pulmonary insufficiency leads to death from progressive atelectasis.
      (2) Cuboidal cells line air spaces, and capability of surfactant production is present but not in sufficient quantity for lung stability.
      (3) Due to a small pulmonary capillary bed, the nutritional blood supply to the developing lung is compromised.

E. Clinical presentation.
1. Almost exclusively premature infants:
   a. Will appear to be a normally grown, healthy premature infant with good Apgar scores at birth.
   b. Usually starts at or soon after birth.
      (1) Resuscitation in the delivery room may be necessary if asphyxia or delay in onset of respiration occurs.
      (2) Use least amount of manual positive pressure needed for chest movement to reduce risk of overdistention, air leaks, or development of pulmonary interstitial emphysema.
2. Increasing respiratory difficulty is seen in the first 3–6 hours.
   a. Symptoms are progressive.
      (1) Tachypnea (>60 breaths/minute) is usually the first sign. Color is maintained.
      (2) Audible expiratory grunt:
         (a) Heard during the first few hours.
         (b) Due to forcing air past a partially closed glottis.
         (c) Used to maintain positive end-expiratory pressure (PEEP) at alveolar level.
         (d) Increases with increasing severity of disease.
      (3) Intercostal and sternal retractions seen as ventilatory effort increases.
      (4) Nasal flaring.
      (5) Cyanosis due to increasing hypoxemia.
3. Oxygen requirements increase to maintain arterial Po_2 at 50–70 mm Hg.
4. Lung compliance decreases.
   a. More physical effort needed to keep terminal airways open.
   b. Paradoxical seesaw respirations are seen.
   c. Pseudopectus deformity (anterior chest wall and sternum collapse) seen if chest wall is unstable.
5. If signs and symptoms are unattended, infant becomes obtunded and flaccid.
   a. Pale gray color obscures severe central cyanosis.
   b. Poor capillary filling time (3–4 seconds).
   c. Progressive edema develops, usually seen in the face, palms, and soles.
6. Oliguria is common in first 48 hours.
7. Breath sounds diminish and lung auscultation usually described as "poor air entry" despite vigorous effort on the infant's part.
8. Rales occur as the disease progresses.
9. Cardiac murmurs are generally not heard until after 24 hours of age.
10. Tachycardia (heart rate 150–160/minute) is common and more prevalent if acidosis and hypoxemia are present.

F. Diagnosis.
1. Criteria.

a. Clinical findings reflect diminished lung stability due to abnormal surface tension properties.
b. Hypoxemia (defined as arterial Po_2 level <50 mm Hg in room air) responding to supplemental inspired oxygen.
c. Chest x-ray shows a diffuse reticulogranular pattern with prominent air bronchogram.
    (1) Central lung markings not prominent.
    (2) Heart border fuzzy and obscured.
    (3) Thymic shadow may be large.
    (4) Uniform granularity or "whiteout" with air bronchogram seen in first few hours indicates severe disease and carries a poor prognosis.
d. Signs and symptoms previously described continue.
e. L/S ratio of <2 or no detectable phosphatidylglycerol in amniotic fluid suggestive of lung immaturity and increased risk of RDS development.
2. Studies.
    a. Chest x-ray.
    b. Arterial blood gases (ABGs).
    c. Complete blood count (CBC).
    d. Other blood studies as needed (e.g., electrolytes, calcium, blood glucose levels).

G. Clinical course.
1. History of disease.
    a. Increasing respiratory distress.
    b. Increasing oxygen requirements.
    c. Decreasing lung compliance.
    d. Improvement 48–72 hours after birth, when type II alveolar cell regeneration occurs and surfactant is produced.
2. Indicators of a good prognosis.
    a. The infant will have a progressive rise in systemic arterial blood pressure over 4–5 days after birth as the child improves clinically (Stahlman, 1986).
    b. Large, more mature infants who did not need ventilation or required <60% fractional inspired oxygen (Fio_2); by 48 hours, these infants experience diuresis and have rapid clinical improvement over 3–4 days.
3. Indicators of a poor prognosis.
    a. Infants with very low birthweight (VLBW) (<1000 g) and gestational age (<28 weeks) who also need ventilator care.
    b. Clinical and biochemical findings (as previously described) that appear quickly after birth in smaller infants.
    c. Continuous positive airway pressure (CPAP) or assisted ventilation due to apnea (unresponsive) or low Pao_2 in oxygen concentrations >60%.
    d. Prolonged ventilatory support.
    e. Development of chronic lung disease.
4. Mortality in the VLBW infants is greater even with prompt recognition and treatment.

H. Differential diagnosis. (Each will be discussed in greater detail later in the chapter.)
1. Pneumonia.
2. Transient tachypnea of the newborn.
3. Anatomical disorders of the respiratory tract.

I. Complications.
1. Pulmonary (to be discussed later in detail).
    a. Acute: air leaks.
    b. Chronic: bronchopulmonary dysplasia (BPD).
2. Cardiovascular.
    a. Patent ductus arteriosus.
    b. Systemic hypotension.

3. Renal: oliguria.
    a. Most likely to follow hypoxia, hypotension, or shock ("pre-renal" renal failure).
    b. VLBW infants have immature renal function with decreased glomerular filtration.
4. Metabolic.
    a. Acidosis.
    b. Hypo- or hypernatremia.
    c. Hypocalcemia.
    d. Hypoglycemia.
5. Hematological.
    a. Anemia.
    b. Disseminated intravascular coagulation (DIC).
6. Neurological.
    a. Seizures.
    b. Intraventricular hemorrhage.
7. Other.
    a. Secondary infection.
        (1) Complication of assisted ventilation or CPAP.
        (2) Generally associated with gram-negative organisms (i.e., *Pseudomonas aeruginosa*, *Aerobacter*, *Klebsiella*, and *Escherichia coli*).
        (3) Difficult to treat in an already damaged lung.
        (4) May produce chronic pneumonia, making weaning difficult and prolonged.
    b. Retinopathy of prematurity (ROP).
    c. Displaced endotracheal tubes.
    d. Thrombus formation or complications of umbilical catheters needed to monitor respiratory status.

J. **Management.**
1. Supportive.
    a. Respiratory.
        (1) Provide warm, humidified oxygen to maintain Pao_2 between 50 and 70 mm Hg (60–80 mm Hg at high altitudes).
        (2) Use of CPAP via nasal prongs or endotracheal tube may be helpful.
        (3) Use of assisted ventilation for profound hypoxemia (Pao_2 <50 mm Hg) and/or hypercapnia ($Paco_2$ >60 mm Hg).
        (4) Chest physiotherapy.
        (5) Use of pulse oximetry and/or transcutaneous monitoring.
        (6) Surfactant replacement therapy.
    b. Chest x-ray for verification of diagnosis.
2. Other.
    a. Temperature stabilization.
    b. Adequate fluid and electrolyte intake.
    c. Restore acid-base balance by use of sodium bicarbonate ($NaHCO_3$) infusion (1–2 mEq/kg diluted 1:1 in sterile water) given no faster than 1 mEq/kg/ minute for metabolic acidosis. Assisted ventilation is used for respiratory acidosis.
    d. Sampling and monitoring of arterial blood gases; serum sodium, potassium, chloride, calcium, bilirubin, and glucose.
    e. Monitor blood pressure for hypotension.
        (1) Maintain hematocrit.
        (2) Volume replacement if indicated.
        (3) Pharmacological agents as indicated (e.g., dopamine or dobutamine).
    f. Administer antibiotics for associated pneumonia and risk of infection from catheters, endotracheal tubes, and any procedures performed on infant. (Refer to Chapter 18.)
    g. Observation for complications.

K. **Prevention of RDS.**
1. Ultimate goal of therapy.
2. Glucocorticoid administration pre-natally.
3. Use of L/S ratio and phosphatidylglycerol determination for timing labor induction or elective cesarean section is an important means of preventing RDS.
4. Use of prudent obstetrical and pediatric judgment to avoid situations leading to pulmonary circulation compromise in the fetus or newborn.
    a. Maternal hypotension.
    b. Oversedation.
    c. Maternal hypoxia.
    d. Fetal distress without prompt delivery.
    e. Delayed resuscitation.
    f. Uncorrected hypoxia or acidosis.
    g. Hypothermia.
    h. Hypovolemia.

L. **Outcome.**
1. Morbidity related to complications of prematurity.
2. Infants with chronic lung disease improve slowly and progressively if they can be kept infection-free; will commonly have episodes of bronchiolitis and occasionally develop pneumonia during the first few years of life; long-term sequelae are related to specific complications (e.g., BPD, IVH, ROP).
3. Very immature infants are showing more developmental sequelae in later follow-up (e.g., perceptual problems, motor delays) (Mayes et al., 1985).
4. Prognosis for normal development is better in infants with fewer complications.
5. Birthweight relationship exists (lower birthweight related to greater morbidity).

PNEUMONIA

A. **Definition:** Infection of the fetal or newborn lung. May be one of two types.
1. Intrauterine.
    a. Due to passage of infecting agent by infection of fetal membranes.
    b. Transplacental transmission.
    c. Aspiration of meconium or infected amniotic fluid during delivery.
2. Neonatal.
    a. Acquired during nursery stay.
    b. Pathogens are generally different from those acquired in utero.
    c. Usually secondary to primary disease elsewhere.
    d. Result by passage from other infants, equipment, or caretakers.

B. **Incidence.**
1. Will vary from center to center as well as to the causative agent.
2. Bacterial pneumonia incidence is comparable with that of sepsis—1 in 2000 in full-term, 1 in 200 with birthweight <2500 g, and 1 in 10 with birthweight <1000 g (Hodson and Truog, 1989).

C. **Etiology.**
1. Risk of infection greatest in prematures.
2. Agents are many.
    a. Bacterial.
        (1) Group B beta-hemolytic streptococci (most common).
        (2) *Escherichia coli.*
        (3) *Staphylococcus aureus.*
        (4) *Staphylococcus epidermidis.*
        (5) *Haemophilus influenzae.*
        (6) *Streptococcus pneumoniae.*
        (7) *Listeria monocytogenes.*
        (8) Other gram-negative organisms.

  b. Viral.
  (1) Cytomegalovirus (CMV).
  (2) Respiratory syncytial virus (RSV).
  (3) Enterovirus.
  (4) Herpesvirus.
  c. Other.
  (1) *Treponema pallidum.*
  (2) *Pneumocystis carinii.*
  (3) *Chlamydia trachomatis* (usually occurs after 3 weeks of age).
  (4) Aspiration pneumonia (associated with feedings).

D. **Pathophysiology.**
1. Intrauterine pneumonia.
  a. Generally follows prolonged rupture of membranes.
  b. Ascending organisms infect amniotic fluid; if mother is in active labor, contamination occurs more rapidly.
  c. Infective organisms may cross the placenta and enter the fetal circulation and cause pneumonia.
  d. Infants usually show signs of generalized illness from birth, but signs of illness may be delayed hours to days if the infective fluid is aspirated during delivery.
2. Neonatal pneumonia.
  a. Occurs days to weeks after birth.
  b. Usual pathogens are coagulase-positive staphylococci, group A streptococci, *Escherichia coli*, and *Staphylococcus epidermidis.*
  c. Will present as a secondary result of a primary disease, such as infection of the cord stump and circumcision wounds.
  d. Pathophysiology would be specific to infecting agent.

E. **Clinical presentation.**
1. Prolonged labor (>24 hours).
  a. Prolonged rupture of membranes (longer than 24 hours).
  b. Maternal fever.
  c. Foul smelling or purulent amniotic fluid.
  d. Fetal tachycardia.
  e. Loss of heart rate pattern variability.
2. Signs/symptoms.
  a. Signs and symptoms are often indistinguishable from those of other forms of respiratory distress and sepsis.
  b. Tachypnea, grunting, retractions, cyanosis, hypoxemia, and hypercapnia.
  c. If severe involvement occurs, shock-like syndrome is seen usually in the first 24 hours of life with recurrent apnea followed by cardiovascular collapse, profound hypoxemia, and persistent pulmonary hypertension. These signs present a poor prognosis.
3. Physical examination.
  a. Physical signs are variable.
  b. In addition to those findings noted previously, localized dullness and rales may be heard.
  c. Diminished breath sounds may be present over one or more areas, or they may be harsh.

F. **Diagnostic evaluation.**
1. History of any previously mentioned contributing factors is suggestive.
2. Infants may require resuscitation in the delivery room.
3. Chest x-rays can be variable. They may show the following:
  a. Unilateral or bilateral alveolar infiltrates.
  b. A more diffuse interstitial pattern.
4. Blood cultures should be obtained, although they are rarely positive unless there is generalized bacterial sepsis.

5. A complete blood count should be obtained.
   a. May show neutropenia.
   b. May have abnormal band to total neutrophil ratio.
6. Urine for latex agglutination test for group B streptococci has proved to be helpful because the results can be obtained faster than cultures.
7. Arterial blood gases (ABGs) should be obtained, since metabolic acidosis may be severe.
8. Tracheal aspirate culture should be considered, especially if the infant is intubated.

G. Differential diagnosis.
1. Respiratory distress syndrome (RDS).
2. Sepsis.

H. Complications.
1. Meningitis.
2. Gram-negative pneumonia may show cardiopulmonary complications similar to those of RDS.
3. Septic shock.
4. Disseminated intravascular coagulation (DIC).
5. Persistent pulmonary hypertension.

I. Management.
1. Antibiotic therapy.
   a. Initially when agent is unknown, coverage should be broad-spectrum antibiotics—i.e., ampicillin and gentamicin. (See Chapter 18 for dosages.)
   b. If an organism is recovered, antibiotics should be based on sensitivity.
2. Maintain temperature.
3. Monitor blood pressure.
   a. Volume expansion up to 30 ml/kg using albumin, whole blood, fresh-frozen plasma, or packed red blood cells for hypotension or hypoperfusion.
   b. Correct hypotension after volume status is corrected with vasopressors such as dopamine (5–15 μg/kg/minute infusion).
4. Oxygen or assisted ventilation to maintain normal ABGs.
5. Correction of metabolic acidosis.
6. Adequate fluid and electrolyte intake.
7. If shock is evident, treatment of DIC may be needed.
8. Monitor glucose.
9. Provide family support.

J. Outcome.
1. Infants who present with serious bacterial disease at birth are more likely to die regardless of quick and appropriate care.
2. Infants with milder bacterial forms will have a more benign course with a good outcome.
3. When pneumonia is caused by viral and other agents, outcome depends on the agent and the overall effect it has on the infant.

RETAINED LUNG FLUID SYNDROMES

A. Definition and clinical presentation.
1. Transient tachypnea of the newborn (TTN).
   a. Usually seen in term/near-term infants, especially with cesarean section or precipitous, stressful delivery.
   b. In the first few hours, tachypnea (respiratory rate up to 120/minute) without significant retractions or rales.
   c. Minimal cyanosis, normal alveolar ventilation based on pH and Pco_2.
   d. Some infants require O_2 of 35–40% to remain pink and well saturated.
   e. May last 3–4 days.
2. RDS, type II (Philip, 1987).

    a. Occurs in near-term infants.

    b. Grunting, retractions, and nasal flaring.

    c. Biochemical changes are minimal.

    d. Course is transient (usually around 24 hours) and benign.

B. Etiology.

1. Delay in removal of lung fluid.
2. Excessive amount of lung fluid.

C. Pathophysiology.

1. Lung fluid is a major component of these syndromes.
2. Fluid is usually forced out by thoracic compression with vaginal delivery.
3. During cesarean section, the forces to expel lung fluid are less, leading to a tendency to retain lung fluid.
4. After delivery, when air breathing begins, fluid removal is primarily by the lymphatic capillaries.
5. Respiratory symptoms are seen when there is a delay in fluid removal or an excessive amount of fluid.

D. Diagnosis.

1. Early signs and symptoms may be difficult to distinguish from those of other respiratory problems; however, they are usually milder.
2. A chest x-ray is helpful, although it may be indistinguishable from other disorders.
    a. Diffuse haziness in both lung fields with clearing at the periphery and streakiness.
    b. Fluid present in the interlobar fissures.
    c. Mild hyperinflation.
3. Diagnosis is frequently one of exclusion.

E. Differential diagnosis.

1. RDS.
2. Pneumonia.
3. Polycythemia (high hematocrit syndrome).

F. Management.

1. Because diagnosis is not conclusive, other disorders should be ruled out.
2. Supportive management.
    a. Oxygen.
    b. Temperature regulation.
    c. Adequate fluid intake.
    d. Maintain ABGs within normal levels.
    e. Maintain blood glucose at normal levels.
3. If respiratory rate is greater than 60, delay feedings to avoid possible aspiration.
4. If anything in history indicates risk of infection, broad-spectrum antibiotics (e.g., ampicillin and gentamicin) should be administered until cultures are negative.

G. Outcome.

1. These syndromes are self-limited.
2. Oxygen requirement and tachypnea decrease steadily over several days. Infant may remain mildly tachypneic beyond the need for oxygen.

PERSISTENT PULMONARY HYPERTENSION OF THE NEWBORN (PPHN)

A. Definition.

1. Persistence of the cardiopulmonary pathway seen in the fetus (Levin et al., 1975).
2. Dominant feature is high resistance in the pulmonary vessels causing obstruction of blood flow through the lungs.
3. Right-to-left shunting through the ductus arteriosus and/or foramen ovale occurs.

B. **Etiology and pathophysiology.**
1. Precipitating factors.
   a. Asphyxia (hypoxia and acidosis) at birth.
   b. Asphyxia during transitional circulatory adaptation.
   3. Hypothermia, hypoglycemia, hypocalcemia, and hypoxia lead to acidosis, which will potentiate vasoconstriction.
2. Etiology based on the mechanism causing increased pulmonary pressure.
   a. Pulmonary vasoconstriction due to asphyxia.
      (1) Classic form of PPHN.
      (2) Infants fall into two groups of pulmonary vasoconstriction:
         (a) Those with normal pulmonary vascular development.
         (b) Those with increased pulmonary vascular smooth muscle (usually associated with chronic fetal hypoxia).
      (3) Causes of PPHN secondary to pulmonary vasoconstriction.
         (a) Obstruction of the airway (i.e., aspiration syndromes, masses, etc.).
         (b) Pneumonia.
         (c) Atelectasis.
         (d) CNS depression.
         (e) Pre-natal pulmonary hypertension.
            i. Fetal systemic hypertension.
            ii. Premature closure of ductus arteriosus (seen with maternal aspirin, prostaglandin inhibitors, phenytoin [Dilantin], lithium, or indomethacin taken in significant amounts).
         (f) Any condition preventing normal circulatory transition at delivery can lead to pulmonary vasoconstriction.
      (4) Most cases of PPHN will fall in this category.
   b. Decreased number of pulmonary vessels.
      (1) Blood is shunted because there are too few vessels for blood to flow through the lungs.
      (2) Contributing conditions.
         (a) Pulmonary hypoplasia.
         (b) Space occupying lesions: lung mass prevents normal development of lung tissue and capillary bed. Examples are diaphragmatic hernia and lung cysts.
         (c) Congenital heart disease: pulmonary atresia or tricuspid atresia may lead to decreased blood flow and vascular underdevelopment.
      (3) These conditions predispose infants to hypoxia causing vasoconstriction in an area of increased pulmonary resistance.
   c. Functional obstruction of the pulmonary vascular bed.
      (1) Associated with hyperviscosity syndrome in utero.
      (2) Polycythemia (hematocrit >65%) may predispose the infant to the above syndrome.
      (3) Usually associated with fetal-fetal transfusions or maternal-fetal transfusions.
      (4) May occur due to chronic fetal hypoxemia.
   d. Research has shown that the presence of leukotrienes may be a major stimulus to pulmonary vasoconstriction (Stenmark et al., 1983).

C. **Clinical presentation.**
1. Usually seen in near-term, term, or post-term infants.
2. History of hypoxia or asphyxia at birth.
   a. Low Apgar scores.
   b. Infant usually slow to breath or difficult to ventilate.
   c. Meconium-stained fluid, nuchal cord, abruptio placentae or any acute blood loss, and maternal sedation are important things to note and be aware of as risk factors for the development of PPHN.
3. Respiratory.
   a. Symptoms seen before 12 hours of age.

   b. Tachypnea.
   c. Retractions if airway is obstructed (e.g., aspiration).
   d. Cyanosis is out of proportion to degree of distress (may not see cyanosis with Pao_2 <50 mm Hg).
   e. Pao_2 is low despite high oxygen concentration administration.
   f. Chest x-ray can be normal unless aspiration or pneumonia present (will see infiltrates in these cases).
4. Cardiovascular.
   a. Blood pressure is usually lower than normal.
   b. EKG will show a right axis deviation.
   c. Systolic murmur heard frequently, usually from a patent ductus arteriosus or foramen ovale.
   d. Echocardiogram shows dilated right side of the heart and evidence of pulmonary hypertension.
   e. Congestive heart failure has been reported occasionally.
5. Metabolic.
   a. Hypoglycemia.
   b. Hypocalcemia.
   c. Metabolic acidosis.
   d. Decreased urine output or coagulopathy due to kidney and liver damage from asphyxia may occur.

D. Diagnosis.
1. It is important to diagnose PPHN but particularly to identify the cause because it may affect treatment.
2. Will have suspicion based on history and clinical course.
3. Because of right-to-left shunting at level of ductus arteriosus, there will be a pre-ductal and post-ductal Pao_2 difference.
   a. Draw simultaneous blood samples for ABGs from the right radial artery (pre-ductal) and an umbilical artery catheter (UAC) (post-ductal).
   b. Difference in Pao_2 of 10 mm Hg or greater documents ductal shunting.
4. Pulmonary pressures can be measured and cardiac defects diagnosed by echocardiography.
5. Chest x-ray may or may not be helpful, but should be taken to rule out other lung pathology.
6. Electrolytes, calcium, glucose levels, and CBC should be checked.

E. Differential diagnosis.
1. Rule out congenital heart disease.
2. Pulmonary disease.
   a. Severe disease may mimic PPHN.
   b. May coexist with PPHN.

F. Complications.
1. Pulmonary.
   a. Air leaks.
   b. Bronchopulmonary dysplasia (BPD).
2. Cardiovascular.
   a. Systemic hypotension.
   b. Congestive heart failure.
3. Renal.
   a. Decreased urine output.
   b. Kidney damage due to asphyxia.
   c. Hematuria.
4. Metabolic.
   a. Hypoglycemia.
   b. Metabolic acidosis.
5. Hematological.
   a. Thrombocytopenia.

　　　　b. DIC.

　　　　c. Hemorrhage (GI, pulmonary, etc.).

　　6. Neurological.

　　　　a. CNS irritability.

　　　　b. Seizures.

　　7. Iatrogenic.

　　　　a. Thrombus formation or complications of invasive monitoring equipment.

　　　　b. Displaced endotracheal tubes.

　　8. Other.

　　　　a. Edema.

　　　　b. Abdominal distention.

　　　　c. Side effects from pharmacological agents used for treatment.

G. Management.

　　1. Main goal is to correct hypoxia and acidosis (major contributing factors) and promote pulmonary vascular dilation as well as support extrapulmonary systems.

　　2. Management will depend on the cause of PPHN.

　　3. Supportive care.

　　　　a. Monitoring vital signs.

　　　　b. Temperature stabilization.

　　　　c. Adequate IV fluid infusion.

　　　　d. Monitoring electrolytes, glucose, calcium, CBC, ABG.

　　　　e. Correction of metabolic abnormalities.

　　　　f. Blood cultures and antibiotics.

　　　　g. Close observation and correction of any complications.

　　4. Specialized monitoring.

　　　　a. Umbilical catheters.

　　　　　　(1) Arterial (UAC): blood gas access, arterial pressure monitoring.

　　　　　　(2) Venous (UVC): central pressure monitoring.

　　　　b. Right radial arterial line.

　　　　c. Transcutaneous monitoring: pre-ductal and post-ductal application.

　　　　d. Pulse oximetry: to evaluate oxygen saturation.

　　5. Oxygen: oxygen is the most potent pulmonary vasodilator.

　　6. Ventilation.

　　　　a. Hyperoxygenation.

　　　　　　(1) Goal is to keep Pao_2 >90 mm Hg.

　　　　　　(2) Danger of retinopathy of prematurity (ROP) is minimal, since most infants are term or near-term.

　　　　b. Hyperventilation.

　　　　　　(1) $Paco_2$ values at 20–25 mm Hg.

　　　　　　(2) Will aid in reducing acidosis and pulmonary artery pressure due to vasodilatory effect of alkalosis.

　　　　c. Maintain pH between 7.45 and 7.55; if hyperventilation alone does not accomplish this goal, use of buffers may be needed (e.g., $NaHCO_3$, THAM).

　　7. Minimal stimulation and handling.

　　　　a. Infants will show marked fluctuations (generally decreases) in their Pao_2 if handled or manipulated.

　　　　b. The pulmonary arteries are very reactive to changes in Pao_2; therefore, any action that causes a decrease in Pao_2 will cause further vasoconstriction (e.g., suctioning, blood sampling, vital signs, ventilator changes).

　　　　c. Suction only as needed to maintain a patent airway.

　　　　d. Consider sedatives/analgesics for procedures or treatments.

　　8. Pharmacological support.

　　　　a. Muscle relaxants.

　　　　　　(1) Used when infant's own respirations interfere with assisted ventilation.

　　　　　　(2) Paralysis prevents resisting the ventilator, reduces pulmonary vascular resistance, and reduces the risk of air leaks and BPD.

(3) Agents used are as follows:
   (a) Curare.
       i. Dosage: 0.3 mg/kg prn.
       ii. Advantage of pulmonary vasodilation effect due to histamine action.
       iii. Disadvantages are hypotension and reduced cardiac output.
       iv. Should be used with sedation.
   (b) Pancuronium bromide (Pavulon).
       i. Dosage: 0.05–0.1 mg/kg every 1–2 hours.
       ii. Shorter acting with fewer cardiovascular side effects than curare.
       iii. If used longer than 2 days, side effects include fluid retention, edema, and ileus.
       iv. Should be used with sedation.
b. Vasopressors.
   (1) Goal is to keep the systemic pressure above normal to decrease shunting.
   (2) Dopamine is the drug of choice.
       (a) Dosage: begin with 2–5 μg/kg/minute via infusion and titrate with blood pressure to a maximum of 20 μg/kg/minute.
       (b) Low doses (2–10 μg/kg/minute) will increase heart rate, cardiac output and renal blood flow, whereas higher doses (15–20 μg/kg/minute) will decrease renal blood flow.
   (3) Dobutamine may also be used for BP support.
       (a) 2–25 μg/kg/minute via continuous infusion and titrate by monitoring BP; optimal BP will vary with gestational age.
       (b) Increased cardiac contractility, cardiac index, oxygen delivery, and oxygen consumption. Cardiac output increases depending on myocardial catecholamine stores.
c. Pulmonary vasodilators.
   (1) Tolazoline (Priscoline).
       (a) Drug of choice.
       (b) Action: alpha-adrenergic blocking agent.
       (c) Effects: dilates pulmonary arteries, decreasing pulmonary vascular resistance; smooth muscle relaxation; increases heart rate; increases cardiac output.
       (d) Dosage: 1–2 mg/kg bolus over 10 minutes followed by 1–2 mg/kg/hour IV infusion into the superior vena cava circulation.
       (e) Adequate blood volume is necessary prior to vasodilator therapy.
       (f) Systemic vasodilation may occur. Vasopressors (e.g., dopamine) may be required to maintain blood pressure.
       (g) There is often an unpredictable response to this drug.
   (2) Isoproterenol (Isuprel).
       (a) Action: dilates the pulmonary arteries and airways, increases cardiac output.
       (b) Tachycardia and systemic hypotension may be seen.
       (c) Dosage: .05–0.5 μg/kg/minute continuous IV infusion.
   (3) Other agents.
       (a) Prostaglandin I_2 (prostacyclin) and nifedipine (calcium channel blocker) may prove to be more specific and effective.
       (b) Require further testing because use in humans is limited and is not recommended at this time.
d. Analgesics/sedatives.
   (1) Chloral hydrate.
       (a) Dosage: 25–50 mg/kg given orally or rectally every 6–8 hours.
       (b) Produces sedative effect.
       (c) Onset of effect may be longer than with IV sedatives.
   (2) Morphine sulfate.
       (a) Dosage: 0.05–0.2 mg/kg IV q 4–6 hours or prn.

        (b) Used for analgesia/sedation.
        (c) Results in histamine release and may cause hypotension.
        (d) May see withdrawal symptoms after prolonged use.
     (3) Fentanyl citrate.
        (a) Dosage: $1-4$ μg/kg q $2-4$ hours IV.
        (b) Used as a sedative for ventilated patients.
        (c) Pulmonary vascular stress responses are decreased, making this a more beneficial drug to use in infants with PPHN.
        (d) May see withdrawal symptoms after prolonged use.
9. Extracorporeal membrane oxygenation (ECMO). (Refer to Chapter 11.) May be utilized if conventional therapy is unsuccessful.

H. Outcome.
1. PPHN mortality is >50%.
2. Long-term neurodevelopmental sequelae are suspect and need further evaluation (Leavitt et al., 1987).
3. Preliminary studies are favorable.

MECONIUM ASPIRATION SYNDROME (MAS)

A. Definition and etiology.
1. Meconium is a mixture of epithelial cells and bile salts found in the fetal intestinal tract.
2. With asphyxia in utero peristalsis is stimulated and relaxation of the anal sphincter occurs, releasing meconium into the amniotic fluid.
3. Aspiration may occur anytime meconium has passed into the amniotic fluid, but the risk increases when repeated episodes of severe asphyxia lead to gasping respirations in utero.

B. Incidence: Meconium-stained amniotic fluid is present in $8-10\%$ of all pregnancies, but severe aspiration is less common.

C. Pathophysiology.
1. Complete or partial airway obstruction can occur.
2. Atelectasis or ball-valve air trapping leading to hyperinflation may be seen.
3. A chemical pneumonitis may develop as a result of aspiration of meconium (probably due to bile salts).
4. Asphyxia and the results of chronic hypoxia may predispose these infants to PPHN.

D. Clinical presentation/diagnosis.
1. Disease of term or post-term infants.
2. Rarely seen in infants <36 weeks' gestation.
3. Frequently vigorous resuscitation is needed in the delivery room due to central depression.
4. Respiratory distress signs are non-specific and may include tachypnea, nasal flaring, and retractions.
5. Respiratory distress may range from mild and transient to severe and prolonged.
6. If there has been prolonged placental insufficiency, infants may appear to be wasted with hanging skin folds (usually around knees, buttocks, and axillae).
7. Nail beds and skin are usually stained a yellow-green color.
8. Chest may appear to be hyperinflated or barrel shaped.
9. Chest x-ray shows hyperexpanded, lucent areas mixed with areas of atelectasis throughout lung fields.
10. Expiration phase of respirations may be prolonged.
11. Rales and rhonchi are common on auscultation.
12. No specific laboratory data are useful for diagnosis of MAS.
13. ABGs will show the following:
    a. Respiratory and metabolic acidosis in severe cases.

b. Low Pao$_2$ even with 100% oxygen administration.

14. Infants who have not had placental insufficiency will not appear to be malnourished but may be mildly to severely stained.

E. Complications.

1. Pulmonary.
   a. Air leaks: common.
   b. Pneumonia.
   c. PPHN.
   d. Bronchopulmonary dysplasia (BPD).
2. Metabolic.
   a. Acidosis.
   b. Hypoglycemia: may be severe and persistent.
   c. Hypocalcemia.
3. Hematological.
   a. Polycythemia.
   b. Hyperviscosity.
4. Neurological: will depend on degree of asphyxia seen.

F. Management.

1. Prevention.
   a. Proper delivery room management.
      (1) Suction nasopharynx, oropharynx, and hypopharynx with delivery of head to remove any meconium before first breath is taken.
      (2) Perform tracheal suction by direct laryngoscopy using direct suction to the endotracheal tube.
      (3) May need repeated intubation and tracheal suctioning to remove excessive meconium.
   b. Respiratory care.
      (1) ABGs to determine degree of respiratory compromise and type of therapy needed.
      (2) Oxygen and/or assisted ventilation.
         (a) Use same parameters for therapy as with RDS. May want to use a lower positive end-expiratory pressure (PEEP) (to avoid inadvertent PEEP) and a higher respiratory rate to induce alkalosis and prevent PPHN.
         (b) May need to keep Po$_2$ high (>90 mm Hg) to avoid PPHN.
      (3) Use of sedatives and paralysis may be necessary if infant is ventilated, as with PPHN.
      (4) Air leaks should be considered if a sudden deterioration occurs.
   c. General care.
      (1) Correction of metabolic abnormalities.
      (2) Blood cultures and antibiotics.
      (3) Close observation and correction of any complication that may arise.

G. Outcome.

1. The prognosis for infants with mild cases of MAS is generally excellent unless complications such as seizures, PPHN, or severe asphyxia occur during the course of the disease.
2. In more severe cases, neurological sequelae are common and death may occur despite vigorous, maximal support.

Bronchopulmonary Dysplasia (BPD)

A. Definition.

1. In 1967, Northway and associates first described the process.
   a. Occurs in infants who receive assisted ventilation for RDS/HMD and develop chronic lung changes.

      b. Changes are described in four stages based on the time that change occurred (from 0 to 30 days of life) and what type of alveolar and bronchial damage and repair occurred.
2. In 1979, Bancalari and colleagues described different criteria.
      a. Oxygen dependency for >28 days.
      b. Required clinical signs associated with changes in the chest x-ray following assisted ventilation.
3. In 1984, Toce and associates offered a scoring system based on clinical and x-ray findings at 21 days of age.

B. Incidence.
1. Incidence figures vary because of the difference in diagnostic criteria.
2. Overall, BPD seems to be decreasing, but the population of infants receiving assisted ventilation has changed since first described (Edwards et al., 1977).
3. Approximately 2.5–6% of ventilated infants develop BPD, and up to 40% of very low birthweight (VLBW) infants are affected (Markestad and Fitzhardinge, 1981; Vohr et al., 1982; Yu et al., 1983).

C. Etiology.
1. Oxygen toxicity is thought to be a major factor in the development of BPD.
      a. Animal studies show reduction in capillary endothelial cells and hypertrophy in remaining cells (Crapo et al., 1980).
      b. With longer exposure, capillary proliferation, stromal edema, and interstitial fibrosis are seen.
      c. The lung contains an antioxidant enzyme system that helps prevent injury from free oxygen radicals and matures lung surfactant with increases before birth in rabbit studies (Frank and Groseclose, 1984).
      d. Overproduction of mucus followed by cessation of production, loss of ciliary action, and epithelial metaplasia has been seen between 1 and 4 days (Boat et al., 1973).
      e. Oxygen can lead to an increase in inflammatory cells found in tracheal secretions (Merritt et al., 1983).
        (1) Cells contain elastase, which can damage lung stroma.
        (2) Alpha-1-protease inhibitor activity decrease thought to be caused by oxidation.
2. Assisted ventilation with positive pressure and barotrauma contributes to BPD development.
      a. Intubation interrupts normal pulmonary function (mucociliary function is damaged; dead space is increased, leading to increased pressure needs).
      b. Low peak airway pressure, even with high oxygen concentration, has shown a lower incidence of BPD development (Taghizadeh and Reynolds, 1976).
      c. Barotrauma is related to the intensity and amount of time exposed to elements of positive-pressure ventilation (peak inspiratory pressure [PIP], inspiratory time, and positive end-expiratory pressure [PEEP]).
3. Increased shunting (left-to-right) via a patent ductus arteriosus (PDA) has been described as a possible cause of BPD.
      a. Improved lung compliance was seen following PDA ligation in infants with RDS.
      b. When PDA is a complication of RDS, the risk of BPD development is increased (Bancalari and Gerhardt, 1986; Nickerson, 1985).
4. Impact of early fluid intake with RDS has been described in relation to BPD development. An increased fluid load during the first 5 days of life was shown in infants with BPD and congestive heart failure (CHF) compared with infants with RDS and PDA without CHF and infants with CHF without BPD (Brown et al., 1978).
5. Nutritional deficiencies have been implicated as contributing to BPD in animal studies. In premature infants this cannot be replicated, but further study is needed.
6. Gestational age plays an important role in the development of BPD.

a. Damage to the developing lung is more likely in infants weighting <1500 g.
b. Damage may occur with less exposure to the previously noted factors in the low birthweight (LBW) infant.

D. Pathophysiology.
1. Process is continuous but divided into stages for classification.
2. Stage I is indistinguishable from RDS. Early interstitial changes can be seen.
3. Stage II shows regeneration and proliferation of the bronchial epithelium; the alveolar epithelium shows necrosis with early fibrosis; chest x-ray shows diffuse haziness.
4. Stage III shows the beginning of chronic disease. There is widespread bronchial and bronchiolar metaplasia; alveoli show signs of emphysema; interstitial edema is present; pulmonary hypertension develops; chest x-ray will show small cysts that are present throughout lung fields but that are prominent in perihilar areas.
5. Stage IV reflects chronic disease with obliterative bronchiolitis and interstitial fibrosis; chest x-ray shows hyperexpansion due to increase in size and number of cysts (will persist for 3–4 months or longer).
6. Northway (1967) proposed time periods when the previous stages were seen, but the changes have been seen by others earlier than first described (Banerjee et al., 1972; Bancalari et al., 1979; Toce et al., 1984; Watts et al., 1977).
7. Continuous process pathologically.

E. Clinical presentation.
1. Predisposing factors.
   a. Oxygen, intubation, and assisted ventilation. (See etiology.)
   b. Gestational age.
   c. Nutritional deficiencies.
   d. Underlying lung disease.
   e. Air leaks.
2. Increase in ventilatory requirements or inability to wean from ventilator.
3. Hypoxia, hypercapnia, and respiratory acidosis.
4. Rales, rhonchi, and wheezing are audible.
5. Retractions evident.
6. Increased secretions are sometimes seen.
7. Bronchospasm.
8. EKG will show right ventricular hypertrophy and right axis deviation.
9. Chest x-ray will show previously noted changes and cardiomegaly.
10. Fluid intolerance evidenced by increase in weight, edema, decrease in urine output despite no change in fluid intake.

F. Diagnosis.
1. Diagnosis is one of exclusion.
2. Differential diagnosis.
   a. Sepsis.
   b. Pneumonia.
   c. Airway obstruction.
   d. PDA.
3. BPD starts earlier than other chronic lung disease in neonates (to be discussed later).
4. Chest x-rays (as previously described) and clinical signs (tachypnea, hypercapnia, hypoxia, rales, etc.) help make the diagnosis but are not conclusive.

G. Complications.
1. Intermittent bronchospasm.
2. Inability to wean from ventilator and/or oxygen.
3. Recurrent infections.
   a. Pneumonia.
   b. Upper respiratory infections.
   c. Otitis media.
4. Congestive heart failure from cor pulmonale.

5. "BPD spells."
   a. Infant becomes irritable, agitated, dusky; has increased respiratory effort, hypoxia, and hypercapnia.
   b. Etiology is unknown but may be due to bronchospasm or increased pulmonary vascular resistance.
6. Gastroesophageal reflux.
7. Developmental delays.

H. Management.
1. Continued respiratory support.
   a. Continue assisted ventilation.
      (1) Weaning should be *slow.*
      (2) Decrease the rate due to the need for high PIP to deliver adequate tidal volume (TV).
   b. After extubation, oxygen is needed to avoid hypoxia.
      (1) Oxygen inhalation alleviates airway constriction seen in infants with BPD (Tay-Uyboco et al., 1989).
      (2) Maintain Pao_2 >55 mm Hg and pH >7.25.
      (3) Pulmonary vascular resistance is decreased.
      (4) Oxygen may enhance growth.
   c. Weaning can be accomplished by use of pulse oximetry, occasional ABGs, capillary blood gases (CBGs), and/or serum bicarbonate levels (to assess compensation).
2. Use of diuretics.
   a. Used to control fluid retention leading to pulmonary edema that is seen with BPD.
   b. Furosemide (Lasix) is used most often.
      (1) Decreases airway resistance and increases both airway compliance and conductance for 1 hour after a single dose.
      (2) Total body water, extracellular water, and interstitial water were significantly decreased 4 hours after a single dose (O'Donovan and Bell, 1989).
      (3) Renal calcification has been reported with daily long-term use (Hufnagle et al., 1983).
      (4) Dosage: 1 mg/kg every 6–24 hours given IV, IM, or PO (Durand and Kao, 1990).
   c. Chlorothiazide (Diuril) (10–20 mg/kg/day divided q 12 hours PO) has been used with results similar to those seen with furosemide (Kao et al., 1984).
   d. Follow serum electrolytes to monitor for hyponatremia, hypokalemia, and metabolic alkalosis.
   e. If an infant responds to diuretic therapy, oral preparations should be used when possible.
3. Use of bronchodilators.
   a. Theophylline (aminophylline) is the most widely used bronchodilator and is given in doses of 2–4 mg/kg every 6 hours.
   b. Reduces airway resistance and increases compliance (Durand and Kao, 1990).
   c. Use of Albuterol (Proventil) in aerosol treatments may be useful in infants with wheezing.
   d. Other bronchodilator aerosols that may be used include cromolyn (Intal) and terbutaline (Brethine).
4. Fluid restriction will help reduce pulmonary edema and right-sided heart failure.
5. Cardiac evaluation for complications.
   a. Cor pulmonale (right ventricular hypertrophy) is a result of pulmonary hypertension and can be seen in BPD infants.
   b. EKG and echocardiography should be performed monthly to evaluate for right ventricular hypertrophy.

6. Optimize nutrition.
   a. Provide increased calories to compensate for increased work of breathing and fluid restriction.
   b. Optimal nutrition is needed for growth and healing of the lungs.
   c. Use of 24 calorie per ounce (or higher) formula is needed to help keep fluid intake low.
7. Chest physiotherapy and suctioning are helpful to loosen and remove bronchial secretions.
8. Evaluate infant for tracheostomy.
   a. Usually done after 6–8 weeks of assisted ventilation and an inability to wean off the ventilator.
   b. Reduces risk of airway complications (e.g., tracheomalacia, bronchomalacia).
   c. Advantages.
      (1) Cannot slip into the bronchus.
      (2) Infant able to feed orally.
      (3) Easily replaced.
      (4) Infant can be handled and held more easily.
      (5) Decreased airway resistance.
   d. Disadvantages.
      (1) Postoperative difficulties such as bleeding, infection, and air leak.
      (2) Long-term commitment to tracheostomy (months to years).
      (3) Delayed speech.
      (4) Skin problems and infection.
      (5) May make home care difficult or even impossible, necessitating prolonged hospitalization.
9. Team approach to care.
   a. Involve parents early in care.
   b. Consistent nursing care.
   c. Detailed care plan outlining infant's personality and developmental care needs.
   d. Utilize occupational therapy and physical therapy as necessary.
   e. The physician, nurses, and parents need to communicate openly and often concerning infant's conditions and plan of care.
10. Use of steroids.
    a. Use in treatment of BPD remains controversial.
    b. May aid by increasing compliance and ability to wean from the ventilator faster.
    c. Main complication in treated infants is high infection rate.
    d. Side effects of steroid therapy include systemic hypertension, glucose instability, and growth failure.
    e. Dexamethasone has been used successfully in controlled studies (Avery et al., 1985; Mammel et al., 1983).

I. Outcome.
1. Mortality rate of 30–40% has been reported.
   a. Most of these infants die while still in nursery.
   b. All have advanced BPD.
   c. Death is due to infection or respiratory failure.
2. After discharge, mortality rate is <10%.
   a. Usually not due to respiratory failure.
   b. Complications such as cor pulmonale or infection are the usual causes of death.
3. Many infants will be discharged home on oxygen.
4. Recurrent pulmonary infections and growth retardation are seen commonly among survivors (Gibson et al., 1988; Markestad and Fitzhardinge, 1981; Yu et al., 1983).
5. Gradual improvement is seen during the first 2 years of life, but pulmonary

function and chest x-rays continue to remain abnormal for many years (Griscom, et al., 1989; Nickerson, 1990).
6. Neurological and developmental sequelae can occur in BPD survivors.
   a. Severe handicaps have been reported as low as 6–10% and as high as 60–80% of infants with BPD (Fitzhardinge and Markestad, 1981; Hakulinen, et al., 1988; Vohr, 1982).
   b. These handicaps are thought to be related to the early neonatal course rather than to BPD.

Chronic Lung Disease in Premature Infants

A. Definition.
1. Changes in pulmonary structure and function without underlying disease.
2. Majority of cases are seen in infants weighing <1500 g.
3. Has been called pulmonary insufficiency of prematurity, chronic pulmonary insufficiency of prematurity (CPIP), and Wilson-Mikity syndrome (W-MS) (Burnard et al., 1965; Krauss et al., 1975; Wilson and Mikity, 1960).
4. W-MS was first described in the late 1950s and early 1960s before the use of assisted ventilation, and CPIP was described in 1975.

B. Incidence. Incidence is unknown because assisted ventilation has become routine in the treatment of symptomatic premature infants. Makes differentiation from BPD difficult.

C. Etiology/pathophysiology.
1. Abnormal distribution of air (overexpansion and atelectasis) due to characteristics of the premature lung best describes pulmonary insufficiency in premature infants.
2. At the end of the first week, the functional residual capacity (FRC) decreases, resulting in hypoxia and hypercapnia.
3. Premature infants respond to the preceding with apnea and atelectasis.
4. In some infants, this will progress to radiographic cystic appearance seen after the first month typical of W-MS.

D. Clinical presentation/diagnosis.
1. These forms of chronic lung disease can be seen in very premature infants with minimal exposure to increased oxygen.
2. Symptoms appear usually at 7–10 days of life.
3. Symptoms seen early are transient cyanosis, hyperpnea, and retractions.
4. Symptoms increase in severity for 2–6 weeks.
5. Chest x-ray shows cystic changes or may be normal.
6. There is increasing O_2 dependency and CO_2 retention.

E. Management.
1. Supportive.
   a. Give oxygen to maintain normal Pao_2.
   b. Chest physiotherapy.
   c. IV fluids.
   d. Employ all other supportive measures mentioned in previous sections (e.g., temperature, electrolytes, etc.).

F. Outcome.
1. Mortality rates of 10–30% have been reported with these forms of chronic lung disease.
2. Generally there is complete clearing by 2–6 months.
3. Often resolves with growth.

Air Leaks

A. **Definition.**
1. Pulmonary air leak describes several conditions that can occur spontaneously or as a secondary cause, usually when assisted ventilation is used.
2. Commonly recognized air leaks. (Refer to Chapter 33.)
   a. Pneumomediastinum: air accumulated in anterior mediastinum.
   b. Pneumothorax.
      (1) Air collection between parietal and visceral pleura.
      (2) May be unilateral or bilateral.
   c. Pneumopericardium: air is trapped between the heart and the pericardial sac.
   d. Pneumoperitoneum: air that enters the peritoneal space via the posterior mediastinal openings in the diaphragm.
   e. Pulmonary interstitial emphysema (PIE).
      (1) Small areas of extra-alveolar air scattered in pulmonary tissue.
      (2) May localize in one lobe or occur diffusely.
      (3) May progress to pneumothorax and/or pneumomediastinum.

B. **Incidence.**
1. Pneumothorax and pneumomediastinum.
   a. Occur spontaneously in 0.5–1% of normal term infants.
   b. Incidence increases to 4% in RDS cases.
   c. Use of CPAP will increase risk to 15% and with assisted ventilation as high as 20–25% (Philip, 1987).
2. There are no statistics for pneumopericardium or pneumoperitoneum. Both conditions are rare; however, the risk increases with the use of assisted ventilation.
3. There are no statistics for PIE, but it is seen frequently with assisted ventilation.

C. **Pathophysiology.**
1. Air leaks are generally iatrogenic, resulting from the use of excessive airway pressure during resuscitation or with assisted ventilation.
2. Can occur spontaneously if there is uneven air distribution at birth.
   a. Some areas are expanded, while others remain collapsed.
   b. Infant will generate pressure to expand unopened areas, leading to greater pressure in already expanded areas, resulting in an air leak.
3. Frequently there is underlying lung disease present.
   a. Obstructive: such as ball-valve air-trapping seen with MAS.
   b. Poor lung compliance: such as seen with RDS.

D. **Clinical presentation/diagnosis.** (See also Chapter 33 for X-ray presentation.)
1. Pneumothorax.
   a. Considered when there is a sudden deterioration in the condition of the infant.
   b. Useful signs include decreased breath sounds on the affected side, hypotension, skin mottling, and shift of the mediastinum (detected by shift of point of maximal cardiac impulse on auscultation) to the unaffected side.
   c. Chest x-ray should be taken as soon as possible.
   d. Transillumination (translucent glow when fiberoptic light is placed against the skin) of the chest wall may confirm presence of pneumothorax without having to wait for a chest x-ray.
   e. If the air leak is small, may be asymptomatic.
2. Pneumomediastinum.
   a. Should be anticipated with MAS.
   b. Signs include increased anteroposterior diameter of chest and indistinct heart sounds.

c. Chest x-ray will show "sail sign" indicating elevation of thymus (surrounded by air).

3. Pneumopericardium.
   a. Immediate presentation with hypotension, muffled heart sound, and bradycardia from cardiac tamponade.
   b. Is life threatening.

4. Pneumoperitoneum.
   a. Must be careful to determine if air on x-ray is from a pulmonary complication or from rupture of abdominal wall.
   b. This complication usually does not require surgical intervention unless it is a result of abdominal wall rupture.
   c. Usually seen in conjunction with a large pneumothorax and pneumomediastinum.

5. Pulmonary interstitial emphysema (PIE).
   a. Difficult to interpret.
   b. Limited to infants with poor lung compliance receiving continuous positive airway pressure or positive-pressure ventilation.
   c. Can only be diagnosed by chest x-ray.
   d. Chest x-ray shows microcystic areas throughout one or both lungs; may show hyperinflated lungs and flattened diaphragm.
   e. May progress to pneumomediastinum and/or pneumothorax.
   f. Hypoxia and hypercapnia are commonly present with FIO_2 and high pressure.

E. Management.

1. Pneumothorax.
   a. If asymptomatic, will often resolve without treatment.
   b. Symptomatic (tension) pneumothorax requires emergency removal of air.
      (1) Thoracentesis (needle aspiration to remove air): may be necessary if infant has acutely deteriorated until a chest tube can be placed.
      (2) Usually accomplished by placement of a thoracostomy tube (multiple-holed tube) in anterior chest and connected to underwater seal drainage system with continuous negative pressure of 10–15 cm H_2O.
      (3) Thoracostomy tube is left in place until air ceases to bubble from the chest tube for at least 24 hours and pneumothorax is resolved by chest x-ray. The chest tube is then clamped and the infant is observed for signs of reaccumulation of air. The chest tube is removed 12–24 hours after the tube has been clamped if the infant remains asymptomatic.
      (4) In asymptomatic infants or non-ventilated infants, administration of 100% oxygen will aid the absorption of the air in the pneumothorax by the pleural capillaries. Due to the toxic effects of oxygen, this treatment is not recommended for pre-term infants.

2. Pneumomediastinum.
   a. Usually is not treated.
   b. If associated with pneumothorax (common occurrence), high oxygen concentration will help resolve as described above.

3. Pneumopericardium.
   a. Emergency treatment is required.
   b. Air removal is accomplished by placement of a long catheter or chest tube into the pericardial sac (there will be a gush of air when sac is entered) with constant application of gentle negative pressure.
   c. The pericardial tube should be connected to underwater drainage, because pneumopericardium may reoccur.

4. Pneumoperitoneum.
   a. Careful diagnosis to determine if air is from rupture of an abdominal origin or from an extension of a pneumothorax.
   b. Surgery is rarely needed due to a pulmonary complication.
   c. If due to an extension of a pneumothorax, treatment will be as above.

d. If diaphragmatic movement is compromised, needle aspiration as previously described will be necessary.
5. PIE.
  a. If unilateral and persistent, intubation of a mainstem bronchus supplying opposite lung may show improvement in condition.
  b. If bilateral, supportive treatment is given (oxygen, ventilation, fluids, etc.).
  c. Minimize positive inspiratory pressure and shorten inspiratory time.
  d. High-frequency ventilation.
  e. Place affected side in dependent position.

F. **Outcome.**
1. Outcome depends on underlying lung pathology.
2. Mortality is high with pneumopericardium, bilateral pneumothoraces, and bilateral PIE.
3. In survivors of bilateral PIE, the risk of chronic lung disease is high.

Pulmonary Hypoplasia

A. **Definition:** defective or inhibited growth of the lungs.

B. **Pathophysiology.**
1. Conditions that compress and limit lung growth are one cause of pulmonary hypoplasia (e.g., diaphragmatic hernia).
2. Conditions that result in oligohydramnios (e.g., renal disorders, amniotic fluid leakage) are associated with pulmonary hypoplasia due to thoracic compression.
3. Associated congenital malformations should be considered, such as renal dysgenesis (Potter's syndrome), phrenic nerve absence, and vertebral and chromosomal anomalies.

C. **Diagnosis.**
1. Often very difficult to diagnose.
2. Any of the above conditions should suggest pulmonary hypoplasia.
3. Usually present with severe respiratory distress.
4. Higher than usual pressures are needed for ventilation. Pneumothorax is common.
5. Hypercapnia may be difficult or impossible to treat early in the infant's course.
6. Chest x-ray will usually show decreased volume of the thorax.
7. May see symptoms of PPHN.

D. **Management.**
1. Cannot prevent development of the problem at present.
2. Treatment is supportive and directed at respiratory failure.
  a. Assisted ventilation.
  b. Treatment of PPHN.
  c. Extracorporeal membrane oxygenation (ECMO) if disorder is reversible.

E. **Outcome.**
1. Degree of hypoplasia determines outcome.
2. Mortality rate is high and may also be affected by cause of the hypoplasia.
3. Management is difficult, but infant can function adequately if treatment and support can be continued until lung growth occurs, although this is rare.

Pulmonary Hemorrhage

A. **Definition.**
1. Localized areas of bleeding into alveoli (generally found at autopsy).
2. Can be a massive generalized bleeding event.

B. Etiology/pathophysiology.
1. Usually occurs as a complication of other disorders, such as:
   a. Pneumonia.
   b. Sepsis.
   c. Hemolytic disease.
   d. Kernicterus.
   e. CNS hemorrhage.
   f. Congenital heart disease.
   g. Patent ductus arteriosus with a large left-to-right shunt.
2. May be due to trauma from improper suctioning technique.

C. Clinical presentation.
1. May present with sudden, severe respiratory distress.
2. Bright red blood can be suctioned from the trachea.

D. Management.
1. Use of assisted ventilation is necessary to maintain gas exchange.
2. Transfusion of whole blood.
3. Identify any clotting abnormalities and treat.
4. Treat underlying disease.

E. Outcome.
1. If bleeding is massive, death will occur quickly despite vigorous management.
2. If hemorrhage is small or isolated, infant will recover and outcome will be more dependent on underlying disease.

Non-Respiratory Causes of Respiratory Distress

A. Upper airway disorders.
1. Choanal atresia.
   a. Protrusion of bone or membrane into nasal passages causing blockage or narrowing.
   b. If condition is bilateral, gasping respirations and cyanosis occur immediately after birth.
   c. Signs of distress are intermittent when condition is unilateral.
   d. Failure to pass a catheter through the nasal passages to the posterior oropharynx will make the diagnosis.
   e. Initially treat by placing infant in prone position with a large oral airway taped securely in place (an endotracheal tube can be used if placement of an oral airway is difficult).
   f. Surgical correction of the problem is necessary and consists of perforation of the obstruction and serial dilation by use of obturators.
2. Micrognathia.
   a. Defined as mandibular undergrowth.
   b. Occurs with certain syndromes such as Pierre-Robin, trisomy 18, trisomy 22, cri du chat 5P.
   c. Airway distress may be alleviated by prone positioning and the head placed downward.
   d. Use of an oral airway or endotracheal tube will provide an open airway.
   e. Humidification will be needed if an endotracheal tube is in place to prevent the drying of secretions.
   f. Surgery may be necessary.
3. Cystic hygroma.
   a. Benign water cysts occurring most frequently in the neck (80%) but can also be found in the groin, axilla, and mediastinum.
   b. Usually seen at birth.
   c. Mass will occupy the submandibular region and may compromise the airway.

d. Symptoms depend on the size and location.
e. Treatment is related to complications.
(1) If infant is asymptomatic, surgical excision is performed between 4 and 12 months of age.
(2) Excision must be performed at an earlier age if the airway is compromised or if recurrent infections occur.
(3) Multiple excisions are usually performed to prevent damage to nerves and vascular structures.
4. Obstruction of larynx or trachea.
a. Stridor is a major symptom and usually requires no specific treatment, but mechanical causes must be ruled out.
b. Direct laryngoscopy will reveal structural abnormalities such as polyps, webs, and granulomas.
c. Hemangiomas of the larynx or trachea may cause obstruction.
d. Extrinsic compression of the upper airway occurs with thyroglossal duct cyst, cervical neuroblastoma, vascular ring, and double aortic arch.
e. Laryngotracheomalacia results from collapse of the larynx and cervical trachea producing stridor; usually self-limiting and resolves by 6–12 months of age, when the tracheal diameter increases and the cartilage matures.
5. Tracheoesophageal fistula. (Refer to Chapter 13.)

B. Thoracic disorders.
1. Cystic adenomatoid malformation.
a. Intrapulmonary mass consisting of multiple small cysts.
b. Respiratory distress may be seen in newborns, or the malformation may cause no symptoms.
c. May be confused with diaphragmatic hernia on x-ray.
d. Treatment of choice is surgical excision of the involved lobe.
2. Bronchogenic cyst.
a. Mucus-producing cyst.
b. May cause tracheal, bronchial, or esophageal obstruction.
c. Distress usually not severe.
d. Treatment is surgical excision.
3. Congenital lobar emphysema.
a. Overdistention of one or more lobes of the lung (upper lobes generally affected, 10% seen in the right middle lobe).
b. Inability of the lung to deflate properly, possibly due to a defect in bronchial cartilage.
c. May produce severe respiratory distress within hours of birth but usually is delayed for weeks or months.
d. Chest x-ray is diagnostic. (Refer to Chapter 33.)
e. Surgical resection is the treatment of choice.
4. Chondrodystrophies.
a. Group of disorders of bone growth resulting in short stature.
b. Respiratory distress may be seen due to small thoracic cavities.
c. Treatment will be based on degree of distress.
5. Neuromuscular disorders.
a. Conditions resulting in hypotonia, such as spinal muscular atrophy and myotonic dystrophy, result in varying degrees of respiratory distress.
b. Management will depend on degree of distress.

C. Central nervous system disorders.
1. Seizures.
2. Hypoxic-ischemic injury.
3. Intracranial hemorrhages.
a. Subdural.
b. Subarachnoid.
c. Periventricular-intraventricular.
d. Intracerebellar.

4. Drugs.
5. Meningitis.
6. Respiratory distress may vary from mild to severe.
7. Treatment related to underlying cause.

D. **Cardiovascular and hematological disorders.**
1. Congenital heart disease.
2. Anemia.
3. Polycythemia.
4. Shock.
5. Sepsis.
6. Respiratory distress may vary from mild to severe.
7. Treatment related to underlying cause.

E. **Diaphragmatic disorders.**
1. Diaphragmatic hernia.
2. Diaphragmatic paralysis.
   a. May be unilateral or bilateral.
   b. Due to phrenic nerve palsy.
   c. Diagnosis made by use of fluoroscopy.
   d. Surgical plication is the treatment.
3. Diaphragmatic eventration.
   a. Incomplete development of diaphragm.
   b. May be symptom-free into adulthood.
   c. In newborns, symptoms may resemble those of diaphragmatic hernia.
   d. Chest x-ray and fluoroscopy will confirm diagnosis.
   e. Treatment consists of plication of the elevated leaf of diaphragm.

F. **Renal disorders.**
1. Pulmonary hypoplasia; results from renal agenesis or renal dysgenesis (see previous section).
2. These conditions are usually untreatable, and death will occur within hours or days.

STUDY QUESTIONS

1. An accurate indicator of lung maturity is:
   a. A lecithin/sphingomyelin ratio <2:1.
   b. The presence of meconium in the amniotic fluid.
   c. The presence of phosphatidylglycerol.

2. Which of the following is associated with persistent pulmonary hypertension of the newborn?
   a. Maternal analgesia.
   b. Neonatal anemia.
   c. Perinatal asphyxia.

3. Respiratory distress syndrome is common in which one of the following conditions?
   a. 38th week in term infants.
   b. Growth-retarded infants.
   c. Infants of diabetic mothers.

4. A cause of transient tachypnea of the newborn is:
   a. Congenital disease.

   b. Pulmonary hypertension.
   c. Retained lung fluid.

5. A contributing cause of meconium aspiration is:
   a. Perinatal stress.
   b. Post-dates.
   c. Pulmonary hypoplasia.

6. A cause of bronchopulmonary dysplasia is:
   a. Congenital anomalies.
   b. Poor nutrition.
   c. Prolonged assisted ventilation.

7. Which of the following is not an air leak?
   a. Pneumothorax.
   b. Pneumatosis intestinalis.
   c. Pulmonary interstitial emphysema.

8. Pulmonary hypoplasia is associated with:
   a. Diaphragmatic hernia.
   b. Hyaline membrane disease.
   c. Polyhydramnios.

Answers to Study Questions

1. c	4. c	7. b
2. c	5. a	8. a
3. c	6. c	

REFERENCES

Argyle, J.C.: Pulmonary hypoplasia in infants with giant abdominal wall defects. Pediatr. Pathol., 9(1):43–55, 1989.

Avery, G.B., Fletcher, A.B., Kaplan, K., and Brudno, D.S.: Controlled trial of dexamethasone in respirator-dependent infants with bronchopulmonary dysplasia. Pediatrics, 75:106–111, 1985.

Bancalari, E., and Gerhardt, T.: Bronchopulmonary dysplasia. Pediatr. Clin. North Am., 33(1):1–20, 1986.

Bancalari, E., Abdenour, G.E., Feller, R., and Gannon, J.: BPD: Clinical presentation. J. Pediatr., 95:819–823, 1979.

Banerjee, C.K., Girling, D.J., and Wigglesworth, J.S.: Pulmonary fibroplasia in newborn babies treated with oxygen and artificial ventilation. Arch. Dis. Child., 47(254):509–518, 1972.

Bartlett, R.H., Andrews, A.F., Toomasian, J.M., et al.: Extracorporeal membrane oxygenation for newborn respiratory failure. Forty-five cases. Surgery, 92:425–433, 1982.

Block, M.F., Kling, O.R., and Crosby, W.M.: Antenatal glucocorticoid therapy for the prevention of respiratory distress syndrome in the premature infant. Obstet. Gynecol., 50(2):186–190, 1977.

Blott, M., and Greenough, A.: Neonatal outcome after prolonged rupture of the membranes starting in the second trimester. Arch. Dis. Child., 63(10 Spec. No.):1146–1150, 1988.

Boat, R., Kleinerman, J., Fanaroff, A., and Matthews, J.: Toxic effects of oxygen on culture of human neonatal respiratory epithelium. Pediatr. Res., 7(7):607–615, 1973.

Brown, E.R., Stark, A., and Sosenko, I.: Bronchopulmonary dysplasia: Possible relationship to pulmonary edema. J. Pediatr., 92:982–984, 1978.

Burnard, E.D., Grattan-Smith, P., Picton-Warlow, C.G., and Grauaug, A.: Pulmonary insufficiency in prematurity. Austral. Pediatr. J., 1:12, 1965.

Caspi, E., Schreyer, P., Weintraub, Z., et al.: Prevention of the respiratory distress syndrome in premature infants by antepartum glucocorticoid therapy. Br. J. Obstet. Gynecol., 83(3):187–193, 1976.

Chernick, V.: Fetal breathing movements and the onset of breathing at birth. Clin. Perinatol., 5:257–268, 1978.

Crapo, J.D., Barry, B.E., Foscue, H.A., and Shelburn, J.: Structural and biochemical changes in rat lungs occurring during exposures to lethal and adaptive doses of oxygen. Am. Rev. Respir. Dis., 122(1):123–143, 1980.

Durand, D.J., and Kao, L.C.: Pharmacologic treatment of bronchopulmonary dysplasia. In Lund, C.H. (Ed.): Bronchopulmonary Dysplasia: Strategies for Total Patient Care. Petaluma, Neonatal Network, 1990, pp. 55–74.

Edwards, D.K., Dyer, W., and Northway, W.H., Jr.: Twelve years experience with BPD. Pediatrics, 59(6):839–846, 1977.

Frank, L., and Groseclose, E.E.: Preparation for birth into an O_2 rich environment: The antioxidant enzymes in the developing rabbit. Pediatr. Res., 18:240–244, 1984.

Gamsu, H.P., Mullinger, B.M., Donnai, P., and Dash, C.H.: Antenatal administration of betamethasone to prevent respiratory distress syndrome in preterm infants: Report of a UK multicentre trial. Br. J. Obstet. Gynecol., 96(4):401–410, 1989.

Gay, J.H., Dailey, W.G.R., Meyer, B.H.P., et al.: Ligation of the patent ductus arteriosus in premature infants. J. Pediatr. Surg., 8:677, 1973.

Gibson, R.L., Jackson, J.C., Twiggs, G.A., et al.: Bronchopulmonary dysplasia. Survival after prolonged mechanical ventilation. Am. J. Dis. Child., 142(7):721–725, 1988.

Griscom, N.T., Wheeler, W.B., Sweezy, N.B., et al.: Bronchopulmonary dysplasia: Radiographic appearance in middle childhood. Radiology, 171(3):811–814, 1989.

Guzzetta, P.C., Randolph, J.C., Anderson, K.D., et al.: Surgery of the neonate. In Avery, G.B. (Ed.): Neonatology: Pathophysiology and Management of the Newborn, 3rd ed. Philadelphia, J.B. Lippincott, 1986, pp. 950–952.

Hakulinen, A., Heinonen, K., Jokela, V., and Kiekara, O.: Occurrence, predictive factors and associated morbidity of bronchopulmonary dysplasia in a preterm birth cohort. J. Perinat. Med., 16(5–6):437–446, 1988.

Halliday, H.L., McClure, G., and Reid, M. (Eds.): Handbook of Neonatal Intensive Care, 2nd ed. London, Bailliere Tindall, 1985.

Hazebroek, F.W., Tibball, D., Bos, A.P., et al.: Congenital diaphragmatic hernia: Impact of preoperative stabilization. A prospective study in 13 patients. J. Pediatr. Surg., 213(12):1139–1146, 1988.

Hodson, W.A., and Truog, W.E.: Critical Care of the Newborn, 2nd ed. Philadelphia, W.B. Saunders Co., 1989.

Hufnagle, K.G., Khan, S.N., Penn, D., et al.: Renal complication of long-term furosemide treatment in preterm infants. Pediatrics, 70:360–363, 1983.

Johnston, P.W., Bashner, B., Liberman, R., et al.: Clinical use of extracorporeal membrane oxygenation in the treatment of persistent pulmonary hypertension following surgical repair of congenital diaphragmatic hernia. J. Pediatr. Surg., 23(10):908–912, 1988.

Kao, L.C., Warburton, D., Cheng, W.H., et al.: Effect of oral diuretics on pulmonary mechanics in infants with chronic BPD: Results of a double-blind crossover trial. Pediatrics, 74:37–44, 1984.

Krauss, A.N., Klain, D.B., and Auld, P.A.M.: Chronic pulmonary insufficiency of prematurity. Pediatrics, 55(1):55–58, 1975.

Langham, M.R., Jr., Krummel, T.M., Greenfield, L.J., et al.: Extracorporeal membrane oxygenation following repair of congenital diaphragmatic hernias. Ann. Thoracic Surg., 44(3):247–252, 1987.

Leavitt, A.M., Watchko, J.F., Bennett, F.C., and Folsom, R.C.: Neurodevelopmental outcome following persistent pulmonary hypertension of the neonate. J. Perinatol., 7(4):288–291, 1987.

Levin, D., Gates, L., Newfeld, E., et al.: Persistence of the cardiopulmonary circulatory pathway: Survival of an infant after a prolonged course. Pediatrics, 56:58–64, 1975.

Lewis, J.M., and Sammons, W.A.H.: Premature Babies: A Different Beginning. St. Louis, C.V. Mosby, 1985.

Liggins, C.G., and Howie, R.N.: A controlled trial of antepartum glucocorticoid treatment for prevention of the respiratory distress syndrome in premature infants. Pediatrics, 50(4):515–525, 1972.

Mammel, M.C., Johnson, D.E., Green, T.P., and Thompson, T.R.: Controlled trial of dexamethasone therapy in infants with bronchopulmonary dysplasia. Lancet, 2:1356–1358, 1983.

Markestad, T., and Fitzhardinge, P.M.: Growth and development in children recovering from BPD. J. Pediatr., 98:597–602, 1981.

Merritt, T.A., Cochrane, C.G., Holcomb, K., et al.: Elastase and alpha-proteinase inhibitor activity during respiratory distress syndrome in the pathogenesis of bronchopulmonary dysplasia: Role of inflammation. J. Clin. Invest., 72:656–666, 1983.

Naulty, C.M., Horn, S., Conry J., and Avery, G.B.: Improved lung compliance after ligation of patent ductus arteriosus in hyaline membrane disease. J. Pediatr., 93:682, 1978.

Nickerson, B.: BPD, chronic pulmonary disease following neonatal respiratory failure. Chest, 87:528–535, 1985.

Nickerson, B.: An overview of bronchopulmonary dysplasia: Pathogenesis and current therapy. In Lund, C.H. (Ed.): Bronchopulmonary Dysplasia: Strategies for Total Patient Care. Petaluma, Neonatal Network, 1990, pp. 1–15.

Northway, W.H., Rosan, R.C., and Porter, D.Y.: Pulmonary disease following respiratory therapy of hyaline-membrane disease. N. Engl. J. Med., 276:357–368, 1967.

O'Donovan, B.H., and Bell, E.F.: Effects of furosemide on body water compartments in infants with bronchopulmonary dysplasia. Pediatr. Res., 26(2):121–124, 1989.

Papageorgiou, A.N., Doray, J.L., Ardila, R., and Kunos, I.: Reduction of mortality, morbidity and respiratory distress syndrome. Pediatrics, 83(4):493–497, 1989.

Patrick, J., Natale, R., and Richardson, B.: Patterns of human fetal breathing activity at 34–35 weeks gestational age. Am. J. Obstet. Gynecol., 132:507–513, 1978.

Philip, A.G.S.: Neonatology: A Practical Guide, 3rd ed. Philadelphia, W.B. Saunders Co., 1987.

Stahlman, M.L.: Respiratory disorders in the newborn. In Avery, G.B., (Ed.): Neonatology: Pathophysiology and Management of the Newborn, 3rd ed. Philadelphia, J.B. Lippincott, 1986, pp. 418–445.

Stenmark, K.R.: Leukotriene C_4 and D_4 in neonates with hypoxemia and pulmonary hypertension. N. Engl. J. Med., 309:77–80, 1983.

Taghizadeh, A., and Reynolds, E.O.R.: Pathogenesis of BPD following hyaline-membrane disease. Am. J. Pathol., 82(2):241–264, 1976.

Tay-Uyboco, J.S., Kwiatkowski, K., Cates, D.B., et al.: Hypoxic airway constriction in infants of very low birth weight recovering from moderate to severe bronchopulmonary dysplasia. J. Pediatr., 115(3):456–459, 1989.

Toce, S.S., Farrell, P.M., Leavitt, L.A., et al.: Clinical and roentgenographic scoring systems for assessing bronchopulmonary dysplasia. Am. J. Dis. of Child., 138:581–585, 1984.

Vohr, B.R., Bell, C.F., and Oh, W.M.: Infants with BPD: Growth pattern and developmental outcome. Am. J. Dis. Child., 136(5):443–447, 1982.

Watts, J.L., Oriagno, R.L., and Brady, J.P.: Chronic pulmonary disease in neonates after artificial ventilation. Distribution of ventilation and pulmonary interstitial emphysema. Pediatrics, 60:273–281, 1977.

Weber, T.R., Connors, R.H., Pennington, D.G., et al.: Neonatal diaphragmatic hernia. An improving outlook with extracorporeal membrane oxygenation. Arch. Surg., 122(5):615–618, 1987.

Wilson, M.G., and Mikity, V.G.: A new form of respiratory disease in premature infants. Am. J. Dis. Child., 99:489–499, 1960.

Yu, V.Y.H., Orgell, A.A., Lim, S.B., et al.: Growth and development of VLBW infants recovering from BPD. Arch. Dis. Child., 58:791–794, 1983.

Robin Kriedeman

Apnea of the Newborn

Objectives

1. Define the six types of apnea.

2. Identify causes of apnea.

3. Describe the pathogenesis of apnea in the premature infant.

4. Describe the evaluation process for an infant with apnea.

5. Discuss management techniques for controlling apnea.

6. Provide guidelines for the use of home monitoring.

Apnea represents one of the most frequently encountered respiratory problems in the pre-term infant. Why some infants begin having "spells" and others do not remains a mystery, though certain factors have a fairly good predictive value. In general, a clinical presentation within the first 24 hours is usually seen as a symptom of some pathology, whereas apnea later in the neonatal period is most often associated with immaturity. The exact pathways have yet to be distinguished, but apnea could be characterized as the result of an immature respiratory control system exposed to physiological demands it is not equipped to handle. This chapter provides a comprehensive review of apnea and discusses causes, evaluation, and treatment of apnea.

Definitions of Apnea

A. **Periodic breathing.**
1. Periods of apnea (5–10 seconds) followed by periods of ventilation (10–15 seconds). The overall respiratory rate is 30–40 breaths/minute, whereas during the ventilatory interval, the respiratory rate is 50–60 breaths/minute (Avery and Fletcher, 1974).
2. Primarily seen in well, premature infants more than 24 hours old.
3. It is not accompanied by cyanosis and/or change in heart rate.
4. Periodic breathing is more frequent the more immature the infant and becomes dramatically less frequent after 36 weeks' gestation.

5. Forty to fifty per cent of premature infants will exhibit periodic breathing in the neonatal period (Rigatto, 1982).

B. **Apnea.**

1. The cessation of respiratory air flow and/or respiratory movements for 20 seconds or longer.
2. The cessation of respiratory air flow is associated with pallor, bradycardia, cyanosis, oxygen desaturation, or a change in level of consciousness (Fanaroff and Martin, 1987).
3. The vast majority of apneic periods occur in infants who are immature and have no organic disease. Approximately 25% of all infants <2500 g and 80% of infants <1000 g experience apnea during their neonatal course.

Types of Apnea

A. Primary apnea.

1. Cessation of respiratory movements following a period of rapid respiratory effort as a result of asphyxia during the delivery process.
2. Exposure to oxygen and/or stimulation during this period will usually induce respirations.

B. Secondary apnea.

1. When asphyxia is prolonged, a period of deep, gasping respirations occurs with a concomitant fall in blood pressure and heart rate. The gasping becomes weaker and slower and then ceases.
2. At this stage, the infant will not respond to stimulation and will require resuscitation.
3. For every minute in secondary apnea prior to resuscitation, there is a 2 minute delay before gasping is re-established and another 2 minutes before onset of rhythmic respirations.
4. Primary and secondary apnea can be indistinguishable at birth (Bloom and Cropley, 1987; Fanaroff and Martin, 1987).

C. Central apnea.

1. A total absence of air flow and respiratory effort (Krauss, 1986).
2. The cause of central apnea in premature infants is unknown.
3. Contributing factors are thought to include the following (Hodson and Truog, 1989):
   a. Chest wall afferent neuromuscular signals and chest wall stability.
   b. Diaphragmatic fatigue.
   c. The immature paradoxical ventilatory response of the neonate to hypoxia.
   d. Altered levels of local neurotransmitters in the brainstem region of the central nervous system.

D. Obstructive apnea.

1. Absence of air flow with continued respiratory effort associated with blockage of the airway, usually at the level of the pharynx (Anderson et al., 1983; Krauss, 1986; Marchal, et al., 1987; Martin et al., 1986).
2. Flexion of the neck may induce airway obstruction.
3. May result from ineffective air flow at the mouth or nose and may be seen with congenital facial anomalies such as macroglossia (Beckwith-Wiedemann syndrome or congenital hypothyroidism) or micrognathia (Pierre Robin syndrome).
4. Ten percent of all apnea is obstructive in origin.

E. Mixed apnea.

1. A combination of central and obstructive apnea.
2. Fifty percent of all apnea is mixed apnea.

F. Idiopathic or "apnea of prematurity."

1. Diagnosed by excluding pathophysiological processes in the premature infant.
2. Typically associated with periodic breathing (Brazy et al., 1987).

3. Recurrent apnea seen in infants <1.5 kg who are premature and show no other abnormalities.
4. Onset is generally on days 2–5 of life and is rare on the first day. Apnea on the first day may be pathological in origin.
5. Events cease by term in 95% of infants.

Pathogenesis Of Apnea in the Premature Infant

A. Immature central respiratory center.
1. There is decreased afferent traffic secondary to:
   a. Poor CNS myelinization.
   b. Decreased number of synapses.
   c. Decreased dendritic arborization (Gerhardt and Bancalari, 1984a).
2. Decreased amounts of neurotransmitters have been measured in apneic infants and may play an important role in respiratory control (Kattwinkel, 1977).
3. Fluctuating respiratory center output has been implicated.

B. Chemoreceptors.
1. Located in the medulla (central), carotid, and aortic bodies (peripheral), chemoreceptors relay information about pH, Po_2, and Pco_2 via the vagus and glossopharyngeal nerves.
   a. Hypoxemia is sensed peripherally and results in stimulation of these chemoreceptors and an increase in alveolar ventilation. Premature infants with apnea fail to respond to hypoxemia as effectively as infants who are not apneic.
   b. Hypercapnia is sensed centrally. Pre-term infants have a diminished response to hypercapnia, which predisposes them to apnea (Anas and Perkin, 1984). A normal response to an increase in arterial Pco_2 is an increase in minute ventilation. Premature infants exhibit a diminished inspiratory effort and a blunted response to carbon dioxide, resulting in hypoventilation and hypercapnia (Korones, 1986). This blunted response to hypoxia further depresses the respiratory center's sensitivity to elevated levels of carbon dioxide.
2. Factors influencing pH, Po_2, and Pco_2 could effect a change in the type and quality of afferent input and concomitantly affect the efferent output.
3. Biphasic response of the premature to hypoxia.
   a. During the first minute of hypoxia, a brief increase in respiratory rate is seen followed in the next 2–3 minutes by a decrease in respiratory rate, periodic breathing, respiratory depression, and apnea (Kattwinkel, 1977; Krauss, 1986; Martin, et al., 1986).
   b. At 7–18 days post-natal age, an infant can maintain the adult response to hypoxemia of sustained hyperventilation (Martin, et al., 1986).
4. Depressed response to hypercapnia.
   a. The premature infant exhibits decreased sensitivity to increased levels of carbon dioxide, requiring higher levels of carbon dioxide to stimulate respirations (Anderson et al., 1983; Kattwinkel, 1977).

C. Thermal afferents.
1. Apnea is increased in an environment that may be too warm for the infant (Kattwinkel, 1977).
2. Thermal receptors in the trigeminal area of the face produce an apneic response to stimulation by a cold gas mixture (Marchal et al., 1987).

D. Mechanoreceptors.
1. Stretch receptors alter the timing of respiration at various lung volumes.
   a. Head's paradoxical reflex: a gasp followed by apnea after abrupt lung inflation.
   b. Hering-Breuer reflex.

(1) Vagally mediated, it acts to inhibit inspiration and/or prolong expiration.

(2) Shortens expiratory time at low lung volumes to maintain lung volumes and concomitantly increase respiratory rate (Marchal et al., 1987; Martin et al., 1986).

(3) Prolongs expiratory time at high lung volumes.

2. Pharyngeal collapse and airway obstruction: produced by negative pharyngeal pressure generated during inspiration (Martin et al., 1986).

3. Intercostal phrenic inhibitory reflex: inward movement of the ribcage during inspiration prematurely ends inspiration (Martin et al., 1986).

E. Protective reflexes.

1. Stimulation of the posterior pharynx with suctioning, endotracheal or gavage tube placement, or gastroesophageal reflux can stimulate apnea (Marchal et al., 1987; Rigatto, 1982).

2. Pulmonary irritant receptors can produce an apneic response to direct bronchial stimulation (Martin et al., 1986).

3. Laryngeal taste receptors can produce an apneic response to various chemical stimuli (Kattwinkel, 1977).

F. Sleep state.

1. Eighty per cent of a neonate's day is spent in sleep.

2. Respiratory depression has been found to occur predominantly during REM or transitional sleep (Anderson et al., 1983).

   a. May be influenced by central mechanisms at the level of the brainstem (Martin et al., 1986).

      (1) May be due to a defect in a sleep-related feedback loop or respiratory command (Kriter and Blanchard, 1989).

      (2) Rigatto (1982) showed that 1–4 week old prematures maintained a hyperventilatory response to hypoxia in quiet sleep but a biphasic response in REM sleep (Anderson et al., 1983).

   b. May be related to paradoxical respirations in which chest wall movements are out of phase resulting in ribcage collapse with abdominal expansion during inspiration. This would lead to a decrease in lung volume and functional residual capacity.

   c. May be related to decreased skeletal muscle tone of the tongue and pharynx during sleep, which could lead to increased resistance and obstruction in the upper airway (Spitzer and Fox, 1986).

Causes of Apnea

A. Prematurity.

B. Hypoxia.

C. Respiratory disorders.

1. Respiratory distress syndrome.
2. Pneumonia.
3. Aspiration.
4. Acidosis.
5. Airway obstruction.
6. Pneumothorax.
7. Atelectasis.
8. Pulmonary hemorrhage.
9. Post-extubation.
10. Congenital anomalies of the upper airway.

D. Cardiovascular disorders.

1. Hypotension
2. Arrhythmias.
3. Congestive heart failure.

4. Patent ductus arteriosus.

E. **Infection.**
1. Sepsis.
2. Pneumonia.
3. Meningitis.
4. Viral infections.
5. Necrotizing enterocolitis.

F. **Central nervous system disorders.**
1. Congenital malformations.
2. Seizures.
3. Asphyxia.
4. Intracranial hemorrhage.
5. Kernicterus.
6. Tumors.

G. **Drugs.**
1. Maternal drugs.
   a. Narcotics.
   b. Analgesics.
   c. Anesthesia.
   d. Beta-blocker hypertensives.
   e. Magnesium sulfate.
2. Neonatal drugs.
   a. Anticonvulsants.
      (1) Phenobarbital, pentobarbital.
   b. Cardiovascular
      (1) Prostaglandin E.
   c. Narcotics/analgesics.
      (1) Fentanyl (Sublimaze), morphine, midazolan hydrochloride (Versed), lorazepam (Ativan).

H. **Metabolic.**
1. Hypocalcemia.
2. Hypoglycemia.
3. Hypomagnesemia.
4. Hyponatremia.
5. Acidosis.
6. Hyperammonemia.

I. **Hematopoietic.**
1. Polycythemia.
2. Anemia.

J. **Reflex stimulation.**
1. Posterior pharyngeal stimulation.
2. Gastroesophageal reflux.

K. **Environmental.**
1. Rapid warming.
2. Hypothermia.
3. Hyperthermia.
4. Elevated environmental temperature.
5. Feeding.
6. Stooling.
7. Painful stimuli.

Evaluation of Apnea

A. **History.**
1. Perinatal risk factors.
   a. Maternal bleeding, drugs, fever, hypertension, prolonged rupture of mem-

branes, polyhydramnios, chorioamnionitis, decreased fetal movements, abnormal fetal presentation.
    b. Fetal hypoxia, asphyxia, trauma.
2. Neonatal risk factors:
    a. Prematurity.
    b. Cardiorespiratory disease.
    c. Metabolic abnormalities.
    d. Temperature instability.
    e. Infection.
    f. Environmental causes.
    g. CNS disorders.

B. **Physical examination.** A complete physical and neurological examination should be performed. Observe for signs of respiratory distress, heart disease, and congenital malformations. Behavior, abnormal tone, or posturing may suggest a neurological focus. An abdominal examination should also be performed, which may reveal symptoms related to obstruction, infection, necrotizing enterocolitis, or congestive heart failure.

C. **Documentation of apneic episodes.** A record of apneic episodes should be maintained as a part of the infant's record. This allows the caregiver to determine a pattern (if any) to the apnea. It may also provide information to precipitating events or specific events that the apnea may be associated with. Information should include the following:
1. Length of apneic episode.
2. Time of apneic episode and any relation to feeding (before, during, or after), sleep procedures, activity, or stooling.
3. Infant's position: prone, supine, head of bed elevated or flat.
4. Associated bradycardia.
5. Associated color change.
6. Type of stimulation needed to resolve the apneic episode.
    a. Self-resolved episode.
    b. Gentle tactile stimulation.
    c. Vigorous tactile stimulation.
    d. Oxygen.
    e. Bag/mask ventilation.

D. **Laboratory work-up.**
1. Basic laboratory work-up: evaluates for infection, respiratory alteration, and basic metabolic problems.
    a. CBC with differential and platelets.
    b. Blood gases.
    c. Glucose, electrolytes, calcium.
    d. Blood culture, spinal tap, urine culture.
2. Extensive laboratory work-up: evaluates for less common causes of apnea.
    a. Toxicology screen.
    b. Urine for metabolic screen (amino acids, organic acids).
    c. Serum ammonia.

E. **Other.**
1. EKG/echocardiogram: may detect cardiac abnormality or conduction disturbances.
2. EEG: may confirm suspected seizures.
3. Chest x-ray: may demonstrate cardiac or respiratory abnormalities.
4. Cranial ultrasound/CT scan: to evaluate the CNS system for structural abnormalities or intracranial hemorrhages.
5. Barium swallow/pH study: to evaluate pharyngeal function or gastroesophageal reflux.
6. Polysomnogram: examines eye movements, muscle activity, end-tidal CO_2, transcutaneous O_2 levels, oral or nasal airway, chest and abdominal wall move-

ment, and cardiorespiratory patterns to detect type of apnea and relate it to sleep state (Kriter and Blanchard, 1989).
7. Pneumogram.
   a. Measures chest wall movement, heart rate, oxygen saturations, nasal air flow by thermistry or carbon dioxide probe, and esophageal pH; it is useful in detecting types of apnea, amount of periodic breathing, bradycardia, and oxygen desaturations (Krauss, 1986; Spitzer and Fox, 1986).
   b. Not proved to have predictive value in distinguishing infants at risk for sudden infant death syndrome (SIDS) (NIH, 1986).

Management Techniques

A. Treat specific disease or underlying cause.

B. Provide needed medical or surgical intervention.

C. Provide environmental temperature at the low end of the neutral thermal zone (Kattwinkel, 1977; Marchal et al., 1987).

D. Avoid triggering reflexes:
1. Vigorous catheter suctioning.
2. Hot or cold to the face.
3. Sudden gastric distention.

E. Maintain infant in prone position whenever possible. Prone positioning is associated with higher oxygen tension, shorter gastric emptying time, and decreased incidence of regurgitation and aspiration (Marchal et al., 1987).

F. Place a neck roll under the infant's neck and shoulders to decrease neck flexion and prevent airway obstruction when in the supine position.

G. Avoid vigorous manual ventilation to prevent intermittent hyperoxia and blunting of CO_2 response of the infant.

H. Cutaneous stimulation increases the number of external stimuli to compensate for decreased afferent signals to the respiratory center (Marchal et al., 1987).
1. Irregularly oscillating water bed.
2. Rocking bed.
3. Touch.

I. Painful stimuli, loud noises, extremely vigorous tactile stimulation, or potent odors should be avoided in attempting to manage apnea.

J. Continuous positive airway pressure (CPAP).
1. Increases end-expiratory lung volumes and splints the upper airway and weak chest wall, thus improving compliance and oxygenation and decreasing respiratory muscle work, so that diaphragmatic movements are less tiring and more effective (Marchal et al., 1987; Martin et al. 1986).
2. Complicates gavage feedings and may increase risk of aspiration.

K. Pharmacological therapy.
1. Methylxanthine therapy (aminophylline/theophylline, caffeine), administered either orally or intravenously. Used to treat apnea of prematurity after pathological causes have been eliminated.
   a. Mechanism of action is unclear but thought to include the following:
      (1) Stimulation of medullary respiratory center via central chemoreceptors.
      (2) Central nervous system excitation.
      (3) Relaxation of bronchial smooth muscle with theophylline.
      (4) Increased respiratory drive and respiratory frequency.
      (5) Increased ventilatory response to carbon dioxide.
      (6) Increased respiratory muscle activity.
      (7) Non-specific inhibition of adenosine receptors.
      (8) Increased skeletal muscle contractility (Blanchard and Aranda, 1986;

Flood, 1989; Kriter and Blanchard, 1989; Loisel, 1987; Marchal et al., 1987).

  b. Pharmacokinetics.

    (1) Half-life of aminophylline/theophylline is approximately 30 hours.

    (2) Half-life of caffeine is approximately 100 hours.

    (3) Both theophylline and caffeine are rapidly absorbed intravenously. Oral absorption of caffeine is rapid. Oral absorption of theophylline is variable (Loisel, 1987).

    (4) Caffeine and theophylline are metabolized in the liver. Metabolism is much slower in the newborn period.

    (5) Theophylline is metabolized to caffeine by a metabolic pathway unique to the premature infant (Loisel, 1987).

    (6) Serum concentrations must be checked to avoid toxic levels.

  c. Dosage:

    (1) Aminophylline:

      (a) Route: IV.

      (b) Loading dose: 5 mg/kg.

      (c) Maintenance dose: 1–2 mg/kg q 8–12 hours.

      (d) Therapeutic level: 5–15 μg/ml.

    (2) Theophylline:

      (a) Route: PO.

      (b) Loading dose: 5 mg/kg.

      (c) Maintenance dose: 1–2 mg/kg q 8–12 hours.

      (d) Therapeutic level: 5–15 μg/ml.

    (3) Caffeine:

      (a) Route: IV or PO.

      (b) Loading dose: 10 mg/kg (20 mg/kg caffeine citrate).

      (c) Maintenance dose: 2.5 mg/kg (5 mg/kg caffeine citrate) q 24 hours.

      (d) Caffeine citrate is preferable over the sodium benzoate preparation because the latter displaces bilirubin from its albumin binding sites (Marchal et al., 1987).

      (e) Therapeutic level: 5–20 μg/ml.

  d. Side effects of methylxanthines include tachycardia, vomiting, GI hemorrhage, jitteriness, seizures, relaxation of lower esophageal sphincter leading to reflux, diuresis and dehydration, hyperglycemia, and hypotension following rapid IV administration.

  e. Caffeine versus theophylline:

    (1) Theophylline is a more potent vasodilator (Kriter and Blanchard, 1989).

    (2) Theophylline appears to cause a more rapid and sustained tachycardia than caffeine (Marchal et al., 1987).

    (3) Caffeine diffuses more rapidly in the CNS (Marchal et al., 1987).

    (4) Caffeine is given only once a day.

    (5) Caffeine has a wider therapeutic index (Blanchard and Aranda, 1986).

    (6) Caffeine may be effective in apnea not responding to theophylline, and vice versa (Blanchard and Aranda, 1986).

    (7) Caffeine has a longer half-life, resulting in smaller changes in its plasma concentration (Loisel, 1987).

2. Doxapram.

  a. Potent respiratory stimulant for apnea refractory to xanthine therapy.

  b. Mechanism of action thought to be stimulation of the peripheral (carotid body) chemoreceptors at low dose (0.5 mg/kg) and a central effect at a higher dose (Blanchard and Aranda, 1986; Marchal et al, 1987).

  c. Increases minute ventilation and tidal volume without an effect on respiratory timing (Martin et al., 1986).

  d. Pharmacokinetics.

    (1) The half-life is approximately 10 hours in the first few days of life and 8 hours at 10 days of age (Blanchard and Aranda, 1986).

    (2) Steady-state levels are reached within 24 hours (Beaudry et al., 1988).

e. Dosage:
  (1) Route: IV (oral dosages of 12 mg/kg every 8 hours have been studied).
  (2) Dose range: 0.5–2.5 mg/kg/hour administered by continuous infusion (Barrington et al., 1987; Beaudry et al., 1988; Blanchard and Aranda, 1986; Hayakawa et al., 1986; Marchal et al., 1987).
  (3) Controversy exists over therapeutic and toxic plasma levels. Guidelines include the following:
    (a) Therapeutic levels: less than 5 mg/liter (Hayakawa et al., 1986).
    (b) Toxic levels: 5 mg/liter (Marchal et al., 1987). Levels greater than 3.5 mg/liter may produce side effects (Marchal et al., 1987).
f. Side effects:
  (1) Jitteriness, irritability, vomiting, seizures, abdominal distention, increased gastric residuals, hyperglycemia, and glycosuria (Hayakawa et al., 1986; Marchal et al., 1987).
  (2) Hypertension, tachycardia, and increased cardiac output.
  (3) Respiratory stimulation increases workload of breathing, therefore increasing oxygen consumption and CO_2 production; also increased tidal volume and respiratory rate.
  (4) Used in the first few days of life can place the infant at risk for intraventricular hemorrhage (IVH).
g. Preparation contains benzyl alcohol. Use in the newborn is not recommended.

L. **Assisted ventilation:** used for apnea resistant to other methods of therapy.

Home Monitoring

A. **Effectiveness of home monitoring.** The Consensus Development Conference on Apnea and Home Monitoring (NIH, 1986) states that cardiorespiratory monitoring is effective in preventing death due to apnea for certain selected infants but is clearly inappropriate for others, with the primary objective being to serve the best interest of the infant based on the infant's history.

B. **Indications for home monitoring.**
1. Prematurity with persistent apnea and bradycardia (Krauss, 1986).
2. Thermistor documentation of apnea (Spitzer and Fox, 1986).
3. Thermistor documentation of increased periodic breathing (greater than 5%) (Spitzer and Fox, 1986).
4. Seizures presenting with apnea (Krauss, 1986).
5. Sibling of SIDS victim (Krauss, 1986; Spitzer and Fox, 1986).
6. Gastroesophageal reflux and other feeding difficulties associated with apnea (Krauss, 1986; Spitzer and Fox, 1986).
7. Pulmonary, cardiac, or neurological problems (Krauss, 1986; Spitzer and Fox, 1986).
8. Apparent life-threatening event (ALTE) (Krauss, 1986; Spitzer and Fox, 1986). ALTE is characterized by some combination of apnea, color change, marked change in muscle tone, choking, or gagging, which is frightening to the observer, who may feel the infant has died. Previously termed "aborted crib death" or "near-miss SIDS" (NIH, 1986).

C. **In-hospital and follow-up family support for home monitoring.**
1. Informed consent (NIH, 1986).
2. Assessment of family (NIH, 1986).
3. Anticipatory guidance to help prepare family for demands of home monitoring (Ariagno, 1984; NIH, 1986).
4. CPR instruction (Ariagno, 1984; NIH, 1986).
5. Thorough explanation of monitor operation (Ariagno, 1984; NIH, 1986).
6. Written instructions for use of monitor (NIH, 1986).
7. Twenty-four hour availability of equipment supporter (Ariagno, 1984).

8. Long-term follow-up plan (Ariagno, 1984).
9. Ongoing medical evaluation of need for continued monitoring (Ariagno, 1984).

STUDY QUESTIONS

1. The sleep state during which apnea predominantly occurs is:
   a. Active sleep.
   b. Quiet sleep.
   c. REM sleep.

2. A common cause of apnea is:
   a. Hypertension.
   b. Sepsis.
   c. Placement of central venous catheter.

3. Methylxanthine therapy for the treatment of apnea may be recommended for:

   a. A premature infant with a low birthweight.
   b. Any infant with a family history of SIDS.
   c. Prior to extubation of any ventilated infant.

4. The percentage of premature infants <1000 g who will experience apnea during the neonatal period is:
   a. 60%.
   b. 70%.
   c. 80%.

Answers to Study Questions

1. c
2. b
3. a
4. c

REFERENCES

Anas, N.G., and Perkin, R.M.: The pathophysiology of apnea in infancy. Perinatology-Neonatology, 8:65–70, 1984.

Anderson, J.V., Jr., Martin, R.J., and Fanaroff, M.B.: Neonatal respiratory control and apnea of prematurity. Perinatology-Neonatology, 7(7):65–70, July 1983.

Ariagno, R.L.: Evaluation and management of infantile apnea. Pediatr. Ann., 13(3):210–217, 1984.

Avery, M.E., and Fletcher, B.D.: The Lung and Its Disorders in the Newborn Infant, 3rd ed. Philadelphia, W.B. Saunders Co., 54–58, 1974, pp.

Barrington, K.J., Finer, N.N., Torok-Both, G., et al.: Dose-response relationship of doxapram in the therapy of refractory idiopathic apnea of prematurity. Pediatrics 80(1):22–27, 1987.

Beaudry, M.A., Bradley, J.M., Gramlich, L.M., and LeGatt, D.: Pharmacokinetics of doxapram in idiopathic apnea of prematurity. Dev. Pharmacol. Ther., 11:65–72, 1988.

Blanchard, P.W., and Aranda, J.V.: Drug treatment of neonatal apnea. Perinatology-Neonatology, 10(2):21–28, 1986.

Bloom, R.S., and Cropley, C.: Textbook of Neonatal Resuscitation. Dallas, American Heart Association, 1987.

Brazy, J.E., Kinney, H.C., and Oakes, W.J.: Central nervous system structural lesions causing apnea at birth. J. Pediatr., 111(2):163–175, 1987.

Fanaroff, A., and Martin, R. (ed.): Neonatal-Perinatal Medicine. St. Louis, C.V. Mosby, 1987, pp. 619–620.

Flood, E.: Caffeine citrate in the NICU. Neonatal Network, 7(5):37–39, 1989.

Gerhardt, T., and Bancalari, E.: Apnea of prematurity: I. Lung function and regulation of breathing. Pediatrics, 74(1):58–62, 1984a.

Gerhardt, T., and Bancalari, E.: Apnea of prematurity: II. Respiratory reflexes. Pediatrics, 7(1):63–66, 1984b.

Hayakawa, F., Hakamada, S., Juno, K., et al.: Doxapram in the treatment of idiopathic apnea of prematurity: Desirable dosage and serum concentrations. J. Pediatr., 109(1):138–140, 1986.

Hodson, W.A., and Truog, W.E.: Critical Care of the Newborn, 2nd ed. Philadelphia, W.B. Saunders Co., 1989, p. 73.

Kattwinkel, J.: Neonatal apnea: Pathogenesis and therapy. J. Pediatr., 90(3):342–347, 1977.

Korones, S.B.: High Risk Newborn Infants: The Basis for Intensive Care Nursing. St. Louis, C.V. Mosby, 1986, pp. 229–231.

Krauss, A.N.: Apnea in infancy: Pathophysiology, diagnosis and treatment. NY State J. Med., 86(2):89–96, 1986.

Kriter, K.E., and Blanchard, J. Management of apnea in infants. Clin. Pharm., 8:577–587, 1989.

Loisel, D.B.: Methylxanthines in the NICU. Neonatal Network, 6(3):23–28, Vol 6 No. 3 1987.

Marchal, F., Bairam, A., and Vert, P.: Neonatal apnea and apneic syndromes. Clin. Perinatol., 14(3):509–529, 1987.

Martin, R.J., Miller, M.J., and Waldemar, A.C.: Pathogenesis of apnea in preterm infants. J. Pediatr., 109(5):733–741, 1986.

Merenstein, G., and Gardner, S.: Handbook of Neonatal Intensive Care. St. Louis, C.V. Mosby, 1989, p. 417.

National Institutes of Health (NIH): Consensus Development Conference statement on infant apnea and home monitoring, 6(6):1–10, 1986.

Spitzer, A.R., and Fox, W.W.: Pediatr. Clin. North Am., 33(3):561–581, 1986.

BIBLIOGRAPHY

Avery, G.: Neonatology: Pathology and Management of the Newborn. Philadelphia, J.B. Lippincott, 1981, pp. 284, 483, 1083.

Bromberger, P., James, H.E., Saunders, B., and Schneider, H.: Sudden infant apnea and insidious hydrocephalus. Childs Nerv. Syst. 4:241–243, 1988.

Caddell, J.L.: Magnesium therapy in premature neonates with apnea neonatorum. J. Am. Coll. Nutr., 7(1):5–16, 1988.

DeMaio, J.G., Harris, M.C., Deuber, C., and Spitzer, A.R.: Effect of blood transfusion on apnea frequency in growing preterm infants. J. Pediatr., 114(6):1039–1041, 1989.

Jamali, F., Barrington, K.J., Finer, N.N., et al.: Doxapram dosage regimen in apnea of prematurity based on pharmacokinetic data. Dev. Pharmacol. Ther., 11:253–257, 1988.

Kelly D., and Shannon, D.C.: Managing apnea in infancy. Perinatology-Neonatology, 38–43, November-December 1979.

Keyes, W.G., Donohue, P.K., Spivak, J.L., et al.: Assessing the need for transfusion of premature infants and role of hematocrit, clinical signs, and erythropoietin levels. Pediatrics, 84(3):412–417, 1989.

Nadkarni, S., Hay, A.W.M., Faye, S., and Congdon, P.J.: The relationship between theophylline, caffeine and heart rate in neonates. Ann. Clin. Biochem., 25:408–410, 1988.

Lacy, T., et al.: Neonatology: Basic Management, On-Call Problems, Diseases, Drugs. Norwalk, CT, Appleton & Lange, 1988–1989, pp. 122–123, 313–314.

Oren, J., Kelly, D.H., and Shannon, D.C.: Pneumogram recordings in infants resuscitated for apnea of infancy. Pediatrics, 83(3):364–368, 1989.

Preston, G.: A practical approach to apnea. Henry Ford Hosp. Med. J., 36(4):204–206, 1988.

Rigatto, H.: Infant Apnea. Pediatr. Clin. North Am., 29(5):1105–1116, 1982.

Rodriques, A.M., Warburton, D., and Keens, T.G.: Elevated catecholamine levels and abnormal hypoxic arousal in apnea of infancy. Pediatrics, 79(2):269–274, 1987.

Rosen, C.L., Glaze, D.G., and Frost, J.D., Jr.: Home monitor follow-up of persistent apnea and bradycardia in preterm infants. AJDC, 140:547–550, 1986.

Saigal, S., Watts, J., and Campbell, D.: Randomized clinical trial of an oscillation air mattress in preterm infants: Effect on apnea, growth and development. J. Pediatr., 109(5):857–864, 1986.

Sims, M.E., Turkel, S.B., Vazirani, M., and Hodgman, J.E.: Factors differentiating postponed neonatal death from survival in low birth weight infants. J. Perinatol., 8(2):88–92, 1988.

Donna J. Rodden

Surfactant Replacement Therapy

Objectives

1. Identify the two components that compose the pulmonary surfactant system.

2. Name the two main active ingredients of endogenous surfactant and their properties.

3. List the five functional characteristics of natural surfactant.

4. Identify the four types of replacement surfactants and describe the properties of each.

5. Discuss and analyze the outcome of three Exosurf studies.

6. List the criteria that qualify an infant for surfactant replacement therapy (SRT) and the recommended dosage.

7. List the administration guidelines for Exosurf.

8. Demonstrate how to prepare Exosurf.

9. Recognize the anticipated responses during the post-dosing period.

10. Describe the administration guidelines for Survanta.

At one time, respiratory distress syndrome (RDS) was the leading cause of death in live-born pre-term infants. The United States recorded approximately 10,000 deaths per year from RDS in the early 1970s. Although surfactant deficiency is the primary cause of RDS, many other factors contribute to respiratory failure in the very premature infant, including lung structure, weak musculature, and decreased pulmonary blood flow. Surfactant replacement therapy has the potential to result in an improved outcome for affected infants by decreasing the complications and severity of RDS. Approximately 5000 babies still die annually of RDS and its complications. Yet, RDS is no longer the leading cause of death in live-born pre-term infants.

The vision of surfactant replacement therapy (SRT) first occurred in the late 1950s, but it was not until the 1970s that clinical trials began. There are four categories of replacement surfactants, each developed from different sources. The different types of surfactant replacement differ in properties and recommendations for administration. There are many clinical trials proving the efficacy and safety of SRT in treating infants who are at risk for developing RDS or have established RDS. Exosurf Neonatal and Survanta are currently the only products with Food and Drug Administration (FDA) approval. With the research in progress, we will have more information on the long-term effects of receiving surfactant. As products receive FDA approval, we will be able to compare the products to one another.

Historical Overview of Surfactant

A. **In 1929, Kurt von Neergaard** was the first to suggest that surface tension played an important role in lung expansion.

B. **Pattle (1955) and Clements (1957)** isolated and reported the function of surfactant.

C. **Avery and Mead (1959)** reported that infants dying of RDS lacked pulmonary surfactant. It was from this work that replacement therapy was envisioned.

D. **Robillard and colleagues (1964) and Chu and associates (1967)** were the first to attempt replacement therapy using dipalmitoylphosphatidylcholine (DPPC) alone. These trials were unsuccessful, owing to the use of only one active ingredient in natural surfactant. From these studies came the understanding that other components in lung lavage besides DPPC were necessary for surfactant function.

E. **Enhorning and Robertson (1972) and Adams and associates (1978)** reported using whole surfactant complexes in animal studies with successful results. This resulted in the possibility of use in clinical trials.

F. **During the 1980s, many investigators began developing replacement surfactants for use in clinical trials.** This is explained in more detail under types of replacement surfactants.

The Pulmonary Surfactant System

A complete pulmonary surfactant system needs both lung surfactant and alveolar type II cells for normal pulmonary function and mechanics (Notter, 1988).

A. **Lung surfactant is mainly lipids, primarily DPPC, which is responsible for decreasing the surface tension at the air-liquid interface in the alveolus.** Surfactant-specific proteins compose 5–10% of the total mass of lung surfactant. These proteins are responsible for absorption and rapid spreading of lung surfactant and have functions in surfactant metabolism (Wright and Clements, 1987).

B. **Alveolar type II cells are important to the pulmonary system because they can synthesize, store, secrete, and recycle lung surfactant** (Notter, 1988). Endogenous production of surfactant by type II cells of the lung normally begins at 24–28 weeks' gestation, with production increasing until term (Shapiro, 1988).

Functional Characteristics of Surfactant

The five functional characteristics of natural surfactant reported by Merritt (1989) are as follows:

A. Reducing surface tension at the air-liquid interface in the alveolus.

B. Decreasing the work of breathing.

C. Increasing alveolar stability on expiration.

D. Decreasing the leakage of proteins and water leading to pulmonary edema.

E. Decreasing atelectasis.

Types of Replacement Surfactants

Replacement surfactants vary in their source, collection technique, processing and composition (Shapiro, 1988; Notter, 1988). Shapiro (1988) has performed an extensive review looking at the various types of replacement surfactants. There are four categories for the different types of surfactants.

A. **Natural human surfactant is obtained from amniotic fluid.** Some properties are as follows:
1. Human in origin.
2. Contains all surfactant proteins.
3. Difficult to harvest large quantities (i.e., amniotic fluid from approximately five cesarean sections will produce enough surfactant to treat one infant).

B. **Whole surfactant is obtained by lung lavage from animal sources.** Because of the following properties, it has not been used much in clinical trials:
1. It contains a large amount of animal protein (10%).
2. During sterilization, the biological activity is severely diminished.

C. **Modified natural surfactants are obtained by extracting surfactant from lung lavage or tissue and chemically modifying it.** Sources for this extract are cows, calves, and pigs. The properties of this form of surfactant include the following:
1. Derived from a natural source.
2. Potent surface tension–lowering ability.
3. Can be sterilized.
4. Contain only 1–2% proteins.
5. Large amounts of surfactant can be obtained easily and inexpensively.
6. There may be immunological reaction to the animal proteins.

D. **Synthetic surfactants.** Two types are as follows:
1. Artificial lung-expanding compound (ALEC). Some of its characteristics are as follows (Ten Centre Study Group, 1987):
    a. Simple in composition (contains DPPC and phosphatidylglycerol [PG]).
    b. Protein-free.
    c. Inexpensive to manufacture.
    d. Questionable surface tension–lowering ability.
    e. A decrease in neonatal mortality for the first 28 days from 27% to 14% when compared with study controls.
    f. A reduction of serious intraventricular hemorrhage from 24% to 16% when compared with study controls.
    g. Less respiratory support in the first 10 days for the ALEC-treated babies compared with the control group.
    h. The effects begin hours after administration, versus immediate effects seen with other products.
2. Exosurf Neonatal. Exosurf Neonatal contains a mixture of DPPC and dispersing and emulsifying agents. Its properties include the following:
    a. Simple in composition.
    b. Inexpensive for the manufacturer to prepare.
    c. Good surface tension–lowering properties, yet not as good as those of surfactant extracts.
    d. A protein-free synthetic formulation.
    e. Additives may have some unidentified adverse biological effects.

Clinical Use of Surfactants

Currently, the only surfactant preparations available for clinical use are Exosurf Neonatal and Survanta. Exosurf was the first to receive FDA approval in August

Table 8–1
RESULTS OF EXOSURF NEONATAL WHEN COMPARED WITH PLACEBO

	Rescue Treatment for Infants 700–1350 g at Birth with Established RDS	Rescue Treatment for Infants Weighing 1250 g or Greater at Birth with Established RDS	Prophylactic Treatment for Infants Weighing 700–1100 g at Birth
Mortality from RDS	66% reduction	66% reduction	50% reduction
Mortality at 1 year from any cause	44% reduction	Not assessed	33% reduction
Pulmonary air leaks	Reduction of pneumothorax and pulmonary interstitial emphysema	Reduction of pneumothorax and pulmonary interstitial emphysema	Reduction of pneumothorax
Lung disease	Reduction in severity of RDS No significant reduction in BPD	42% reduction in BPD	No significant reduction in BPD
Incidence of apnea	Increased	Increased	Increased
Nosocomial infections, sepsis, and deaths from sepsis	No change	No change	No change
Days on intermittent mandatory ventilation (IMV)	No significant difference	Decreased number of days on IMV	No significant difference

1990. It has shown significant benefit for infants with RDS (Nightingale, 1990). Table 8–1 is a summary of some research findings.

EXOSURF NEONATAL

Based on information from completed clinical trials, recommendations for use are as follows (Burroughs Wellcome Co., 1990):

A. The prophylactic treatment criteria are used on infants who are at risk of developing RDS as a preventive measure.
1. Criteria:
    a. Intubated and mechanically ventilated.
    b. Infants with a birthweight <1350 g.
    c. Infants with a birthweight >1350 g with evidence of pulmonary immaturity.
2. Treatment:
    a. Three doses of 5 ml/kg of Exosurf Neonatal administered 12 and 24 hours from the first dose if the infant remains mechanically ventilated during this time.

B. The rescue treatment criteria are used in treating infants with established RDS in the rescue mode.
1. Criteria:
    a. Infants who have developed RDS.
        (1) The respiratory distress is not attributable to causes other than RDS (i.e., pneumonia, meconium aspiration, and transient tachypnea of the newborn [TTN]).
        (2) Chest radiograph findings consistent with diagnosis of RDS (reticulogranular pattern, enlarged heart, and the presence of an air bronchogram).
2. Treatment:
    a. Two 5 ml/kg doses of Exosurf Neonatal 12 hours apart while the infant is on mechanical ventilation.

Table 8–2
SUMMARY OF ADMINISTRATION GUIDELINES

	Exosurf	Survanta
Criteria		
Prophylaxis	Intubated and mechanically ventilated	Intubated
	Birthweight <1350 g	Birthweight <1250 g
	Birthweight >1350 g and lung immaturity	Birthweight >1250 g and lung immaturity
Rescue	RDS on x-ray	RDS on x-ray
	Intubated and mechanically ventilated	Intubated and mechanically ventilated
Administration		
Amount	5 ml/kg in two divided doses	4 ml/kg in four divided doses
Frequency	Prophylaxis: three doses 12 hours apart	Four doses in 48 hours with at least 6 hours
	Rescue: two doses 12 hours apart	between doses
Common Acute Effect		
During administration	Transient bradycardia	Transient bradycardia
	O_2 desaturation	O_2 desaturation
Post-administration	Increased lung compliance	Increased lung compliance
	Hyperoxia	Hyperoxia

The risk of developing respiratory distress syndrome (RDS) increases as gestational age decreases, occurring in three out of four infants born at less than 30 weeks (Reynolds and Wallander, 1989).

Administration Guidelines (Table 8–2)

The dose should be administered as early as possible and after documented RDS develops. Administration does not need to be in the delivery room. The priority is to stabilize the infant by ensuring correct endotracheal tube placement, assessment of cardiac/pulmonary status, and satisfactory oxygen saturation (Sao$_2$) of >90%.

A. **Stabilize the infant:**
1. Correct endotracheal tube placement.
2. Adequate oxygenation (Sao$_2$ > 90%).
3. Placement of intervascular line and indwelling arterial line.

B. **Weigh the infant to determine correct initial dose.** Use this weight for subsequent doses.

C. **Ensure correct endotracheal tube placement** by observing symmetrical chest movements and listening for equal breath sounds.

D. **Obtain x-ray** for RDS documentation, endotracheal tube placement, and indwelling line position.

E. **Suction the endotracheal tube to decrease the necessity of having to do so after dosing.**

F. **Use continuous electrocardiogram and transcutaneous oxygen saturation monitoring to continuously assess response to the procedure.**

G. **Change ventilator settings.**
1. The infant on very low ventilator settings may need the settings changed during or before dosing.
2. If the infant is very labile, ventilator settings may need to be changed before dosing.
   a. Recommendations include the following:
      (1) Set peak inspiratory pressure (PIP) to visualize chest excursion. Usually, pre-treatment PIP is adequate.
      (2) Increase fraction of inspired oxygen (Fio$_2$) by 20% to minimize any transient deterioration in oxygenation.

(3) Minimum ventilator rate should be 25 breaths/minute to allow greater ease in administration.

H. **Prepare the suspension.** Pre-packaged kits of Exosurf Neonatal are equipped with a 10 ml vial of sterile powder, a 10 ml vial of sterile water, and endotracheal tube adapters (sizes 2.5 mm ID through 4.5 mm ID). These kits should be stored at room temperature in a dry place.
1. Draw up 8 ml of the 10 ml of sterile (preservative-free) water provided, using an 18 or 19 gauge needle.
2. Remove metal circular seal on the Exosurf vial top.
3. Cleanse rubber stopper with alcohol swab.
4. Insert needle from sterile water syringe into Exosurf vial.
5. Allow the vacuum in the vial to draw the 8 ml of sterile water into the vial. If there is no vacuum, DO NOT USE! It is the force of the vacuum that mixes the preparation.
6. Without removing the needle, aspirate as much of the 8 ml back out of the vial and suddenly release the syringe plunger (to allow vigorous mixing and Exosurf activation). Repeat the above three or four times. Check to make sure the suspension is a cloudy homogenous liquid. If there are any large flakes or particulate material, continue mixing. If the large flakes or particulate are persistent, the vial should not be used.
7. Once reconstituted, the suspension is stable for up to 12 hours at room temperature or refrigerated. If the suspension seems to have separated, gently shake or swirl the vial to resuspend the preparation.

I. **Draw up 5 ml/kg of Exosurf from below the froth while maintaining the vacuum.** Do not use more than 8 ml from the 10 ml vial mixture.

J. **Attach endotracheal tube adapter** with side port, and maintain the endotracheal tube erect.

K. **Attach Exosurf-filled syringe** to the side port.

L. **Administer two half-doses of 2.5 ml/kg each** while maintaining mechanical ventilation.
1. Place the infant in the midline position.
2. Instill the first half-dose in small amounts over 30–60 inspiratory cycles. Slow the rate of dosing if any of the following occur:
   a. Decrease in heart rate.
   b. The infant becomes dusky or agitated.
   c. Transcutaneous oxygen saturation falls more than 15%.
   d. Reflux of Exosurf occurs in the endotracheal tube. If necessary, increase the PIP, ventilator rate, and FiO_2.
3. Turn infant 45 degrees to the right; hold for 30 seconds.
4. Return to the midline position and instill the second half-dose, using the same procedure as with the first half-dose.
5. Turn the infant 45 degrees to the left for 30 seconds.
6. Return to midline position.
7. Remove the syringe and RECAP THE SIDEPORT.
8. Listen for equal breath sounds to confirm correct placement of the endotracheal tube. The breath sounds will be coarse and wet.
9. There should be minimal handling of the infant for 2 hours post-dose.
10. Do not suction for at least 2 hours after dosing unless there are clinical signs of mucous plugging.
11. Monitor the infant closely (see below).
12. Obtain arterial blood gases every 1–2 hours for the first 6 hours.

Anticipated Response During the Post-dosing Period

After giving the dose, it is imperative that an experienced clinician be at the bedside for at least 60 minutes to respond immediately to any changes the infant might have. Exosurf Neonatal can rapidly affect lung compliance and oxygenation. Some changes must be made without waiting for confirmation from blood gases. During the clinical trials, these responses have been reported:

A. **Improved chest expansion.** After dosing, chest expansion can improve; if so, decrease PIP immediately. This may prevent an air leak from occurring.

B. **Improved color of infant and transcutaneous oxygen saturation >95%.** To avoid hyperoxia, decrease the FIO_2 in repeated small increments to get an O_2 saturation of 92–95%.

C. **Hypocapnia.** Hypocapnia will be evidenced by arterial or transcutaneous CO_2 readings of <35 torr. To correct this problem, decrease the ventilator rate.

D. **Pulmonary hemorrhage.** The incidence of pulmonary hemorrhage increases in babies who are <700 g and who are treated with Exosurf (10% versus 2% in the placebo group). This complication usually occurs within the first 2 days of life. Pulmonary hemorrhage is most frequent in infants who are younger in gestational age, of lower birth weight, are male, or had an untreated patent ductus arteriosus (PDA). Care should be given to:
1. Aggressively diagnose and treat PDA during the first 2 days of life.
2. Decrease the FIO_2 instead of ventilator pressures during the first 24–48 hours after dosing in those at risk for pulmonary hemorrhage.
3. Minimal decreases in the positive end-expiratory pressure (PEEP) for at least 48 hours after dosing.

E. **Mucous plugs.** Exosurf is a mucolytic agent. There may be an increase in secretions after dosing. In rare situations (3/1000), the increase in mucus has resulted in obstructing the endotracheal tube. If, after dosing, the infant's ventilation becomes impaired, a mucous plug may be the cause, as evidenced by increase in the partial pressure of carbon dioxide (PCO_2), difficulty in passing a suction catheter, and having desaturation spells. If suctioning does not clear the endotracheal tube, remove the blocked tube immediately and reintubate.

Special Considerations When Deciding to Treat with Exosurf

A. **In infants <700 g, consider the potential risks and benefits of giving Exosurf.** In this weight group, overall mortality did not differ significantly between the Exosurf treatment group and placebo groups.

B. **Characteristics of SRT.** Generally, SRT has decreased mortality, allowed lower FIO_2 and ventilator settings over the first 3 days of life, and decreased air leak complications; other problems of prematurity (e.g., PDA, intraventricular hemorrhage [IVH], and chronic lung disease [CLD]) occur at a rate similar to those of untreated infants.

SURVANTA

Survanta is a modified natural surfactant extracted from minced bovine lung, supplemented with DPPC, tripalmitin, and palmitic acid. Listed are a few studies published using Survanta.

A. **A prevention protocol gave one dose of Survanta or air/placebo** (Soll et al., 1990).
1. Patients were screened according to the following:
   a. Estimated fetal weight between 750 and 1250 g.
   b. Estimated gestational age of 24–30 weeks.
   c. Documentation obtained regarding maternal glucocorticoid therapy for prevention of RDS.
   d. Necessary placement of an endotracheal tube and a heart rate >100 beats/minute within the first 15 minutes of life.

2. Exclusion criteria:
   a. Intratracheal drugs given to resuscitate the infant.
   b. Lung maturity documented by a lecithin/sphingomyelin ratio.
   c. Maternal history of either heroin or methadone use during pregnancy.
   d. Major congenital anomalies.
3. This study evaluated the average arterial/alveolar (a/A) ratio, FIO_2, and mean airway pressure (MAP) during the 72 hours after treatment and the clinical status at 7 and 28 days of life. Study results showed that infants receiving Survanta had the following:
   a. A significant decrease in the FIO_2 at 72 hours after treatment.
   b. No differences in the a/A ratio and MAP at 72 hours after treatment.
   c. Less critical radiographic changes at 24 hours of age.
   d. No differences in clinical status at days 7 and 28.

B. **A rescue treatment using one dose of Survanta or air/placebo** was published by Horbar and colleagues (1989).
1. The criteria for entry were as follows:
   a. Infant weight was between 750 and 1750 g.
   b. Diagnosis of RDS between 3 and 6 hours after birth.
   c. The infant was receiving assisted ventilation.
   d. The infant had an FIO_2 requirement of 40% or greater and a PO_2 of 80 mm Hg or less.
   e. Normal blood pressure.
   f. Post-ductal arterial catheter in place.
   g. The infant's blood glucose concentration was 40 mg/dl or greater.
   h. No sign of seizure activity.
   i. Ability to administer Survanta within 8 hours of birth.
2. Study results showed the infants who received Survanta had the following:
   a. A reduction in the severity of RDS during the 72 hours after treatment.
   b. No significant differences in the clinical status on day 7 or day 28 after treatment.
   c. A decrease in the frequency of pneumothorax.
   d. No significant long-term improvement in clinical status or reduction in neonatal mortality.

C. **A rescue treatment for infants with hyaline membrane disease (HMD) administered multiple doses of Survanta or air/placebo** (Couser, 1990).
1. The criteria used for this study were as follows:
   a. Estimated infant weight of 600–1250 g.
   b. Gestational age of 23–29 weeks.
   c. Heart rate >100 beats/minute.
2. The following procedure was used for administering Survanta or air:
   a. The infant was intubated and weighed immediately after birth.
   b. The first dose was given in the delivery room within 15 minutes after birth.
   c. Up to three additional doses were given in the first 48 hours if the infant:
      (1) Remained ventilated.
      (2) Required an FIO_2 of 30% or greater.
      (3) Had radiographic findings consistent with HMD.
      (4) Required a minimum of 6 hours between doses.
3. Exclusion criteria:
   a. Lung maturity documented by a lecithin/sphingomyelin ratio of >2:1.
   b. Maternal use of either heroin or methadone during pregnancy.
   c. Major congenital anomalies.
4. Study results showed that infants receiving Survanta had the following:
   a. Improved lung compliance at 24 hours of age and at 7 days of age.
   b. Improved oxygenation during the first 72 hours of life.
   c. A decrease in the MAP requirements during the first week of life.
   d. Long-term effects are unknown. These infants were followed for the first 7 days of life only.

Recommendations for Use

Based on information from completed clinical trials, recommendations for use are as follows (Ross Laboratories, 1991):

A. **The prevention treatment criteria are used as a preventive measure for infants who are at risk of developing RDS.**
1. Criteria:
   a. Intubated.
   b. Infants with a birthweight <1250 g.
   c. Infants with evidence of surfactant deficiency.
2. Treatment:
   a. Give first dose preferably within 15 minutes of birth. Infant does not need to be mechanically ventilated for the first dose.
   b. Four doses can be administered in the first 48 hours of life.
   c. Repeat doses can be given 6 hours after the preceding dose if the infant remains intubated, mechanically ventilated, and requires at least 30% inspired oxygen to maintain a Pao_2 less than or equal to 80 torr.
   d. Radiographic confirmation of RDS should be obtained before administering additional doses.

B. **The rescue treatment criteria are used in treating infants with established RDS in the rescue mode.**
1. Criteria:
   a. Chest radiograph finding consistent with diagnosis of RDS (reticulogranular pattern, enlarged heart, and the presence of an air bronchogram).
   b. Intubated and mechanically ventilated.
2. Treatment:
   a. Give dose as soon as possible, preferably by 8 hours of age.
   b. Four doses can be administered in the first 48 hours of life.
   c. Repeat doses can be given 6 hours after the preceding dose if the infant remains intubated, mechanically ventilated, and requires at least 30% inspired oxygen to maintain a Pao_2 less than or equal to 80 torr.

Administration Guidelines for Survanta

A. **Prepare Survanta for dosing.**
1. Remove the vial from a 2–8°C refrigerator, warm at room temperature for 20 minutes or warm in the hand for at least 8 minutes. DO NOT USE ARTIFICIAL WARMING METHODS.
2. Inspect for discoloration prior to administration. The color should be off-white to light brown.
3. Swirl the vial gently to redisperse if settling has occurred. DO NOT SHAKE.
4. Unused, unopened vials that have been warmed may be returned to the refrigerator within 8 hours and stored for future use. Drug should not be warmed and returned to the refrigerator more than once.
5. Vials are for single dose only and should be entered only once.

B. **Administer Survanta in four equal doses of 1 ml/kg each through a 5.0 Fr feeding tube.**
1. Cut the 5.0 Fr feeding tube so it will extend just beyond the end of the endotracheal tube above the infant's carina.
2. Determine the total dose of Survanta (4 ml/kg) based on the infant's birthweight.
3. Slowly draw up the entire contents of the vial into a plastic syringe through a large-gauge needle (eg, at least 20 gauge). Each vial contains 8 ml of solution.
4. Attach the pre-measured 5 Fr catheter to the syringe.
5. Fill the catheter with Survanta.
6. Discard the excess through the catheter so that only the total dose to be given remains in the syringe.

7. Ensure proper placement and patency of the endotracheal tube prior to administration.
8. Adjust ventilator settings to maintain appropriate oxygenation and ventilation.
   a. In clinical trial, the infant's ventilator settings were changed to a rate of 60 breaths/minute, inspiratory time 0.5 second, and FIO_2 1.0 immediately prior to giving the first rescue dose.
   b. Manual hand-bag ventilation should not be used to administer repeat doses.
9. Briefly disconnect the infant from the ventilator or Ambubag.
10. Insert the catheter through the endotracheal tube.
11. Position the infant. Give each quarter-dose with the baby in a different position:
    a. Head down, body turned to the right.
    b. Head down, body turned to the left.
    c. Head up, body turned to the right.
    d. Head up, body turned to the left.
12. Gently inject 1 ml through the catheter over 2–3 seconds.
13. After each quarter-dose, remove the catheter, hold the infant in the position, and manually or mechanically ventilate for at least 30 seconds or until stable. Give 60 breaths/minute and pressures that are adequate for air exchange and chest wall movement.
14. Reposition the infant for instillation of the next quarter-dose, using the same procedures.
15. No suctioning for 1 hour post-dosing unless signs of airway obstruction occur.

C. **Acute clinical effects may occur during or following dosing.** It is imperative that an experienced clinician be at the bedside for at least 60 minutes to respond immediately to any changes the infant might have. Responses that have been reported during and following the dosing procedure include the following:
1. Improved chest expansion.
2. Improved color of infant and transcutaneous oxygen saturation.
3. Bradycardia.
4. Decreased oxygen saturation.
5. Endotracheal tube reflux.
6. Pallor.
7. Vasoconstriction.
8. Hypotension.
9. Endotracheal tube blockage.
10. Hypertension.
11. Hypercapnia.
12. Apnea.

Conclusion

Since the discovery of endogenous surfactant and its functions, intense research has led to the development of artificial surfactant preparations, which have proved effective in the management of RDS in the newborn. The effects of surfactant replacement therapy (SRT) include stabilization of alveoli, prevention of epithelial disruption during ventilation, and reduction of leakage of serum macromolecules into the alveolus. Clinical trials have proved that infants who receive SRT have a decrease in mortality, decrease in severity of RDS, and reduced risk of pneumothorax and pulmonary interstitial emphysema. Although there are benefits of SRT, there are some complications of prematurity that are not improved by SRT. These include the incidence of patent ductus arteriosus, periventricular hemorrhage–intraventricular hemorrhage (PVH-IVH), and bronchopulmonary dysplasia (BPD).

Although SRT in the NICU is an exciting development, there may be another side to the story. The question has been raised as to what will be the effect on the cost of health care and its resources. Will there be an increased incidence of infants who would have died and now survive with neurological and developmental handicaps after receiving surfactant? Short-term (1 year) follow-up studies show no increase in handicap among surfactant-treated infants compared with controls; however, long-term results are not available. A report stated that infants who receive SRT compared with the controls have higher total hospital cost, probably owing to the increased survival of the treated infants. The pre-term infant already is one of the largest health care consumer groups.

Besides treating infants with RDS, there is interest in treating other neonatal conditions such as meconium aspiration syndrome and pneumonia with surfactant. Outside the nursery investigators are interested in treating adult respiratory distress syndrome (ARDS) with surfactant. ARDS is a complex disease that results in a surfactant deficiency state. Unlike neonatal RDS, ARDS generally does not begin with surfactant deficiency. Animal studies suggest that SRT might be useful in ARDS.

SRT will remain a clinical treatment for RDS. There is still a need to acquire more information about agents that regulate the individual surfactant components and the mechanism by which they work. Gaining further information on surfactant will enrich our basic knowledge and also will aid in clinical decisions. Some unanswered questions include: Is one type of surfactant better than another? When is the best timing for the first dose? Is it best to give it preventively or in the rescue mode? How many doses are optimal, and what are the indications for repeating the doses? There is much research that needs to be done to optimize surfactant therapy in the pre-term infant.

STUDY QUESTIONS

1. Which of the following statements regarding the pulmonary surfactant system is correct?
   a. Alveolar type II cells can synthesize, store, secrete, and recycle lung surfactant.
   b. Endogenous production of surfactant by type II cells of the lung normally begins at term.
   c. Lung surfactant is mainly protein.

2. A functional characteristic of natural surfactant is:
   a. Decreases the work of breathing.
   b. Decreases the incidence of neonatal apnea.
   c. Decreases length of hospitalization.

3. What is the recommended dosage of Exosurf for prophylactic treatment of RDS?
   a. Four ml/kg or 100 mg/kg given in four divided doses.
   b. Three doses of 5 ml/kg administered 12 and 24 hours from the first dose.
   c. Two 5 ml/kg doses given 12 hours apart.

4. After dosing with surfactant, a trained clinician must be present to recognize and respond to which anticipated response?
   a. Hypercapnia.
   b. Improved chest expansion.
   c. Intraventricular hemorrhage.

Answers to Study Questions

1. a
2. a
3. b
4. b

REFERENCES

Adams, F.H., Towers, B., and Osher, A.B.: Effect of tracheal instillation of natural surfactant in premature lambs in clinical and autopsy findings. Pediatr. Res., 12:841–848, 1978.

Avery, M.E., and Mead, J.: Surface properties in relation to atelectasis and hyaline membrane disease. Am J Dis Child, 97:517–523, 1959.

Burroughs Wellcome Co.: Produce Monograph: Synthetic Lung Surfactant for the Treatment of Neonatal Respiratory Distress Syndrome, 1990. (Available from Burroughs Wellcome Co., Research Triangle Park, NC 27709.)

Chu, J., Clements, J.A., and Cotton, E.K.: Neonatal pulmonary ischemia: Clinical and physiologic studies. Pediatrics, 40:709–782, 1967.

Clements, J.A.: Surface tension of lung extracts. Proc. Soc. Exp. Biol. Med., 95:170–172, 1957.

Couser, R.J.: Effects of exogenous surfactant therapy on dynamic compliance during mechanical breathing in preterm infants with hyaline membrane disease. J. Pediatr., 116(1):119–124, 1990.

Enhorning, G., and Robertson, B.: Lung expansion in the premature rabbit fetus after tracheal digestion of surfactant. Pediatrics, 50:58–66, 1972.

Horbar, J.D., et al.: A multicenter randomized, placebo-controlled trial of surfactant therapy for respiratory distress syndrome. N. Engl. J. Med., 320(15):959–965, 1989.

Merritt, T.A., Hallman, M., Spragg, R., et al.: Exogenous surfactant treatments for neonatal respiratory distress syndrome and their potential role in the adult respiratory distress syndrome. Drugs, 38(4):591–611, 1989.

Nightingale, S.L.: From the Food and Drug Administration. JAMA, 264(14):1802, 1990.

Notter, R.H.: Biophysical behavior of lung surfactant: Implications for respiratory physiology and pathophysiology. Semin. Perinatol., 12(3):180–212, 1988.

Pattle, R.E.: Properties, function and origin of the alveolar lining layer. Nature, 175:1125–1126, 1955.

Reynolds, M.S., and Wallander, K.A.: Use of surfactant in the prevention and retreatment of neonatal respiratory distress syndrome. Clin. Pharm., 8:559–576, 1989.

Robillard, E., Alarie, Y., Dagenais-Perusse, P., et al.: Microaerosol administration of synthetic dipalmitoyl lecithin in the respiratory distress syndrome: A preliminary report. Can. Med. Assoc. J., 90:55–66, 1964.

Ross Laboratories: Produce Monograph: Survanta Beractant Intratracheal Suspension, 1991. (Available from Ross Laboratories, Columbus, OH 43216).

Shapiro, D.L.: The development of surfactant replacement therapy and the various types of replacement surfactants. Semin. Perinatol., 12(3):174–179, 1988.

Soll, R.F., et al.: Multicenter trial of single-dose modified bovine surfactant extract (Survanta) for prevention of respiratory distress syndrome. Pediatrics, 85(6):1092–1102, 1990.

Ten Centre Study Group: Ten Centre trial of artificial surfactant (artificial lung expanding compound) in very premature babies. Br. Med. J., 294:991–996, 1987.

Wright, J.R., and Clements, J.A.: Metabolism and turnover of lung surfactant. Am. Rev. Respir. Dis., 135:426–444, 1987.

BIBLIOGRAPHY

Ballard, P.L.: Hormonal regulation of pulmonary surfactant. Endocr. Rev., 10(2):165–181, 1989.

Hallman, M., Merritt, T. A., and Schneider, H.: Isolation of human surfactant from amniotic fluid and a pilot study of its efficacy in respiratory distress syndrome. Pediatrics, 71:473–482, 1983.

Holm, B.A., and Matalon, S.: Role of pulmonary surfactant in the development and treatment of adult respiratory distress syndrome. Anesth. Analg., 69(6):805–818, 1989.

Merritt, T.A., Hallman, M., Bloom, B.T., et al: Prophylactic treatment of very premature infants with human surfactant. N. Engl. J. Med., 315(13):785–790, 1986.

Perelman, R.H., and Farrell, P.M.: Analysis of causes of neonatal death in the United States with specific emphasis on fatal hyaline membrane disease. Pediatrics, 70:570–575, 1982.

Weaver, T.E., and Whitsett J.A.: Structure and function of pulmonary surfactant proteins. Semin. Perinatol., 11(3):213–220, 1988.

Joanne R. Kilb
Stephen Kilb

Assisted Ventilation

Objectives

1. Identify the terms and abbreviations of FRC, TV, VC, and TLC and how these relate to the neonate.

2. Apply the concepts of elastic recoil, compliance, resistance, gas trapping, inadvertent PEEP, work of breathing, ventilation-perfusion ratio, and mean airway pressure in relation to the neonate.

3. Distinguish clinical symptoms of respiratory distress in the neonate. Contrast different monitoring methods used in the newborn, comparing the advantages and disadvantages of each method.

4. List the potential causes of respiratory and metabolic acidosis and alkalosis in a newborn. Identify guidelines of ranges of pH, PaO_2, $PaCO_2$, and HCO_3, and base excess in different respiratory disease states in the neonate.

5. Evaluate blood gas data to determine a neonate's acid-base status.

6. Identify several treatment modalities available for infants experiencing respiratory distress.

7. Describe the various types of mechanical ventilation.

8. List nursing interventions required to care for ventilated infants based on the theories of mechanical ventilation.

9. Recognize the appropriate use of common medications frequently encountered in caring for ventilated, critically ill neonates.

Caring for an infant requiring assisted ventilation and oxygen support can be a challenge. An understanding of the basic physiology and concepts governing the use of oxygen and mechanical ventilatory support should provide the necessary knowledge to meet this challenge. The focus of this chapter is to provide the basic knowledge used in caring for the infant requiring conventional ventilation or oxygen therapy. Newer therapies such as high-frequency ventilation, extracorporeal membrane oxygenation (ECMO), and surfactant are covered in separate chapters.

Physiology

A. **Definitions** (values from Goldsmith and Karotkin, 1988, p. 436).
1. Functional residual capacity (FRC): the volume of gas left in the lungs after normal expiration (30 ml/kg).
2. Tidal volume (TV): the volume of air entering the airway and lungs with each single breath at rest (6–8 ml/kg).
3. Vital capacity (VC): the amount of air maximally inspired and maximally expired (40 ml/kg).
4. Total lung capacity (TLC): the amount of air contained by the lung after the end of maximal inspiration (newborn 63 ml/kg).

B. **Concepts.**
1. Elastic recoil: the natural tendency for stretched objects to recoil to their resting state of volume. During inhalation, alveoli will stretch to a certain point, and during exhalation, the alveoli will return to their original size in an infant with normal lungs.
2. Compliance: the elasticity of the lung. It refers to the relationship between a given change in volume and the pressure required to produce that change. An infant with severe hyaline membrane disease will have decreased compliance (because of lack of surfactant) requiring increased pressures to provide a given volume of gas.
3. Resistance: the result of friction in moving parts (Goldsmith and Karotkin, 1988). It refers to the relationship between a given change in pressure and a given change in flow. Resistance to gas in a 2.5 mm endotracheal tube is higher than in a 3.5 mm endotracheal tube because of the narrow lumen of the smaller tube. It takes greater pressure to force air through this small tube. There are many sources of resistance in the newborn—nasal passages, glottis, trachea, and main bronchi. If an infant is intubated, the endotracheal tube is also a source of resistance.
4. Gas trapping: more gas enters the lung than leaves the lung. A partially occluded endotracheal tube can cause gas trapping.
5. Inadvertent positive end-expiratory pressure (PEEP): a result of gas trapping whereby volume and pressure increase in the distal airways through end-expiration.
6. Work of breathing: the pressure generated to overcome the resistance forces opposing volume expansion and gas flow into and out of the lungs during respiration. Surfactant decreases the work of breathing in the neonate.
7. Ventilation-perfusion ratio: the oxygen content in the blood depends partly on the ratio between alveolar ventilation and capillary blood flow ($\dot{V}_A/Q$) (Goldsmith and Karotkin, 1988, p. 226). For example, in a term infant with pneumonia, there are areas of the lung with exudate that are not ventilating properly, thus preventing adequate gas exchange. The blood is not exchanging gas because underventilation is causing a low ventilation-perfusion ratio. Figure 9–1 depicts more examples concerning the effects of various ventilation-perfusion ratios on blood gas tensions.
8. Mean airway pressure (MAP): the average pressure delivered to the proximal airways from the beginning of one inspiration to the beginning of the next. Several parameters from conventional ventilation contribute to increasing MAP. These include increasing peak inspiratory pressure, reversing the inspiratory/expiratory ratio, increasing PEEP, increased inspiratory time, and increasing the inspiratory flow rate. All of these parameters help to improve oxygenation by increasing MAP. MAP is felt to be the major determinant of oxygenation (Goldsmith and Karotkin, 1988, p. 63)

C. **Laws.**
1. Boyle's law: volume of a gas (V) is inversely proportional to the pressure (P) to which it is subjected at a constant temperature. $P_1V_1 = P_2V_2$.

V_A/Q Relationships

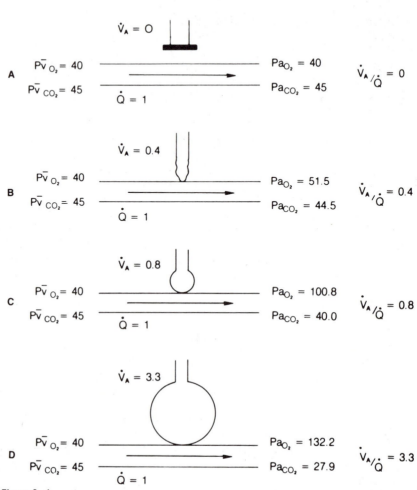

Figure 9–1

Effects of various ventilation-perfusion ratios on blood gas tensions. *A,* Direct venoarterial shunting ($\dot{V}A/\dot{Q}$ = 0). Venous gas tensions are unaltered, and arterial blood has the same tension as venous blood. *B,* Alveolus with a low $\dot{V}A/Q$ ratio. Only partial oxygenation and CO_2 removal take place in this alveolus owing to underventilation in relation to perfusion. *C,* Normal alveolus. *D,* Underperfused alveolus with high $\dot{V}A/Q$ ratio. Note that although the oxygen tension is 32 mm greater than alveolus *C,* this results in only a slightly higher saturation and oxygen content. (From Thibeault, D.W., and Gregory, G.A. Neonatal Pulmonary Care. Norwalk, CT, Appleton-Century-Crofts, 1986.)

2. Dalton's law: states that in a gas mixture, the pressure exerted by each individual gas is independent of any of the pressures exerted by other gases in the mixture. Oxygen has its own partial pressure compared with carbon dioxide in the mixture of gases we call air.
3. Henry's law: the weight of a gas absorbed by a liquid with which it does not combine chemically is directly proportional to the partial pressure of the gas to which the liquid is exposed (and its solubility in the liquid) (Levitzky, 1986).
4. Laplace's law: states that the pressure needed to stabilize an alveolus is directly proportional to twice the surface tension and inversely proportional to the radius of the structure. In the neonate, surface tension increases with decreased amounts of surfactant and decreases with adequate amounts of surfactant. With each inspiration, alveoli in the lung have differing volumes. Larger alveoli

require less distending pressure to open, whereas smaller alveoli require greater pressure to open. Surfactant's effectiveness in reducing surface tension increases as the radius of the alveoli get smaller and decreases as the radius of the alveoli get bigger.

D. **Control of breathing.** See Table 9–1 (Goldsmith and Karotkin, 1988) for a complete review of factors affecting the control of breathing in the neonate.

Table 9–1
FACTORS AFFECTING CONTROL OF VENTILATION IN THE SPONTANEOUSLY BREATHING NEONATE

A. Neurological Factors
1. "Maturity" of the central nervous system (CNS)
   a. Degree of *myelination*, which largely determines speed of impulse transmission and response time to stimuli affecting ventilation
   b. Degree of *arborization* or dendritic interconnections (synapses) between neurons, allowing summation of excitatory potentials coming in from other parts of the CNS, and largely setting the neuronal depolarization threshold and response level of the respiratory center
2. Sleep state (i.e., rapid eye movement or REM sleep vs. quiet or non-REM sleep)
   a. *REM sleep* is generally associated with irregular respirations (both in depth and frequency), distortion and paradoxical motion of the rib cage during inspiration, inhibition of Hering-Breuer and glottic closure reflexes, and blunted response to CO_2 changes
   b. *Quiet sleep* is generally associated with regular respirations, a more stable rib cage, and a directly proportional relationship between Pco_2 and degree of ventilation
3. Reflex responses
   a. *Hering-Breuer reflex*, whereby inspiratory duration is limited in response to lung inflation sensed by stretch receptors located in major airways. Not present in adult humans, this reflex is very active during quiet sleep of newborn babies but absent or very weak during REM sleep.
   b. *Head's reflex*, whereby inspiratory effort is further increased in response to rapid lung inflation. Thought to produce the frequently observed "biphasic sighs" of newborns that may be crucial for promoting and maintaining lung inflation (and therefore breathing regularity) after birth
   c. *Intercostal-phrenic reflex*, whereby inspiration is inhibited by proprioception (position-sensing) receptors in intercostal muscles responding to distortion of the lower rib cage during REM sleep
   d. *Trigeminal-cutaneous reflex*, whereby tidal volume increases and respiratory rate decreases in response to facial stimulation

   e. *Glottic closure reflex*, whereby the glottis is narrowed through reflex contraction of the laryngeal adductor muscles during respiration, thereby "breaking" exhalation and increasing subglottic pressure (as with expiratory "grunting")

B. Chemical Drive Factors (Chemoreflexes)
1. *Response to hypoxemia (falling PaO_2) or to decrease in O_2 concentration breathed* (mediated by peripheral chemoreceptors in carotid and aortic bodies):
   a. Initially there is increase in depth of breathing (tidal volume), but subsequently (if hypoxia persists or worsens), there is depression of respiratory drive, reduction in depth and rate of respiration, and eventual failure of arousal
   b. For the first week of life at least, these responses are dependent on environmental temperature, i.e., keeping the baby warm
   c. Hypoxia is associated with an increase in periodic breathing and apnea
2. *Response to hyperoxia* (increase in FiO_2 breathing causes a transient respiratory depression, stronger in term than in pre-term infants
3. *Response to hypercapnia (rising $PaCO_2$ or [H^+]) or to increase in CO_2 concentration breathed* (mediated by central chemoreceptors in the medulla):
   a. Increase in ventilation is directly proportional to inspired CO_2 concentration (or, more accurately stated, to alveolar CO_2 tension), as is the case in adults
   b. Response to CO_2 is in large part dependent on sleep state: in quiet sleep, a rising $PaCO_2$ causes increase in depth and rate of breathing, whereas during REM sleep, the response is irregular and reduced in depth and rate. The degree of reduction closely parallels the amount of rib cage deformity occurring during REM sleep
   c. Ventilatory response to CO_2 in newborns is markedly depressed during behavioral activity such as feeding, and easily depressed by sedatives and anesthesia

From Goldsmith, J.P., and Karotkin, E.H.: Assisted Ventilation of the Neonate, 2nd ed. Philadelphia, W.B. Saunders Co., 1988, p. 28.

Treatment Modalities

A. Oxygen therapy.
1. Oxyhood: consists of warm, humidified oxygen at a measured concentration.
   a. Indications: cyanosis, hypoxemia, apnea, and respiratory difficulty.
   b. Complications and disadvantages: hyperoxia leading to lung tissue injury and retinal damage, confining movement, and temperature instability. Adequate flow is required to wash out CO_2 build-up.
2. Nasal cannula: consists of humidified 100% oxygen at a set flow rate delivered via a cannula with the flow directed into the nares.
   a. Indications: low oxygen requirement oxyhood, prolonged oxygen requirement (bronchopulmonary dysplasia [BPD]), transfer or transport of infant, or need for something less confining than oxyhood.
   b. Complications and disadvantages: same as with oxyhood; pressure-related tissue damage due to improper or infrequent changing. Unable to measure exact concentration of oxygen. Malposition, displacement of the cannula leading to hypoxemia.
3. Continuous positive airway pressure (CPAP).
   a. Mask CPAP: consists of positive pressure (2–8 cm) with or without oxygen via face mask. Requires a tight seal around nose and mouth.
      (1) Indications: alveolar collapse, apnea, respiratory difficulty, or pulmonary edema.
      (2) Advantages: short-term use to assist with alveolar expansion and to inhibit alveolar collapse (atelectasis); does not require intubation.
      (3) Disadvantages: requires a constant seal to remain effective, infants may fight or struggle against mask, causes gastric distention.
      (4) Complications: pulmonary hyperexpansion potentially leading to air leaks (pneumothorax, etc.), aspiration of stomach contents, ineffective ventilation with further or increasing respiratory difficulty.
   b. Nasal CPAP: consists of nasal prongs or single nasopharyngeal tube that delivers 2–8 cm of positive pressure with or without oxygen.
      (1) Indications: same as with mask CPAP, prolonged mask CPAP (if mask CPAP is required for more than a few minutes).
      (2) Advantages: attached to infant via soft velcro straps and does not require constant attention to maintain a face mask seal. Does not require intubation; same as with face mask CPAP.
      (3) Disadvantages: less positive pressure in delivery if infants open their mouth; same as with mask CPAP.
      (4) Complications: same as with mask CPAP; pressure-related tissue damage from prolonged or improper use.
   c. Endotracheal CPAP: continuous positive pressure delivery via an endotracheal tube.
      (1) Indications: same as with nasal and mask CPAP; access to direct pulmonary suctioning; upper airway obstruction; central nervous system disorders; occasionally used just prior to extubation from ventilator.
      (2) Advantages: pressure and oxygen remain constant.
      (3) Disadvantages: requires intubation by a skilled provider, endotracheal tube may be malpositioned and/or become dislodged.
      (4) Complications: trauma secondary to tube placement; port of entry for pathogens; increased risk of pulmonary air leaks; hypoventilation; mucous plugging; prolonged use may contribute to subglottic stenosis; laryngomalacia; or tracheomalacia.
4. Assisted ventilation: consists of aiding the infant with ventilation using mechanical support.
   a. Indications: hypoxemia, hypercapnia, and/or acidemia related to respiratory failure, pulmonary insufficiency, cardiovascular collapse, CNS disease, or surgery.

   b. Advantages: consistent delivery of assisted ventilation and O_2 therapy to promote respiratory homeostasis. Lessens work of breathing.
   c. Disadvantages: same as with endotracheal CPAP; involves radiation of infant to validate tube placement; requires continuous monitoring of heart rate, respiratory rate, and oxygen saturations.
   d. Complications: same as with endotracheal CPAP; hyperventilation; BPD; and retinopathy of prematurity (ROP).

B. **Types of assisted ventilation.**

1. Intermittent negative-pressure ventilation (INPV): provides the ability to ventilate by chest wall movement and eliminates the need for intubation. However, does require a sealed chamber or jacket type device, which severely limits the access to the infant for purposes of monitoring. Using this method of ventilation will affect thermoregulation in the neonate. Almost never used in treating neonates with respiratory problems.
2. Intermittent positive-pressure ventilation (IPPV).
   a. Volume ventilator: administers a predetermined volume of gas regardless of pulmonary compliance and resistance. Rate can be set or used as an assist mode at the infant's own respiratory rate.
   b. Pressure-limited ventilator: administers a predetermined pressure at the termination of inspiration regardless of the volume of gas delivery. A decrease in lung compliance could result in hypoventilation.
   c. Time-cycled, pressure-limited ventilator: administers a predetermined pressure of gas but allows for adjustment in the duration of inspiration and expiration. Also allows for spontaneous respiratory effort of the infant, thereby facilitating a gradual reduction of support.
   d. Bag and mask ventilation: delivery of positive pressure and oxygen via face mask. Maximum pressure can be preset to prevent excessive pressure. Does not require intubation and can be very effective for short-term use.

C. **Care of the ventilated patient.**

1. Airway management: prior to any respiratory treatment modality, the airway should be kept open and free of secretions. Endotracheal intubation should only be performed by a skilled provider and an assistant. (Refer to Chapter 34.)
2. Initiating assisted ventilation. Once the decision has been reached to place an infant on a ventilator and the endotracheal tube is appropriately placed and secured, the following ventilator parameters must be determined:
   a. Rate. The most commonly used ventilator in the NICU is the time-cycled, pressure-limited IPPV, owing to the ability to adjust peak pressure, PEEP, inspiratory time, and rate. Infants without respiratory failure have a resting respiratory rate of about 40/minute, whereas infants with respiratory failure may have a respiratory rate of 0–100/minute or greater. The goal of mechanical ventilation is one of assisting with the infant's respiratory effort to promote adequate ventilation. Therefore, a beginning ventilator rate of 30–40/minute for an infant with respiratory failure should be adequate. The ventilator rate will affect the ability to blow off CO_2.
   b. Peak inspiratory pressure (PIP). To determine the appropriate PIP requires careful and skilled assessment, as the complications of excessive PIP can be deleterious. Auscultation of breath sounds to assess aeration and compliance is necessary. Experimenting with an anesthesia bag and mask to find the best rate and pressure may be useful and allows the clinician to determine the infant's ventilating needs. Visual inspection of chest wall movement in conjunction with a pressure gauge reading from the anesthesia bag may guide your assessment. A beginning PIP of 20 cm is appropriate for most pre-term infants, with increases or decreases as needed. Be aware that the flow rate will affect the amount of PIP required. PIP will affect the Pao_2.
   c. Positive end-expiratory pressure (PEEP). This is essential to maintain the functional residual capacity and prevent alveolar collapse. This is especially important when ventilating infants with surfactant deficiency, owing to

their propensity towards collapse. Physiological PEEP is estimated at 2 cm. Therefore, infants with a tendency for collapse should start at 4 cm and have adjustments as needed. PEEP will effect PaO_2 and PCO_2.

   d. Inspiratory/expiratory time ratio (I/E ratio). The determination of the proper I/E ratio should be based on the underlying reason for ventilation. Physiologic I/E ratio in a non-disease state is equal to 1:2 or 1:3, meaning a short inspiratory time and a long expiratory time. This type of ratio would best benefit an infant with unknown cause of distress or with CNS or congenital heart disease. An I/E ratio of 1:1 would be best for infants requiring a high ventilator rate and lower PIP, such as with pulmonary interstitial emphysema. Finally, an inverse I/E ratio of 3:1 – 2:1 would be appropriate for treating infants requiring higher mean airway pressure (MAP) to maintain the PaO_2, such as with the acute stages of meconium aspiration with resulting persisting pulmonary hypertension (Goldsmith and Karotkin, 1988). The I/E ratio will affect the PaO_2 and PCO_2.

   e. Flow rate. Low flow of 5 – 10 liters/minute: accomplishments are more physiologic respiration or sine type waveform. The inspiratory pressure gradually builds to a peak just prior to expiration. High flow of 10 liters/minute or greater accomplishes a rapid peak pressure and maintains it until expiration, thus being more consistent with a square type waveform. Flow rate will affect PaO_2.

   f. Mean airway pressure (MAP). This is defined as the average distending pressure throughout a complete respiratory cycle. The MAP can be calculated using a specific formula, but it is most often digitally displayed by the ventilator. The desired effect of an increased MAP is improved oxygenation. Increasing the MAP can be achieved by manipulating the PEEP, PIP, I/E ratio, and flow rate. Although the desired effect of an increased PaO_2 is achieved, there is also an increase in barotrauma to the lungs. Close attention to the MAP during ventilation is essential, especially once the underlying disease begins to resolve.

Monitoring During Therapy

A. **Physical assessment.**

1. Observation: one of the most valuable tools in assessing an infant's respiratory status. Does the infant appear to be comfortable while breathing, or does the baby show signs and symptoms of distress by grunting, flaring, and retracting? Silverman and Anderson (1956) developed a screening tool of five signs/symptoms to assess respiratory distress in the newborn (Fig. 9–2). Assess the skin color of the infant. Skin color should be uniformly pink. Skin color that is blue, dusky, or pale needs to be evaluated further. A dramatic change in skin color needs to be investigated immediately to rule out a pneumothorax versus a mechanical obstruction. Observe the infant's respiratory rate. Is it within the normal range (40–60 breaths/minute)? When observing the respiratory rate, consider variables such as environment, temperature, and the infant's state of activity/inactivity, which can increase or decrease the respiratory rate. Observe if the chest rises symmetrically; if asymmetrical, suspect a possible pneumothorax, diaphragmatic hernia, or phrenic nerve palsy.

2. Auscultation. Listen to the breath sounds carefully to determine differences in the upper and lower lung fields and differences in the left from the right lung fields. Is aeration equal bilaterally? Are rales or rhonchi evident? A finding in a ventilated infant may be louder breath sounds on the right; if present, suspect that the endotracheal tube has slipped into the right bronchus. However, this may also represent a pneumothorax and should be evaluated. Rule out other noises and their points or origin. Bowel sounds heard in the chest are an indication of a diaphragmatic hernia.

SILVERMAN-ANDERSEN RETRACTION SCORE

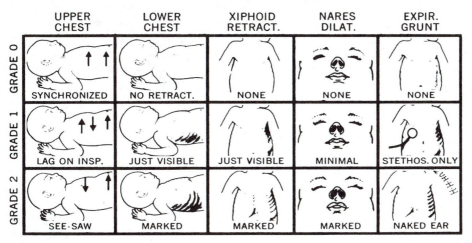

Figure 9-2
Silverman and Anderson scale to assess respiratory distress in the newborn. (Adapted from Silverman, W.A., and Anderson, D.H.: Reproduced by permission of Pediatrics, *17*:1-10, copyright 1956.)

B. Pulse oximetry.

1. Pulse oximetry is a non-invasive and continuous method of measuring hemoglobin oxygen saturation. Using red and infrared light, the saturation of O_2 bound to hemoglobin is determined by a digital readout displayed by the monitoring device. The main advantage of pulse oximetry is the short response time in determining the O_2 saturation in a neonate. It also reduces the number of invasive blood gas measurements necessary for a particular infant. It can be used in various settings outside of the NICU (i.e., in neonatal transport, delivery room care, and surgery).

2. An accurate reading is dependent on several factors, a primary factor being the perfusion status of the infant. It has been documented that accuracy decreased with low-perfusion states (Fanconi, 1985). Phototherapy, motion artifact, dyes (baby footprints), and vasoconstricting drug (dopamine) can affect saturation readouts. Pulse oximetry *does not eliminate* the need for blood gas analysis. When an infant's acid-base balance is in question, blood gas determination then needs to be made. Pulse oximetry helps to assess an infant's oxygenation status. Continuous saturations >96% may indicate that an infant is ready to be weaned from O_2 therapy, depending on the acute or chronic nature of the infant's disease. Wasunna and Whitelow (1987) have suggested that saturations >92% may be associated with hyperoxia in the pre-term infant. Table 9-2 gives guidelines of percentage parameters for O_2 saturation monitoring.

C. Transcutaneous monitoring.

1. Transcutaneous monitoring (TCM) of Po_2 is a non-invasive method that measures through a heated electrode the oxygen flow across the skin (skin Po_2). The advantage of TCM is the same as for the pulse oximeter. TCM reduces the number of invasive blood gas measurements and also can be used in various settings outside the NICU. The TCM also has several disadvantages. The readout on the TCM is not immediate—a warming period is required (10-20 minutes), and after about 4-6 hours, the TCM begins to lose its measurement reliability, thus requiring change of the probe. The TCM requires frequent calibration during use. The electrode has been reported to cause burns in premature infants and skin breakdown in the very low birthweight preterm infant from the probe adhesive. Also, the readout time of the transcutaneous Po_2 values lags 5-10 seconds behind the Pao_2 value but the correlation be-

Table 9-2
PRACTICAL HINTS FOR O_2 SATURATION MONITORING

Acceptable Limits	Acute	Chronic
	87-95%	*90-95%*
Oxygen management parameters	Wean from O_2 when infant stable and StcaO$_2$ readings are consistently >95% every 15 minutes to ½ hour	Wean from O_2 when infant stable and StcaO$_2$ readings are consistently >95% every 12-24 hours
Blood gas requirements	When StcaO$_2$ < 85% or >97% consistently over 15 minutes to ½ hour Monitoring and EKG heart rate not correlating and perfusion status poor	When StcaO$_2$ <87% or >95% consistently over 1 hour

From Dziedzic, K., and Vidyasagar, P.: Clin. Perinatol., *16*(1):179-197, 1989.

tween the Pao$_2$ value and the transcutaneous Po$_2$ value is as high as .98 (Peabody, 1978). This correlation can change if the infant is in overt shock, with transcutaneous Po$_2$ values much lower (Rooth et al., 1987). TCM should be used for trending measurements. The TCM does not replace the need for arterial blood gases.

2. Transcutaneous Pco$_2$ monitoring. Transcutaneous Pco$_2$ monitoring can be of benefit when monitoring those infants with respiratory problems characterized by hypercapnia. It's also beneficial in determining complications due to pneumothorax or mechanical obstruction before clinically evident by the infant. Correlation with transcutaneous Pco$_2$ is fairly accurate, but transcutaneous Pco$_2$ can overestimate Paco$_2$ (Herrell et al., 1980).

D. **Blood gas measurement.** Blood gas measurement is the standard method for monitoring oxygenation and acid-base balance in the ill newborn. Different methods are available for obtaining the blood sample, with umbilical arterial catheterization the most commonly used method. Other methods for sampling include indwelling peripheral arterial catheters, intermittent arterial puncture, and capillary sampling. Arterial samples are preferred over capillary samples (heelstick or fingerstick) because arterial samples are more reliable in obtaining an accurate Pao$_2$ value. Capillary samples are useful in infants with chronic lung disease to follow Pco$_2$ and pH. All of these methods are invasive, with the potential for major complications.

Medications Used During Ventilation Therapy

A. **Bronchodilators.**
1. Aminophylline (theophylline). Relaxes smooth muscle, thereby increasing blood flow to the lungs. Does stimulate cardiac muscle, which increases cardiac output. Increases vital capacity.

    a. *Dosage:*   Loading dose is 5-6 mg/kg. Maintenance dose is 2.5-5.0 mg/kg/day given every 6, 8, or 12 hours.

    b. *Administration:*   IV drip, IV, PO.

    c. *Monitoring:*   Trough levels obtained 1/2 hour prior to a dose 48-72 hours after initiating therapy. Therapeutic range is 7-10 μg/ml for apnea, 10-20 μg/ml for bronchodilatation (Young and Mangum, 1990).

    d. *Considerations:* Consider holding dose if the heart rate exceeds 180/minute. Signs of toxicity include GI upset, tachycardia, poor weight gain, hyper-reflexia, and seizures.

2. Albuterol/terbutaline: achieves bronchodilatation effects similar to those of aminophylline but with less cardiovascular stimulation. Also enhances the clearance of mucociliary secretions (Goldsmith and Karotkin, 1988).

    a. *Dosage:*   Aerosol: 0.1–0.5 mg/kg/dose every 2–6 hours in a nebulized solution. Oral: 0.1–0.3 mg/kg/dose every 6–8 hours (Young and Mangum, 1990).

    b. *Monitoring:*   Serum concentration levels not determined; monitor heart rate and respiratory effects.

    c. *Considerations:*   Aerosol preparation is diluted with normal saline prior to use. Oral syrup is generally well tolerated. Signs of toxicity include tachycardia, arrhythmia, tremors, and irritability.

3. Isoproterenol (Isuprel). Decreases pulmonary artery pressure and resistance with minor cardiac effects, thereby increasing blood flow to the lungs. Not entirely beta$_2$-selective; therefore, tachycardia may be noted.

    a. *Dosage:*   0.05–0.5 μg/kg/minute. May be given as continuous IV drip, IV, or directly into the endotracheal tube undiluted or mixed with normal saline.

    b. *Monitoring:*   Frequent vital signs, as this agent will increase the heart rate; central venous pressure line preferred; check blood glucose concentration, because this drug will increase insulin production.

    c. *Considerations:*   Usually reserved for infants with severe BPD and reactive airway disease in which bronchospasms significantly alter ventilation-perfusion. Signs of toxicity include arrhythmia, tachycardia leading to congestive heart failure, diminished venous return, and hypoglycemia.

B. **Diuretics.**

1. Furosemide (Lasix): specific action is on the ascending loop of Henle, affecting chloride transport, causing loss of not only chloride but also sodium, potassium, and calcium. This will increase the pH of the urine.

    a. *Indications:*   Respiratory distress syndrome (RDS)/patent ductus arteriosus: associated with an increase in pulmonary blood flow causing congestive heart failure. The goal is to cause diuresis, which will decrease vascular resistance and improve ventricular function. In BPD, furosemide improves pulmonary compliance and decreases ventilator and oxygen requirements when an acute onset of pulmonary edema is obvious. Has been used in the treatment of a pre-term infant with RDS in whom a diuresis has not been appreciated.

    b. *Dosage:*   1–2 mg/kg/dose; can be given IV, IM, or PO.

    c. *Monitoring:*   Measure urinary output and specific gravity to gauge the response. Determine serum electrolyte values to monitor sodium, potassium, and calcium losses.

    c. *Considerations:*   Known to be ototoxic, with transient and permanent hearing loss reported; renal calculi reported with chronic use.

2. Spironolactone (Aldactone). Exerts an inhibitory effect on the aldosterone regulating mechanism, causing an increase in sodium loss but sparing potassium.

    a. *Indications:*   Infants with BPD and/or congenital heart defects resulting in congestive heart failure (CHF).

b. *Dosage:* 1–3 mg/kg/day given PO once a day.

c. *Monitoring:* Serum electrolytes 2 or 3 days after initiating therapy. May cause hyperkalemia secondary to decreased urinary loss. Monitor urine output and specific gravity.

d. *Considerations:* May cause rashes, vomiting, and diarrhea. Use with caution in infants with impaired renal function.

3. Chlorothiazide (Diuril). Inhibits sodium reabsorption in the distal renal tubule. Known to have a potentiating effect when used with furosemide; thought to be calcium sparing.

a. *Indications:* Infants with refractory edema related to BPD and/or CHF.

b. *Dosage:* 10–20 mg/kg/day given PO every day or twice a day.

c. *Monitoring:* Serum electrolytes, owing to increased loss of sodium, potassium chloride, and bicarbonate. Displaces bilirubin at the binding sites. Monitor urine output and specific gravity.

d. *Considerations:* Best response seen if used in conjunction with Lasix or Aldactone. May cause electrolyte disturbances and hyperglycemia, and should be used with caution in infants with impaired renal function.

4. Hydrochlorothiazide (HydroDIURIL). Essentially the same as chlorothiazide; see above.

a. *Dosage:* 1–2 mg/kg/day given PO every day or twice a day.

C. **Corticosteroids.**

1. Dexamethasone (Decadron). Considered experimental as a long-acting anti-inflammatory medication used to treat lung injury in chronic lung disease.

a. *Indications:* Short-term use to decrease laryngeal edema secondary to prolonged intubation. Long-term use in ventilator-dependant infants with radiographic evidence of BPD.

b. *Dosage:* Short-term use: 0.5 mg/kg/day given IV or PO twice a day. Long term use: 0.5 mg/kg/day IV or PO for 3–7 days, then decrease dose to 0.3 mg/kg/day for 3–7 days. This dose is then decreased by 10% every 5 days until 0.1 mg/kg/day is reached; then give every other day for 1 week. (Avery et al., 1985).

c. *Monitoring:* Serum electrolytes and glucose.

d. *Considerations:* Experimental use in treating infants with BPD. Known side effects include hyperglycemia, hypertension, and poor weight gain. Can cause immunosuppression, thus diminishing response to infection. Osteoporosis and renal calculi have been reported when used in conjunction with Lasix.

D. **Cardiovascular agents.**

1. Dopamine. Catecholamine drug with dose-dependent interactions. *Low dose* (2–5 µg/kg/minute) will decrease vascular resistance in renal blood flow and increase urine output. *Intermediate dose* (5–15 µg/kg/minute) increases contractility of the heart and increases cardiac output and blood pressure. *High dose* (>15µg/kg/minute) will increase pulmonary systemic resistance. Not recommended in neonates, owing to decreased renal blood flow at high doses (Young and Mangum, 1990).

a. *Indications:* Shock (cardiogenic, hypovolemic, or septic) and significant persisting CHF.

b. *Dosage:* As above; begin at low end of dosage range for desired effect and increase as needed.

c. *Monitoring:* Heart rate, blood pressure, perfusion, and urine output frequently.

d. *Considerations:* Most commonly used to treat hypotension (persisting) and/or congenital heart disease in neonates. Cardiology consultation is advised. Signs of intolerance are tachycardia or arrhythmia.

2. Dobutamine. Synthetic catecholamine drug very similar to dopamine but with fewer beta-2 effects. Increases cardiac output with less tachycardia and arrhythmia.

a. *Indications:* Shock-like cardiac output failure; hypotension.

b. *Dosage:* 2–25 μg/kg/minute by continuous IV infusion.

c. *Monitoring:* Same as with dopamine.

d. *Considerations:* May cause hypotension in a patient who is hypovolemic. Best to begin at low-dose range and increase as needed. Signs of toxicity occur with high end of dosage range.

3. Tolazoline (Priscoline). Potent systemic vasodilator; alpha-adrenergic blocker; antihypertensive at high doses.

a. *Indications:* Persistent pulmonary hypertension of the newborn (PPHN). Used to decrease pulmonary vascular resistance and increase blood flow to the lungs.

b. *Dosage:* Test dose, 1–2 mg/kg/ IV over 10 minutes. Infusion, 0.2–4.0 mg/kg/hour IV in vein that empties into superior vena cava (any vein in upper extremities and scalp) (Young and Mangum, 1990).

c. *Monitoring:* Recommend pre- and post-administration Pao_2; if an increase of Pao_2 by 20–40 is not appreciated after test dose is given, continuous infusion is not likely to be of benefit. Monitor vital signs, especially blood pressure, closely. Measure urine output.

d. *Considerations:* Antihypertensive drug can cause hypotension. Have volume support on hand. Often will be used in conjunction with dopamine and dobutamine due to the hypotensive effect. Cardiology consultation is advised prior to use. Signs of toxicity include hypotension and GI disturbances. Caution is advised in patient with impaired renal function.

E. **Paralyzing agents.**
1. Pancuronium (Pavulon). Classified as a neuromuscular blocker. This drug promotes muscle relaxation and paralysis.

a. *Indications:* Infants who require moderate to high ventilatory support, to decrease O_2 consumption and cerebral blood flow fluctuations.

b. *Dosage:* 0.1 mg/kg/dose IV push slowly every 1–2 hours.

c. *Monitoring:* Vital signs, especially BP; relaxes smooth muscle — vasodilation and resulting hypotension.

d. *Considerations:* *Must* have mechanical ventilator support in place prior to use. Need to provide frequent clearing of airway, as secretions build up without swallow reflex. Signs of toxicity include tachycardia and blood pressure change (hypotension or hypertension).

F. **Drugs for pain/sedation.**
1. Morphine sulfate: narcotic analgesic.

   a. *Indications:* Analgesia or sedation.

   b. *Dosage:* 0.05–0.2 mg/kg slow IV push every 4–6 hours; 10–15 μg/kg/hour IV continuous infusion.

   c. *Monitoring:* Heart rate, blood pressure, and respiratory rate; GI status for diminished function; decreases GI motility, may cause abdominal distention.

   d. *Considerations:* Depresses respiratory center. Causes decreased GI motility and hypotension. Can be addictive. Can be reversed with naloxone (Narcan).

2. Fentanyl (Sublimaze). Narcotic analgesic.

   a. *Indications:* Analgesia, sedation.

   b. *Dosage:* 1–4 μg/kg/dose slow IV push; IV drip, 1–5 μg/kg/hour.

   c. *Monitoring:* Same as with morphine.

   d. *Considerations:* Same as with morphine.

3. Midazolam (Versed). Short-acting synthetic benzodiazepine.

   a. *Indications:* Sedative.

   b. *Dosage:* 0.07–0.2 mg/kg slow IV push; 2–8 μg/kg/minute continuous IV infusion.

   c. *Monitoring:* Same as with morphine.

   d. *Considerations:* Short-acting Valium derivative, used in conjunction with ventilator therapy. Monitor respiratory rate closely. Known to cause seizures after rapid infusion. Signs of toxicity would include respiratory depression.

4. Pentobarbital (Nembutal). Short-acting barbiturate; provides no analgesia.

   a. *Indications:* Sedation.

   b. *Dosage:* 2–6 mg/kg IV slowly.

   c. *Monitoring:* Heart rate, respiratory rate, and blood pressure.

   d. *Considerations:* Short-term IV sedation. Does not cause respiratory depression at this dose range.

5. Chloral hydrate. Effective sedative and/or hypnotic; provides no analgesia.

   a. *Indications:* Sedation, sleep prior to procedure, test, or surgery.

   b. *Dosage:* Sedation: 25–50 mg/kg/dose PO, give every 6 hours prn. Hypnotic: 50–75 mg/kg/dose PO, 1 hour prior to procedure.

   c. *Monitoring:* Vital signs and sleep state; little value in monitoring serum drug levels.

   d. *Considerations:* Known GI irritant; should be diluted with formula. Chloral hydrate is not an analgesic, and excitement may be noted if painful stimuli are experienced.

6. Acetaminophen (Tylenol). Contains analgesic and antipyretic properties.

   a. *Indications:*   Fever and analgesia.

   b. *Dosage:*   10–15 mg/kg/dose. PO or suppository, prn every 6–8 hours.

   c. *Monitoring:*   Vital signs and signs of pain (tachycardia, tachypnea, and irritability).

   d. *Considerations:* Non-narcotic analgesic. Relief in infants with minor procedure-oriented pain. Will not affect respiratory drive. Signs of toxicity are liver injury, rash, fever, thrombocytopenia, leukopenia, and neutropenia.

Nursing Care

A. **Airway management.** Primary goal: airway, once established, should be kept patent and free of secretions.
1. Airway (nasopharyngeal, endotracheal, tracheostomy, etc.): should be secured in place, and verification of airway should be confirmed immediately after being placed, either by x-ray or by physical assessment.
2. Care of the different airways.
   a. Oxyhood: warm, humidified O_2 only via hood to prevent heat loss. Cleaned and changed per unit protocol.
   b. Nasal cannula: removed and cleaned of secretions every 4–6 hours prn. Inspect surrounding tissue for pressure-related injury. Change according to unit protocol.
   c. Nasopharyngeal or nasal prong CPAP: cleared of secretions every 2–4 hours. Inspect surrounding tissue for pressure-related injury. Water-based lubricant may aid in placing tubes and help maintain a seal. Change tubes per unit protocol.
   d. Endotracheal tube: securing device (i.e., tape etc.) should be changed prn to prevent tube from being dislodged. Scheduled replacement of tube remains a controversy.
   e. Tracheostomy: securing tracheostomy tape is changed using aseptic technique, as needed. Tube is changed weekly; inspect site for signs of tissue pressure and/or necrosis. Family members need to be included in this procedure, thus facilitating potential discharge.
3. Suctioning of airway. Provide continuous patency.
   a. Non-tracheal tubes. Suctioning of the mouth, nose, and tubes should be performed on an as-needed basis. The presence of a foreign body in the mouth or nose will cause slight increase in secretions. Suctioning can coincide with the cleaning or changing of these tubes.
   b. Tracheal tubes (endotracheal tube, tracheostomy). The amount of secretion in these tubes will be disease related. Infants with resolving RDS, PDA, BPD, and pneumonia are more likely to require frequent suctioning, owing to an increased production of mucus. However, patients with early-stage RDS, CNS disease, and most congenital heart disease (CHD) will not be very mucus producing and require less suctioning. The need for suctioning of the tracheal tube should be an integral part of your assessment of the ventilated patient.

B. **Equipment function.**
1. All infants requiring mechanical ventilation should be placed on an FDA-approved ventilator that plainly displays rate (intermittent mandatory ventilation [IMV]), pressure, PEEP, tidal volume (when applicable), inspiratory time, I/E ratio, and O_2 concentration. Mean airway pressure (MAP) is optional, as it can be calculated.

2. All mechanical ventilators should have alarms activated to alert caregivers of ventilator malfunction or disconnection.
3. All mechanical ventilators should have pre-set pressure relief valves to ensure against administration of excessive peak inspiratory pressure/PEEP.
4. All mechanical ventilators should have frequently scheduled inspections by licensed respiratory therapists. Inspections are usually performed every 1–2 hours and documented.
5. All ventilator tubing is changed at scheduled intervals as designated by hospital policy.
6. All infants requiring O_2 therapy should have O_2 concentration analyzed on scheduled intervals by a licensed respiratory therapist, and analysis should be documented in the permanent record.
7. Continuous oxygen analysis is preferred, including alarm capability to notify caregivers if the prescribed oxygen concentration is no longer within a specified range.
8. The following equipment is to be located in the immediate area of all infants requiring mechanical ventilation. This equipment should be checked for proper functioning and replaced as needed at scheduled intervals.

Laryngoscopes with sterile blades:
Size 0 for infants <4 kg
Size 1 for infants >4 kg

Sterile endotracheal tubes (Bloom and Cropley, 1987):
Size 2.5, <1000 g
Size 3.0, 1000–2000 g
Size 3.5, 2000–3000 g
Size 4.0, >3000 g
Sterile stylette (plastic coated)
Suctioning sterile tubing and catheters (gauge set at 80–100 mm Hg)
Sterile orogastric (nasogastric) tubes:
Size 5 Fr, <1 kg
Size 8 Fr, > kg

Anesthesia bag and mask: capable of delivering 90–100% O_2 and O_2 source

Tape, scissors, and benzoin

C. **Monitoring.**
1. All infants receiving oxygen therapy should be considered as potential candidates for mechanical ventilation and therefore should require the following monitoring equipment:
   a. Heart rate monitor with audible beat-to-beat capability and alarming device for bradycardia (<100/minute) or tachycardia (>180/minute). Monitor should provide visual display of EKG and actual heart rate.
   b. Respiratory monitor: visual display of respiratory wave pattern and actual respiratory rate. Should include alarm device for apnea and tachypnea. Respiratory rate trend mode is optional but preferred.
   c. Peripheral (cuff) BP monitoring performed on a scheduled interval and documented on the permanent record.
   d. Oxygen analyzer: continuous preferred, intermittent mandatory alarm device for O_2 concentration greater than or less than desired range.
   e. Pulse oximetry: continuous preferred, intermittent mandatory scheduled check and documentation of peripheral O_2 saturations. Continuous pulse oximetry will have alarm device to alert if O_2 saturations are less than or greater than desired range. All infants requiring mechanical ventilation should have all the monitoring as listed above and based on their clinical condition:
      (1) Arterial access (usually via an umbilical artery catheter) for:
         (a) Blood gas sampling.

(b) Blood pressure monitoring.
(2) Transcutaneous Po_2 and Pco_2 monitor (optional if arterial access is available, recommended if access is limited or not available). Visual display of transcutaneous Po_2 and Pco_2 readings. Alarm device for Po_2 values and Pco_2 values that are designated as out of the desired range. Frequently, connected to a graphic recorder that enables the caregiver to access Po_2 and Pco_2 trends.
(3) Pulse oximetry.
(4) Physical assessment and monitor inspection performed by the primary caregiver on a scheduled interval. Documentation of assessment on the permanent record.

Weaning from the Ventilator

A. **Indications.**
1. Clinical signs consistent with beginning resolution.
2. Hyperventilation.

B. **Techniques.** Reducing the mechanical ventilatory oxygen support for an infant involves a process of evaluating several respiratory parameters. An ongoing assessment of the following is instrumental in a successful withdrawal of ventilatory support.
1. Physical assessment of respiratory status (i.e., breath sounds, aeration, compliance, rate, etc.). Cardiovascular status: heart rate, blood pressure, presence of murmur, color, and perfusion. Neurological status: presence of spontaneous respirations, tone, reflex irritability, etc.
2. Radiological evaluation: chest x-ray consistent with improving aeration and ventilation. No air leak, atelectasis, infiltrates.
3. Laboratory evaluation of fluid, electrolyte, and hematological stability.
4. Blood gas analysis: if all of the above mentioned categories are stable and improving, reduction of ventilatory support by the NNP or MD in accordance with blood gas values is possible. Pao_2: if values are within the desired range, do not adjust PIP, PEEP inspiratory time, O_2 concentration, or flow rate. If values are above the desired range, reduce the PIP, Fio_2, inspiratory time, PEEP, or flow rate in that order, then reassess. $Paco_2$: if values are within the desired range, do not adjust the IMV (rate). If values are lower than the desired range, decrease the IMV, then reassess. PIP, PEEP, inspiratory time, and flow rate are the parameters that influence the amount of barotrauma to the lungs. Oxygen toxicity is also injurious to lung tissue. Therefore, PIP and O_2 are initially lowered before the other parameters. Hyperventilation to achieve alkalosis is not uncommon in treating certain pulmonary complications in the newborn. Lowering the $Paco_2$ to <20 has been associated with changes in cerebral blood flow. In certain circumstances, one may benefit the infant by reducing the IMV (rate) initially prior to lowering PIP or Fio_2. The etiology of the lung disease should guide you in your attempts to wean ventilator support.

C. **Extubating from mechanical ventilation.**
1. Once low ventilator parameters have been attained (IMV <30/minute, PIP <18, and Fio_2 $<30\%$), the decision of when to extubate should be contemplated. An assessment of the infant's ability to sustain respiration without ventilator support is made. Endotracheal CPAP is sometimes used as a trial period off the ventilator. In this way, should the infant not tolerate being off the ventilator, only the ventilator needs manipulation to re-establish ventilation; the infant need not be disturbed. At other times, especially when dealing with premature infants with resolving RDS, extubation to nasal prong CPAP and O_2 and then to oxyhood or nasal cannula will be performed. Frequently infants will self-extubate and have a strong enough respiratory drive to remain extu-

bated. When one reaches these decisions, it is best to know each infant's respiratory status, disease process, and overall clinical condition.

D. Nursing care.
1. The airway management, equipment function, and monitoring of the infant as discussed above in nursing care remain unchanged during this period of ventilator support reduction.
2. Frequent assessment of the infant's vital signs, blood pressure, O_2 saturations, and behavior patterns is essential. Documentation of this assessment will facilitate the appropriate changes in ventilator needs.
3. Immediate notification of the primary caregiver (MD, resident, NNP) of respiratory or cardiovascular decompensation is essential during this weaning period.
4. Adequate preparation for extubation prior to the event will add to the success of withdrawing ventilator support.
   a. Have all equipment required for intubation.
   b. Endotracheal tube, nasopharyngeal tube, and oral suctioning performed prior to extubation.
   c. Have post-extubation equipment (oxyhood, nasopharyngeal tube, NP, CPAP, etc.) already set up prior to extubation.
   d. Blood gas determination within 1 hour after extubation.
   e. Consider chest x-ray if respiratory or cardiovascular decompensation occurs after extubation (looking for atelectasis).
   f. Continue frequent physical assessment every 1–2 hours for 24 hours after extubation.
   g. Appropriate explanation to family members regarding plan of extubation prior to the event is necessary.

Blood Gas Interpretation

The purpose of obtaining blood gases in a neonate is to determine if the baby is adequately ventilating and/or perfusing (Goldsmith and Karotkin, 1988). Blood gases are the basis for analyzing if oxygenation is adequate and for deducing what the acid-base balance is in a particular neonate. In analyzing oxygenation, look at the Pao_2 value; to evaluate the acid-base balance, look at the pH, $Paco_2$, base excess, and bicarbonate values. Acceptable blood gas values (modified from Goldsmith and Karotkin) give parameters for Pao_2, $Paco_2$, pH, HCO_3, and base excess values (Table 9–3). If a capillary sample is obtained, the one parameter that will change is the Pao_2 value. A 40–50 mm Hg value is usually acceptable. Check in your unit for standards concerning acceptable parameters in blood gas interpretation.

A. Respiratory/metabolic acidosis and alkalosis. Primary changes in $Paco_2$ reflect a respiratory component to an acidosis-alkalosis, whereas primary changes in HCO_3 reflect a metabolic component to acidosis-alkalosis.
1. Respiratory acidosis raises $Paco_2$ and lowers pH.

Table 9–3
ACCEPTABLE BLOOD GAS VALUES

	<28 weeks	38–40 wk	Term Infant with Pulmonary Hypertension	Infant with BPD
Pao_2	50–65	50–70	>100	60–80
$Paco_2$	40–50	40–50	<30	45–60
pH	>7.28	>7.30	>7.5	7.35–7.45
HCO_3	18–24	20–24	>24	>20

Data from Goldsmith and Karotkin, 1988.

Causes	Mechanism
CNS Depression	
Maternal narcotics during labor, asphyxia, severe intra-cranial bleeding, neuromuscular disorder, CNS dys-maturity (apnea of prematurity).	
Decreased Ventilation-Perfusion Ratio	
Obstructed airways, meconium aspiration, choanal atresia, bloody mucus, blocked endotracheal tube, external compression of airway.	Decrease in alveolar ventilation
Decreased Lung Compliance	
HMD, chronic pulmonary insufficiency	
Injuries to Thoracic Cage	
Diaphragmatic hernia, phrenic nerve paralysis, and pneumothorax	
Iatrogenic (inadequate mechanical ventilation	

2. Metabolic acidosis lowers HCO_3, pH, and base excess (negative value).

Causes	Mechanism
Decreased tissue perfusion	Increase in lactic acid production
Sepsis, CHF	
Renal failure	Increase in organic acids
Renal tubular acidosis	Loss of base
Diarrhea	Loss of base

3. Respiratory alkalosis lowers Pa_{CO_2} and raises pH

Causes	Mechanism
Iatrogenic (mechanical ventilation)	
Hypoxemia	Increase in alveolar ventilation
CNS irritation (pain)	

4. Metabolic alkalosis raises HCO_3, pH, and base excess (positive value).

Causes	Mechanism
Gastric suctioning	Loss of acid
Severe vomiting	Loss of acid
Diuretic therapy	Loss of H^+ ion via kidney
Iatrogenic (gave too much HCO_3)	Adding a base
Exchange transfusion	Citrate in anticoagulant is metabolized

B. **Compensation/correction of acidosis-alkalosis.** Compensation occurs in response to a primary disturbance in acid-base equilibrium whereby the change in the pH is relieved. Compensation is a change in the system not originally affected by the primary disturbance. Correction is a change in the system originally affected by the primary disturbance by some intervention, using available therapy by the clinician.

1. Compensated respiratory acidosis is characterized by the retention of bicarbonate as a result of adjustment in renal function. The primary disturbance is the accumulation of carbon dioxide, thus increasing carbonic acid concentration. The kidneys respond to this disturbance by holding on to HCO_3. This compensation by the kidney can take several days if not corrected by ventilation therapy. When fully compensated, the pH is near normal and $Paco_2$ values and HCO_3 are increased.
2. Compensated metabolic acidosis is characterized mainly by hyperventilation. Hyperventilation is the compensatory mechanism activated by the primary disturbance of an accumulation of acid that devours the available base. CO_2 excreted through the lungs lowers the carbonic acid concentration to match the lower available bicarbonate. When fully compensated, the pH is near normal and the $Paco_2$ and the serum HCO_3 values are both low.
3. Compensated respiratory alkalosis is characterized by the kidneys increasing their secretion of bicarbonate to restore the bicarbonate/carbonic acid ratio to normal. The primary disturbance is caused by hyperventilation with excessive elimination of CO_2. When fully compensated, the pH is near normal, but $Paco_2$ and serum HCO_3 are at the lower end of normal.
4. Compensated metabolic alkalosis is characterized by hypoventilation to diminish the elimination of CO_2. The primary disturbance is the accumulation of bicarbonate; by retaining CO_2, the appropriate reaction between sodium bicarbonate and carbonic acid is restored. When compensated, the pH is almost normal but the $Paco_2$ and serum bicarbonate values are elevated. See Table 9–4 concerning uncompensated and compensated acidosis-alkalosis.
5. Correction of acidosis-alkalosis. A correction of acidosis or alkalosis can be achieved sooner if one manipulates ventilation settings or gives bicarbonate to achieve a desired value. If you increase your pressure or rate on the ventilator, you will blow off CO_2. If you decrease the rate or pressure, you will encourage retention of CO_2. If you have an infant with severe metabolic acidosis, consider giving sodium bicarbonate 2 mEq/kg slow IV push (Young and Mangum, 1990) (no faster than 1 mEq/kg/minute). For acute correction of HCO_3 base deficit, take your base deficit × (wt in kg) × (0.3). You can estimate the base deficit by subtracting the infant's bicarbonate value from the normal value of 24. In giving HCO_3, dilute (1:1) with sterile H_2O, give slowly (no faster than 1 mEq/kg/minute to avoid hyperosmolarity), and be sure you have adequate ventilation.

Table 9–4
UNCOMPENSATED/COMPENSATED ACIDOSIS-ALKALOSIS

Disturbance	Blood pH	Blood PCO_2	Blood HCO_{33}
Normal	7.35–7.45	35–45	20–24
Respiratory acidosis			
Uncompensated	▼⁻	▲	N
Fully compensated	N	▲	▲⁺
Metabolic acidosis			
Uncompensated	▼⁻	N	▼
Fully compensated	N	▼⁻	▼
Respiratory alkalosis			
Uncompensated	▲⁺	▼	N
Fully compensated	N	▼	▼⁻
Metabolic alkalosis			
Uncompensated	▲⁺	N	▲
Fully compensated	N	▲⁺	▲

Abbreviations: N, normal; ▲, high; ▲⁺, highest; ▼, low; ▼⁻, lowest.

C. Interpreting a blood gas. When interpreting a blood gas, you need to:
1. Evaluate the pH and decide if there is an acidosis or alkalosis.
2. Evaluate the $Paco_2$ value to determine if there is a respiratory component.
3. Evaluate the HCO_3 or base excess to evaluate if there is a metabolic component.
4. Evaluate the Pao_2 value and determine if there is hypoxia.
5. Now that you have interpreted the gas, what are you going to do about it? Decide what event is occurring to affect these values and what specific clinical disorder(s) is known to produce this type of event. What are the possible buffer responses, and what corrective measures can you initiate? For example, 1 day old Baby Boy Smith with an estimated gestational age of 29 weeks has moderate RDS. His blood gas values have been relatively stable the last few hours. You receive gas values obtained before his much needed endotracheal tube suctioning with the following results: pH, 7.27; $Paco_2$, 57; Pao_2, 60; HCO_3, 20; and base excess of -4. From these values, you know he has an acidosis with a respiratory component. The specific event causing this might be a partially obstructed airway from mucus. Possible suctioning of this baby might help his pH and his $Paco_2$. You suction this infant and follow-up with another gas determination to decide if there is any improvement.

STUDY QUESTIONS

1. Which of the following methods gives the most accurate assessment in evaluating Pao_2?
   a. Arterial blood gases.
   b. Pulse oximetry.
   c. Transcutaneous Po_2 monitoring.

2. Baby Jones has the following arterial blood gas results: pH, 7.29; Pao_2, 78; $Paco_2$, 36; HCO_3, 17.6; base excess, -7.6. You suspect:
   a. Metabolic acidosis.
   b. Respiratory acidosis.
   c. Respiratory alkalosis.

3. Baby Smith has these arterial blood gas results: pH, 7.47; Pao_2, 89; $Paco_2$, 40; HCO_3, 32.5; base excess, $+5$. You suspect:
   a. Metabolic acidosis.
   b. Metabolic alkalosis.
   c. Respiratory alkalosis.

4. Surfactant properties include all but which one of the following:
   a. Improves lung compliance.
   b. Increases the work of breathing.
   c. Provides alveolar stability.

5. Compensated metabolic acidosis is characterized by:
   a. Hyperventilation.
   b. Hypoventilation.
   c. Kidneys increasing their secretions of HCO_3.

6. Possible causes for respiratory acidosis in a neonate include all but which one of the following:
   a. CNS depression.
   b. Decreased tissue perfusion.
   c. Obstructed airway.

7. The preferred method of treatment in correcting a severe metabolic acidosis in a ventilated neonate includes which one of the following:
   a. Give 5% albumin 10 ml/kg.
   b. Give $NaHCO_3$ 2 mEq/kg slow IV push.
   c. Increase ventilator rate.

8. Urinary loss of which of the following electrolytes is most commonly seen with the use of furosemide:
   a. Cl^-, Ca^{++}, K^+, Mg^{++}.
   b. NA^+, K^+, CL^-, Ca^{++}.
   c. Na^+, PO_4, CL^-, Ca^{++}.

9. Which of the following diuretics is the most Ca^{++} sparing:
   a. Aldactone.
   b. Diuril.
   c. Lasix.

10. Dopamine will improve renal blood flow and urine output at which of the following doses?
   a. $2-5$ $\mu g/kg/minute$.
   b. $10-15$ $\mu g/kg/minute$.
   c. >15 $\mu g/kg/minute$.

11. Which of the following is an appropriate paralyzing drug for the newborn?
    a. Fentanyl.
    b. Morphine.
    c. Pancuronium.

12. The most commonly used mechanical ventilator in the NICU is:
    a. Pressure-controlled, positive-pressure ventilator.
    b. Time-cycled, positive-pressure ventilator.
    c. Volume ventilator.

13. A low flow of 5-10 liters/minute on a time-cycled pressure ventilator will achieve which type of respiratory wave form?
    a. Block wave.
    b. Sine wave.
    c. Square wave.

14. Mean airway pressure is defined as:
    a. The amount of distending pressure remaining after the expiratory phase is complete.
    b. The average distending pressure throughout a complete respiratory cycle.
    c. The highest amount of pressure exerted at the peak of inspiration.

15. The drug tolazoline would be most appropriate in treating an infant with which of the following disease entities?
    a. BPD.
    b. PDA.
    c. Persistent pulmonary hypertension (PPHN).

Answers to Study Questions

1. a	6. b	11. c
2. a	7. b	12. b
3. b	8. b	13. b
4. b	9. b	14. b
5. a	10. a	15. c

References

Avery, G.B., Gletcher, A. B., Kaplan, M., and Brudno, D.S.: Controlled trial of dexamethasone in respirator-dependent infants with bronchopulmonary dysplasia. Pediatrics, *75*:106, 1985.

Bloom, R.S., and Cropley, C.: Textbook of Neonatal Resuscitation. American Heart Association–American Academy of Pediatrics, 1987.

Goldsmith, J.P., and Karotkin, E.H. (eds.): Assisted Ventilation of the Neonate, 2nd ed. Philadelphia, W.B. Saunders Co., 1988.

Herrell, N., Martin, R.J., Pultusker, M., et al.: Optimal temperature for the measurement of transcutaneous carbon dioxide tension in the neonate. Pediatr., *97*(1):114–117, 1980.

Livitzky, M.G.: Pulmonary Physiology, 2nd ed. New York, McGraw-Hill, 1986.

Peabody, J.L.: Clinical limitations and advantages of transcutaneous oxygen electrodes. Acta Anaesthesiol. Scand., *68*:76–82, 1978.

Wasunna, A., and Whitelow, G.L.: Pulse oximetry in preterm infants. Arch. Dis. Child., *62*:957–971, 1987.

Young, T.E., and Mangum, O.B.: Neofax. A Manual of Drugs Used in Neonatal Care, 3rd ed. Columbus, OH, Ross Laboratories, 1990.

Bibliography

Avery, G.B.: Neonatology: Pathophysiology and Management of the Newborn, 3rd ed. Philadelphia, J.B. Lippincott, 1987.

Broughton, J.O.: Understanding Blood Gases. Ohio Medical Products, Reprint #456, 1971.

Carlo, W.A., and Chatburn, R.L. (eds.): Neonatal Respiratory Care, 2nd ed. Chicago, Year Book Medical Publishers.

Courtney, S.E., Weber, K.R., Breakie, L.A., et al.: Capillary blood gases in the neonate. A reassessment and review of the literature. Am. J. Dis. Child., *144*(2):168–172, 1990.

Dziedzic, K., and Bidyasagar, D.: Pulse oximetry in neonatal intensive care. Clin. Perinatol., *16*(1):177–197, 1989.

Epstein, M.F., Cohen, A.R., Felman, H.A., and Raemer, D.B.: Estimation of Paco$_2$ by two non-invasive methods in the critically ill newborn infant. J. Pediatr., *106*(2):282–286, 1985.

Pernoll, M., Benda, G.I., and Babson, S.G.: Diagnosis and Management of the High Risk Fetus and Neonate, 5th ed. St. Louis, C.V. Mosby, 1986.

Roberts, R.J.: Drug Therapy in Infants. Philadelphia, W.B. Saunders Co., 1984.

Rooth, G., Huch, A., and Huch, R.: Transcutaneous oxygen monitors are reliable indicators of arterial oxygen tension (if used correctly). Pediatrics, *79*(2):283–286, 1987.

Scanlon, J.W., Nelson, T., Grylack, L.J., and Smith, Y.F.: A System of Newborn Physical Examination. Baltimore, University Park Press, 1979.

Sendak, M.J., Harris, A.P., and Donham, R.T.: Use of pulse oximetry to assess arterial oxygen saturation during newborn resuscitation. Crit. Care Med., *14*(8):739–740, 1986.

Thibeault, D.W., and Gregory, G.A. (eds.): Neonatal Pulmonary Care. Norwalk, CT, Appleton-Century-Crofts, 1986.

Peggy Cohen Gordin

High-Frequency Ventilation

Objectives

1. Describe the mechanisms of gas exchange involved in spontaneous, conventional, and high-frequency ventilation.

2. Choose the appropriate assessment techniques to monitor and examine patients receiving high-frequency ventilation.

3. Analyze patient changes that occur during high-frequency ventilation for early identification of potential complications.

The term *high-frequency ventilation (HFV)* refers to several forms of mechanical ventilation that have shown promise in the treatment of severe neonatal respiratory failure complicated by air leaks. In some cases, HFV appears to provide adequate ventilation for patients with poor pulmonary compliance while generating lower airway pressures than conventional mechanical ventilation. This chapter reviews the general concepts behind HFV, the care of neonates receiving two major types of HFV in clinical use, and some of the early outcome data from HFV studies on the neonatal population.

Physiology of High-Frequency Ventilation

A. Gas exchange mechanisms in spontaneous and conventional mechanical ventilation.
1. Convection (bulk flow) in large airways goes to approximately the eighth bronchial generation.
2. Molecular diffusion occurs in terminal airways and alveoli.
3. Alveolar ventilation is the result of the respiratory rate multiplied by the tidal volume delivered, less the anatomical deadspace volume ($V_A = RR \times$ [tidal volume $-$ deadspace volume]).

B. Gas exchange mechanisms in HFV.
1. HFV uses tidal volumes that may be less than or equal to the anatomical deadspace volume.
   a. Applying the gas exchange theories for conventional ventilation, alveolar ventilation during HFV should be zero.

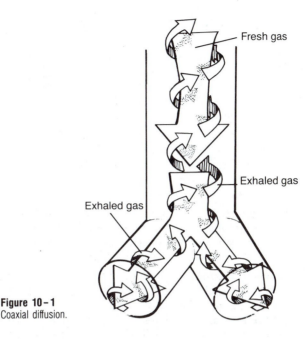

Figure 10-1
Coaxial diffusion.

b. Alternative theories for gas exchange have been proposed to explain how HFV works.
   (1) Augmented (facilitated) diffusion: diffusion of gas molecules occurs higher up in the airways.
   (2) Coaxial diffusion: fresh gas travels down the center of the airway, whereas CO_2 elimination occurs along the periphery of the airway (Fig. 10-1).
   (3) Entrainment: gas molecules from higher up in the airway are pulled into the area of low pressure created behind a high-velocity gas entry point such as a jet cannula port (Fig. 10-2).
   (4) Inter-regional gas mixing: gases in the periphery of the lung may move between alveolar units to provide better matching of ventilation and perfusion.

C. **Effectiveness of gas exchange.** All forms of HFV appear to produce adequate gas exchange at lower peak airway pressures, theoretically reducing the risk of barotrauma.

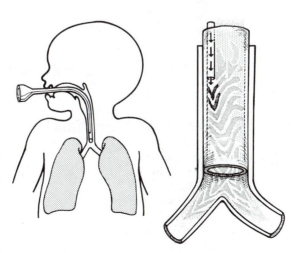

Figure 10-2
Entrainment during high-frequency jet ventilation (HFJV). Gas molecules near the jet orifice are "entrained," or dragged along with the jet pulse, whereby additional volume is delivered to the patient without substantially increasing static airway pressure. (From Harris, T. R.: *In* Goldsmith, J. R., and Karotkin, E. H. (eds.): Assisted Ventilation of the Neonate, 2nd ed. Philadelphia, W. B. Saunders Co., 1988.)

Types of HFV and Terminology

A. **High-frequency positive-pressure ventilation.**
1. Use of conventional ventilators at rapid rates (60–150 breaths/minute).
2. Technique often used for anesthesia insufflation during bronchoscopies and other airway procedures, and for conventional ventilation of infants with persistent pulmonary hypertension.

B. **High-frequency jet ventilation (HFJV).**
1. Technique that delivers rapid, high-velocity pulses from a pressurized gas source directly into the trachea via a small cannula (100–900 "breaths"/minute).
2. Expiration is passive.

C. **High-frequency oscillatory ventilation (HFOV).**
1. System that generates a very rapid vibration gas in the airway using a piston or vibrating diaphragm (400–2400 "breaths"/minute).
2. Expiratory phase is usually active, assisted by the oscillating device.

D. **High-frequency flow-interrupted ventilation (HFFI).**
1. Class of high-frequency ventilators that use a variety of mechanisms to interrupt the gas flow to the patient.
2. May be classified as an oscillator (Mammell and Boros, 1988), but gas flow is unidirectional (expiration is passive); some authors classify as a jet (Spitzer et al., 1988).

Indications for Use of HFV

A. **Severe lung disease that is unresponsive to conventional ventilation.** HFV is used as a "rescue" therapy when conventional support appears to be failing.

B. **Pulmonary air leaks, pulmonary interstitial emphysema, pneumothorax, bronchopleural fistulas, and pneumopericardium.**
1. Most successful application in clinical trials to date.
2. Rate of gas flow through chest tubes is decreased during HFV compared with conventional ventilation (Gonzalez et al., 1987).

C. **Hypoplastic lungs, diaphragmatic hernia.**
1. Limited success; may be an "intermediate" step prior to extracorporeal membrane oxygenation (ECMO).
2. Theoretical appeal owing to lower pressures needed to produce adequate gas exchange.

D. **Persistent pulmonary hypertension, meconium aspiration.**
1. Used primarily as rescue therapy, with mixed success. Interruption of gas flow occurs further back from patient's airway than with jet ventilation.
2. Theoretical advantage. May achieve excellent CO_2 removal with less barotrauma.
3. May be used as "intermediate" step prior to ECMO.

High-Frequency Oscillatory Ventilation: Clinical Application

A. **Ventilator design.**
1. Piston or vibrating diaphragm that moves a small volume of gas toward and away from patient.
2. Continuous fresh gas flow eliminates CO_2 build-up and delivers oxygen.
3. Low-pass filter allows continuous gas flow to escape while maintaining vibration of gas in the airway.

4. Proximal airway pressure is monitored by the ventilator, but clinical relevance is questionable because it probably does not reflect alveolar pressure.

B. **Parameters.** Parameters to be set and/or monitored during HFOV are different from those used with conventional ventilators.
1. Stroke volume: volume of gas displacement produced by the vibrating device; affects CO_2 elimination.
2. Mean airway pressure: affects oxygenation.
3. Amplitude: size of the pressure wave produced by the oscillator (another way to describe the volume delivered).
4. Sighs: conventional breaths given periodically to recruit alveoli and minimize atelectasis.
5. Fractional inspired oxygen concentration (FIO_2): set on the ventilator as with conventional ventilation.

C. **Patient care and assessment.**
1. No special endotracheal tube is required.
2. Suctioning procedure is performed as usual.
3. Assess chest wall vibration rather than breath sounds to determine effectiveness of ventilator settings and lung compliance changes.
4. Vibration may interfere with electrical monitoring of heart rate and respiratory rate.
   a. Use pulse from arterial line or pulse oximeter for heart rate monitoring if necessary.
   b. Respiratory rate cannot be monitored.
5. Sighs help to reduce microatelectasis and improve oxygenation.

D. **Complications and problems.**
1. Microatelectasis, poor oxygenation.
2. Increased incidence of intraventricular hemorrhage in collaborative trial of HFV using oscillator for treatment of respiratory distress syndrome in pre-term infants (HIFI Study Group, 1989).

High-Frequency Jet Ventilation: Clinical Application

A. **Ventilator design: Bunnell Life Pulse** (neonatal jet ventilator approved for use in severe airleak by the FDA).
1. Servo-controlled driving pressure: continuously adjusts the pressure of the gas supply to the jet cannula to maintain desired peak airway pressure.
2. Solenoid valve: opens and closes gas supply to the jet cannula.
3. Humidification system is built in-line.
4. Proximal airway pressures are monitored and continuously displayed; used in servo-control of pressure delivery.
5. Conventional ventilator is used in tandem to provide gas for entrainment, positive end-expiratory pressure (PEEP), and background ventilation (sighs).

B. **Parameters.** Parameters to be set and/or monitored by clinician are similar to those of conventional ventilator.
1. Peak inspiratory pressure (PIP): set on jet and conventional ventilator.
   a. Jet PIP is usually initially set at the same PIP required during conventional ventilation, and the conventional ventilator PIP is lowered by $2-5$ cm H_2O.
   b. If the PIP of conventional breaths is higher than the jet, they will interrupt the jet.
2. Servo-pressure: driving pressure is internally adjusted by the ventilator as patient compliance and pressure settings change; follow as trend data.
   a. Lower servo-pressure reflects worsening lung disease, airway obstruction, tension pneumothorax, or kinked ventilator tubing.
   b. Higher servo-pressure may indicate that lung compliance is improving or a leak in the patient/system (e.g., pneumothorax being continuously evacuated by chest tubes).

3. PEEP: set on the conventional ventilator, displayed on the jet ventilator; value displayed may be lower than value set, owing to where and how it is measured.
4. Jet valve on-time: percentage of time valve is open; similar to inspiratory time, usually 0.02 seconds.
5. Rate: set on jet and conventional ventilator.
   a. Jet rate usually 400–500/minute; Bunnell default setting of 420/minute appears to be most effective for that ventilator.
   b. Conventional intermittent mandatory ventilation (IMV) rate is usually set between 5 and 20 breaths/minute to provide background ventilation (sigh breaths), which helps to prevent atelectasis.
6. FiO_2: set on jet and conventional ventilator.

C. **Patient care and assessment.**
1. Patient must be re-intubated with special endotracheal tube that has jet port and pressure monitoring port built in (Fig. 10–3).
2. Suctioning may be performed with HFJV running or with manual ventilation as usual.
   a. Placing jet ventilator on stand-by mode during suctioning may prevent airway damage due to shearing force of opposing positive and negative pressures.
   b. Suctioning with the jet ventilator on may help decrease respiratory decompensation during the procedure in some patients.
   c. If suctioning is performed with the jet ventilator running, suction must be applied as the catheter is inserted as well as when withdrawn to prevent over-pressurization of the circuit and alveolar rupture.
3. Humidification of gases is very important with HFJV to prevent obstruction of the endotracheal tube.
   a. The jet port should be irrigated with 0.5 ml normal saline solution or air every 3–4 hours.
   b. The main port of the endotracheal tube is suctioned as usual.
4. The tubing to the conventional ventilator must never be kinked, as over-pressurization of the circuit and alveolar rupture may occur if expiratory gas cannot escape.
5. Vibration of the chest wall is an indicator of lung compliance, airway patency, and effectiveness of ventilator settings.
   a. Chest wall vibration must be assessed after head position changes to ensure

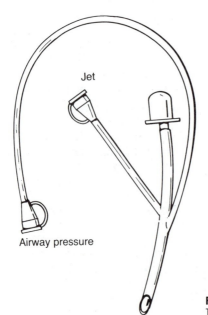

Jet

Airway pressure

Figure 10–3
Triple-lumen endotracheal tube.

that the jet port on the endotracheal tube has not been occluded by the tracheal wall.

b. Sudden decrease in chest wall vibration may indicate a plugged endotracheal tube or a pneumothorax.

6. Vibration may interfere with electrical monitoring of heart rate and respiratory rate.
   a. Use pulse from arterial line or pulse oximeter to monitor heart rate if necessary.
   b. Respiratory rate cannot be monitored.
7. Jet ventilation is more efficient at CO_2 elimination than at oxygenation.
   a. Increasing the background ventilation rate may improve oxygenation.
   b. The pressure difference between PIP and PEEP is the major determinant of ventilation.
   c. Mean airway pressure is the major determinant of oxygenation.
8. Patients are generally weaned to a low PIP and then switched back to conventional ventilation prior to extubation.

D. **Complications and problems.**
1. Airway obstruction, including decreased chest wall vibration, increased P_{CO_2}, and decreased servo-pressure.
2. Necrotizing tracheobronchitis (inflammatory injury to tracheal mucosa):
   a. Has been reported in patients receiving HFJV, as well as other forms of mechanical ventilation at high rates.
   b. Signs: increasing frequency of mucous plugs, bloody or necrotic material aspirated with suctioning, and airway obstruction.
   c. Extent determined by bronchoscopy or on post-mortem examination.
3. Microatelectasis and poor oxygenation may occur after prolonged HFJV, necessitating return to conventional ventilation.
4. Air-trapping occurs at very high rates or with excessive jet valve on-times.

Summary of Research and Outcome Data

A. **Treatment of RDS complicated by air leak** (Carlo et al., 1984; Carlo et al., 1987; Frantz et al., 1983; Mammell and Boros, 1988; Marchak et al., 1981).
1. Short-term trials (48 hours or less) have shown adequate or improved gas exchange at lower airway pressures with both HFJV and HFOV.
2. Greatest success with HFV has been achieved in the treatment of severe air leak syndromes.

B. **Prevention of bronchopulmonary dysplasia (BPD).**
1. Published studies on HFJV thus far have not been designed to look at the long-term effects on morbidity (Mammell and Boros, 1988).
   a. Many published trials have been rescue protocols: severe lung damage already assumed to be present.
   b. Short-term trials have focused only on whether technique is an effective alternative to conventional mechanical ventilation.

C. **Treatment of hypoplastic lungs/diaphragmatic hernia** (Mammell and Boros, 1988).
1. Small numbers reported within rescue protocols using both HFJV and HFOV.
   a. Temporary improvement in gas exchange at lower airway pressures.
   b. Poor overall survival.

D. **Treatment of persistent pulmonary hypertension** (Spitzer et al., 1988).
1. There is a published report that is part of a rescue protocol: 30 patients with persistent pulmonary hypertension from a variety of causes, 67% survival.

E. **Overall outcomes and follow-up data.**
1. HFOV: multicenter collaborative trial for treatment of respiratory failure in pre-term infants (HIFI Study Group, 1989).
   a. No difference in incidence of BPD or mortality with HFOV.

b. Increased incidence of intraventricular hemorrhage and periventricular leukomalacia with HFOV.
2. HFJV: multicenter trial for early treatment of pulmonary interstitial emphysema (PIE); limited data regarding outcomes and follow-up after long-term use.
   a. Encouraging results in early treatment of PIE with HFJV (Keszler et al., 1991).
   b. Necrotizing tracheobronchitis and other airway damage may be greater with long-term use than with other forms of mechanical ventilation (Mammell and Boros, 1988).
   c. Data from Children's Hospital of Philadelphia do not show any increase in incidence of intraventricular hemorrhage compared with similar patients treated with conventional ventilation (Spitzer et al., 1988).

STUDY QUESTIONS

1. High-frequency ventilation (HFV) is defined as mechanical ventilation at rapid rates using:
   a. Convective gas transport.
   b. Entrainment to produce gas exchange.
   c. Small tidal volumes.

2. A useful physical assessment parameter during high-frequency ventilation is:
   a. Auscultation of breath sounds.
   b. Chest wall vibration.
   c. Respiratory efforts.

3. After repositioning a patient receiving HFJV, the nurse notices that suddenly chest wall vibration has decreased and the transcutaneous CO_2 is rising. A likely cause of this is:
   a. Kinked conventional ventilator tubing.
   b. Obstruction of the jet cannula port.
   c. Tension pneumothorax.

4. Microatelectasis is a complication of HFV that results in:
   a. Hypercapnia.
   b. Increased chest wall vibration.
   c. Poor oxygenation.

Answers to Study Questions

1. c   3. b
2. b   4. c

REFERENCES

Carlo, W. A., Chatburn, R. L., and Martin, R. J.: Randomized trial of high-frequency jet ventilation versus conventional ventilation in respiratory distress syndrome. J. Pediatr., 110:275–282, 1987.

Carlo, W. A., Chatburn, R. L., Martin, R. J., et al.: Decrease in airway pressure during high-frequency jet ventilation in infants with respiratory distress syndrome. J. Pediatr., 104:101–107, 1984.

Frantz, I. D., Werthammer, J., and Stark, A. R.: High-frequency ventilation in premature infants with lung disease: Adequate gas exchange at low tracheal pressure. Pediatrics, 71:483–488, 1983.

Gonzalez, F., Harris, T., Black, P., and Richardson, P.: Decreased gas flow through pneumothoraces in neonates receiving high-frequency jet versus conventional ventilation. J. Pediatr., 110:464–466, 1987.

HIFI Study Group: High-frequency oscillatory ventilation compared with conventional mechanical ventilation in the treatment of respiratory failure in preterm infants. N. Engl. J. Med., 320(88):93, 1989.

Keszler, M., Donn, S. M., Bucciarelli, R. L., et al.: Multicenter controlled trial comparing high-frequency jet ventilation and conventional mechanical ventilation in newborn infants with pulmonary interstitial emphysema. J. Pediatr., 119:85–93, 1991.

Mammell, M. C., and Boros, S. J.: High frequency ventilation. In Goldsmith, J. P., and Karotkin, E. H. (eds.): Assisted Ventilation of the Neonate, 2nd ed. Philadelphia, W. B. Saunders Co., 1988, pp. 190–199.

Marchak, B. E., Thompson, W. K., Duffy, P., et al.: Treatment of RDS by high-frequency oscillatory ventilation: A preliminary report. J. Pediatr., 99:287–292, 1981.

Spitzer, A. R., Davis, J., Clarke, W. T., et al.: Pulmonary hypertension and persistent fetal circulation in the newborn. Clin. Perinatol., 15(2):389–413, 1988.

Jan Nugent

Extracorporeal Membrane Oxygenation (ECMO) in the Neonate

Objectives

1. Discuss history and related mortality statistics for neonatal ECMO.

2. Discuss indications and contraindications for ECMO.

3. Discuss the criteria used to determine an infant's need for ECMO.

4. Review the technical and mechanical aspects of the ECMO procedure.

5. Review the physiology of extracorporeal circulation.

6. Discuss the general care given to infants undergoing the ECMO procedure and the support provided to their families.

7. Review follow-up and outcome of ECMO survivors.

Extracorporeal membrane oxygenation (ECMO) is the process of prolonged cardiopulmonary bypass (extracorporeal circulation) that provides cardiorespiratory support for infants in reversible, profound respiratory, and/or cardiac failure. Despite recent advances in ventilatory management, respiratory failure remains the most frequent cause of neonatal death. ECMO is used as a "rescue" therapy for the 2–5% of critically ill infants who fail to respond to maximal conventional ventilatory, medical, and surgical treatments.

ECMO: A Historical Perspective

A. **John Gibbon (1937) invented the first heart-lung machine** and was the first physician to use the technology to perform cardiac surgery successfully. This prototype required direct exposure of the blood to oxygen and a roller pump.

B. **Development of a membrane lung by Clowes (1956)** allowed for separation of the blood and gas phases and dramatically reduced complications (thrombocytopenia, hemolysis, organ failure) due to direct exposure of blood to oxygen.

C. **The development of silicone rubber by Kammermeirer (1957)** made the membrane lung feasible for long-term support.

D. Kolobow (1969 to 1970) demonstrated the safe use of extracorporeal support for up to 7 days in lambs, using a coiled silicone membrane lung.

E. Prolonged ECMO support for moribund neonates in respiratory failure was attempted in 1965–1971. Bartlett began extensive clinical studies and reported improvements in survival and morbidity (Bartlett, 1984, 1986; Bartlett and Gazzaniga, 1978, 1980; Bartlett et al., 1982, 1985).

F. First survivor in 1975.
1. 55% survival rate in 1981 (Bartlett et al., 1982).
2. 100% survival rate in 1985 (Bartlett et al., 1985).

G. Bartlett's success prompted clinical trials at various centers throughout the United States.
1. These centers reported results similar to those of Bartlett's.
2. O'Rourke and colleagues, in a prospective clinical trial, demonstrated that overall survival of ECMO-treated infants was 99% compared with 60% of infants treated with conventional mechanical therapy (O'Rourke et al., 1989).
3. Neonatal ECMO Registry Report (1991) lists over 3000 infants treated since 1975, with overall survival rate of 83%.

Criteria for Use of ECMO

A. Respiratory or cardiac pathology must be acute and reversible within 7–14 days.
1. Respiratory distress syndrome.
2. Meconium aspiration syndrome.
3. Persistent pulmonary hypertension of the newborn.
4. Congenital diaphragmatic hernia.
5. Sepsis.
6. Life support prior to or after cardiac surgery.

B. Cranial and cardiac ultrasound are performed to rule out intracranial hemorrhage and cyanotic congenital heart disease.

C. Final selection is based on objective criteria predictive of >80% mortality (Table 11–1). To achieve specificity, each ECMO center must determine its own mortality indicators and criteria.

D. Contraindications to ECMO include the following (Nugent, 1991):
1. Cyanotic congenital heart disease (except infants requiring stabilization and life support prior to or after surgery).
2. Irreversible pulmonary damage (bronchopulmonary dysplasia).
3. Intracranial hemorrhage.
4. Birthweight of <2 kg.
5. Gestational age of <35 weeks (these infants and those <2 kg at birth have significant incidence of intracranial hemorrhage during ECMO).

Venoarterial (VA) Perfusion

A. Technique.
1. Drains unoxygenated blood from the right side of the heart through catheter placed in right atrium via right internal jugular vein.
2. Oxygenated blood is returned through the right common carotid artery into the ascending aorta.

B. Advantages.
1. Provides both respiratory and cardiac support by decompressing pulmonary circulation; decreases pulmonary artery and pulmonary capillary filtration pressure and supports circulation by augmenting the pumping action of the heart.

Table 11–1
CRITERIA PREDICTIVE OF POTENTIAL MORTALITY

1. Newborn pulmonary insufficiency index (NPII). The NPII score is a single-number cumulation of oxygen requirement, acidosis, and time. This score assesses the severity of an infant's respiratory distress in the first day of life. In the past, the NPII was used effectively as a measure of high mortality risk (>80%). Since the advent of induced alkalosis as a treatment of persistent pulmonary hypertension of the newborn (PPHN), the NPII has not been applicable (Chapman et al., 1988).

2. Alveolar-arterial gradient >620 mm Hg for 12 hours. Alveolar-arterial oxygen difference ($AaDO_2$) is a measure of alveolar efficiency in transporting oxygen to pulmonary capillaries. Use of this criterion assumes that the baby is ventilated with 1.0 FIO_2 and that the $PACO_2 = PaCO_2$. The following calculation is used:

$$AaDO_2 = (FIO_2)\ (713) - PaO_2 - PaCO_2$$

The numerical value 713 assumes an atmospheric pressure of 760 mm Hg minus vapor pressure (47 mm Hg); PaO_2 and $PaCO_2$ are measured by assaying arterial blood gases. Retrospective reviews demonstrate that an $AaDO_2 > 620$ for 12 consecutive hours correlates with >80% mortality (Beck et al., 1986).

3. Acute deterioration despite optimal therapy: either a $PaO_2 < 40$ mm Hg, or a $pH \leq 7.15$ for 2 hours (Chapman et al., 1988).

4. Lack of response to treatment of PPHN: two of the following indications for 3 hours: $PaO_2 < 55$ mm Hg; $pH < 7.4$; hypotension (Chapman et al., 1988).

5. Severe barotrauma. Co-existence of four of the following:

    Interstitial emphysema
    Pneumothorax
    Pneumopericardium
    Pneumoperitoneum
    Subcutaneous emphysema
    Persistent air leak for 24 hours
    Mean airway pressure of ≥ 15 cm H_2O (Chapman et al., 1988)

6. Congenital diaphragmatic hernia with respiratory failure: $PaO_2 < 80$ mm Hg or $FIO_2 > 0.8$ twenty-four hours after surgery (Chapman et al., 1988). $PaCO_2 > 40$ mm Hg (2 hours after surgery), with ventilation index (mean airway pressure × respiratory rate) >1000 (Bohn et al., 1989).

7. Oxidation index. The oxidation index can be utilized to predict mortality and incidence of bronchopulmonary dysplasia. The oxygenation index is calculated by dividing the product of the FIO_2 (times 100) and the mean airway pressure by the post-ductal PaO_2:

$$\frac{\text{Mean airway pressure} \times FIO_2 \times 100}{\text{Post-ductal } PaO_2}$$

Retrospective data demonstrate that an oxidation index ≥ 40 correlates with a predicted mortality risk of 80–90%; an index ≥ 25–40 correlates with a 50–60% mortality (Cordiz et al., 1987).

2. Positive-pressure ventilation can be reduced to minimal parameters (peak inspiratory pressure [PIP], 16–18 cm H_2O; positive end-expiratory pressure [PEEP], 3–4 cm H_2O; rate, 10–20/minute; FIO_2, 21%).
3. Requires less surgical time and lower pump flows than venovenous (VV) route.

C. **Risks.**
1. Emboli (air or particulate) could be infused directly into the arterial circulation.
2. Ligation of carotid artery may affect cerebral perfusion.

Circuit Components (Fig. 11–1)

A. **Cannulas.**
1. Remove deoxygenated venous blood and return oxygenated blood to the arterial circulation.

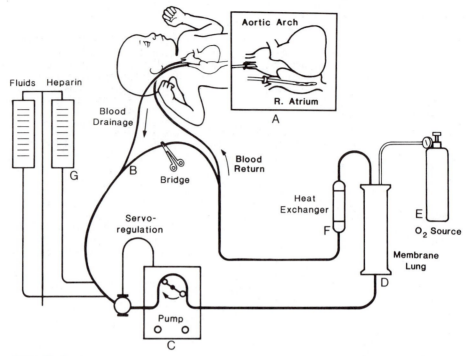

Figure 11–1
Components of ECMO circuit: cannulas, PVC tubing, roller head pump, membrane oxygenator (lung), gas source, heat exchanger, and infusion pumps.

2. Venous cannula must be capable of delivering total cardiac output (120–150 ml/kg/minute) to the membrane lung; cannulas of largest possible internal diameter (10–12 Fr) are inserted.
3. Prior to insertion, the infant is paralyzed to prevent respiratory movement and air embolism and systemically heparinized to prevent clotting of cannulas and circuit.
4. Venous cannula tip is positioned in the right atrium, in order to drain blood flow from the inferior and superior venae cavae; arterial cannula tip reaches just to the aortic arch.

B. Polyvinylchloride (PVC) tubing.
1. Has Leur lock connectors, stopcocks, infusion sites, and silicone bladder.
2. Provides for circulation of blood through components of circuit; removal of blood (venous side of circuit); and administration of parenteral fluids, medications, and blood products (venous side of circuit).
3. Only platelets are infused on the arterial side of circuit.
4. Follow same precautions and guidelines for safe administration of medications and blood products directly into patients when placing into circuit.

C. Bladder box assembly.
1. Fail-safe alarm system.
2. Collapsible silicone bladder distends with returning venous blood.
3. Inadequate flow (decreased venous return) into the ECMO circuit causes the bladder to collapse, which triggers a microswitch and audible alarm and stops the roller head pump.
4. Upon re-expansion of the bladder, the microswitch re-engages the pump and normal pump operation continues.
5. See Table 11–4 for causes of decreased venous return.

6. Adequate venous return is critical for maintaining cardiorespiratory support; the cause for decreased return must be recognized and corrected immediately.
7. Servo-regulation of ECMO flow can also be achieved by transducers placed in-line in the circuits. Pre-membrane (venous) pressure and post-membrane (arterial) pressure may be monitored continuously to signal extracorporeal flow problems prior to collapse of the silicone bladder. This allows for early detection and timely intervention.
   a. Rise in pre-membrane pressure indicates decreased venous return.
   b. Rise in post-membrane pressure indicates membrane oxygenator or heat exchanger malfunction.

D. **Roller head pump.**
1. Compresses and displaces the blood in the PVC tubing placed in the pump raceway.
2. Pushes blood forward, creates gentle suction in the venous cannula, and assists left ventricular function when using VA bypass.
3. Digital display indicates circuit flow in cubic centimeters per minute.
4. Electrically powered; must be hand cranked or attached to battery pack if power failure occurs.

E. **Membrane oxygenator (Sci Med/Kolobow).**
1. Solid silicone polymer membrane envelope with plastic space screen wrapped spirally around a spool, and encased in a silicone rubber sleeve.
2. Membrane oxygenators are oxygenators of choice, because they eliminate the damaging blood-gas interface, ensure constant blood volume, and are relatively easy to operate.

F. **Heat exchanger.**
1. Located downstream from the oxygenator.
2. Re-warms blood to 37.2°C (normothermic) prior to returning to the infant's circulation.
3. Heat loss occurs from cooling effect of ventilating gases inside the oxygenator and circuit exposure to ambient air temperature.

G. **Bubble-detector.**
1. Placed distal (patient side) to heat exchanger.
2. When air (bubble) is detected, the roller head pump is shut off and flow to the patient ceases.

H. **Activated clotting time (ACT) machine.**
1. Used to intermittently monitor (every 30–60 minutes) the infant's ACT.
2. Infusion pump is used to continuously infuse a heparin solution (100 U/ml) into the ECMO circuit.
3. Heparin solution is titrated to keep the ACT within the desired range (180–250 seconds).
4. To control the amount of heparin that is administered, no heparin is added to any other medications or fluids (an exception may be the fluids being infused into umbilical or peripheral arterial lines).
5. Factors that influence heparin requirements are thrombocytopenia, abnormal clotting studies, and urinary output.

Blood Gas Monitoring Device

A. **Fiberoptic technology** allows for continuous monitoring of arterial pH, Pao_2, base excess/bicarbonate, Pvo_2, $Pvco_2$, and venous saturation (Svo_2).

B. **Arterial values** monitor the membrane oxygenator function.

C. **Venous values** monitor the adequacy of extracorporeal perfusion in meeting the infant's metabolic needs.

Physiology of Extracorporeal Circulation*

A. Blood flow.

1. VA bypass is instituted by draining venous blood into the ECMO circuit; a like amount of oxygenated blood is returned to the arterial circulation.
2. As bypass flow increases, flow through the pulmonary artery decreases faster than bypass flow, and reduces total flow in the systemic circulation, causing peripheral and pulmonary hypotension.
3. Blood volume replacement is required for optimal tissue perfusion.
4. ECMO perfusion is non-pulsatile (pulse contour decreases as flow rate increases); kidneys interpret this as inadequate flow and promote the release of renin and aldosterone, which causes sodium retention, extracellular fluid expansion, and decreased total body potassium.
5. Total patient flow is the sum of ECMO flow and pulmonary blood flow; adequate flow is reached when oxygen delivery and tissue perfusion result in normoxia, normal pH, normal venous oxygen saturation (Svo_2), and normal organ function.
6. Total gas exchange and support are achieved at a flow rate of 120–150 ml/kg/minute.

B. Gas exchange.

1. The membrane lung has two compartments divided by a semipermeable membrane: ventilating gas is on the one side, and blood is on the other.
2. Oxygen diffuses into the blood, owing to a pressure gradient between the 100% oxygen in the gas compartment and the low oxygen pressure in the venous blood.
3. Carbon dioxide diffuses from the blood compartment to the gas compartment as a result of a pressure gradient between venous carbon dioxide pressure and the ventilating gas. Carbon dioxide transfer rate is six times greater than oxygen transfer. The ventilating gas mixture is usually enriched with carbon dioxide to prevent hypocapnia.

C. Blood-surface interface.

1. During ECMO, 80% of the cardiac output is exposed to a large artificial surface each minute.
2. Clot formation is prevented by systemic heparinization; platelet destruction is minimized by pre-exposure of the circuit to albumin.
3. Platelets show the greatest effect of exposure to a foreign surface, as evidenced by decreased platelet count (thrombocytopenia) and function.
4. Hemolysis is negligible, and survival of red cells is not altered.
5. All types of white cells decrease in concentration, and phagocytic activity is significantly decreased.
6. After cessation of ECMO, platelets and white blood cell counts return to normal.

Care of the Infant

A. Cannulation.

1. Cannulation and initiation of bypass occur in the NICU under local anesthesia with the operating room staff in attendance.
2. See Table 11–2 for nursing responsibilities and interventions.

B. During ECMO "run."

1. Bypass is gradually instituted until approximately 80% (120–150 ml/minute) of cardiac output is diverted through the ECMO circuit.

---

*Extensive reviews are available in Nugent, 1991; Bartlett and Gazzaniga, 1980.

Table 11-2
NURSING RESPONSIBILITIES AND INTERVENTIONS FOR ECMO

Responsibility	Intervention
Obtain and document baseline physiological data	Record weight, length, head circumference
	Draw blood samples for complete blood count (CBC), electrolytes, calcium, glucose, BUN, creatinine, PT/PTT, platelets, arterial blood gases
	Record vital signs: heart rate; respiratory rate; systolic, diastolic, mean blood pressure; temperature
Ensure adequate supply of blood products for replacement	Draw type and crossmatch samples for two units of red cells, fresh-frozen plasma
	Keep one unit of packed cells and fresh-frozen plasma always available in the blood bank
Maintain prescribed pulmonary support	Maintain ventilator parameters
	Administer muscle relaxants if indicated
Assemble and prepare equipment	Prepare infusion pumps to maintain arterial lines and infusion of parenteral fluids and medications into the ECMO circuit
	Place the infant on a radiant warmer with the head positioned at the foot of the bed to provide thermoregulation and access for cannulation
	Attach infant to physiological monitoring devices for heart rate, intra-arterial blood pressure, transcutaneous oxygen, etc.
	Insert urinary catheter and nasogastric tube; place to gravity drainage
	Remove intravenous lines just prior to heparinization (optional)
	Prepare loading dose of heparin (100 U/kg)
	Prepare heparin solution for continuous infusion (100 U/ml/D_5W)
	Prepare paralyzing drug (pancuronium bromide, 0.1 mg/kg; or succinylcholine, 1-4 mg/kg)
	Assist in insertion of arterial line (umbilical or peripheral)
	Administer prophylactic antibiotic
Monitor cardiopulmonary status	Monitor heart rate and intra-arterial blood pressure continuously
	Obtain blood gases after paralysis and during cannulation as indicated by the infant's response to the procedure
Be prepared to administer cardiopulmonary support	Have available medications and blood products to correct hypovolemia, bradycardia, acidosis, cardiac arrest
Administer medications	Give loading dose of heparin systemically when vessels are dissected free and are ready to be cannulated. Give paralyzing drug systemically just prior to cannulation of internal jugular vein if infant has not been previously paralyzed
Reduce ventilator parameters to minimal settings	Once adequate bypass is achieved, reduce peak inspiratory pressure (PIP) to 16-20 cm H_2O, positive end-expiratory pressure (PEEP) to 4 cm H_2O, ventilator rate to 10-20 breaths/minute, and FIO_2 to 21%
Monitor and document physiological parameters	Record hourly: heart rate, blood pressure (systolic, diastolic, mean), respirations, temperature, transcutaneous Po_2, CO_2, oxygen saturation, ACT, ECMO flow

Continued

Table 11–2
NURSING RESPONSIBILITIES AND INTERVENTIONS FOR ECMO (*Continued*)

Responsibility	Intervention
	Measure hourly and accurately intake and output of all body fluids (urine, gastric contents, blood); measure every 4 hours urine pH, protein, glucose, specific gravity; hematest all stools
	Assess hourly: color, breath sounds, heart tones, murmurs, cardiac rhythm, arterial pressure waveform, peripheral perfusion
	Perform hourly neurological check, including fontanel tension; pupil size and reaction; level of consciousness; reflexes, tone, and movement of extremities
	Record ventilator parameters hourly
	Assess weight and head circumference daily
	Draw arterial blood gases from umbilical or peripheral line hourly
	All other blood specimens are drawn from the ECMO circuit: electrolytes, calcium, platelets, Chemstrip, hematocrit every 4–8 hours, CBC, PT/PTT, BUN, creatinine, total and direct bilirubin, plasma hemoglobin, fibrinogen, fibrin split products, blood culture as indicated
Administer medications	Remove air bubbles and double-check dosages before infusion
	Administer no medications IM or by venipuncture
	Place all medications and fluids into the venous side of the ECMO circuit
	Prepare and administer the arterial line (umbilical or peripheral) infusion
	Administer parenteral alimentation
Provide pulmonary support	Perform endotracheal suctioning based on individual assessment and need
	Maintain patent airway; be alert to extubation or plugging
	Obtain daily chest films and tracheal aspirant culture as indicated
	Maintain ventilator parameters
Prevent bleeding	Avoid all of the following: rectal probes, injections, venipunctures, heel sticks, cuff blood pressures, chest tube stripping, restraints, chest percussion
	Avoid invasive procedures. Do not change nasogastric tube, urinary catheters, or endotracheal tube unless absolutely necessary; use pre-measured endotracheal tube suction technique
	Observe for blood in the urine, stools, endotracheal or nasogastric tubes
Maintain excellent infection control	Change all fluids and tubing daily
	Change dressings daily and prn
	Clean urinary catheter site daily
	Maintain strict aseptic and hand-washing technique
	Use universal barrier precautions
Provide physical care	Keep skin dry, clean, and free from pressure points
	Give mouth care prn

Table 11-2
NURSING RESPONSIBILITIES AND INTERVENTIONS FOR ECMO (*Continued*)

Responsibility	Intervention
Provide pain management, sedation, stress reduction	Provide range of motion as indicated
	Turn child side to side every 1-2 hours
	Minimize noise level
	Cluster patient care to maximize sleep periods
	Administer analgesia: fentanyl, 9-18 μg/kg/hour (increased dosage required due to fentanyl binding to membrane oxygenator)
	Manage iatrogenic physical dependency by following a dose reduction regimen (reduce dose 10% every 4 hours) (Caron and Maguire, 1990)
Be alert to complications and emergencies	See Tables 11-4 and 11-5

Reprinted by permission of Neonatal Network, Acute Respiratory Care of the Neonate, 1991.

2. At maximum flow, blood gases should normalize and Svo_2 is maintained >70%.
3. Svo_2 is an excellent indicator of adequate flow, because it is a measure of tissue perfusion and efficiency of extracorporeal circulation in meeting metabolic demands.
4. Ventilator parameters are reduced to minimal settings; vasopressor therapy and chemical paralysis are usually discontinued; enteral feedings are withheld; and blood loss is quantified and replaced.
5. See Tables 11-3 to 11-5 for nursing interventions, ECMO specialist responsibilities, and complications and emergencies.

C. Weaning/decannulation.
1. Signs of improvement and indicators that the infant is ready to be weaned are as follows:
   a. Improvement of lung fields on chest x-ray.
   b. Clinical findings: weight loss, improved breath sounds, rising Pao_2 on fixed ECMO flow, improvement in lung compliance.
2. Once improvement has been ascertained, flow rate is decreased slowly in 10-20 ml increments until ECMO support is no longer needed to maintain adequate gas exchange at low ventilator settings.
3. When flow rate is 50 ml/kg/minute, a state of "idling" is achieved; the infant remains at this lowest possible flow for 4-8 hours.
4. If improvement in lung function remains stable, cannulas are clamped, heparin infusion is switched to the infant, and the circuit is recirculated via a bridge. If blood gases deteriorate, the cannulas are unclamped and ECMO support resumes.
5. Decannulation proceeds if blood gas values remain satisfactory.
6. Prior to decannulation, the infant is paralyzed and ventilator parameters are increased to compensate for loss of spontaneous respiratory function.
7. Under local anesthesia, the cannulas are removed. The internal jugular vein is ligated. The integrity of the carotid artery will dictate if carotid reconstruction is to be performed. Approximately 30-40% of ECMO survivors will meet the criteria for reanastomosis of the right common carotid artery.
8. After decannulation, the infant is weaned as tolerated from the ventilator and routine NICU care is resumed.

Table 11-3
ECMO SPECIALIST RESPONSIBILITIES AND INTERVENTIONS

Responsibility	Intervention
Maintain and monitor ECMO circuit	Check circuit carefully for air, clots, tightness of connectors, stopcocks
	Check bladder box alarm function
	Monitor pump arterial and venous blood gases each shift to assess oxygenator function. Pump arterial Po_2 <100 mm Hg, CO_2 retention, or leaking membrane indicates oxygenator failure
Assess infant	Check cannula placement and stability Assess breath sounds, neurological status Observe volume of fluid and blood drainage
	Monitor vital signs and lab values
Maintain prescribed parameters: pH, 7.35–7.45 PaO_2, 60–80 mm Hg $PaCO_2$, 35–45 mm Hg MAP, 45–55 mm Hg Hct, 45–55% Platelets, 70,000–100,000 SvO_2 > 70% SaO_2 > 90%	Maintain infant's systemic arterial blood gases by adjusting sweep gas and pump flow Maintain mean arterial blood pressure (MAP), hematocrit (Hct), and platelets by infusion of appropriate blood products
ACT, 180–250 seconds	Assess ACT hourly or prn; titrate heparin infusion to maintain parameters
Assist nurse in care	Draw all blood samples from circuit except systemic arterial blood gases
	Coordinate recording of intake and output with nurse
	Assist in all position changes Administer and monitor all medications, blood products, and fluids placed into the pump circuit
Be prepared to deal with pump emergencies. See Tables 11–4 and 11–5.	

Reprinted by permission of Neonatal Network, Acute Respiratory Care of the Neonate, 1991.

Table 11-4
ECMO COMPLICATIONS

Complication	Rationale and Treatment
Electrolyte/glucose/fluid imbalance	Sodium requirements decrease 1–2 mEq/kg/day; potassium requirements increase to 4 mEq/kg/day secondary to action of aldosterone
	Calcium replacement may be required if citrate-phosphate-dextrose anticoagulated blood is used; reduce dextrose concentration of maintenance and heparin infusions if hyperglycemia occurs
	Maintain total fluid intake at 100–150 ml/kg/day
	Fluid intake should balance output; furosemide may be required if positive fluid balance occurs
Central nervous system deterioration: cerebral edema, intracranial hemorrhage, seizures	This significant complication of ECMO can be related to pre-ECMO hypoxia, acidosis, hypercapnia, or vessel ligation
	Drug of choice for seizures is phenobarbital
	Serial EEGs and cranial ultrasound evaluation may be required
Generalized edema	Extracellular space is enlarged by systemic distribution of crystalloid solution in the prime and action of aldosterone and antidiuretic hormone

Table 11-4
ECMO COMPLICATIONS (*Continued*)

Complication	Rationale and Treatment
Renal failure	Furosemide or hemofiltration may be indicated if edema causes brain or lung dysfunction
	Acute tubular necrosis results from pre-ECMO hypotension and hypoxia
	Monitor output and indicators of renal failure: blood urea nitrogen (BUN), creatinine
	Increase renal perfusion by increasing pump flow and use of dopamine (5 μg/kg/minute)
	Hemodialysis may be added to the circuit if necessary
Bleeding/thrombocytopenia	This is the most frequent cause of death
	Large foreign surface of ECMO circuit lowers platelet function and count
	This is most common in infants requiring surgery or chest tubes
	Minimize with good control of ACT (180-200 seconds) and judicious use of platelets and fresh-frozen plasma
	All surgical procedures must be performed with electrocautery
Decreased venous flow return/hypovolemia	Infants must have adequate circulating volume to obtain adequate rates
	This is manifested by collapsing silicone bladder triggering bladder box alarm; decrease in extracorporeal flow rate, arterial pressure, arterial pulse amplitude, and SvO_2
	Blood sampling, wound drainage, or peripheral dilatation may account for hypovolemia
	Check for pneumothorax, partial venous catheter occlusion or malposition, which may decrease venous drainage and return
	Replace volume with packed cells, fresh-frozen plasma
	Treat pneumothorax with chest tube placement
	Raise level of bed to enhance gravity drainage of venous blood
Hypervolemia/hypertension	This is caused by overinfusion of blood products, which causes a larger percentage of blood to flow through malfunctioning lungs. It can also be caused by renal ischemia and release of renin/angiotensin
	It is manifested by widening pulse amplitude and decreasing systemic oxygenation at a fixed extracorporeal flow rate
	Treat overinfusion by removing blood from the circuit. Renal hypertension may dictate use of captopril or labetalol
Patent ductus arteriosus	Left-to-right shunting may occur, causing increased blood flow to lungs, necessitating high pump flows without expected increase in PaO_2
	Ligation may be indicated because weaning will not be successful
Mechanical	See Table 11-5

Reprinted by permission of Neonatal Network, Acute Respiratory Care of the Neonate, 1991.

Table 11-5
CIRCUIT EMERGENCY PROCEDURES

Circuit Emergencies	
Air embolism Tubing rupture Oxygenator malfunction Decannulation Pump failure ↓ Come off bypass	Power failure Gas source failure ↓ Provide back-up Power/gas source
Circuit Emergency Procedures	
Nurse Ventilation Anticoagulation Chemical resuscitation Replace blood loss	*ECMO Specialist* Clamp catheters Open bridge Remove gas source Repair circuit

Data from Nugent, 1991.

Parental Support

A. **The ECMO candidate's parents are in crisis;** they are aware that ECMO is a method of last resort with no guarantee of positive result; the technology is overwhelming.

B. **Parents need concise, accurate information** about their child's condition and required procedures.

C. **Parent-to-parent support, utilizing parents of "ECMO graduates,"** is efficacious and a positive experience.

D. **Parents should have access to their infant.** The ECMO candidates have an increasingly bright outcome, and every effort should be made to encourage involvement and bonding.

Follow-up and Outcome

A. **Critical scrutiny of survivors is essential to assess the value and safety of ECMO.** Survivors should be periodically evaluated for the following:
1. Growth and development.
2. Cardiorespiratory development.
3. Cerebrovascular status.
4. Neurological and psychological functioning.

B. **Early follow-up studies** reported normal physical growth and development; adequate cerebral blood flow; neurological competence appropriate for age in 83% in one study, 75% in another (Krummel et al., 1984).

C. **Long-term follow-up study of children ages 4-9 years** demonstrated 75% normalcy rate (Towne et al., 1984).

D. **A relatively current study demonstrated a 90% normalcy rate for ECMO survivors at 1 year of age.** Poor outcome was associated with major intracranial hemorrhage and chronic lung disease (Glass et al., 1989).

E. **Differentiation between pre-existing deficits and those secondary to ECMO therapy is difficult.** Morbidity and mortality rates have and will continue to improve because of extensive experience with the technique, case selection, and earlier intervention.

STUDY QUESTIONS

1. A clinical indication for use of ECMO is:
   a. bronchopulmonary dysplasia.
   b. persistent pulmonary hypertension of the newborn.
   c. respiratory distress syndrome in the very low birthweight infant.

2. A contraindication for use of ECMO is:
   a. congenital diaphragmatic hernia.
   b. intraventricular hemorrhage.
   c. meconium aspiration.

3. Final selection criteria is based on:
   a. absence of intracranial hemorrhage.
   b. criteria predictive of >80% mortality.
   c. presence of reversible pulmonary pathology.

4. Venoarterial perfusion:
   a. does not provide cardiac support.
   b. drains unoxygenated blood from the right atrium.
   c. returns oxygenated blood to the left atrium.

5. A significant complication related to the rise of ECMO is:
   a. hypoglycemia.
   b. hyperkalemia.
   c. thrombocytopenia.

6. Poor outcome in ECMO survivors is associated with:
   a. birthweight <2500 g.
   b. intracranial hemorrhage.
   c. thrombocytopenia.

Answers to Study Questions

1. b   3. b   5. c
2. b   4. b   6. b

REFERENCES

Bartlett, R.: Extracorporeal oxygenation in the neonate. Hosp. Pract., 4:139–151, 1984.

Bartlett, R.: Respiratory support: Extracorporeal membrane oxygenation in newborn respiratory failure. *In* Welch, K., et al. (eds.): Pediatric Surgery. New York, Year Book Medical Publishers, 1986, pp. 74–77.

Bartlett, R., and Gazzaniga, A.: Extracorporeal circulation for cardiopulmonary failure. Curr. Probl. Surg., *12*(5):1–96, 1978.

Bartlett, R., and Gazzaniga, A.: Physiology and pathophysiology of extracorporeal membrane circulation. *In* Ionesue, J. (ed.): Techniques in Extracorporeal Circulation. Boston, Butterworths, 1980, pp. 1–43.

Bartlett, R., et al.: Extracorporeal membrane oxygenation for newborn respiratory failure. Forty-five cases. Surgery, 92:425–433, 1982.

Bartlett, R., et al.: Extracorporeal circulation in neonatal respiratory failure: A prospective randomized study. Pediatrics, 76(4):479–487, 1985.

Beck, R., Andersen, K., and Pearson, G.: Criteria for extracorporeal membrane oxygenation in a population of infants with persistent pulmonary hypertension of the newborn. J. Pediatr. Surgery., 21:297–302, 1986.

Bohn, D., et al.: Ventilatory predictors of pulmonary hypoplasia in congenital diaphragmatic hernia, confirmed by morphologic assessment. J. Pediatr., *111*:423–431, 1989.

Caron, E., and Maguire, D.: Current management of pain, sedation and narcotic physical dependency of the infant on ECMO. J. Perinat. Neonat. Nurs., 4:63–74, 1990.

Chapman, R., Toomasian, J., and Bartlett, R.: Extracorporeal Membrane Oxygenation Technical Specialist Manual. Ann Arbor, MI, University of Michigan Press, 1988.

Cordiz, R., Cillery, R., and Bartlett, R.: Extracorporeal membrane oxygenation in pediatric respiratory failure. Pediatr. Clin. North Am., 34:39–46, 1987.

Glass, P., Miller, M., and Short, B.: Morbidity for survivors of extracorporeal membrane oxygenation: Neurodevelopmental outcome at 1 year of age. Pediatrics, 83:72–78, 1989.

Krummel, T., et al.: The early evaluation of survivors after extracorporeal membrane oxygenation for neonatal pulmonary failure. J. Pediatr. Surg., 19:585–590, 1984.

Neonatal ECMO Registry Report, 1/1/91.

Nugent, J.: Extracorporeal membrane oxygenation in the newborn. In Nugent, J. (ed.): Acute Respiratory Care of the Newborn. Petaluma, CA, Neonatal Network, 1991.

O'Rourke, P., et al.: Extracorporeal membrane oxygenation and conventional medical therapy in neonates with persistent pulmonary hypertension of the newborn: A prospective randomized study. Pediatrics, 84:957–963,1989.

Towne, B., Lott, I., and Hicks, D.: Long-term follow-up of newborns with persistent pulmonary hypertension in the newborn. Clin. Perinatol., 11:410–414, 1984.

NEONATAL PATHOPHYSIOLOGY: MANAGEMENT AND TREATMENT OF COMMON DISORDERS

Margaret Crockett

Cardiovascular Disorders

Objectives

1. Describe how to differentiate between cyanosis that is cardiac in origin and that which is pulmonary in origin.

2. Name the major classifications of congenital heart disease; list two anomalies in each.

3. Define and describe hemodynamics and resulting clinical signs and possible treatment of tetralogy of Fallot, coarctation of the aorta, patent ductus arteriosus (PDA), ventricular septal defect (VSD), atrial septal defect (ASD), and hypoplastic left heart.

4. Describe basic medical rationale for care of the newborn with suspected or identified cardiac defect.

5. Describe basic surgical rationale for treatment of major cardiovascular defects.

6. List signs and symptoms of congenital heart abnormalities of the newborn.

7. Describe a cardiac catheterization and list the major postoperative nursing concerns.

8. List the signs and symptoms of PDA and the current medical and surgical interventions.

9. Discuss the treatment modalities employed in congestive heart failure, including the use and risk/benefit to the neonate.

10. Define the three classifications of shock and list one cause under each category.

Until the twentieth century, there was limited clinical interest in congenital heart disease. In the majority of cases, the anomaly was incompatible with life; in the others, no treatment existed either to remedy the condition or to relieve its symptoms. Today, with advances in medical and surgical therapy, the survival and quality of life of infants with congenital heart disease have markedly improved.

Advances in angiography, echocardiography, and radionuclide imaging, coupled with a more complete understanding of newborn physiology, have lead to improvements in diagnostic capabilities without undue risk. Additionally, the advent of deep hypothermia with circulatory arrest permits the total correction of many forms of congenital heart disease in the neonatal period. In some cases, early intervention is essential to prevent long-term morbidity and/or early mortality.

In this chapter, topics considered to be of interest to the neonatal nurse are covered. For more in-depth coverage, standard pediatric cardiology texts should be consulted.

Cardiovascular Embryology and Anatomy

CARDIAC DEVELOPMENT (Hazinski, 1983a; Moore, 1988)

A. The majority of fetal cardiac development occurs between the 3rd and 7th week of fetal life.

1. 3rd week of fetal life: a single cardiac tube is formed from two endothelial

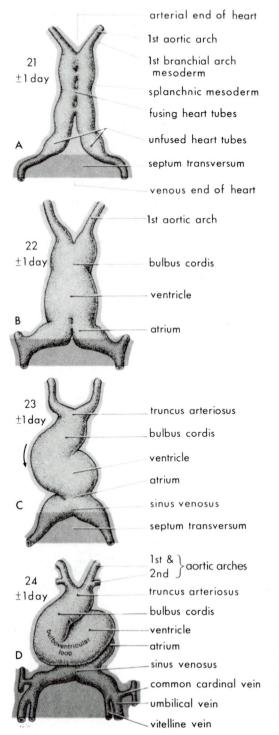

arterial end of heart

1st aortic arch

1st branchial arch mesoderm

splanchnic mesoderm

fusing heart tubes

unfused heart tubes

septum transversum

venous end of heart

21 ±1 day

A

1st aortic arch

bulbus cordis

ventricle

atrium

22 ±1 day

B

truncus arteriosus

bulbus cordis

ventricle

atrium

sinus venosus

septum transversum

23 ±1 day

C

1st & 2nd } aortic arches

truncus arteriosus

bulbus cordis

ventricle

atrium

sinus venosus

common cardinal vein

umbilical vein

vitelline vein

24 ±1 day

D

Figure 12–1
Sketches of ventral views of the developing heart (20–25 days), showing fusion of the endocardial heart tubes to form a single heart tube. Bending of the heart tube to form a bulboventricular loop is also illustrated. (From Moore, K.: The Developing Human, 4th ed. Philadelphia, W.B. Saunders Co., 1988, p. 292.)

tubes (endocardial heart tubes). A fusion of the two tubes occurs cranially to caudally.

2. With elongation of the cardiac tube, it expands and loops to the right (Fig. 12–1). A malrotation results in cardiac malposition, i.e., dextrocardia or corrected (*L*) transposition (Hazinski, 1983a).

3. Cardiac separation occurs between the 5th and 6th week.

   a. Atrial septum and foramen ovale are formed from two septa and endocardial cushions.

     (1) An initial septum (septum primum) grows from the top of the common atrium extending toward the endocardial cushions (Fig. 12–2*A*), leaving an opening (ostium primum between the rim of the septum primum and the endocardial cushions.

     (2) Perforation occurs high in the septum primum to form the ostium secundum; growth of the endocardial cushions eliminates the ostium primum.

     (3) A second septum (septum secundum) appears to the right of the septum primum and grows to overlap the ostium secundum. Thus, the flapped opening, the foramen ovale, is created (Fig. 12–2*C*).

   b. Ventricular separation.

     (1) Results from fusion of the endocardial cushions (forming the membranous portion of the ventricular septum) and dilatation and fusion of the ventricles (creating the muscular ventricular septum) (Fig. 12–3).

   c. Endocardial cushion tissue forms the atrioventricular values.

     (4) Tricuspid valve: between right atrium and ventricle.

     (2) Mitral valve: between left atrium and ventricle.

   d. Abnormal development during cardiac separation can lead to the following:

     (1) Ventricular septal defect (VSD), atrial septal defect (ASD), endocardial cushion defect (atrioventricular [A-V] canal).

     (2) Absence, deformation, stenosis, or atresia of tricuspid and/or mitral valves.

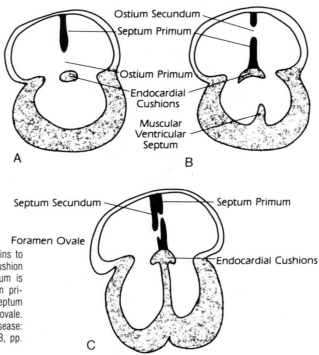

Figure 12–2

Atrial septation. *A*, Septum primum begins to form, extending toward endocardial cushion (note ostium primum). *B*, Ostium primum is closed and perforation forms in septum primum (called ostium secundum). *C*, Septum secundum forms, creating the foramen ovale. (From Hazinski, M.F.: Congenital heart disease: Part I. Neonatal Network, February 1983, pp. 34–35.)

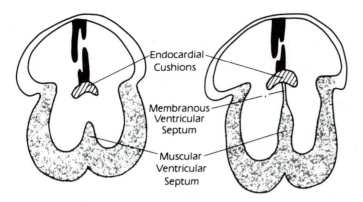

Figure 12–3
Ventricular septation (with muscular and membranous septum). (From Hazinski, M.F., Congenital heart disease: Part I. Neonatal Network, February 1983, pp. 34–35.)

GREAT VESSEL DEVELOPMENT

A. **A single vessel (truncus arteriosus)** extends from the ventricles until the 4th week of fetal life.

B. **5th week:** ridges appear within the vessel or trunk. These ridges extend and spiral, separating the truncus arteriosus into the aorta and pulmonary artery (Fig. 12–4).
1. Swellings at the base of the truncus appear and fuse to form the right and left ventricular outflow tracks.
2. The semilunar valves (aortic and pulmonic valves) develop from three ridges of tissue at the opening to the aorta and pulmonary trunk.

C. **Developmental abnormalities of truncal separation include:**
1. Persistent truncus arteriosus.
2. Tetralogy of Fallot.
3. Pulmonary and/or aortic valve atresia or stenosis.
4. Transposition of the great vessels (D-transposition).

CIRCULATORY DEVELOPMENT

A. **Heart contractions begin by 22 days;** the atrium and ventricle muscle layers are continuous. Contractions result in a wave-like peristalsis. The initial circulation is an ebb-and-flow type.

B. **Coordinated contractions** established by the 4th week of gestation provide a unidirectional flow.

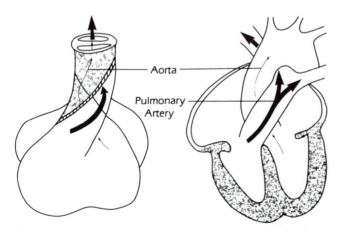

Figure 12–4
Closing of the truncus arteriosus and division into the pulmonary artery and aorta. (From Hazinski, M.F.: Congenital heart disease: Part I. Neonatal Network. February 1983, p. 35.)

C. **Establishment of fetal circulation.** With completion of atrial and ventricular separation, development of valves between chambers and outflow tracks, and separation of the truncus arteriosus into the great vessels, fetal circulation is established.

D. **Fetal circulation is anatomically and physiologically different from adult circulation.** For a full discussion of fetal circulation and cardiopulmonary adaptation at birth, see Chapter 3.

CARDIOVASCULAR PHYSIOLOGY

A. Normal circulation (Fig. 12–5).
1. Oxygen-poor blood enters the right atrium and passes through the tricuspid valve into the right ventricle, where it is pumped through the pulmonary artery to the lungs.
2. As the blood flows through the lungs, it gives up carbon dioxide and gains oxygen.
3. Oxygen-rich blood returns from the lungs through the pulmonary veins. It enters the left atrium, then passes through the mitral valve into the left ventricle, which pumps it through the aortic valve and into the aorta.
4. The aorta then delivers oxygenated blood to all body organs and tissues.

B. Cardiac depolarization.
1. Is the result of the electrical discharge across the myocardial cell (total net movement of ions across the cell wall). Cardiac depolarization is measured by the electrocardiograph (EKG).
2. Shortening of muscle fibers (contraction) usually follows cardiac depolarization (Guyton, 1976). Strength of cardiac (ventricular) contraction is measured by blood pressure or arterial pulse palpation.
3. Cardiac electrical activity does not ensure adequate cardiac function.
   a. Congenital defects or surgical injury to the conduction system may result in arrhythmias or heart block.
   b. Electrolyte disturbance, i.e., altered fluid composition surrounding the cells, can effect electrical activity.
      (1) Hypo- and hyperkalemia.
      (2) Hypo- and hypercalcemia.
      (3) Hypoxia.
      (4) Acidosis.

C. Cardiac output (CO).
1. CO is the volume of blood ejected by the heart in 1 minute. Approximations vary from 120 to 200 ml/kg/minute.
2. Cardiac output = stroke volume × heart rate (liters/minute).
   a. As heart rate fluctuates, so will cardiac output.
      (1) Normal full-term newborns can vary their heart rate range from 59 to 220/minute in a monitored 24 hour period (Southall et al. 1977).
      (2) Significant or persistent bradycardia will result in a drop in the neonate's cardiac output.
   b. Tachycardia seems to be an effective mechanism for improving cardiac output as long as the tachycardia does not compromise diastolic filling time and decrease coronary artery perfusion (Hazinski, 1983b).
3. Stroke volume is relatively fixed at 1.5 ml/kg and is affected by three factors: pre-load, contractility, and afterload (Zaritsky, 1984).
   a. Pre-load: the volume of blood in the ventricles before contraction.
      (1) Clinically, pre-load is a measurement of pressure rather than volume in the ventricles before contraction.
      (2) Increasing the volume in the ventricles, consequently lengthening the myocardial fibers before contraction, should result in improved stroke volume (Frank-Starling law) (Patterson and Starling, 1914). The new-

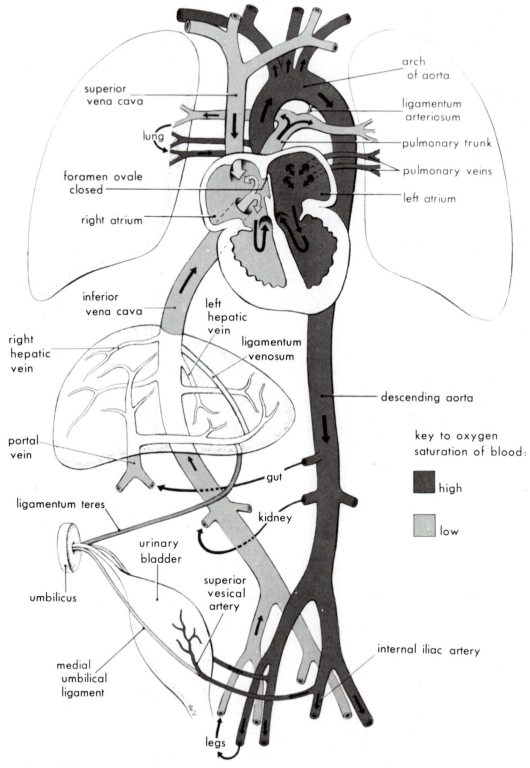

Figure 12–5

A simplified representation of the neonatal circulation. The adult derivatives of the fetal vessels and structures that become non-functional at birth are also shown. The arrows indicate the course of the neonatal circulation. The organs are not drawn to scale. After birth, the three shunts that short-circuited the blood during fetal life cease to function, and the pulmonary and systemic circulations become separated. (From Moore, K.: The Developing Human, 4th ed. Philadelphia, W.B. Saunders Co., 1988, p. 327.)

born's smaller portion of contractile mass, less compliant myocardium, and normal maximization of myocardial fiber length make it unlikely that the neonate with low cardiac output will respond favorably to volume infusion (Hazinski, 1983b).
   b. Contractility: speed of ventricular contraction.
      (1) Cardiac cycle consists of ventricular contraction (systole) followed by ventricular relaxation (diastole). As contraction time decreases, relaxation time (diastole) increases with an increase in ventricular filling volume (pre-load) prior to contraction.
      (2) Ventricular contractility cannot be clinically measured.
      (3) Contractility in neonates is influenced by the following:
         (a) Exogenous catecholamine (dopamine/dobutamine) use increases blood pressure and cardiac output (Crockett and Tappero, 1989).
         (b) Acidosis and hypoxia appear to depress contractility. Myocardial response to catecholamines is impaired by acidosis.
   c. Afterload: the resistance to blood leaving the ventricle.
      (1) Dependent on systemic vascular resistance (SVR) and pulmonary vascular resistance (PVR); if SVR or PVR increases, afterload increases.
      (2) The neonate's myocardium is very sensitive to increased afterload; with small increases in afterload, stroke volume can fall significantly (Friedman, 1973).
      (3) Afterload can be reduced by intravenous infusions of vasodilators, e.g., nitroglycerin and nitroprusside. Tolazoline and dobutamine can be used to decrease PVR (Hazinski, 1983b).
4. Concepts of blood flow
   a. Flow $\alpha = \dfrac{\text{Pressure}}{\text{Resistance}}$
   b. Blood flow will always take the path of least resistance.
   c. If heart action (pressure) remains unchanged but vasoconstriction or dilatation or obstruction to flow (resistance) changes, flow will change (i.e., cardiac output will vary).
   d. PVR starts to fall after delivery and reaches adult levels by 2 months (Hazinski, 1983a). This process is influenced by prematurity, low birthweight, and hypoxia episodes.

Congenital Heart Disease (CHD)

OCCURRENCE

CHD occurs in 7.5–8.0:1000 live births (<1%) (Freed, 1984a, b).

A. **Unknown causes: 85%.** Probably an inherited predisposition combined with environmental predisposition at a critical period during cardiac development.

B. **Genetic factors.**
1. Chromosomal abnormalities: 8%.
   a. Incidence of congenital heart disease varies with chromosomal abnormality.
      (1) 50% of trisomy 21.
      (2) 90% of trisomy 18 and 13.
      (3) 25–50% of chromosome deletion syndromes 18, 13, 5, and 4.
   b. Single mutant gene syndromes: 3%.
      (1) Both autosomal dominant and recessive syndromes have been associated with CHD.

C. **Environmental factors: 2%.**
1. Maternal ingestion of teratogenic drugs.

a. Thalidomide dramatically illustrated the extraordinarily deleterious effects of prescribed drug on a developing fetus.

2. Anticonvulsants.
   a. All teratogenic syndromes induced by anticonvulsants have associated congenital cardiac defects.
   b. Hydantoin ingestion has a 7–10% risk for classic fetal hydantoin syndrome, with ventricular and septal defects, coarctation of the aorta, and PDA being the most frequent cardiac malformations (Harned, 1990).
   c. Pentobarbital has no confirmed specific embryopathy but may potentiate the effects of other drugs taken concurrently.

3. Anticoagulants.
   a. Warfarin (Coumadin) causes abortion or fetal embryopathic development in the 6th to 9th week of gestation. Cardiac malformations have been identified, but no consistent cardiac defect has been noted.
   b. Heparin, owing to its larger molecular weight, does not cross the placenta.

4. Antineoplastic medications.
   a. Aminopterin: cardiac manifestations include dextroposition but are not as prominent as other defects resulting from drug ingestion.
   b. In general, the disorders for which antineoplastics are utilized are serious enough to preclude pregnancy.

5. Lithium.
   a. Leads to defects such as Ebstein's anomaly, ASD, and tricuspid atresia.

6. Trimethadione:
   a. Increased incidence of transposition of the great vessels, tetralogy of Fallot, and hypoplastic left heart syndrome.

7. Drugs of abuse.
   a. Alcohol: fetal alcohol syndrome is accompanied by a variety of cardiac lesions: i.e., VSD with or without subpulmonic and subaortic stenosis, coarctation of the aorta, aortic regurgitation, and ASD.
   b. Amphetamine-induced congenital cardiac conditions, especially septal defects, PDA, and transpositions, have been suggested (Nora et al., 1970).

D. **Maternal disease/viral infections** (Table 12–1).
1. Rubella is the only viral illness that produces clinically significant heart disease (peripheral pulmonic stenosis and patent ductus arteriosus).

E. **Exposure to environmental hazards** such as radiation, heat, and gases may produce teratogenic effects, but there are no specific associated cardiac malformations.

SEX PREFERENCES ASSOCIATED WITH CARDIAC LESIONS (Flyer and Lang, 1981)

A. Males.
1. Coarctation of the aorta.
2. Aortic stenosis.
3. Transposition of the great vessels (TGV).

B. Females.
1. Atrial septal defect (ASD).
2. Patent ductus arteriosus (PDA).

Approach to Diagnosis of Cardiac Disease

HISTORY

A. Gestational age.
1. Pre-term:
   a. Much more likely to have pulmonary problems resulting in cyanosis than CHD, but do have higher incidence of:

Table 12-1
CLASSIFICATION OF MATERNAL DISEASES AFFECTING THE FETAL CARDIOVASCULAR SYSTEM

Category I: Maternal Diseases that Directly Affect the Fetal Cardiovascular System (Excluding Teratogenic Effects)
Pheochromocytoma Hyperthyroidism Diabetes mellitus Collagen vascular disease (e.g., Ro antibody) Smoking Rubella Cytomegalovirus Enterovirus infection Toxoplasmosis Listeriosis Maternal group B streptococcal colonization with fetal invasion Syphilis Inherited metabolic diseases
Category II: Maternal Diseases that May Indirectly Affect the Fetal Cardiovascular System as a Result of Abnormalities of Uteroplacental Function
Neoplastic diseases Diabetes mellitus Maternal cardiac disease Anemia (including the hemoglobinopathies) Hypertensive disorders Collagen vascular disease (e.g., lupus anticoagulant and systemic lupus erythematosus) Renal disease (associated with hypertension) Smoking Asthma Cholestatic jaundice of pregnancy Cytomegalovirus Bacterial infections
From Katz, V., and Bowes, W.: Maternal diseases affecting the fetal cardiovascular system. *In* Long, W. (ed.): Fetal and Neonatal Cardiology. Philadelphia, W.B. Saunders Co., 1990, p. 135.

     (1) PDA.
     (2) Left-to-right shunts, e.g., VSD or atrioventricular (A-V) canal.
2. Term.
   a. Majority of infants with CHD are full-term babies.

B. **Maternal disease** (see Table 12-1).
1. Infants of uncontrolled diabetic mothers (IDM) have an increased risk of:
   a. TGV.
   b. VSD.
   c. PDA (Fletcher, 1981).
2. Viral and bacterial illnesses may directly and indirectly affect the fetal cardiovascular system (see Table 12-1).

C. **Congenital diseases or syndromes may have associated cardiac anomalies.**
The following associations have been noted.
1. Trisomy 13: PDA and/or VSD.
2. Trisomy 18: VSD, PDA.
3. Trisomy 21: ASD, VSD, A-V canal, PDA.
4. Turner's syndrome: coarctation of the aorta.
5. DiGeorge's syndrome: PDA, peripheral pulmonary stenosis.
6. Rubella syndrome: PDA, peripheral pulmonic stenosis.
7. Fetal alcohol syndrome: VSD, ASD, tetralogy of Fallot.

D. **Mode of delivery.**
1. Vaginal delivery usual for CHD, with initial good APGAR scores.
2. History of cesarean section and poor Apgar scores more indicative of asphyxia and respiratory distress.

E. **Pre-natal diagnosis with the use of ultrasonography** may identify the infant with congenital heart disease prior to delivery.

CLINICAL PRESENTATION

A. **Cyanosis** (in the 1st week may be sole evidence of a heart lesion).
1. With cardiovascular problems, cyanosis is unexpected or gradual in onset.
2. Cyanosis observation.
   a. Dependent on hemoglobin (Hgb) levels; 3.5–5% desaturation of Hgb is necessary before cynanosis becomes apparent.
   b. Will be influenced by presence of anemia or polycythemia and the levels of 2,3-diphosphoglycerate.
3. Differentiation between central and peripheral cyanosis.
   a. Peripheral cyanosis results from sluggish movement of blood through the extremities and increased tissue oxygen extraction.
      (1) Persists from birth and can last several days.
      (2) Does not involve mucous membranes.
      (3) May be caused by peripheral vasomotor instability.
   b. Central cyanosis results from blood leaving the heart desaturated.
      (1) Seen as bluish discoloration of tongue and mucous membranes reflecting arterial desaturation.
      (2) Central cyanosis may present difficulties in differential diagnosis between respiratory and cardiac origin.

B. **Respiratory pattern.**
1. Useful in the differentiation of cyanosis.
2. Tachypnea (>60 bpm) without respiratory distress is associated with congestive heart failure. In the absence of cyanosis, may indicate a left-to-right shunt lesion.
3. Hyperpnea (increased respiratory depth) is observed in congenital heart lesions resulting in diminished pulmonary blood flow.
4. Crying may exacerbate cyanosis in newborns with CHD due to increased tissue demands for oxygen.

C. **Heart sounds.**
1. S_1 (first heart sound) represents closure of the mitral and tricuspid valves at the end of atrial systole.
   a. Best heard at cardiac apex (5th intercostal sternal border).
   b. S_1 is accentuated with the following:
      (1) Cardiac output increased.
      (2) Increased flow across atrioventricular valves.
      (3) Specific conditions such as:
         (a) PDA.
         (b) VSD with increased mitral flow.
         (c) Total anomalous pulmonary venous connection (TAPVC).
         (d) Arteriovenous malformation.
         (e) Tetralogy of Fallot.
         (f) Anemia.
         (g) Fever.
   c. Conditions decreasing S_1 include the following:
      (1) Decreased atrioventricular conduction.
      (2) Congestive heart failure (CHF).
      (3) Myocarditis.
2. S_2 (second heart sound) occurs at the end of ventricular systole from closure of aortic and pulmonic valves.
   a. Heart sounds heard best at upper left sternal border.
   b. A split S_2 is a normal occurrence, reflecting closure of aortic valve prior to the pulmonic valve.
      (1) Increases on inspiration.

     (2) Single S_2 is often heard in the first 2 days of life due to increased pulmonary vascular resistance (PVR).

     (3) Splitting of S_2 is influenced by:

        (a) Abnormalities of aortic or pulmonic valves.

        (b) Conditions altering PVR or SVR.

  c. Conditions widening the S_2 are influenced by:

     (1) ASD.

     (2) TAPVC.

     (3) Tetralogy of Fallot.

     (4) Pulmonary stenosis.

     (5) Ebstein's anomaly.

  d. Absent S_2 splits occur in the following:

     (1) Pulmonary atresia and severe pulmonary stenosis.

     (2) Aortic stenosis/atresia.

     (3) Persistent pulmonary hypertension.

     (4) L-transposition of the great vessels (TGV).

     (5) Truncus arteriosus.

3. S_3 (third heart sound).

  a. Follows S_2 and is a low-pitched, broad sound.

  b. Prominent in situations of increased atrioventricular flow and increased ventricular filling (Moller, 1990; Johnson, 1990).

     (1) Left-to-right shunts, e.g., ASD, VSD, PDA.

     (2) Anemia.

     (3) Mitral valve insufficiency.

4. S_4 (fourth heart sound).

  a. Rarely heard in the newborn.

  b. Indicative of primary myocardial disease.

5. Ejection clicks.

  a. Are abnormal (except during first 24 hours of life) and indicate cardiac disease.

  b. Audible for short duration after S_1.

  c. Associated with dilation of the great vessels or deformity of aortic or pulmonic valve.

  d. Conditions associated with ejection clicks include the following:

     (1) Aortic valve stenosis.

     (2) Truncus arteriosus.

     (3) Tetralogy of Fallot (severe).

     (4) Pulmonary valve stenosis.

     (5) Hypoplastic left heart.

     (6) Coarctation of the aorta.

6. Murmurs.

  a. Murmurs result from turbulence of blood flow and may be due to:

     (1) Abnormal valves.

     (2) Septal defects.

     (3) Regurgitated flow through incompetent valves.

     (4) High blood flow across normal structures.

  b. Physiological murmurs have been noted in 60% of newborns in the first 48 hours of life (Baudo and Rowe, 1961; Engle, 1981). Generally, these murmurs are from:

     (1) Transient left-to-right flow via ductus arteriosus.

     (2) Increased flow over pulmonary valve associated with fall in PVR.

     (3) Mild bilateral peripheral pulmonary arterial stenosis possible, owing to size and pressure differences between the main pulmonary trunk and the left and right pulmonary arterial branches (Johnson, 1990).

  c. Evaluation of murmurs includes the following:

     (1) Intensity of sound.

        (a) Murmurs are graded. Those less than grade III/VI generally present no hemodynamic problems (Moller, 1990) (Table 12–2).

Table 12-2
GRADING OF MURMURS

Grade I   Soft; requires extended listening
Grade II   Soft; heard immediately
Grade III   Moderate intensity; no thrill
Grade IV   Loud; often with thrill or palpable vibration at murmur site
Grade V   Loud; thrill present; audible with stethoscope partially off the chest
Grade VI   Loud; audible with stethoscope off chest

(2) Location within cardiac cycle.
  (a) Systolic: heard during ventricular systole, i.e., between S_1 and S_2.
    i. Identified as early, mid-, or late systolic.
    ii. Pansystolic (holosystolic): murmurs present for duration of systole. Heard in mitral or tricuspid insufficiency, VSD.
    iii. Ejection murmurs: turbulence of blood flow leaving the heart; noted in aortic or pulmonic valve stenosis, tetralogy of Fallot, ASD, and total anomalous pulmonary venous connection (TAPVC).
  (b) Diastolic: heard during period of ventricular filling, i.e., between S_2 and S_1.
    i. Early: results from aortic or pulmonic valve insufficiency.
    ii. Mid: increased blood flow across normal mitral or tricuspid valves.
    iii. Late: associated with stenotic mitral or tricuspid valves.
  (c) Continuous: audible throughout cardiac cycle but can be louder in systole or diastole.
    i. PDA is a classic example of a continuous murmur.
(3) Quality of sound.
  (a) Pitch (reflects frequency of vibrations).
    i. High-pitched sound generally reflects valve insufficiency on left side of heart, whereas a low-pitched sound reflects right-sided valve insufficiencies.
  (b) Other descriptive terms (have less precise meaning).
    i. Harsh.
    ii. Blowing.
    iii. Musical.
(4) Location on chest of murmur's maximum intensity.
(5) Absence of murmur does not indicate absence of significant cardiac disease.

D. Peripheral pulses.
1. Palpate simultaneously on each side and in turn all extremities and carotid.
2. Should be synchronous with equal intensity.
3. Discrepancies, e.g., upper greater than lower extremities, raise possibility of abnormal aortic arch.
4. Weak pulses indicate low systemic output as seen in the following:
  a. Obstruction of left side of heart, e.g., hypoplastic left heart or severe aortic stenosis.
  b. Myocardial failure.
  c. Shock.

E. Blood pressure.
1. Normal values.
  a. Normal full-term: mean systolic, 70–75 mm Hg (range, 55–90); mean diastolic, 40–45 mm Hg (range 30–55).
  b. Premature infant's blood pressure varies with size and gestational age.
    (1) 1000 g infant: systolic mean, 50 mm Hg. Diastolic mean: 30 mm Hg.

2. Blood pressure values may be affected by body temperature, activity, and posture (Johnson, 1990).
3. Upper extremities systolic blood pressure > 20 mm Hg above lower extremities is suggestive of:
   a. Coarctation of the aorta.
      (1) PDA may mask these pressure differences.
   b. Aortic arch abnormalities.
      (1) Additionally, blood pressure differences between upper extremities are seen with aortic arch abnormalities.
      (2) To evaluate: simultaneously measure blood pressure in both arms and one leg. Either leg can be evaluated, since the blood supply to both legs comes from the descending aorta below the level of the defect.
4. Neonatal hypertension is defined as a systolic blood pressure > 90 mm Hg and a diastolic pressure > 60 in a full-term neonate.
   a. Premature infants: systolic > 80 mm Hg; diastolic > 50 mm Hg.
   b. Renal vein thrombosis secondary to high umbilical artery catheter placement is the most common cause of hypertension.

F. **Congestive heart failure (CHF).**
1. Is typically associated with congenital heart lesions. The timing of CHF appearance may assist in diagnosis of the lesion (Tables 12–3 and 12–4).
2. See below for other causes and clinical manifestations of CHF.
3. Late-onset CHF may result from bronchopulmonary dysplasia (BPD) or other pulmonary stressors. (Refer to Chapter 6.)

DIAGNOSTIC ADJUNCTS

A. **Arterial blood gases** are primarily used to help differentiate lung disease versus heart disease as the etiology of cyanosis.
2. $Paco_2$: generally normal in CHD and elevated in pulmonary parenchymal disease.
2. Hyperoxygen test.
   a. Sample arterial Po_2 with infant breathing 100% oxygen versus room air.
      (1) Umbilical artery sample may detect right-to-left shunts via PDA. The lowered Pao_2 is a reflection usually of lung disease and not primary heart disease.
      (2) Administration of oxygen to infants with cardiac disease resulting in high pulmonary blood flow and CHF will improve oxygen levels, i.e., increased Pao_2, through decreased PVR and increased pulmonary blood flow.
      (3) The most accurate assessment of cardiac versus pulmonary disease can be made if the right radial or temporal (pre-ductal) and umbilical artery samples (post-ductal) are taken simultaneously.

Table 12–3
CAUSES OF CONGESTIVE HEART FAILURE IN THE FIRST WEEK OF LIFE

Disease	History	Pulses	EKG	Precordium
Transient myocardial ischemia	+			
Dysrhythmias	±			
Arteriovenous fistula	−	Increased		
Coarctation of the aorta (interrupted aortic arch)	−	Asymmetrical		
Aortic stenosis	−	Decreased	LVH	
Hypoplastic left heart syndrome	−	Decreased	RVH	Hyperactive
Myocarditis	−	Decreased	RVH	Decreased

From Freed, M.: Congenital cardiac malformations. *In* Taeusch, H.W., Ballard, R.A., and Avery, M.E. (eds.): Schaffer & Avery's Diseases of the Newborn, 6th ed. Philadelphia, W.B. Saunders Co., 1991, p. 629.

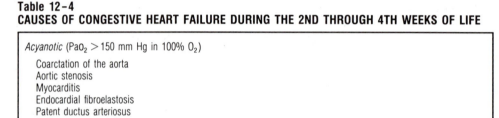

Table 12-4
CAUSES OF CONGESTIVE HEART FAILURE DURING THE 2ND THROUGH 4TH WEEKS OF LIFE

Acyanotic ($PaO_2 > 150$ mm Hg in 100% O_2)

 Coarctation of the aorta
 Aortic stenosis
 Myocarditis
 Endocardial fibroelastosis
 Patent ductus arteriosus
 Aortopulmonary window
 Anteriovenous fistula
 Ventricular septal defect
 Atrioventricular canal defects

Cyanotic ($PaO_2 < 150$ mm Hg in 100% O_2)

 Hypoplastic left heart syndrome
 Total anomalous pulmonary venous return
 Truncus arteriosus
 Transposition and a ventricular septal defect
 Tricuspid atresia and a ventricular septal defect
 Single ventricle

From Freed, M.: Congenital cardiac malformations. *In* Taeusch, H. W., Ballard, R. A., and Avery, M. E. (eds.): Schaffer & Avery's Diseases of the Newborn, 6th ed. Philadelphia, W.B. Saunders Co., 1991, p. 630.

  (4) Use of pre- and post-ductal transcutaneous oxygen monitoring ($TCPO_2$) provides a non-invasive evaluation for cardiac versus pulmonary disease.
 b. Pre-ductal PaO_2 rises in 100% oxygen ≥ 250 torr indicate lung disease; rises of ≤ 100 torr are consistent with cardiac disease (Flyer and Lang, 1981).

B. Chest x-ray is used to:
1. Rule out pulmonary parenchymal disease.
2. Identify increased pulmonary markings as seen in lesions with left-to-right shunting.
3. Evaluate cardiac size and shape.
 a. Cardiomegaly: Defined as cardiac: thoracic ratio > 0.6.
 b. See Chapter 33 for chest x-ray findings in heart disease.

C. Electrocardiography (EKG).
1. Reflects abnormal hemodynamic burdens placed on the heart.
2. Used to determine severity of disease by assessing the degree of atrial or ventricular hypertrophy.
 a. Right ventricular predominance is normal shortly after birth. (In utero, the right ventricle does most of the cardiac work.)
3. Changes in S-T segments or T-waves may suggest myocardial ischemia.
 a. Tall peaked P-waves are common in right-sided heart failure.
 b. Wide notched P-waves are seen with left-sided heart failure.
4. EKG is the major diagnostic tool for evaluating arrhythmias and the impact of electrolyte imbalances (e.g., potassium and calcium) on electrical conductivity.
5. Normal electrocardiogram values in term neonates:
 a. Heart rate: 125–135 in first week.
 b. Normal sinus rhythm: P-wave precedes QRS complex.
 c. P-wave: duration 0.04–0.08 second.
 d. P-R interval: 0.08–0.14 second.
  (1) Prolonged interval is seen in first-degree heart block (usually benign).
 e. QRS complex: duration 0.03–0.07 second.
  (1) Prolonged indicates interventricular conduction delay.
 f. Premature infants have higher resting heart rates with greater variation. P-wave duration is shorter. P-R and QRS intervals are decreased (0.10 and 0.04 second, respectively).

D. Echocardiography.
1. Provides rapid, non-invasive, and painless evaluation of heart anatomy and flow by use of ultrasonic sound waves.
   a. M-mode (single dimension) permits evaluation of anatomical relationships of heart and vessels including relative sizes of each.
   b. Two-dimensional (real-time) echocardiography has greater versatility, providing more specific information regarding anatomical relationships.
   c. Contrast echocardiography is accomplished by rapid injection of saline in a vein while conducting ultrasonography. Allows for greater evaluation of flow patterns throughout the heart; identifies presence of shunts.
2. Although heart echocardiography allows for rapid bedside diagnosis of heart lesions and differentiation from other abnormalities (e.g., sepsis, persistent fetal circulation), it does not replace cardiac catheterization as a diagnostic tool.

E. Cardiac catheterization.
1. An invasive procedure to obtain data (e.g., O_2 saturation and pressure measurements) for definitive diagnostics or in preparation for cardiac surgery.
   a. May be used in palliative treatment (e.g., balloon atrial septostomy in transposition of the great vessels (TGV).
   b. Usually reserved for cyanotic heart lesions.
   c. For acyanotic heart lesions, catheterization can be delayed until full effect of medical management of CHF is seen.
2. Procedure involves advancing a catheter from right inguinal area into inferior vena cava and into the heart.
   a. Umbilical vein may be used instead of the femoral artery.
   b. If balloon septostomy is anticipated, a large vessel will be needed.
   c. Pressure measurements are made of all chambers and outlet tracks.
3. Concomitant angiography (injection of contrast medium) is often performed to maximize cardiac information.
4. Complications.
   a. Mortality risk $<0.5\%$ (Cohn et al., 1985).
   b. High sodium content of contrast medium contributes to myocardiac depression and exerts an osmotic effect, temporarily increasing intravascular volume.
   c. Hemorrhage with catheter insertion or removal may lead to:
      (1) Hypotension.
      (2) Shock.
      (3) Cardiac tamponade if bleeding is in the pericardial sac.
   d. Dysrhythmias are not uncommon (e.g., premature atrial and ventricular beats and tachycardia), owing to catheter manipulation.

F. Laboratory data.
1. CBC with differential.
   a. Rules out anemia or polycythemia as cause of CHF.
   b. Decreased neutrophils and presence of left shift may indicate sepsis. Group B beta-hemolytic streptococci can mimic hypoplastic left heart syndrome.
2. Blood glucose/Dextrostix.
   a. Used to evaluate hypoglycemia as potential cause of cardiomyopathy.
3. Electrolytes (especially potassium and calcium).
   a. Both potassium and calcium are major cations in electrical conductivity. Alterations can adversely affect cardiac contractility.

Congenital Heart Lesions: Acyanotic

PATENT DUCTUS ARTERIOSUS

A. Incidence (4th most common lesion).
1. In term gestations, occurs 1:10,000 live births.

2. In pre-term gestations (Freed, 1984a):
   a. Incidence is inversely related to gestational age.
   b. 20% of infants >1500 g.
   c. 40% of infants <1000 g.
3. Occurs three times more commonly in females than in males.

B. **Anatomy:** persistent patency of the ductus arteriosus after birth (Fig. 12–6).
1. Fetal patency of this structure is functional, serving to divert blood away from fluid-filled lungs toward the placenta for oxygen gas exchange.
2. Patency is influenced by several factors.
   a. Increased oxygen tension is a potent stimulant of smooth muscle contraction: decreases patency.
   b. Lack of ductal smooth muscle (e.g., in prematures) prolongs patency.
   c. Prostaglandins inhibit closure of ductus.

C. **Hemodynamics.**
1. As PVR falls and SVR rises, a left-to-right shunt via the PDA results in blood flows from the aorta into the pulmonary artery, increasing pulmonary blood flow. The increased pulmonary artery pressure and increased left ventricular pressure/volume lead to bilateral CHF.
2. Because left-to-right flow is dependent on a drop in PVR, infants with pulmonary disease (e.g., hyaline membrane disease) will show symptoms when lung disease improves. Prior to this time, PVR greater than SVR leads to a right-to-left shunt via the patent ductus (commonly referred to as persistent pulmonary hypertension of the newborn [PPHN]).

D. **Clinical features.**
1. Characteristically becomes evident at end of the first week of life.
2. Small PDA:
   a. CHF: increased pulmonary vasculature and cardiomegaly.
   b. Bounding peripheral pulses and active precordium.
   c. Murmur may be "silent" in 10–20% of the pre-terms in spite of hemodynamically significant shunt (Clyman, 1990).

E. **Management.**
1. Dependent on whether shunt is hemodynamically significant.
   a. In prematures, the PDA may prolong ventilator use beyond the dictates of the initial lung disease. Early intervention may prevent lung complication of ventilator use.

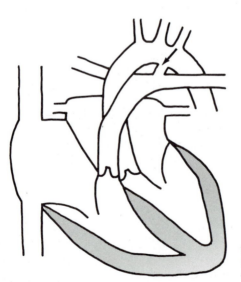

Figure 12–6
Patent ductus arteriosus (PDA). (Redrawn courtesy of G.G. Janos, M.D., 1989.)

2. Criteria for hemodynamically significant ductus arteriosus include the following (Freed, 1984a):
   a. Heart rate >170 beats/minute.
   b. Respiratory rate >70/minute.
   c. Hepatomegaly >3 cm below costal margin.
   d. Bounding pulses >96 hours on continuous positive airway pressure (24 cm H_2O).
   e. Radiographic findings of cardiomegaly (cardiothoracic ratio >.60), pulmonary edema, and increased pulmonary vascularity. These "typical" signs may be absent if infant is receiving positive-pressure ventilation (Clyman, 1990).
3. Conservative measures are generally employed initially:
   a. Fluid restriction.
   b. Diuretics: employed with fluid restriction may lead to electrolyte imbalance, dehydration, and caloric deprivation.
   c. Digitalis.
      (1) In the less than 1250 g infant, has little to no benefit and is frequently toxic.
      (2) In combination with indomethacin, increased susceptibility to digoxin toxicity.
   d. Positive end-expiratory pressure (PEEP) has been found useful in reducing the left-to-right shunt via the PDA.
   e. High hematocrit decreases the PDA shunting and improves systemic oxygen delivery under conditions of decreased perfusion.
4. Indomethacin management:
   a. As a prostaglandin inhibitor, indomethacin can constrict and close the PDA in some prematures.
   b. Dosage: 0.2–0.3 mg/kg given up to three times 8–12 hours apart (Freed, 1984a).
   c. Complications:
      (1) Transient decreased renal function.
      (2) Increased incidence of occult blood loss via gastrointestinal tract.
      (3) Inhibition of platelet function for 7–9 days with potential for intracerebral hemorrhage.
   d. Ductus reopens in 30% of the patients treated with indomethacin (Clyman, 1990).
   e. Contraindications:
      (1) Significant renal failure.
      (2) Frank renal or gastrointestinal bleeding.
      (3) Necrotizing enterocolitis is not a contraindication, but surgical ligation is more rapid and certain resolution of PDA results in prompt decrease in bowel ischemia from the PDA.
      (4) Sepsis: proven or strongly suspected.
5. Surgical management involves ligation of the PDA.
   a. Surgery carries almost negligible risk.
   b. Potential for surgical complications of bleeding with prior indomethacin (risk dependent on time from dose to surgical intervention).

VENTRICULAR SEPTAL DEFECT (VSD)

A. **Incidence:** At 1:3000 live births, VSDs are the most common of all congenital heart diseases.

B. **Anatomy:** abnormal opening in the septum between the right and left ventricle. Sizes range from pinhole to almost complete absence of the ventricular septum (Fig. 12–7).

C. **Hemodynamics:**
1. The degree of hypertrophy of ventricles and pressure relationships are depen-

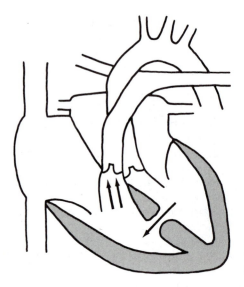

Figure 12-7
Ventricular septal defect (VSD). (Redrawn courtesy of G.G. Janos, M.D., 1989.)

dent on the size of the defect. A small defect allows pressure differences between ventricles.
2. PVR less than SVR results in a left-to-right shunt, producing increased pulmonary blood flow and decreased pulmonary compliance.
3. Excessive pulmonary artery blood flow eventually results in pulmonary artery hypertrophy and stenosis.
4. The high pulmonary artery pressure can delay pulmonary arterioles' maturation.

D. **Clinical features:**
1. Clinical features are size dependent.
2. Small VSD:
   a. Asymptomatic.
   b. High-pitched pansystolic murmur along left sternal border.
3. Moderate VSD: asymptomatic except for murmur and recurrent respiratory infection.
4. Large VSD:
   a. Present at 1-2 months of age with CHF, pulmonary infection, and increased precordial activity.
   b. Loud, blowing pansystolic murmur at left lower sternal border (LLSB).
   c. Chest x-ray: cardiac enlargement and increased pulmonary vascular markings.

E. **Management:**
1. Small defects often close spontaneously; 20% of large defects get smaller or close.
2. With mild CHF, management is with digoxin, diuretics, and anticongestives.
3. Treatment of significant CHF with poor weight gain despite pharmacological management is as follows:
   a. Palliative: surgical banding of pulmonary artery to reduce pulmonary blood flow and decrease CHF.
   b. Surgical: repair by suturing defect or patching defect.
   c. Current trend is earlier surgical repair rather than palliative banding with delayed repair.

F. **Prognosis.** Prognosis is excellent, with spontaneous closure the norm and operative closure required in only 2% of the defects. Late operative mortality is 2.3% (Rosenthal and Bank, 1990). Later course may be complicated by conduction abnormalities, aortic and/or tricuspid insufficiency.

ATRIAL SEPTAL DEFECT (ASD)

A. **Incidence:** 1 : 5000 live births.

B. **Anatomy:** septal defect between right and left atria. Defect may be an ostium secundum defect, patent foramen ovale, or partial endocardial cushion defect (Fig. 12–8).

C. **Hemodynamics:**
1. In early newborn period, right ventricle pressure greater than left ventricle pressure, so no shunt or small right-to-left.
2. As PVR decreases, left-to-right shunt develops with concomitant right ventricular hypertrophy.

D. **Clinical features:**
1. In isolated defect, the patients are generally asymptomatic and unrecognized. If diagnosed in infancy, 50%–100% are symptomatic.
2. CHF from left-to-right shunt and mitral valve insufficiency.
3. "Failure to thrive."
4. Recurrent respiratory infections.
5. Systolic murmur at second left intercostal space, persistent split S_2 if shunt large, diastolic murmur heard at LLSB.
6. Chest x-ray: large pulmonary artery blood flow with enlargement of right atrium and ventricle.

E. **Management:**
1. If asymptomatic, follow without early operative repair; spontaneous ASD closure is possible.
2. ASD with CHF: treat medically with anticongestive therapy and delay surgical repair.
3. ASD with intractable CHF: early surgical repair, i.e., suturing or patching of the defect.

F. **Prognosis:**
1. Spontaneous closure occurs in 25–50% of secundum ASDs during the first year (Moreau and Graham, 1990).
2. Operative mortality is about one-third, with good long-term results in survivors.

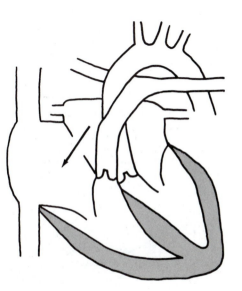

Figure 12–8
Atrial septal defect (ASD). (Redrawn courtesy of G.G. Janos, M.D., 1989.)

ENDOCARDIAL CUSHION DEFECT (A-V CANAL)

A. **Incidence:** 1 : 9000 live births. Most common heart defect in Down syndrome.

B. **Anatomy:**
1. Endocardial cushions form the lower portion of the atrial septum, the upper portion of the ventricular septum, and septal portions of the mitral and tricuspid valves.
2. A wide range of defects exist from simple cleft of the mitral and/or tricuspid valves to complete absence of the lower atrial and upper ventricular septa with common atrioventricular valve (i.e., atrioventricular canal [AVC]) (Fig. 12–9).

C. **Hemodynamics:**
1. With PVR less than SVR, blood dependently shunts left-to-right via the ASD and VSD.
2. The higher pressure of the left ventricle creates obligatory left-to-right shunting via the A-V valve (A-V valve regurgitation).
   a. Blood flows: left ventricle—mitral portion of the A-V valve—left atrium—ASD—right atrium.

D. **Clinical features:**
1. Isolated ostium primum atrial defect: rarely identified in the neonatal period.
2. Isolated ventricular defect: see clinical features of VSD above.
3. Complete A-V canal:
   a. A-V valve regurgitation controls age of presentation.
      (1) Severe: Seen at 1-2 weeks of age with CHF.
      (2) Valves competent: seen 1st or 2nd month of life.
   b. Active precordium with a thrill at the left lower sternal border (LLSB).
   c. Murmurs are variable; usually loud pansystolic at LLSB.
   d. Chest x-ray: cardiomegaly, bilateral atrial and ventricular hypertrophy, increased pulmonary markings.

E. **Management:**
1. Medical management of CHF.
2. Palliative pulmonary artery banding to increase PVR.
   a. Risky: mortality, 30–40% (Freed, 1984a, b)
   b. Does not influence obligatory A-V valve shunting.
3. Primary repair with closure of atrial and ventricular septal defects and mitral and tricuspid valve reconstruction.

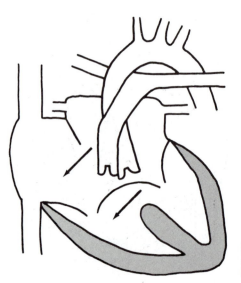

Figure 12–9
Atrioventricular canal (AVC). (Redrawn courtesy of G.G. Janos, M.D., 1989.)

F. **Prognosis.**
1. Dependent on details of anatomical form, presence of significant associated anomalies and non-cardiac anomalies, and significant pulmonary obstructive vascular disease.
2. Best results are seen with ostium primum defect or common atrium; long-term prognosis is good.
3. Outlook for complete A-V canal without operation is poor (46% and 85% mortality by 6 and 24 months, respectively) (Feldt et al., 1990).
4. Mortality of surgical repair varies, with a reported range of 0.6–20% (Chin and Keane, 1982; Sand and Pacifico, 1990).

COARCTATION OF THE AORTA

A. **Incidence:** 1 : 700 live births.
1. Most common congenital heart defect presenting in the second week of life.
2. Male dominance of 2 : 1.

B. **Anatomy:** constriction of the aorta distal to the left subclavian artery (Fig. 12–10).
1. Usually occurs at insertion site of ductus arteriosus.
2. Pre-ductal coarctation associated with hypoplasia of the aortic arch and intra-cardiac defects.

C. **Hemodynamics:**
1. Isolated coarctation: obstruction to left ventricular outflow leads to increased left ventricular, left atrial, and pulmonary venous pressures; pulmonary venous congestion develops.
2. Coarctation with VSD: elevated left ventricular pressure shunts blood left-to-right via VSD, causing pulmonary overload.
3. Pre-ductal coarctation is dependent on PDA for distal aorta and lower body blood flow.

D. **Clinical features:**
1. Congestive heart failure (CHF) with hepatomegaly.
2. Decreased pulses and blood pressures in the lower extremities.
   a. Decreased blood pressure in left arm indicative of left subclavian artery as site of coarctation.

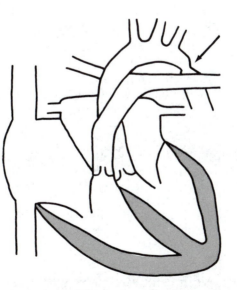

Figure 12–10
Coarctation of the aorta. (Redrawn courtesy of G.G. Janos, M.D., 1989.)

    b. Decreased blood pressure in right arm: right subclavian arises below coarctation (rare).

    c. Pulses that "wax and wane" are related to increase or decrease in PDA blood flow.

3. Heart sounds.

    a. Post-ductal: no murmur or short systolic ejection in axilla or back.

    b. Pre-ductal with VSD: harsh pansystolic murmur at LLSB.

    c. Gallop rhythm may be noted.

4. Chest x-ray: enlarged heart with left ventricular hypertrophy (LVH) and pulmonary vascular congestion.

E. Management:

1. Medical management of CHF.

2. Prostaglandin E_1 to dilate ductus arteriosus (pre-ductal lesion).

3. Isolated post-ductal coarctation: control CHF first, then delayed surgical correction.

4. Surgical correction: two common repairs.

    a. Resection of abnormal segment and reanastomosis; *or*

    b. Subclavian patch across area of obstruction.

    c. With associated anomalies, approaches vary with type of defect.

F. Prognosis:

1. Estimated mortality rate of symptomatic untreated coarctations may be as high as 84%.

2. Outcome is dependent on complexity of coarctation, with mortality rates at 1 month ranging from 0% for simple coarctation to 14% for complex coarctation (Beekman and Rocchini, 1990).

3. Long-term prognosis after coarctation repair is determined by presence of residual or recurrent coarctation, persistence of pulmonary hypertension, and residual cardiovascular lesions.

    a. 25–60% incidence of reoccurrence following resection and end-to-end anastomosis has been reported for repair in infancy.

    b. Left subclavian flap operation has reported an incidence of 0–13% for significant recoarctation, with one report of a 25% reoperation rate (Beekman and Rocchini, 1990).

    c. Potential residual complications include persistent hypertension, Horner's syndrome, and mesenteric vasculitis.

AORTIC STENOSIS

A. Incidence: 1 : 24,000 live births.

B. Anatomy: aortic valve is stenotic with valve cusps thickened or deformed, and the myocardium is hypertrophied.

1. Stenosis may also occur above or below the valve (Fig. 12–11).

C. Hemodynamics:

1. Obstruction to left ventricular outflow leads to increased left ventricular pressures and hypertrophy.

    a. If severe in utero, blood flow through ventricle is decreased, resulting in left ventricular hypoplasia and left-sided heart syndrome.

D. Clinical features.

1. Asymptomatic at birth.

2. Heart sounds: systolic murmur along left sternal border radiating to right upper sternal border.

3. CHF symptoms may be delayed by weeks; progress rapidly following onset.

4. Chest x-ray: cardiomegaly (may be massive) with or without pulmonary venous engorgement.

E. Management:

1. Initially, CHF and acidosis management.

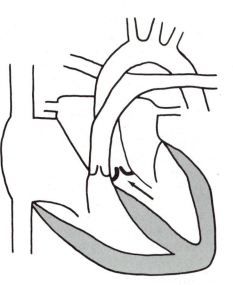

Figure 12–11
Aortic stenosis (AS). (Redrawn courtesy of G.G. Janos, M.D., 1989.)

2. Surgery involves aortic valvotomy.
3. If neonates present in CHF, they usually remain in failure and operative relief is necessary.

F. Prognosis.
1. High operative risk secondary to ventricular hypoplasia and myocardial hypertrophy.
2. Aortic stenosis is the most common cause of sudden death in children with heart disease.

HYPOPLASTIC LEFT HEART

A. Incidence: 1:6000 live births.
B. Anatomy:
1. Hypoplastic left ventricle and ascending aorta.
2. Atresia or hypoplastic mitral and aortic valves (Fig. 12–12).

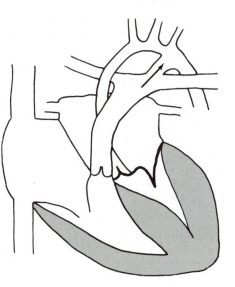

Figure 12–12
Hypoplastic left heart. (Redrawn courtesy of G.G. Janos, M.D., 1989.)

C. Hemodynamics:
1. Obstruction of blood flow through the left side of the heart due to hypoplastic aorta and ventricle leads to pulmonary venous congestion and edema.
2. Blood supply to the descending aorta and to aortic arch and coronary arteries (retrograde flow) is dependent on the PDA.

D. Clinical features.
1. Asymptomatic at birth.
2. Tachypnea and dyspnea with increasing pulmonary blood flow.
3. CHF usually presents at 24–48 hours of life.
4. Cyanosis is rarely permanent despite mixing of systemic and pulmonary circulations.
5. As PDA closes, low output signs occur:
   a. Severe mottling.
   b. Gray pallor of skin.
   c. Markedly diminished pulses.
6. Chest x-ray: cardiomegaly with increased pulmonary blood flow and pulmonary venous congestion.

E. Management:
1. Previously a uniformly fatal lesion; management has been comfort and family support.
2. Surgical procedures have been tried. Currently, the two notable ones are as follows:
   a. Norwood: a two-stage procedure involving the creation of an aorta–to–pulmonary artery anastomosis (palliative stage) and the establishment of a subclavian artery–to–pulmonary artery anastomosis (Fontan's procedure/corrective stage).
   b. Heart transplantation.
   c. Availability of either technique is limited.
   d. If surgical treatment is contemplated, prostaglandin E_1 is used to maintain ductal patency.

Congenital Heart Lesions: Cyanotic

TRANSPOSITION OF THE GREAT VESSELS (TGV)

A. Incidence: 1 : 5000 live births.
   a. Predominance in males 2 : 1.

B. Anatomy: position of the great arteries are reversed—i.e., the pulmonary artery arises from the left ventricle and the aorta from the right ventricle. Without other intracardiac defects (e.g., VSD, ASD), independent parallel circuit exists (Fig. 12–13).
1. "D" presentation: aorta is situated to the left of the pulmonary artery.

C. Hemodynamics:
1. Oxygenated blood returning from the lungs enters the left atrium and ventricle, exiting via the pulmonary artery back to the lungs.
2. Desaturated blood returns to the right atrium and ventricle, leaving via the aorta to perfuse the body.
3. Mixing of oxygenated and unoxygenated blood occurs at the ductus arteriosus (as long as patency exists) or through any existing septal defects (ASD, VSD).
   a. Mixing is required for survival.
   b. Shunting occurs from left to right through septal defects or PDA, ameliorating degree of cyanosis and hypoxia.

D. Clinical features:
1. Cyanosis is present within the first 24 hours of life and becomes progressively more intense.

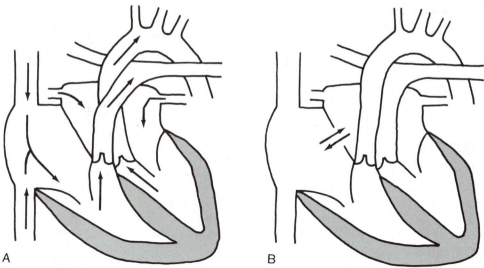

Figure 12–13
Transposition of the great vessels (TGV). *A*, Normal anatomy. *B*, Appearance of the heart with TGV. (Redrawn courtesy of G.G. Janos, M.D., 1989.)

2. Heart sounds: prominent murmurs uncommon; VSD (if present) will have loud murmur.
3. Chest x-ray: normal usually; heart may have "egg-on-side" appearance. Pulmonary vasculature may be increased or decreased.

E. Management:
1. Correction of metabolic derangements.
2. Prostaglandin E_1 to maintain patency of the PDA until palliative surgery performed.
3. Palliation choice is a balloon septostomy.
   a. A balloon catheter is inserted in the femoral or umbilical vein; it is advanced across the foramen ovale into the left atrium, and the balloon is inflated and pulled across the atrium, creating as ASD.
   b. Rapidly improves systemic and pulmonary circulation admixing, thus increasing Pao_2 (30s) and saturation (70s).
4. Corrective surgery:
   a. Physiological correction (Mustard or Senning): creates a baffle at the atrium to divert systemic venous blood into the left ventricle and pulmonary artery and pulmonary venous blood into the right ventricle and aorta. This can be delayed 6 months.
   b. Anatomical correction (arterial switch operation): detaches aorta, pulmonary artery, and coronary arteries, reattaching to "normal" ventricles. Procedure is generally performed within first 2 weeks of life.

F. Prognosis:
1. Changes in medical operative management make short-term data potentially misleading and long-term data out of date.
2. Multicenter data from January 1985 to June 1986 indicate that survival rates for all procedures (i.e., atrial and arterial switches) is as follows (Freed and Castaneda, 1990):
   a. 94% at 1 week.
   b. 90% at 1 month.
   c. 84% at 1 year.
3. Complications/residual effects include dysrhythmias, myocardial ischemia, and aortic and/or pulmonic supravalvular stenosis.

TETRALOGY OF FALLOT

A. **Incidence:** 1:5000 live births. Most common cyanotic heart lesion.

B. **Anatomy:** classified as a combination of four defects, although No. 3 and No. 4 below are consequences of No. 1 and No. 2 (Fig. 12–14).
1. Pulmonary stenosis: obstruction of outflow tract.
2. VSD.
3. Aorta overrides VSD.
4. Right ventricular hypertrophy.

C. **Hemodynamics.**
1. Dependent on degree of pulmonary stenosis.
2. In severe pulmonary stenosis, blood flow passes right-to-left via the VSD with resulting hypoxia and cyanosis.
3. Mild pulmonary stenosis: blood flows left-to-right via VSD with CHF resulting.
4. Mild to moderate pulmonary stenosis: blood flow via VSD may be minimal as long as PVR and SVR are balanced. With crying, right-to-left shunting occurs.

D. **Clinical features:**
1. Presentation is a function of the degree of pulmonary stenosis.
2. Severe obstruction presents in first days of life with severe cyanosis.
3. Milder pulmonary obstruction presents in first days of life with mild cyanosis.
4. Chest x-ray: normal heart size with decreased pulmonary markings if hypoxia exists. Classic picture is that of a boot.
5. Traditional "TET spells" (paroxysmal dyspnea and severe cyanosis) are unusual in the first months of life.

E. **Management:**
1. Palliative treatments all involve creation of systemic-pulmonary shunts:
    a. Waterston: shunt between ascenting aorta and right pulmonary artery (largely abandoned).
    b. Potts: shunt between descending aorta and left pulmonary artery. Abandoned owing to tendency for pulmonary vascular obstructive disease development.
    c. Blalock-Taussig: shunt between subclavian and pulmonary artery.

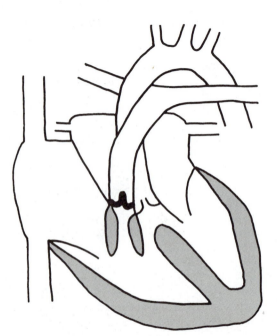

Figure 12–14
Tetralogy of Fallot (TOF). (Redrawn courtesy of G.G. Janos, M.D., 1989.)

2. Corrective surgery involves closure of the VSD using a patch and eliminating the pulmonary stenosis by resection. The pulmonary outflow tract may be enlarged by a patch.
   a. If no complicating anatomical features exist, definitive repair is delayed beyond 6 months.
   b. If child is symptomatic before 6 months of age, a Blalock-Taussig procedure is generally performed, with full correction at 3–4 years of age. According to Freed (1984a, b), there is a reported mortality of 10% for corrective operations within the first year of life and 5% for operations delayed beyond 1 year.
   c. Complications/residual effects: decreased or absent pulses in affected arm, inadequate shunt, CHF secondary to large shunt.

PULMONARY STENOSIS

A. **Incidence:** 1 : 14,000 live births.

B. **Anatomy:** narrowed opening in pulmonary valve as a consequence of pulmonary valve cusp fusions (Fig. 12–15).

C. **Hemodynamics:**
1. In utero, right ventricular hypoplasia can develop, depending on the degree of pulmonary valve stenosis and subsequent decrease in right ventricular blood flow.
2. After birth, the combination of right ventricular hypoplasia and severe pulmonary valve stenosis redirects blood flow right-to-left at the atrial level via the foramen ovale. Pulmonary blood becomes dependent on a left-to-right flow via the PDA.
3. In mild stenosis, the pulmonary blood flow is not excessively restricted and is PDA independent. As PVR decreases, atrial right-to-left shunt will decrease and systemic hypoxia improve.

D. **Clinical features:**
1. Mild pulmonary stenosis: loud systolic murmur at left upper sternal border is the only finding.
2. Moderately severe stenosis:
   a. Murmur is less prominent. Murmur of tricuspid insufficiency may be noted.
   b. Cyanosis is present and increases with PDA closure.
   c. Hepatomegaly.
3. Chest x-ray: mild cardiomegaly with diminished pulmonary blood flow.

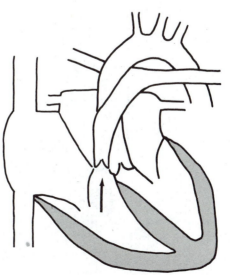

Figure 12–15
Pulmonary stenosis (PS). (Redrawn courtesy of G.G. Janos, M.D., 1989.)

E. **Management:**
1. Cyanotic neonate:
    a. Initial management with oxygen, bicarbonate, and prostaglandin E$_1$.
    b. Surgical valvotomy only treatment.
2. Non-cyanotic neonate: conservative management includes catheterization at 6–12 months if stenosis severe, with subsequent surgery if right ventricular pressure exceeds systemic.

F. **Prognosis:** operative mortality for pulmonary valvotomy irrespective of right ventricular chamber size is less than 25% (Braunlin, 1990).

PULMONARY ATRESIA

A. **Incidence:** 1 : 14,000 live births.

B. **Anatomy:** complete obstruction of the pulmonic valve resulting in a hypoplastic right ventricle and tricuspid valve (Fig. 12–16).

C. **Hemodynamics:**
1. Venous blood returning to the right atrium goes across the foramen ovale into the left atrium, left ventricle, and out the aorta.
2. Blood flow to the lungs is derived entirely from a left-to-right shunt at the ductus arteriosus, which is generally small and tortuous. As the PDA closes, severe hypoxemia ensues.
3. Regurgitant blood flow occurs at the tricuspid valve.

D. **Clinical features.**
1. Mild cyanosis at birth progressing to intense cyanosis by 24 hours.
2. Heart sounds.
    a. PDA murmur is present.
    b. Systolic harsh murmur heard at the left and right sternal borders reflects the tricuspid insufficiency.
    c. Chest x-ray: heart size increased with decreased pulmonary markings.

E. **Management:**
1. Initial treatment is use of oxygen and bicarbonate for metabolic acidosis and prostaglandin E$_1$ to dilate the ductus arteriosus.

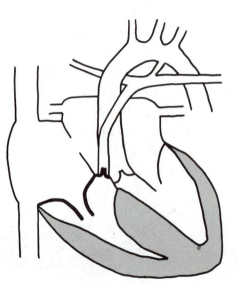

Figure 12–16
Pulmonary atresia. (Redrawn courtesy of G.G. Janos, M.D., 1989.)

2. Mild right ventricle hypertrophy: surgical valvotomy may be effective.
3. With severe hyperplasia of right ventricle and tricuspid valve, initial palliation is variable.
   a. Systemic-to-pulmonary shunt plus the following (see Tetralogy of Fallot: management):
      (1) Atrial septectomy.
      (2) Pulmonary valvotomy.
      (3) Right ventricular outflow tract reconstruction and pericardial patching.
      (4) Modified Fontan operation: attachment of the right atrium to the pulmonary artery may be possible.

F. Prognosis.
1. The operative outlook for pulmonary atresia with intact ventricular septum is poor.
2. Reported survival rates range from 20% to 36%, depending on extent of defect, size of right ventricle, and operative procedure (Braunlin, 1990; Gutgesell, 1990).

TRICUSPID ATRESIA

A. Incidence: 1:18,000 live births.

B. Anatomy: failure of tricuspid valve development with associated patent foramen ovale (Fig. 12–17).
1. VSD usually presents with a hypoplastic right ventricle.
2. Pulmonary atresia or stenosis is possible.
3. Transposition of the great vessels occurs in 30% of the cases.

C. Hemodynamics:
1. Systemic venous blood returns to the right atrium, passing through the foramen ovale into the left atrium and left ventricle. Left ventricular outflow is via the aorta, with pulmonary blood flow being supplied by the lungs.
2. In the presence of a VSD, some of the blood entering the left ventricle shunts across into the hypoplastic right ventricle and out the pulmonary artery, or the aorta in the case of coexisting transposition. If severe pulmonary stenosis or atresia is present, blood flows as though the VSD did not exist. (See C.1 above.)

D. Clinical features:
1. Cyanosis presents soon after birth with isolated defect or coexisting VSD and pulmonary outflow track obstruction. Increasing cyanosis occurs with ductus closure.

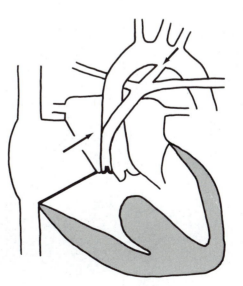

Figure 12–17
Tricuspid atresia. Arrows identify shunting through patent foramen ovale and patent ductus arteriosus. (Redrawn courtesy of G.G. Janos, M.D., 1989.)

2. CHF ensues with large VSD and absent pulmonary stenosis (usually in the first month of life).
3. Murmur: absent, unless associated with pulmonary stenosis or VSD.
4. Chest x-ray: heart size variable, depending on degree of pulmonary stenosis, but generally is non-diagnostic.

E. **Management:**
1. Primary treatment: oxygen, bicarbonate, and prostaglandin E_1 for severe hypoxia.
2. Palliative treatment:
   a. Systemic–to–pulmonary artery shunt. (See Tetralogy of Fallot.)
   b. Large VSD/no pulmonary stenosis: pulmonary artery banding is performed to control CHF.
3. Reparative surgery:
   a. Connection of the right atrium to either the right ventricular outflow track or the pulmonary artery (Fontan) (dependent on right atrium to force blood into the lungs).

F. **Prognosis:**
1. Untreated, the prognosis for tricuspid atresia is only 10–20% survival to 1 year of age (Rao, 1990).
2. With the advent of the Fontan procedure, survival rates have moved from 50–65% (Freed, 1984a) to approach 90% and above (Driscoll and Danielson, 1990; Rao, 1990).

TRUNCUS ARTERIOSUS

A. **Incidence:** 1:33,000 live births.

B. **Anatomy:** a single large, great vessel arises from both ventricles, overriding a VSD (Fig. 12–18).

C. **Hemodynamics:**
1. Both ventricles pump blood into the common trunk supplying systemic and pulmonary circulation. As PVR drops, preferential shunting to the pulmonary circulation occurs, increasing blood flow to the lungs and workload of the left ventricle.
2. If pulmonary arteries are stenotic or hypoplastic, blood flow to the lungs is restricted.

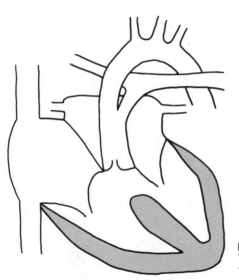

Figure 12–18
Truncus arteriosus. (Redrawn courtesy of G.G. Janos, M.D., 1989.)

D. Clinical features:
1. CHF with bounding pulses.
2. Intermittent cyanosis: severe cyanosis with pulmonary artery stenosis.
3. Heart sounds: systolic ejection click with single S_2.
4. Chest x-ray: Cardiomegaly with increased pulmonary markings. (Exception: If pulmonary artery stenosis exists, decreased pulmonary markings are seen.)

E. Management.
1. Pharmacological management of CHF with cardiac glycosides and diuretics rarely suffices alone.
2. Early surgical repair is the treatment of choice.
   a. Homograft between the right ventricle and the pulmonary artery.
   b. VSD closure.
   c. Left ventricle alone connects with the aorta.

F. Prognosis.
1. Mortality ranges from 10 to 20% if no truncal regurgitation exists (Graham and Gutgesell, 1990).
2. Multiple reoperations for conduit or homograft, truncal valve replacement, and potential myocardial problems influence subsequent mortality and morbidity (Stranger, 1990).

TOTAL ANOMALOUS PULMONARY VENOUS CONNECTION (TAPVC)

A. Incidence: 1 : 17,000 live births.

B. Anatomy: pulmonary veins have no connection with the left atrium but drain into the right atrium either directly or indirectly via a systemic venous channel.
1. Presence of a patent foramen ovale (PFO) or true ASD is required for survival (Fig. 12–19).
2. Varying degrees of pulmonary venous obstruction occur.

C. Hemodynamics:
1. Oxygenated blood from the lungs drains into the right atrium, mixing with the systemic venous return. Part of this flow passes into the left atrium via the PFO

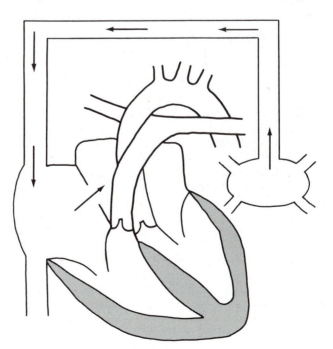

Figure 12–19
Total anomalous pulmonary venous connection (TAPVC). (Redrawn courtesy of G.G. Janos, M.D., 1989.)

or ASD into the left ventricle and out the aorta. With the normal decrease in pulmonary vascular resistance, pulmonary blood flow will increase.

2. If obstruction to pulmonary venous return exists, the resulting increase in pulmonary vascular resistance leads to pulmonary edema and diversion of blood from the pulmonary artery to the aorta via the PDA. Closure of the PDA then increases the right-to-left atrial shunting.

D. Clinical features:
1. Non-obstructed:
   a. CHF.
   b. Mild cyanosis.
   c. Heart sounds: systolic ejection murmur at LSB and mid-diastolic at LLSB; wide split S_2 may be present but generally non-specific.
   d. Chest x-ray: right ventricle dilatation, prominent pulmonary markings; "snowman" appearance.
2. Obstructed:
   a. Cyanosis predominates.
   b. Chest x-ray: normal size with pulmonary venous congestion.

E. **Management:** immediate surgical correction.
1. Cardiac catheterization is omitted to speed time to operation, with surgery based on echocardiography.
2. Anomalous veins are detached and transplanted to the left atrium; the ASD is repaired.

F. **Prognosis:**
1. One multicenter report lists the overall mortality for surgical correction of TAPVC as 27% (Krabill and Lucas, 1990).
2. The long-term prognosis is excellent, as TAPVC is closer to a surgically "curable" condition than most congenital cardiac lesions.

Congestive Heart Failure

ETIOLOGY

A. Congestive heart failure (CHF) refers to a set of clinical signs and symptoms that indicate a dysfunctional myocardium
1. Under these conditions, cardiac output is unable to meet the body's metabolic requirement.
2. Right and/or left ventricular end-diastolic pressures are elevated, impeding systemic and/or pulmonary venous returns.

B. Although structural congenital heart defects are the most common cause of CHF, other causes should be considered:
1. Timing of detection is often quite helpful in predicting causes, as the diseases causing CHF characteristically show up at certain ages. Tables 12–3 and 12–4 indicate conditions associated with CHF and their time of onset.
2. Congestive heart failure in utero that is detected at birth may be due to the following:
   a. Profound anemia: erythroblastosis fetalis or twin-to-twin transfusion.
   b. Arrhythmia: superventricular tachycardia or congenital heart block.
   c. Intrauterine infection with myocarditis.
   d. Arteriovenous malformations (AVM).
   e. Absent pulmonary valve.
   f. Premature ductus arteriosus closure: maternal use of prostaglandin inhibitor.
   g. Volume overload: twin-to-twin or mother-to-infant transfusion.

CLINICAL FEATURES

A. **Common signs include:**
1. Tachypnea (60 – 100 respirations/minute at rest).
2. Tachycardia (150 – 180 beats/minute at rest).
3. Cardiomegaly.
   a. Changes in cardiac contour.
   b. Diminished or engorged pulmonary vasculature.
4. Hepatomegaly (3 – 5 cm below coastal margin) is one of the most useful signs.
5. Pulmonary rales and bronchi.
6. Fatigue or difficulty with feeding.

B. **Less common signs.**
1. Edema: usually not obvious unless CHF present for some time.
2. Inappropriate sweating.
3. Gallop rhythm.
4. Altered pulses (quite variable, depending on underlying etiology).
5. EKG may indicate the following:
   a. Hypertrophy of one or more chambers.
   b. Abnormal mean QRS axis.
   c. Rhythm disturbances.
6. Symptoms of CHF can be characterized as those resulting from pulmonary venous or systemic venous congestion or compensatory mechanisms (Table 12 – 5) and have variable severity (Table 12 – 6).

MANAGEMENT OF CHF

A. **General measures** (appropriate for any heart disease).
1. Semi-Fowler's or prone position to maximize diaphragmatic excursion and lung expansion.

Table 12 – 5
MANIFESTATIONS OF CONGESTIVE CARDIAC FAILURE IN NEONATES AND INFANTS

Alterations of myocardial performance/initiation of compensatory mechanisms
    Cardiomegaly
    Tachycardia
    Diminished peripheral pulsations and perfusion
    Excessive sweating
    Poor feeding and growth retardation
    Gallop rhythm ± murmur
    Cardiogenic shock: hypotension; tachycardia; poor capillary refill; cool, mottled extremities; decreased output; metabolic acidosis

Results of pulmonary venous congestion
    Tachypnea
    Rales
    Dyspnea
    Pulmonary edema
    Hypoxemia

Results of systemic venous congestion
    Hepatomegaly
    Periorbital edema
    Jugular venous distention: difficult to appreciate in the neonate
    Ascites and anasarca: rare, present in hydrops, following cardiac operation or asphyxia

From Monaco, M., and Gay, W.: Congenital cardiac failure. *In* Moller, J., and Neal, W. (eds.): Fetal, Neonatal and Infant Cardiac Disease. Norwalk, CT, Appleton & Lange, 1990, p. 909.

Table 12-6
GUIDELINES FOR ASSESSING THE SEVERITY OF CONGESTIVE HEART FAILURE IN THE NEONATE AND YOUNG INFANT

1. Mild congestive cardiac failure—presence of any three of the following:
   a. Cardiomegaly (cardiothoracic ratio on chest radiograph of greater than .60), the most reliable sign of the presence of cardiac dysfunction.
   b. Persistent tachycardia (heart rate of greater than 150/minute at rest).
   c. Tachypnea with mild degrees of exertion or at rest (respiratory rate greater than 60/minute).
   d. Scattered rales at base of lungs (retractions will often be present but can be seen in large left-to-right shunts without failure).
2. Moderate congestive cardiac failure—mild congestive cardiac failure criteria are met with the addition of one of the following:
   a. Gallop rhythm.
   b. Hepatomegaly (liver greater than 3 cm below costal margin in the absence of significantly hyperaerated lungs with depressed diaphragm).
   c. Pulmonary edema (with interstitial and alveolar edema radiographically).
3. Severe congestive cardiac failure—presence of cardiogenic shock (hypotension; oliguria; poor capillary refill; cool, mottled extremities; acidosis).

From Monaco, M., and Gay, W.: Congenital cardiac failure. *In* Moller, J., and Neal, W. (eds.): Fetal, Neonatal and Infant Cardiac Disease. Norwalk, CT, Appleton & Lange, 1990, p. 912.

2. Decrease oxygen consumption.
   a. Maintain neutral thermal environment.
   b. Avoid unnecessary stresses, e.g., heelsticks, radial sticks.
   c. Sedation: for infant agitation.
   d. Consider assisted ventilation to reduce work of breathing.
3. Provide supplemental O_2. The amount is dictated by the Pao_2 and the presence of congenital heart disease with admixing of arterial and venous blood.
4. Correct acidosis and any metabolic derangements (e.g., hypoglycemia or hypocalcemia).

B. **Specific measures.**
1. Fluid and nutritional support.
   a. During acute phase, volume intake is reduced, generally to two-thirds maintenance levels.
   b. Use of polycose or medium-chain triglyceride (MCT) oil enhances caloric content without significant volume increase.
2. Pharmacological therapy.
   a. Digoxin therapy (Table 12-7).
      (1) Maximizes cardiac output; not as effective in premature babies.
      (2) Digitalize patient (Table 12-7) and observe for bradycardia (discontinue if heart rate under 100 beats/minute).
         (a) Arrhythmias or heart block.
         (b) Hypokalemia.
         (c) Toxicity occurs more frequently in premature infants, owing to a longer serum half-life for digoxin than in term or older infants.
   b. Diuretic therapy.
      (1) Used to eliminate excessive intravascular fluid.
      (2) Furosemide (Lasix), 1-2 mg/kg every 12 hours IV or 1-3 mg/kg every 12 hours PO).
         (a) In severe CHF, IV route is preferable for its rapid onset of action.
         (b) Hypokalemia and hypochloremia are side effects that can result in metabolic alkalosis.
         (c) Urinary losses of calcium occur, placing infant at risk for nephrocalcinosis.
         (d) Use contraindicated in renal failure.
      (3) Ethacrynic acid (Edecrin), 1 mg/kg IV.
         (a) Has similar renal action to furosemide.
         (b) Reported problems include gastrointestinal side effects and ototoxicity (Freed, 1980).

Table 12-7
DIGOXIN DOSAGES AND COMMON SIDE EFFECTS

Digitalizing Schedule	

Pre-term infant
    IV route: 20-30 μg/kg total dose
    PO route: 30-40 μg/kg total dose
Term infant
    IV route: 30-40 μg/kg total dose
    PO route: 40-50 μg/kg total dose
	Total dose is usually divided into three doses, giving one-half, then one-fourth, then one-fourth of the total dose every 8 hours. Check EKG rhythm strip for rate, P-R interval, and dysrhythmias before each dose.

Maintenance Schedule	

Pre-term infant
    IV route: 8-10 μg/kg/day
    PO route: 10-12 μg/kg/day
Term infant
    IV route: 10-12 μg/kg/day
    PO route: 12-14 μg/kg/day
	Total dose should be divided twice a day. Allow 12-24 hours between last digitalizing and first maintenance doses. It takes about 6 days to "digitalize" a patient with maintenance doses alone. The sign of digitalis effect is usually prolongation of the P-R interval. The first sign of digitalis toxicity is usually vomiting, dysrhythmias, or bradycardia.

From Daberkow, E., and Washington, R.: Handbook of Neonatal Intensive Care, 2nd ed. St. Louis, C.V. Mosby, 1989, p. 436.

(4) Chlorothiazide (Diuril), 20-40 mg/kg/day in two oral doses.
    (a) Administered when less acute oral diuresis is required.
    (b) Does not produce the profound potassium losses seen with furosemide.
    (c) may reduce urinary calcium losses seen with furosemide.
  c. Inotropic agents.
    (1) May be necessary in severe CHF or cardiogenic shock.
    (2) Most commonly used are isoproterenol, dopamine, and dobutamine.

C. **Cardiology consult to rule out or establish presence of congenital heart lesion.** Cardiac catheterization, angiocardiography and surgery may be indicated.

Shock

ETIOLOGY

A. **Shock refers to a state of inadequate circulating blood volume resulting in reduced perfusion and oxygenation to the tissues.** Several varieties of shock are recognized.

B. **Hypovolemic shock may be caused by the following:**
1. Blood loss from placental abnormalities, e.g., umbilical cord rupture, abruptio placentae, twin-to-twin transfusion syndrome.
2. Acute blood loss from post-natal hemorrhage.
3. Plasma and fluid losses.
  a. Skin integrity losses (e.g., myelomeningocele, gastroschisis).
  b. Pleural effusions (e.g., erythroblastosis fetalis or non-immune hydrops).
  c. Body water loss via persistent vomiting, diarrhea, or evaporative skin losses.

C. **Cardiogenic shock may be caused by the following:**
1. Myocardial failure from severe hypoxemia, hypoglycemia, and/or acidemia.
2. Congenital heart lesions.
3. Cardiac arrhythmias.
4. Restriction of cardiac function by:
  a. Tamponade.
  b. Tension pneumothorax.
  c. Excessive levels of ventilatory distending pressures.
5. Myocarditis: often associated with sepsis.

D. **Distributive shock:**
1. Results from impaired peripheral arterial resistance usually caused by sepsis (i.e., release of bacterial toxins).
2. Typically associated with gram-negative organisms; however, a gram-positive organism may be the causative agent.

CLINICAL INDICATIONS

A. **Signs of shock are frequently non-specific.** (Cardiogenic shock may be indistinguishable from CHF.)

B. **Cardiopulmonary status changes.**
1. Tachycardia.
2. Tachypnea and/or apnea.
3. Poor peripheral perfusion.
    a. Pallor (especially with blood loss).
    b. Capillary refill time (CRT) > 3 seconds.
4. Hypotension.

C. **Decreased urinary output.**

D. **Metabolic disturbances.**
1. Metabolic acidosis.
2. Hypoglycemia.
3. Hypothermia.

E. **Evidence of coagulation defects.**

F. **Indicators of blood volume** (or effective blood volume) are as follows:
1. Change in hematocrit readings.
2. Response to fluid challenge of 10 mg/kg of saline, while monitoring blood pressure and urine output.
3. Positive Kleihauer-Betke test is indicative of fetal-to-maternal transfusion in utero. This test examines the maternal blood for the presence of fetal RBCs.

G. **Indicators of cardiac function.**
1. See cardiopulmonary patterns (point B above).
2. Echocardiogram establishes anatomical defects and/or specific myocardial function abnormalities.
3. Central venous pressure (CVP) is generally elevated.

H. **Indicators of septic shock.**
1. Signs of sepsis or positive cultures.
2. Normal blood pressure, in the face of prominent hypoperfusion.
3. Edema or sclerema from capillary protein and fluid leakage.
4. Oliguria, proteinuria.
5. Persistent pulmonary hypertension of the neonate (PPHN) is commonly seen.

MANAGEMENT

A. **Shock management depends largely on the prevailing pathogenesis.** A large proportion of the care is supportive.

B. **Supportive care.**
1. Maintain oxygenation and ventilation as dictated by arterial blood gases.
    a. Ventilatory support if concurrent pulmonary disease exists.
    b. Tolazoline may be useful in pulmonary hypertension with hypoxemia.
        (1) Use cautiously in septic shock; systemic hypotension likely.
    c. Provide neutral thermal environment to decrease oxygen consumption.
    d. Decrease external stress (i.e., handling, peripheral blood draws).
2. Promptly treat acidosis to avoid adverse effects on myocardial contractility. Sodium bicarbonate is often necessary.
3. Maintain fluid and electrolyte balance.

C. Specific therapies.

1. Increase blood volume and red cell mass.
   a. Maintains blood pressure and maximizes oxygen content.
   b. Treatment of acute blood loss may require large volume transfusion.
   c. Monitoring arterial blood pressure essential; central venous pressure monitoring should ideally be included.
   d. *Caution:* In cardiogenic shock, added volume may increase the myocardial workload.
2. Treat the infectious process in septic shock.
   a. Antibiotics should be initiated.
   b. Exchange transfusion with fresh whole blood (controversial) provides neutrophils and removes bacterial toxins.
   c. Neutrophil transfusion to augment cellular immunity (controversial).
3. Maximize cardiac output.
   a. Inotropic agents are useful in cardiogenic shock to increase cardiac output and support circulation. Start early in septic shock if evidence of oliguria, hypotension, or acidosis exists.
   b. Isoproterenol (Isuprel): increases heart rate and increases contractility (beta-1-adrenergic effects). Simultaneous effects produce bronchodilation and smooth muscle relaxation (beta-2-effects). Usual dose is .05–0.5 (mcg)μ/kg/minute. Observe for arrhythmias such as premature ventricular contractions (PVCs).
   c. Dopamine (Intropin): increases cardiac contractility and cardiac output. Effects are dose dependent. At low doses (1–5 μg/kg/minute IV), selective vasodilatation of the renal, mesenteric, cerebral, and coronary vascular beds occurs with little effect on heart rate or blood pressure. With moderate doses (6–10 μg/kg/minute), increased BP and improved tissue perfusion can be observed. Beneficial effects are dependent largely on an adequate blood volume. Correct hypovolemia prior to dopamine infusion. At higher doses (> 10 μg/kg/minute IV), vasoconstriction occurs, consisting of vasoconstriction of the pulmonary vasculature, increased right ventricular afterload, reduction in pulmonary blood flow, right-to-left shunting through fetal structures, and increased hypoxemia. Tachycardia, dysrhythmias, and ectopic beats can occur as a consequence of dopamine infusion.
   d. Dobutamine (Dobutex): increases cardiac contractility while exerting limited effects on vasculature. Cardiac output increases depending on myocardial catecholamine stores. A dose of 2–5 μg/kg/minute IV is a reasonable starting dose, with high dose considered 10 μg/kg/minute or greater (Crockett and Tappero, 1989).
   e. Digitalis should be considered and used selectively, especially in the face of hypoxia or toxic myocardiopathy (see Table 12–7).
4. Correct any tension pneumothorax or cardiac tamponade.

STUDY QUESTIONS

1. The establishment of a separate pulmonary and systemic circulatory system occurs in which cardiac lesion?
   a. Coarctation of the aorta.
   b. Tetralogy of Fallot.
   c. Transposition of the great vessels.

2. Blood flow to the lungs is increased when which cardiac lesion is present?
   a. Aortic atresia.
   b. Pulmonary stenosis.
   c. Ventricular septal defect.

3. The cyanosis seen with tetralogy of Fallot results from:
   a. Equalization of ventricular pressures.
   b. Left-to-right ventricular shunt.
   c. Right-to-left ventricular shunt.

4. Which of the following cardiac lesions results in a right-to-left shunt?
   a. Endocardial cushion defect.
   b. Pulmonary stenosis.
   c. Ventricular septal defect.

5. An alteration in which of the following would be expected to have greatest impact on the preterm child's cardiac output?
   a. Afterload.
   b. Contractility.
   c. Heart rate.

6. A false statement regarding neonatal heart murmurs is:
   a. Absence of a murmur rules out significant heart disease.
   b. Murmurs in the first 2 days of life are a common finding in neonates.
   c. Murmurs of grade III/IV or less generally present no hemodynamic problems.

7. In transposition of the great vessels, cyanosis develops rapidly and may increase abruptly with closure of the:
   a. Atrial septal defect.
   b. Ductus arteriosus.
   c. Ventricular septal defect.

8. Which substance is administered to ensure continued patency of the ductus arteriosus?
   a. Oxygen.
   b. Prostaglandin E_1.
   c. Thromboplastin.

9. Which of the following usually results from mixing of arterial and venous blood in the left side of the heart of the infant?
   a. Congestive heart failure.
   b. Cyanosis.
   c. Murmur.

10. In neonates with cardiac disease, evidence of cyanosis is most directly related to:
    a. A lower than normal hemoglobin value.
    b. Discrepancies between hemoglobin and hematocrit values.
    c. The amount of desaturated hemoglobin.

11. Presentation of bounding pulses is expected in:

    a. Coarctation of the aorta.
    b. Hypoplastic left heart.
    c. Patent ductus arteriosus.

12. An uncommon clinical sign of congestive heart failure is:
    a. Edema.
    b. Hepatomegaly.
    c. Tachypnea.

13. A decrease in pulmonary blood flow occurs with:
    a. Coarctation of the aorta.
    b. Tetralogy of Fallot.
    c. Ventricular septal defect.

14. Pulmonary venous congestion is the hemodynamic consequence of:
    a. Hypoplastic left heart.
    b. Pulmonary atresia.
    c. Tetralogy of Fallot.

15. Blood flow leaving the lungs and entering the right atrium either directly or indirectly, via a systemic venous route, describes the hemodynamics of:
    a. Total anomalous pulmonary venous connection.
    b. Transposition of the great vessels.
    c. Truncus arteriosus.

16. The hemodynamic consequences of a complete endocardial cushion defect is best expressed by which one of the following?
    a. Blood flows from the aorta to the pulmonary artery.
    b. Blood flows freely among all chambers of the heart.
    c. Blood flows via a single great vessel to supply systemic and pulmonary circulations.

17. Of the following commonly employed management measures for congestive heart failure, which one is least effective in premature infants?
    a. Digoxin therapy.
    b. Diuretic therapy.
    c. Fluid restriction.

Answers to Study Questions

1. c	7. b	13. b
2. c	8. b	14. a
3. c	9. b	15. a
4. b	10. c	16. b
5. c	11. c	17. a
6. a	12. a	

REFERENCES

Beekman, R., and Rocchini, A.: Coarctation of the aorta and interruption of the aortic arch. *In* Moller, J., and Neal, W. (eds.): Fetal, Neonatal and Infant Cardiac Disease. Norwalk, CT. Appleton & Lange, 1990, pp. 497–521.

Braudo, M., and Rowe, R.: Auscultation of the heart: Early neonatal period. Am. J. Dis. Child., *101*:575–586, 1961.

Braunlin, E.: Pulmonary atresia and pulmonary stenosis with hypoplastic right ventricle. *In* Moller, J., and Neal, W. (eds.): Fetal, Neonatal and Infant Cardiac Disease. Norwalk, CT, Appleton & Lange, 1990, pp. 671–687.

Chin, A.J., and Keane, J.F., et al.: Repair of complete common atrioventricular canal in infancy. J. Thorac. Cardiovasc. Surg., *84*:437–445, 1982.

Clyman, R.: Medical treatment of patent ductus arteriosus in premature infants. *In* Long, W. (ed.): Fetal and Neonatal Cardiology. Philadelphia, W.B. Saunders Co., 1990, pp. 682–690.

Cohn, Jr., Freed, M., et al.: Complications and mortality associated with cardiac catheterization in infants under one year. Pediatr. Cardiol., 6:123–131, 1985.

Crockett, M., and Tappero, E.: Dopamine and dobutamine: Neonatal indications and implications. Neonatal Network, 7(5):16, 1989.

Driscoll, D., and Danielson, G.: Tricuspid atresia. *In* Moller, J., and Neal, W. (eds.): Fetal, Neonatal and Infant Cardiac Disease. Norwalk, CT, Appleton & Lange, 1990, pp. 689–699.

Engle, M.: Heart sounds and murmurs in diagnosis of heart disease. Pediatr. Ann., *10*(3):84–93, 1981.

Feldt, R., Edwards, W., Hagler, D., and Puga, F.: Endocardial cushion defect. In Moller, J., and Neal, W. (eds.): Fetal, Neonatal and Infant Cardiac Disease. Norwalk, CT, Appleton & Lange, 1990, pp. 411–432.

Fletcher, A.: The infant of the diabetic mother. *In* Avery, G. (ed.): Neonatology: Pathophysiology and Management of the Newborn, 2nd ed. Philadelphia, J.B. Lippincott, 1981, p. 295.

Flyer, D., and Lang, P.: Neonatal heart disease. *In* Avery, G. (ed.): Neonatology: Pathophysiology and Management of the Newborn, 2nd ed. Philadelphia, J.B. Lippincott, 1981, pp. 438–472.

Freed, M.: Cardiac disorders. *In* Graef, J., and Crone, T. (eds.): Manual of Pediatric Therapeutics, 2nd ed. Boston, Little, Brown, 1980, pp. 229–246.

Freed, M.: Congenital cardiac malformations. *In* Avery, M.,Taeusch, H., (eds.): Schaffer's Diseases of the Newborn, 5th ed. Philadelphia, W.B. Saunders Co., 1984a, pp. 243–290.

Freed, M.: General considerations. *In* Avery, M., Taeusch, H. (eds.): Schaffer's Diseases of the Newborn, 5th ed. Philadelphia, W.B. Saunders Co., 1984b, pp. 224–243.

Freed, M., and Castaneda, A.: Transposition of the great arteries. *In* Moller, J., and Neal, W. (eds.): Fetal, Neonatal and Infant Cardiac Disease. Norwalk, CT, Appleton & Lange, 1990, pp. 523–554.

Friedman, W.: The intrinsic physiologic properties of the developing heart. *In* Friedman, W., Lesch, M., and Sonnenblick, E. (eds.): Neonatal Heart Disease. New York, Grune & Stratton, 1973, pp. 21–49.

Graham, T., and Gutgesell, H.: Conotruncal abnormalities. *In* Long, W. (ed.): Fetal and Neonatal Cardiology. Philadelphia, W.B. Saunders Co., 1990, pp. 561–570.

Gutgesell, H.: Pulmonary valve abnormalities. *In* Long, W. (ed.): Fetal and Neonatal Cardiology. Philadelphia, W.B. Saunders Co., 1990, pp. 551–560.

Guyton, A.: Textbook of Medical Physiology, 5th ed. Philadelphia, W.B. Saunders Co., 1976, pp. 61–73.

Harned, H.: Teratogenic agents. *In* Long, W. (ed.): Fetal and Neonatal Cardiology. Philadelphia, W.B. Saunders Co., 1990, pp. 595–603.

Hazinski, M.: Congenital heart disease in the neonate. Part I: Epidemiology, cardiac development and fetal circulation. Neonatal Network, 1(4):29–42, 1983a.

Hazinski, M.: Congenital heart disease in the neonate. Part II: Perinatal circulatory changes, postnatal circulation, and cardiovascular physiology. Neonatal Network, 1(5):32–46, 1983b.

Hazinski, M.: Congenital heart disease in the neonate. Part III: Common congenital heart failure. Neonatal Network, 1(6):8–19, 1983c.

Hazinski, M.: Congenital heart disease in the neonate. Part IV: Cyanotic heart disease. Neonatal Network, 2(1):12–25, 1983d.

Hazinski, M.: Congenital heart disease in the neonate. Part VII: Common congenital heart defects producing hypoxemia and cyanoses. Neonatal Network, 2(6):36–48, 1984.

Hazinski, M.: Congenital heart disease in the neonate. Part VIII. Neonatal Network, 3(2):7–19, 1984.

Heyman, M.A., and Rudolph, A.M.: Effects of congenital heart disease on fetal and neonatal circulations. Progr. Cardiovasc. Dis., *15*:115, 1972.

Johnson, G.: Clinical examination. *In* Long, W. (ed.): Fetal and Neonatal Cardiology. Philadelphia, W.B. Saunders Co., 1990, pp. 223–235.

Krabill, K., and Lucas, R.: Total anomalous pulmonary venous connection. *In* Moller, J., and Neal, W. (eds.): Fetal, Neonatal and Infant Cardiac Disease. Norwalk, Ct, Appleton & Lange, 1990, pp. 571–585.

Lynch, T.: Cardiovascular conditions in the newborn. *In* Streeter, N. (ed.): High-Risk Neonatal Care. Rockville, MD, Aspen, 1988, pp. 163–227).

Martin, J.: Cyanosis of the newborn infant. J. Pediatr., *77*(3):485, 1970.

Moller, J.: Physical examination. *In* Moller, J., and Neal, W., (eds.): Fetal, Neonatal and Infant Cardiac Disease. Norwalk, CT, Appleton & Lange, 1990, pp. 167–177.

Moreau, G., and Graham, T.: Atrial septal defect. *In* Moller, J., and Neal, W. (eds.). Fetal, Neonatal and Infant Cardiac Disease. Norwalk, CT, Appleton & Lange, 1990, pp. 403–410.

Nora, J., Vargo, T., Nora, A., et al.: Dexamphetamine: A possible environmental trigger in cardiovascular malformations (letter). Lancet, *1*:1290–1291, 1970.

Patterson, S.W., and Starling, J.: On the mechanical factors which determine the output of the ventricles. J. Physiol., *48*:357, 1914.

Rao, P.: Tricuspid atresia. *In* Long, W. (ed.): Fetal and Neonatal Cardiology. Philadelphia, W.B. Saunders Co., 1990, pp. 525–540.

Rosenthal, A., and Bank, E.: Ventricular septal defect. *In* Moller, J., and Neal, W. (eds.): Fetal, Neonatal and Infant Cardiac Disease. Norwalk, CT, Appleton & Lange, 1990, pp. 371–390.

Sand, M., and Pacifico, A.: Repair of atrioventricular septal defects. *In* Long, W. (ed.): Fetal and Neonatal Cardiology. Philadelphia, W.B. Saunders Co., 1990, pp. 780–788.

Southall, D., Orrell, M., and Talbot, J.: Study of cardiac arrhythmias and other forms of conduction abnormality in newborn infants. Br. Med. J., *2*:597–599, 1977.

Stanger, P.: Truncus arteriosus. *In* Moller, J., and Neal, W. (eds.): Fetal, Neonatal and Infant Cardiac Disease. Norwalk, CT, Appleton & Lange, 1990, pp. 587–602.

Versmold, M., et al.: Aortic blood pressure monitoring during the first 12 hours of life in infants with birth weight of 610 to 4220 grams. Pediatrics, *67*:607–613, 1981.

Patricia Beachy

Gastrointestinal Disorders

Objectives

1. Identify three abdominal wall defects.

2. Discuss common diagnostic tests used for gastrointestinal disorders.

3. Describe the symptoms of diaphragmatic hernia.

4. List seven possible causes of necrotizing enterocolitis.

5. Discuss the binding process for bilirubin in the newborn.

6. Compare and contrast physiological with non-physiological jaundice.

7. Define "hydrops."

8. Discuss the methods used to determine the etiology of hydrops.

Gastrointestinal Embryonic Development

A. **Week 3.** Liver bud is present. Mesentery forming.

B. **Week 4.** Intestine present. Esophagus and stomach distinct.

C. **Weeks 5 and 6.** Intestine elongates and rotates. Stomach rotates.

D. **Week 7.** Circular muscular layer present. Duodenum temporarily occluded. Intestinal loops herniate into umbilical cord.

E. **Week 8.** Villi present. Small intestine rotates within umbilical cord.

F. **Weeks 9 and 10.** Intestine re-enters abdominal cavity and continues rotation.

G. **Week 12.** Muscular layers of intestine present. Active transport of amino acids begins. Pancreatic islet cells appear. Bile appears.

H. **Weeks 13 and 14.** Peristalsis detected.

I. **Week 16.** Meconium present.

J. **Week 24.** Ganglion cells detected in rectum.

K. **Week 34.** Sucking and swallowing become coordinated.

L. **Weeks 36–38.** Maturity of GI system completed.

M. Weeks 5–40. Intestine elongates approximately 100-fold. The small intestine is six times the length of the colon (Avery and Martin, p. 895).

Functions of the Gastrointestinal Tract

A. Absorption and digestion of nutrients.

B. Maintenance of fluid and electrolyte balance.

C. Protection of host from toxins and pathogens.

Disorders of the Gastrointestinal Tract: Abdominal Wall Defects

A. Omphalocele.
1. Definition. An omphalocele is the herniation of abdominal viscera into the umbilical cord usually covered by a peritoneal sac and with the umbilical arteries and veins inserting into the apex of the defect (Fig. 13–1).
2. Etiology. Uncertain, but it may be caused by the incomplete closure of the anterior abdominal wall or incomplete return of the bowel into the abdomen.
3. Incidence. 1 in 5000 to 1 in 6000 live births.
4. Diagnosis. Made on inspection. The defect can be small; therefore, any umbilical cord that is unusually fat should be inspected carefully before clamping to be certain it is not a very small omphalocele.
5. Common characteristics.
   a. Approximately 10% will also have intestinal atresia.
   b. The sizes of omphaloceles differ, but large defects may include the stomach, liver, and spleen as well as the intestines.
   c. A rupture of the omphalocele may occur prior to or at the time of delivery, exposing the viscera to amniotic fluid.
6. Associated anomalies, include the following:
   a. Cardiac defects (15–25%).
   b. Neurological anomalies.

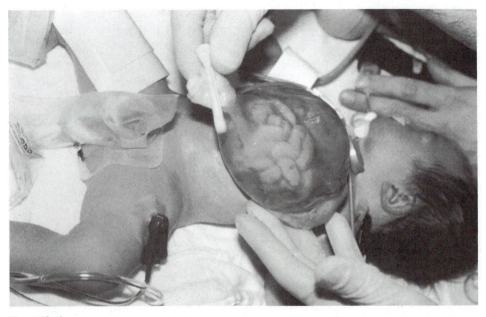

Figure 13–1
Omphalocele.

   c. Genitourinary anomalies.

   d. Skeletal anomalies.

   e. Chromosomal anomalies (67%).

   f. Malrotation of intestine.

   g. Beckwith-Wiedemann syndrome.

B. **Gastroschisis.**

1. Etiology. Unclear, theories include a failure of closure of the lateral fold of the abdominal wall or intrauterine vascular accident involving the omphalomesenteric artery with subsequent disruption of the umbilical ring causing herniation of abdominal contents.

2. Incidence: 1 in 10,000 to 1 in 15,000 live births.

3. The gastroschisis defect is smaller than the omphalocele and is usually placed to the right of the umbilicus (Fig. 13–2).

4. Diagnosis is made by inspection.

5. Common characteristics.

   a. No sac covers the gastroschisis.

   b. Gastroschisis usually includes the small and large intestine and rarely the liver.

   c. The intestine is usually thickened, edematous, and inflamed because it has been exposed to amniotic fluid.

6. Associated anomalies: approximately 10% of affected children have bowel stricture and atresia. Other anomalies are uncommon.

Care of the Neonate with an Abdominal Wall Defect (Omphalocele and Gastroschisis)

A. At the time of delivery, cover exposed bowel with warm, moist dressings. (Sterile normal saline is recommended. Also, cover the dressing in plastic to prevent evaporative heat loss.) Position the infant on his or her side to prevent intestinal vascular compromise. Handling should be kept to a minimum and done only with sterile gloves.

B. The infant is made NPO and an orogastric tube should be passed and put on intermittent low suction for gastric decompression. Bowel distended with air can restrict normal blood flow and further compromise the bowel.

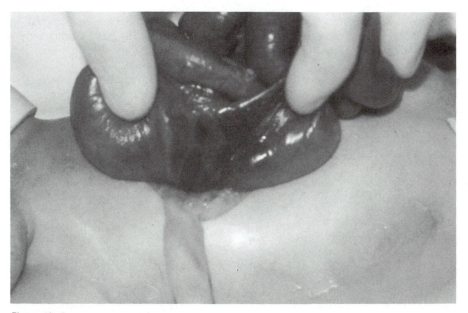

Figure 13–2
Gastroschisis.

C. **Begin IV fluid and electrolyte therapy and antibiotics** as soon as possible. IV fluids are usually increased to approximately 150 ml/kg/day due to increased fluid loss through exposed bowel.

D. **Blood work should be performed**, including Hct, electrolytes, blood type and cross, pH and blood gases, and clotting studies.

E. **Assess the infant carefully** for associated anomalies, syndromes, or deformations.

F. **All newborns with abdominal wall defects require surgical repair.** The types of repair include the following:
1. Primary repair: all intestine is returned to the abdominal cavity, and the fascia and skin are closed.
   a. The infant may require prolonged respiratory support secondary to increased intra-abdominal pressure.
2. Staged reduction: not all the organs are returned to the abdominal cavity during the first surgery; the organs remaining outside the cavity are covered by a Silastic material, forming a sac that is reduced daily.
   a. This minimizes the stress on the respiratory and vascular system by allowing these systems to slowly adjust to the increased pressure of the organs as they are slowly returned to the abdominal cavity.
   b. The reduction is usually accomplished over a period of up to 10 days, after which infection becomes a major consideration.
   c. The abdominal wall is closed after the reduction is completed.
3. Skin flap closure: only the skin is pulled over the exposed organs.
   a. This method is not a long-term solution and is used when the fascia cannot be initially repaired.
4. Non-surgical repair: the defect is painted with Mercurochrome and alcohol and allowed to air dry and epithelialize.
   a. This is uncommon and used only if the infant cannot tolerate surgery or if the reduction fails.

G. Postoperative care.
1. Complications to watch for include sepsis, intestinal obstruction, respiratory distress, and skin necrosis over repaired defect.
2. Continuous monitoring of oxygen saturation, urine output, and blood pressure. Other parameters to watch closely include fluid and electrolyte balance, pH, and clotting times.
3. The infant will require gastric suction after surgery until gastric output is minimal. Parenteral fluids should be replaced with physiologic IV solutions that account for gastric losses (i.e., gastric contents suctioned should be measured every 4 hours, and parenteral fluids increased an equal amount).
4. Appropriate pain management should be initiated (see Appendix B).
5. Feeding is begun very slowly when gastric output is minimal and bowel tones are active.
   a. A low-osmol feeding such as half-strength formula, breast milk, or Pedialyte is usually preferred. Feedings are frequently stopped and started over a period of time.
   b. Most infants will be maintained on hyperalimentation for a period of time until feeding is established.

Prune-belly Syndrome

A. **Definition:** Prune-belly syndrome is the congenital absence of the abdominal musculature.

B. **Incidence is 1 in 35,000 to 1 in 50,000 live births.**
1. Approximately 95% of affected infants are male.

C. **Etiology:** Unclear but may be the result of a generalized developmental defect of abdominal parietes and mesenchyma. The condition is rarely familial, and no cytogenic abnormality has been discovered.

D. **Associated anomalies include the following:**
1. Pulmonary hypoplasia.
2. Intestinal malrotation.
3. Imperforate anus.
4. Hydronephrotic dysplastic kidneys.
5. Cryptorchidism.
6. Urinary tract malformation.

E. **Treatment of infant with prune-belly syndrome.**
1. Surgery may be required to repair associated defects in the renal and urinary systems.
2. No surgical correction of the abdominal wall musculature is possible.
3. Prognosis is related to the extent of the associated renal and urinary defects.

Disorders of the Gastrointestinal Tract: Intestinal Obstruction

Obstruction occurs because of an intrinsic or extrinsic blockage and can be found anywhere from the esophagus to the anus.

A. **Esophageal atresia, tracheoesophageal fistula (TEF).**
1. Incidence: varies between 1 in 800 and 1 in 5000 live births.
2. 30–40% of affected infants have associated anomalies (see 6.c., Preoperative care).
3. Types of TEFs include the following:
  a. Esophageal atresia with tracheoesophageal fistula (85% of cases).
  b. Esophageal atresia without tracheoesophageal fistula (5% of cases).
  c. H-type tracheoesophageal fistula (7% of cases).
  d. Rare upper pouch TEF (rare) (Fig. 13–3).
4. Clinical presentation.
  a. Clinical presentation is dependent on the type of tracheal/esophageal anomaly.
  b. Infant has an inability to swallow saliva which leads to an increase in saliva.
  c. Gastric tube cannot be passed.
  d. Choking or cyanosis with feedings.
  e. Recurrent pneumonia.
5. Diagnosis.
  a. History of polyhydramnios.

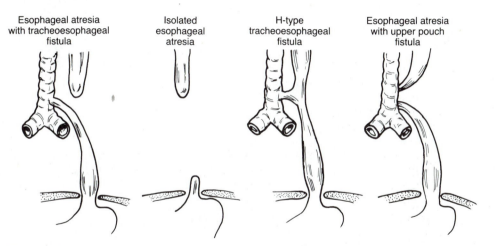

Esophageal atresia with tracheoesophageal fistula   Isolated esophageal atresia   H-type tracheoesophageal fistula   Esophageal atresia with upper pouch fistula

Figure 13–3
Esophageal malformations.

b. The gastric tube will stop in the esophageal pouch (will most likely not pass beyond 10 cm).

c. The x-ray should show the gastric tube curled in the upper esophageal pouch. Air in the gastrointestinal tract indicates the presence or a TEF. A gasless abdomen indicates an isolated esophageal atresia. (Refer to Chapter 33.)

6. Preoperative care.
   a. The head of the bed should be in a 30 degree upright position.
   b. A sump catheter on low constant suction should be left in the upper pouch to suction oral secretions.
   c. Assess the infant for associated anomalies (30–40% of infants will have associated anomalies). The most common associated anomalies include the following:
      (1) Cardiac defects (primarily atrial septal defects and ventricular septal defects) (15%).
      (2) Imperforate anus (10%).

7. Surgical repair.
   a. Primary repair is the anastomosis of the proximal and distal esophagus.
   b. Delayed repair is when repair is postponed due to pneumonia or other coexisting life-threatening problems.
   c. Staged repair is used with infants whose initial surgery finds the two esophageal ends are too far apart for primary anastomosis.
      (1) These infants will have a gastrostomy for feeding after the first surgery.
      (2) Anastomosis may be attempted after 4–6 weeks when the esophageal ends grow closer together. Prior to surgery, suction to the pouch must continue, or a spit fistula is created.

8. Postoperative care.
   a. Intubation with low-pressure ventilation protects the tracheal suture line.
   b. Frequent, careful suctioning of the posterior pharynx with a measured catheter should be performed.
   c. Hyperalimentation and antibiotics are commonly used postoperatively.
   d. Appropriate pain management should be initiated (see Appendix B).
   e. There is usually a thoracic drain in place postoperatively; note the color, consistency, and amounts of fluid drainage. Saliva indicates an esophageal leak.
   f. A gastrostomy tube may be placed for gastric decompression and later feedings.
   g. A gastric tube should not be passed, due to the potential for perforating or damaging the repair.
   h. Barium esophagram is usually performed to establish the presence or absence of a leak before feedings are begun.

9. Postoperative complications.
   a. Respiratory distress.
   b. Pneumonia.
   c. Sepsis.
   d. Leaking of anastomosis.
   e. Dismotility of lower esophageal segment.
   f. Unilateral diaphragmatic paralysis.

10. Long-term considerations include the following:
    a. Dilatation of the esophagus may be necessary if anastomotic stricture occurs (15%).
    b. The infants may have some stridor or a "brassy" cough from tracheomalacia. This is occasionally severe enough to require a tracheostomy.
    c. Gastroesophageal reflux is common.

B. **Pyloric stenosis.**
1. Definition: Hypertrophy of the pyloric musculature.
2. Incidence: 1 of every 500 births.
   a. Males are more likely to be affected than females (4 : 1).

3. Symptoms may occur from the first week of life up to 5 months after birth.
4. Clinical presentation.
   a. Non-bilious vomiting.
   b. Dehydration.
   c. Hypochloremic and hypokalemic alkalosis.
5. Diagnosis.
   a. Presence of non-bilious projectile vomiting, dehydration, and hypochloremic hypokalemic alkalosis.
   b. Visible peristaltic waves in epigastrium.
   c. Palpable pyloric "olive."
   d. Confirmation by ultrasound.
   e. Upper GI contrast study.
6. Preoperative care: Mainly concerned with correcting the hypokalemia, hypochloremia, and dehydration.
7. Postoperative care: Follow routine wound care, pain management guidelines and maintain NPO status for 6–8 hours after surgery.

C. Malrotation.
1. Etiology: Occurs when the fixation of the mesentery of the small bowel has not developed normally. The intestine is subject to torsion on the axis of the superior mesenteric artery.
2. Incidence: Unknown; however, more males are affected than females.
3. Associated anomalies.
   a. Eventration of the diaphragm.
   b. Diaphragmatic hernia.
4. Clinical presentation of acute cases includes:
   a. Bilious vomiting. This is suggestive of malrotation with volvulus formation and needs immediate confirmation.
   b. Abdominal distention.
   c. Blood per rectum.
   d. Signs of shock and sepsis.
5. Clinical presentation of "less acute cases" includes:
   a. Failure to thrive.
   b. Intermittent bilious vomiting.
   c. Abdominal tenderness.
6. Diagnosis.
   a. Presence of symptoms.
   b. X-ray shows evidence of duodenal obstruction and scanty gas distributed through the rest of the bowel. An airless abdomen is an ominous sign.
   c. Contrast upper GI x-ray showing distended stomach and a beak-like narrowing at the pylorus; also gastric mucosa folds are seen on the x-ray.
7. Preoperative care.
   a. Malrotation with volvulus is considered a surgical emergency; the primary goal of preoperative care is to get the infant to the OR as fast as possible; surgery is aimed at release of strangulation of the bowel.
8. Postoperative care.
   a. IV therapy and antibiotics, hyperalimentation.
   b. Routine wound and stoma care.
   c. Appropriate pain management should be initiated (see Appendix B).
   d. The infant should remain NPO until the return of bowel function (usually in 3–7 days).
9. Operative mortality is less than 15%. Morbidity and prognosis depend on the amount of bowel resected.

D. Duodenal atresia.
1. Incidence: Approximately 1 in every 10,000 live births. Females are more commonly affected than males.
2. Etiology: Unknown, but it may result from a failure of recannulization of the GI tract in the second month of fetal life.

3. Associated malformation anomalies (found in 70% of all cases):
   a. Down syndrome (30%).
   b. Intestinal malrotation.
   c. Congenital heart disease.
   d. Renal anomalies.
   e. Tracheoesophageal abnormalities.
   f. Annular pancreas.
4. Clinical presentation.
   a. Bilious vomiting (85%).
   b. Abdominal distention.
   c. Child may pass meconium in first 24 hours of life, then bowel movements cease.
5. Diagnosis.
   a. History of polyhydramnios.
   b. Pre-natal diagnosis by ultrasound.
   c. Presence of bilious vomiting.
   d. X-ray showing "double bubble" pattern. (See Chapter 33.)
6. Preoperative care.
   a. IV therapy
   b. Blood cultures and antibiotics.
   c. A gastric tube should be passed and maintained on intermittent low-pressure suction.
7. Surgery is performed to remove the atretic portions and reanastomose the remaining ends.
8. Postoperative care.
   a. Continue IV (hyperalimentation) and antibiotics.
   b. Appropriate pain management should be initiated (see Appendix B).
   c. NPO 7–10 days, because delayed gastric emptying is common.
   d. Most infants will have a gastrostomy tube in place postoperatively.
9. Prognosis: Excellent. Long-term outcome primarily dependent on associated anomalies/malformations.

E. **Jejunal/ileal atresia.**
1. Incidence: 1 in every 5000 live births. Males and females are equally affected.
2. Etiology: Unknown but is believed to result from an insult to the small bowel in fetal life.
3. Associated conditions include the following:
   a. Intrauterine growth retardation (IUGR).
   b. Additional intestinal obstructions are present in 6–20% of all cases.
4. Clinical presentation.
   a. Bilious vomiting.
   b. Abdominal distention.
   c. Three-quarters of all infants with jejunal atresia will not pass meconium.
   d. Jaundice.
5. Diagnosis.
   a. Presence of symptoms.
   b. History of polyhydramnios.
   c. X-rays showing dilated loops of bowel and multiple air-fluid levels. (Refer to Chapter 33.)
6. Preoperative care.
   a. Pass a gastric tube. This should be maintained on low intermittent suction.
   b. IV fluids.
   c. Blood cultures and antibiotics.
7. Surgery.
   a. Primary anastomosis is performed if the proximal and distal portions of bowel are comparable in size.
   b. Stomas are created if there is a large discrepancy in size. After stomas are healed, irrigation at the small distal stoma will usually help to dilate it so it can be surgically anastomosed to the proximal bowel.

8. Postoperative care.
   a. Continue NPO until normal bowel function is restored (usually 3–7 days).
   b. Appropriate pain management should be initiated (see Appendix B).
   c. Continue IV therapy (hyperalimentation) and antibiotics.
9. Complications.
   a. Meconium ileus.
   b. Peritonitis.
10. Prognosis is excellent, with return to normal bowel function usually occurring within 10 days.

F. Meconium ileus.
1. Incidence: 90% of children with meconium ileus have cystic fibrosis.
2. Etiology.
   a. Meconium is sticky and hyperviscous secondary to hyposecretion of pancreatic enzymes. This abnormal meconium creates an intraluminal obstruction, usually of the distal small bowel.
3. Two types of meconium ileus exist.
   a. Simple meconium ileus.
      (1) Mid-level obstruction with a proximal dilated intestine.
      (2) Thick, tar-like, tenacious meconium with small grape-like pellets of meconium.
      (3) Clinical presentation is usually within 24–48 hours. This includes the following:
         (a) Failure to pass meconium.
         (b) Abdominal distention.
         (c) Bilious vomiting.
         (d) Palpable, rubbery loops of bowel.
   b. Complicated meconium ileus.
      (1) This type of meconium ileus is complicated because of its association with mechanical problems such as the following:
         (a) Volvulus.
         (b) Intestinal necrosis and perforation.
         (c) Meconium peritonitis or pseudocyst formation.
4. Non-surgical management.
   a. A hypertonic contrast enema (Gastrografin or Hypaque) procedure may be successful in dislodging the meconium obstruction and allowing for normal intestinal activity in 25–60% of patients.
   b. Complications of non-surgical management include the following:
      (1) Hypovolemic shock secondary to rapid fluid shift due to hypertonic solution used for enema.
      (2) Intestinal perforation.
5. Preoperative care.
   a. NPO.
   b. Gastric decompression.
   c. IV fluids.
   d. Blood cultures and antibiotics.
6. Surgical management.
   a. Used with complicated meconium ileus and when non-surgical intervention has failed.
      (1) All compromised intestine is resected and stomas are created.
   b. Postoperative care.
      (1) Continue NPO and gastric decompression until normal bowel function is restored (approximately 3–7 days)
      (2) Appropriate pain management should be initiated (see Appendix B).
      (3) Begin to irrigate stomas with Gastrograffin around postoperative day 3.
7. Postoperative complications.
   a. Volvulus.
   b. Gangrene.
   c. Perforation.

8. Prognosis is primarily related to signs and symptoms of cystic fibrosis.

G. Meconium plug syndrome.

1. Pathogenesis is not clear; results from diminished colonic motility and meconium clearance. It is commonly associated with the following:
   a. Infants of diabetic mothers (IDM): probably due to the increased glycogen production leading to decreased bowel motility.
   b. Infants with hypermagnesemia: usually occurs after a woman is treated with $MgSO_4$ for pregnancy-induced hypertension; the decreased bowel motility is secondary to myoneural depression.
   c. Systemic sepsis.
2. Clinical presentation is usually within the first 3 days of life.
   a. Multiple dilated loops of bowel on physical examination.
   b. Bilious vomiting.
   c. Abdominal distention.
3. Diagnosis.
   a. Presence of symptoms.
   b. X-ray will show multiple distended loops of bowel. (Refer to Chapter 33.)
   c. Water-soluble contrast enema will show an intraluminal plug; such an enema will commonly dislodge the plug, and no further interventions will be required.
4. A biopsy for Hirschsprung's disease and sweat test for cystic fibrosis will allow these disorders to be ruled out; 15% of meconium plug patients have Hirschsprung's disease.

H. Imperforate anus.

1. Incidence: 1 in 5000 live births.
2. Etiology: Failure of differentiation of the urogenital sinus and cloaca during embryological development.
3. 50% of the babies with imperforate anus have associated anomalies. There is a wide spectrum of abnormalities of anorectal development; 10% of these children have esophageal atresia with tracheoesophageal fistula.
4. Imperforate anus is classified as high or low, depending on if the imperforation occurs above or below an imaginary line drawn from the symphysis pubis to the coccyx.
5. High imperforate anus with sacral anomaly can be associated with lack of innervation of the bowel/bladder (which causes incontinence).
   a. Diagnosis is made by physical inspection, x-ray, and ultrasound.
   b. Surgical intervention is always necessary, with the procedure dependent on the level of the anorectal pouch. High and intermediate pouches are treated with a colostomy and a definitive pull-through procedure performed after the infant is approximately 8 months/18 pounds.
6. Low imperforate anus.
   a. Diagnosis is made by physical inspection, x-ray, and ultrasound. An infant with anal stenosis or imperforate anal membrane may have a normal appearing rectum and the condition detected only after the absence of stooling is noted.
   b. Surgical intervention is always necessary, with the procedure dependent on the level of the anorectal pouch. A low pouch can usually be repaired by anoplasty with good results.
7. Preoperative care:
   a. NPO.
   b. Gastric decompression.
   c. IV fluids.
8. Postoperative care:
   a. Continue NPO and gastric decompression until normal bowel function is restored.
   b. Appropriate pain management should be initiated (see Appendix B).
9. Postoperative complications depend on the level of the defect, whether there is innervation of the bowel, and what type of repair is performed.

10. Prognosis is excellent with low imperforate anus; however with high imperforate anus, 50% or more of these children will experience bowel incontinence and may require additional surgery.

I. Hirschsprung's disease.

1. Incidence: 1 in 8000 live births. Males are affected four times more often than females.
2. Etiology: Thought to be related to the interrupted migration of neuroblasts before the 12th wk of gestation. This causes a lack of intestinal ganglion cells, which prevents effective peristalsis and leads to functional constipation.
3. Associated anomalies: Not common but may include colonic atresia or imperforate anus. 2% of patients have a chromosomal anomaly.
4. Clinical presentation.
   a. The early symptom is failure to pass meconium within 24–48 hours after birth.
   b. The late symptom is the inability to stool normally. Abnormal stooling since birth is a common symptom of Hirschsprung's disease. As the obstruction continues, the infant may develop enterocolitis, which presents with fever, abdominal distention, and diarrhea. The infant usually becomes symptomatic in the first several weeks and then develops diarrhea, abdominal distention, and/or vomiting. In advanced cases, urinary obstruction may occur secondary to mechanical compression of the ureters and bladder.
5. The most common complication is acute bacterial enterocolitis caused by bacterial invasion leading to sepsis.
6. The diagnosis is suggested by a barium enema that shows a non-distensible rectal ampulla with a dilated bowel above. The diagnosis is confirmed by rectal biopsy showing the absence of ganglion cells and the presence of excess non-myelinated nerves.
7. Treatment is surgery. Initially, a colostomy is created. At 8 months to 1 year, a pull-through procedure is performed with an end-to-end anastomosis at the anus. The overall results are good in 90% of cases.
8. Postoperatively, it is important to closely observe for shock and recurrent necrotizing enterocolitis.

J. Diaphragmatic hernia.

1. Definition: A herniation of abdominal organs into the thoracic cavity through a defect in the diaphragm.
2. Etiology: failure of diaphragmatic closure or early return of intestine prior to diaphragmatic closure. Diaphragmatic hernia can be both a sporadic and a familial disorder.
3. Incidence: 1 in 4000 live births.
4. Associated anomalies: Reported to be as high as 50%. The central nervous system is most frequently involved. Cardiovascular anomalies, skeletal, gastrointestinal, genitourinary, and other defects are all associated with diaphragmatic hernia.
5. The herniation of the intestine into the chest results in hypoplasia of the lung. Displacement of the mediastinum into the chest may also cause hypoplasia of the other lung.
6. 85% of diaphragmatic hernias occur on the left.
7. The defect can vary from a small slit to the complete absence of the diaphragm on the affected side.
8. Clinical presentation.
   a. Drastically decreased air exchange compromise secondary to hypoplasia and compression.
   b. Hypoperfusion and hypoxia secondary to right-to-left shunting through the ductus arteriosus, foramen ovale, and intrapulmonary shunts.
   c. Respiratory distress at birth or shortly after birth, including cyanosis, decreased breath sounds on one side of the chest.
   d. Heart tones may be shifted from their normal point of maximum intensity.
   e. Hypoxia and respiratory acidosis.

f. A scaphoid abdomen.

g. X-ray examination with air-filled loops of intestine within the chest and a mediastinal shift. (Refer to Chapter 33.)

9. Immediate treatment and preoperative care:

a. Respiratory support, including intubation and positive-pressure ventilation if needed. (Pneumothorax is more common in the contralateral chest.)

b. Gastric decompression should be performed as soon as possible to prevent entrance of air into the herniated intestine.

c. Preparation for surgery needs to be accomplished quickly; two primary considerations are as follows:

(1) Establishment of adequate perfusion and oxygen status.

(2) Correction of acid-base imbalances.

10. This is considered a surgical emergency, and correction should take place as soon as possible.

a. Primary closure of the diaphragmatic defect is usually possible.

b. When primary closure is not possible, a synthetic patch or muscle flap can be used to close the diaphragmatic defect.

11. Postoperative special considerations:

a. Gastric decompression should continue until the bowel is functioning (approximately 7–10 days).

b. Appropriate pain management should be initiated (see Appendix B).

c. A chest tube for drainage should be placed on water seal (without suction) to prevent acute mediastinal shifts.

d. Pulmonary management should be carried out very carefully, owing to hypoplastic lungs, potential pulmonary hypertension, and potential for pneumothorax. If pulmonary management fails, consider extracorporeal membrane oxygenation (ECMO). ECMO might also be considered preoperatively to achieve acid-base stability prior to surgery.

e. Blood pressure and perfusion may be especially problematic, and vasopressors such as dopamine and/or dobutamine may be required.

12. Survival rate depends on the preoperative status—i.e., a 40–60% chance of survival is expected if the symptoms are noted within the first 8 hours of life. Later onset of symptoms increases the survival rate.

K. Necrotizing enterocolitis (NEC).

1. Definition: Necrotizing enterocolitis is an acquired disease that affects the GI system, particularly that of premature infants. It is characterized by areas of necrotic bowel, both small and large intestine.

2. Incidence: 1–15% of all admissions to the NICU.

3. Etiology: Unclear; suggested causes include one or more of the following:

a. Infection.

b. Hypertonic feeding. 90–95% of all infants who get NEC have had enteral feedings.

c. Asphyxia/hypoxia. During asphyxia, blood is shunted away from the gut to the brain, heart, and kidneys to protect them.

d. Hypovolemia.

e. Hypothermia.

f. Umbilical line.

g. Exchange transfusion.

h. Severe stress.

i. Hypotension.

4. Clinical assessment includes any or all of the following findings:

a. Abdominal distention.

b. Gastric aspirates.

c. Bilious vomiting.

d. Bloody stools.

e. Lethargy.

f. Apnea/bradycardia.

    g. Hypoperfusion.

    h. Hypotension secondary to third-space fluid loss from the intravascular space into the extracellular (third-space) compartment.

    i. Temperature instability.

    j. Visible loops of bowel.

5. Laboratory findings include the following:

    a. Leukocytosis/leukopenia.

    b. Thrombocytopenia.

    c. Electrolyte imbalances.

    d. Acidosis.

    e. Hypoxia.

    f. Hypercapnia.

    g. Presence of blood in stools.

    h. Carbohydrate malabsorption, reflected in a positive Clinitest, may be an early sign of NEC.

    i. Disseminated intravascular coagulation (DIC).

6. X-ray findings:

    a. Pneumatosis intestinalis (air within the wall of the intestine). (Refer to Chapter 33.)

    b. Air into the portal venous system. (Refer to Chapter 33.)

    c. Pneumoperitoneum (free air in the abdomen). (See Chapter 33.)

7. Non-surgical medical treatment for necrotizing enterocolitis includes the following:

    a. NPO status.

    b. Gastric decompression.

    c. Evaluation and correction of thrombocytopenia, electrolyte imbalances, acidosis, and hypoxia.

    d. Antibiotics.

    e. Serial x-rays, (usually every 6 hours).

    f. Respiratory support as needed.

    g. Circulatory support as needed to prevent hypotension. Fresh-frozen plasma, dopamine and/or dobutamine should be considered.

    h. Fresh-frozen plasma for DIC; consider use of vitamin K.

    i. Careful monitoring of intake and output.

    j. Frequent abdominal girth measuring.

    k. Watch blood glucose carefully.

8. Surgical treatment is used if medical management is not possible or fails, or if the following conditions exist:

    a. Pneumoperitoneum.

    b. Progressive acidosis.

    c. Progressive thrombocytopenia.

    d. Leukopenia.

    e. Progressive pneumatosis.

    f. Fixed dilated loop of bowel.

    g. Abdominal wall edema/erythema.

9. The surgical procedure.

    a. Resection of obvious necrotic bowel.

    b. Creation of stomas most common (it is rare to have a primary anastomosis).

    c. If a large amount of bowel appears to be involved, at the initial exploration, bowel resection is limited to obviously necrotic bowel and a second exploration is performed within 12–24 hours to re-evaluate bowel viability.

10. Postoperative care includes the following:

    a. A central venous line is placed for hyperalimentation.

    b. Maintenance of fluid and electrolyte balance.

    c. Antibiotics (both a penicillin derivative and an aminoglycoside).

    d. Gastric decompression.

    e. Appropriate pain management (see Appendix B).

    f. Observation of stomas for color and drainage.

    g. NPO status until the bowel is functioning, then begin the slow resumption of feedings with a diluted formula.

11. Prognosis.
    a. Necrotizing enterocolitis is a frequent cause of death for newborns undergoing surgery (30–40% mortality).
    b. Gastrointestinal sequelae include strictures (20%), enteric fistulas, and short bowel syndrome (malabsorption and diarrhea).

Hyperbilirubinemia

A. Natural history.
1. 25–50% of all newborns develop clinical jaundice.
2. Most newborns will appear jaundiced when their serum bilirubin concentration is greater than 7 mg/dl.
3. 61% of all healthy term newborns will have a maximum bilirubin level over 12.9 mg/dl.
4. 3% of all term newborns will have a maximum bilirubin level over 15 mg/dl.

B. Origin of bilirubin.
1. Produced from the breakdown of heme-containing proteins.
    a. Major heme-containing protein is red cell hemoglobin (produces 75% of all bilirubin). Catabolism of 1 g of hemoglobin produces 34 mg of bilirubin.
    b. A small percentage (approximately 25%) of bilirubin comes from the breakdown of hemoglobin.
2. Normal newborns will produce 6–10 mg of bilirubin/kg/day.
3. Newborns have a greater red cell mass per kg than adults.
4. The normal lifespan of bilirubin in a newborn is 80–90 days (bilirubin lifespan in adults is 120 days).

C. Bilirubin metabolism.
1. Bilirubin is bound to albumin for transport in the blood to the liver. This bound or unconjugated bilirubin does not usually enter the CNS system and is non-toxic.
2. Within the liver cells, bilirubin is bound to ligandin, Z-protein, and glutathione S-transferase for transport to the smooth endoplastic reticulum for conjugation.
3. Phenobarbital is sometimes given because it increases the concentration of ligandin.
4. Unconjugated bilirubin is converted to water-soluble bilirubin by conjugation in the liver cell.
5. After conjugation, bilirubin is excreted into the bile.
6. Conjugation is limited in the fetus because there is limited fetal hepatic flow. Most bilirubin is cleared by the placenta into the maternal circulation.
7. Small amounts of bilirubin can normally be found in amniotic fluid between 12 and 37 weeks' gestation. Increased amounts of bilirubin in the amniotic fluid may indicate hemolytic disease in the newborn or fetal intestinal obstruction below the bile ducts.

D. Physiological hyperbilirubinemia.
1. Hyperbilirubinemia is considered physiological when bilirubin levels are up to 12 mg/dl by 3 days of life. (In premature babies, the peak may be 10–12 mg/dl on day 5 of life.)
2. Usually caused by an increased bilirubin load in the liver, difficulty clearing the bilirubin from the plasma, and impaired conjugation and excretion of bilirubin.
3. Physiological jaundice is due to a combination of the following:
    a. Increased RBC volume (as compared with adults).
    b. Decreased survival of fetal RBCs.
    c. Increased bilirubin from cell breakdown.
    d. Increased reabsorption of bilirubin from the intestine.
    e. Early feeding decreases serum bilirubin by decreasing the reabsorption of

bile caused by increased gut motility. Feeding introduces bacteria into the gut, which contributes to the conversion of bilirubin to urobilin, a substance that cannot be reabsorbed.
   f. Decreased ligandin.
   g. Decreased caloric intake.
   h. Binding of the Y- and Z-proteins by other anions.
   i. Defective conjugation.
   j. Decreased excretion of bilirubin (Table 13–1).
4. Treatment of physiological jaundice.
   a. There is no evidence that healthy term infants without a pathological cause of jaundice are at risk for brain damage, even with levels in the 20–24 mg/dl range (Maisels and Newman, 1990).
   b. A bilirubin level of 15–17 mg/dl at day 4 of age can be safely followed without phototherapy (Maisels and Newman, 1990).

E. **Non-physiological jaundice.** (For blood in compatibilities, see Chapter 17.)
1. Conditions that suggest non-physiological jaundice include the following:
   a. Clinical jaundice before 36 hours of age.
   b. Serum bilirubin level increasing by greater than 5 mg/dl/day.
   c. A serum bilirubin level greater than 17 mg/dl in a breast-fed term infant.
   d. Clinical jaundice persisting after 8 days in term or 14 days in pre-term infants.
2. Patient history that may suggest non-physiological jaundice:
   a. ABO/Rh incompatibilities, investigate history for previous sibling with jaundice or anemia (suggests blood group incompatibility with the mother).
   b. History of liver disease in the family.
      (1) Galactosemia.
      (2) Alpha-1-antitrypsin deficiency.
      (3) Tyrosinosis.
      (4) Hypermethioninemia.
      (5) Gilbert's disease.
      (6) Crigler-Najjar syndrome (I and II).
      (7) Cystic fibrosis.
   c. Maternal illness during pregnancy.
      (1) Viral.
      (2) Toxoplasmosis.
   d. Maternal drugs (Table 13–2).
      (1) Sulfonamides.
      (2) Nitrofurantoin.
      (3) Antimalarials.
   e. Labor and delivery history.
      (1) Trauma leading to extravascular bleeding.
      (2) Use of oxytocin.
      (3) Asphyxia.
         (a) Inability of liver to process bilirubin.
         (b) Intracranial hemorrhage.
      (4) Delayed cord clamping may lead to polycythemia.
      (5) Prematurity (see Table 13–1).
   f. Breast-feeding.
      (1) Breast milk jaundice is found in approximately 1% of breast-fed infants.
      (2) Bilirubin levels may rise as high as 30 mg/dl by 14 days of life.
      (3) If breast-feeding is stopped, levels decrease rapidly within 48 hours (when breast-feeding is begun again, bilirubin levels may increase slightly, but not to previous high levels).
      (4) Mothers who have had one infant with breast milk jaundice have a 70% recurrence rate in future pregnancies.
      (5) Overall, infants who are breast-fed have slightly higher bilirubin levels than infants who are bottle-fed.

Table 13-1
CAUSES OF NEONATAL HYPERBILIRUBINEMIA

Overproduction	Undersecretion	Mixed	Uncertain Mechanism
Fetal-maternal blood group incompatibility (e.g., Rh, ABO)	**Metabolic and Endocrine Conditions**	Sepsis	Chinese, Japanese, Korean, and American Indian infants
Hereditary spherocytosis (eliptocytosis, Somatocytosis)	Galactosemia	Intrauterine Infections:	Breast milk jaundice
Non-spherocytic hemolytic anemias	Familial non-hemolytic jaundice types I and II (Crigler-Najjar syndrome)	Toxoplasmosis	
G-6-PD deficiency and drug	Gilbert's disease	Rubella	
Pyruvate kinase deficiency	Hypothyroidism	CID	
Other red cell enzyme deficiencies	Tyrosinosis	Herpes simplex	
Alpha-thalassemia	Hypermethioninemia	Syphilis	
Delta-beta thalassemia	Drugs and hormones:	Hepatitis	
Acquired hemolysis due to vitamin K, nitrofurantoin, sulfonamides, antimalarials, penicillin, oxytocin?, bupivacaine, or infection	Novobiocin	Respiratory distress syndrome	
	Pregnanediol	Asphyxia	
	Lucey-Driscoll syndrome	Infant of diabetic mother	
	Infants of diabetic mothers	Severe erythroblastosis fetalis	
	Prematurity		
	Hypopituitarism and anencephaly		
Extravascular Blood	**Obstructive Disorders**		
Petechiae	Biliary atresia		
Hematomas	Dubin-Johnson and Rotor's syndrome		
Pulmonary, cerebral, or occult hemorrhage	Choledochal cyst		
	Cystic fibrosis (inspissated bile)		
Polycythemia	Tumor or band (extrinsic obstruction)		
Fetal-maternal or fetal-fetal transfusion	Alpha-1-antitrypsin deficiency		
Delayed clamping of the umbilical cord	Parenteral nutrition		
Increased Enterohepatic Circulation			
Pyloric stenosis			
Intestinal atresia or stenosis, including annular pancreas			
Hirschsprung's disease			
Meconium ileus and/or meconium plug syndrome			
Fasting or hypoperistalsis from other causes			
Drug-induced paralytic ileus (hexamethonium)			
Swallowed blood			

Abbreviations: G-6-PD, glucose-6-phosphate dehydrogenase; CID, cytomegalovirus inclusion disease, as in TORCH.

Modified from Poland, R. L., and Nostrea, E. Jr.: Neonatal hyperbilirubinemia. *In* Klaus, M. H., and Fanaroff, A. (eds.): Care of the High Risk Neonate, 3rd ed. Philadelphia, W. B. Saunders Co., 1986, Chap. 11; Cloherty, J. P.: Hyperbilirubinemia. *In* Cloherty, J. P., and Stark, A. (eds.): Manual of Neonatal Care, 3rd ed. Reprinted with permission from Boston, Little, Brown and Company, Copyright 1991, pp. 298-335.

F. **Management of hyperbilirubinemia.**
1. Management of hyperbilirubinemia in low birthweight infants is determined by clinical status, age, weight, and history.
2. Management is tied to etiology.
   a. Assess feedings for volume and calories and increase if needed.

Table 13–2
DRUGS THAT CAUSE SIGNIFICANT DISPLACEMENT OF BILIRUBIN FROM ALBUMIN IN VITRO

Sulfonamides
Moxalactam
Fusidic acid
Radiographic contrast media for cholangiography (sodium iodopamide, sodium ipodate, iopanoic acid, meglumine
  ioglycamate)
Aspirin
Apazone
Tolbutamide
Rapid infusions of albumin preservatives (sodium caprylate and N-acetyltryptophan)
Rapid infusions of ampicillin
Long-chain free fatty acids (FFA at high molar ratios of FFA : albumin)

From Roth, P., and Polin, R.A.: Controversial topics in kernicterus. *Clin. Perinatol.*, *15*:970, 1988.

    b. Assess pharmacological status of the baby. If any drugs are being utilized that inhibit bilirubin binding with protein, consider discontinuing their use (see Table 13–2).
    c. Begin phototherapy if age and weight of the baby are appropriate.
    d. For infants less than 1500 g, begin phototherapy at a bilirubin concentration of approximately 5 mg/dl.
    e. For infants between 2.0 and 2.5 kg, begin phototherapy at bilirubin levels of 13–15 mg/dl.
    f. Term infants who are not sick: begin phototherapy between 17 and 20 mg/dl.
    g. In hemolytic disease, phototherapy is begun immediately.
    h. Phototherapy should be begun if there is an abnormally fast rise in the bilirubin level.

G. **Phototherapy.**
1. The amount of iridescence is critical to the effectiveness of phototherapy. The most effective lights are blue lights with high energy output (425–574 nm). Cool white lamps with a nm of 380–700 are usually adequate for treatment. A combination of blue and white lights is often used because they are effective without being so blue that they make the baby look cyanotic.
2. Lamps should be changed after 2000 hours of use because of decreased energy output.
3. All lamps should be covered with Plexiglas to protect the infant from ultraviolet light.
4. Mechanism for phototherapy action.
    a. Photoisomerization and photo-oxidation of tissue bilirubin take place when the baby is exposed to 420–460 nm of light. This leads to more polar, water-soluble bilirubin products that may then be excreted in the bile and urine.
    b. Infants under phototherapy need to have as much skin exposed as possible.
    c. All infants under phototherapy need to have the eyes covered with eye-patches to protect them from the strong light.
    d. Turn the infant frequently to allow all areas of the skin to be exposed.
    e. Temperature control is important to monitor whether the infant is in an open crib, an Isolette, or an overhead warmer.
    f. Home phototherapy is an option that decreases the length of time an otherwise healthy newborn needs to spend in the hospital. Temperature control and fluid intake need to be monitored carefully with these infants.
    g. Monitor fluids carefully.
        (1) Phototherapy increases insensible water loss.
        (2) Phototherapy may cause diarrhea with further fluid loss.

H. **Exchange transfusion.**
1. The decision to perform an exchange transfusion should be made taking into

Table 13–3
SERUM BILIRUBIN LEVEL (mg/dl) AS A CRITERION FOR EXCHANGE TRANSFUSION

	Birthweight (g)				
	<1250	*1250–1499*	*1500–1999*	*2000–2499*	*≥2500*
Standard risk	13	15	17	18	20
High risk	10	13	15	17	18

Reproduced by permission of Pediatrics, Vol. 75, p. 417, copyright 1985.

consideration the bilirubin level, how quickly the level is rising, the gestational age of the infant, and the age (in hours and days) of the infant (Table 13–3).

2. Early exchange transfusion is indicated in babies with significant hemolytic disease such as hydrops fetalis particularly with cord bilirubin levels greater than 4.5 mg/dl with cord hemoglobin under 11 g/dl.

3. Procedure for exchange transfusion.
   a. Sick infants should always be treated for hypoglycemia, acidosis, and temperature control before beginning an exchange transfusion.
   b. The infant is restrained in the warmer and placed on a cardiorespiratory monitor. Oxygen and suction should be available at the bedside.
   c. Ideally, an umbilical artery catheter and umbilical venous catheter are placed (see Chapter 34 for procedure).
   d. The initial blood removed should be sent to the lab for CBC, bilirubin, calcium, and blood cultures.
   e. The rate of exchange is usually 2–4 ml/minute.
   f. Accurate recording of blood volumes exchanged is essential during the procedure.
   g. Watch carefully for hypocalcemia. Symptoms include the following:
      (1) Irritability.
      (2) Tachycardia.
      (3) Prolonged Q-T interval.
   h. Calcium gluconate should be administered if the infant is hypocalcemic. Normal dose is 1 ml of 10% solution.
   i. Always have a resuscitation cart nearby during an exchange transfusion.

4. Complications of exchange transfusions:
   a. Embolization.
   b. Thrombosis.
   c. Necrotizing enterocolitis.
   d. Electrolyte imbalance.
   e. Overheparinization.
   f. Thrombocytopenia.
   g. Infection.
   h. Cardiac arrhythmias and arrest.
   i. Hypoglycemia.

5. Post-exchange care.
   a. Phototherapy should be continued after exchange transfusion.
      (1) Recheck bilirubin levels every 4 hours.
      (2) Check blood glucose levels frequently.
      (3) Observe closely for signs of complications such as infection, electrolyte imbalance, necrotizing enterocolitis, thrombosis, etc.

I. Conjugated hyperbilirubinemia (direct).

1. Causes of elevated conjugated bilirubin (see Table 13–1).
   a. Liver cell injury:
      (1) Cholestatic jaundice related to use of hyperalimentation.
      (2) Infection.
         (a) Viral.

(b) Bacterial.
(c) Parasitic.
(3) Inherited disorders.
b. Excessive bilirubin load.
c. Bile flow obstruction.
(1) Biliary atresia.
(2) Extrahepatic obstruction (choledochal cyst, trisomy 13 or 18, or polysplenia).
(3) Intrahepatic obstruction (choledochal cyst, bile duct stenosis, bile duct rupture, tumors, cystic fibrosis).
d. Maternal/fetal blood group incompatibility (i.e.: ABO, Rh). (See Chapter 17.)
2. Management of conjugated hyperbilirubinemia.
a. A thorough examination to evaluate for hepatomegaly, splenomegaly, petechiae, chorioretinitis, and microcephaly should be performed.
b. Assess liver function tests (AST, ACT), PT, PTT, and serum albumin levels.
c. Test for ABO and Rh incompatibility. (See Chapter 17).
d. Management is related to the causative factor(s).

Hydrops Fetalis

A. **Definition:** generalized subcutaneous edema in fetus/neonate. Usually accompanied by ascites and pleural and/or pericardial effusions.

B. **Etiology.**
1. Hematological.
a. Rh incompatibility (isoimmune hemolytic disease).
b. Alpha-thalassemia.
c. Glucose-6-phosphate dehydrogenase deficiency.
d. Chronic fetal-maternal or twin-to-twin transfusion.
e. Hemorrhage.
f. Bone marrow failure.
2. Cardiovascular.
a. Heart block.
b. Paroxysmal auricular tachycardia, atrial flutter.
c. Cardiac malformation.
3. Renal.
a. Nephrosis.
b. Renal vein thrombosis.
c. Renal hypoplasia.
d. Urinary obstruction.
4. Infection.
a. Syphilis.
b. Rubella.
c. Cytomegalovirus (CMV).
d. Congenital hepatitis.
e. Toxoplasmosis.
f. Parvovirus.
5. Pulmonary.
a. Diaphragmatic hernia.
b. Intrathoracic mass.
c. Cystic adenomatoid malformations.
d. Pulmonary lymphangiectasia.
6. Placenta/cord (uncommon).
a. Cholangioma.
b. Umbilical vein thrombosis.
c. Arteriovenous malformation.

    7. Maternal conditions.
      a. Toxemia.
      b. Diabetes.
    8. Gastrointestinal.
      a. In utero volvulus.
      b. Atresia.
      c. Meconium peritonitis.
    9. Chromosomal.
      a. Turner's syndrome.
      b. Trisomy 13, 18, 21.
      c. Triploidy.
      d. Aneuploidy.
  10. 30% of all cases of hydrops are of unknown or rare miscellaneous causes.

C. Diagnosis.
1. Vigorous pre-natal diagnosis is essential.
2. Ultrasound.
3. Echocardiography.
4. Serological testing for isoimmunization and infection.
5. Chromosomal testing.

D. Management.
1. Fetal transfusion (for isoimmune hemolytic anemia).
2. Maternal digitalis (for heart rhythm abnormalities).
3. Delivery.

E. Immediate neonatal conditions.
1. Resuscitation is frequently required.
2. Paracentesis may be required for difficulties with ventilation.
3. Thoracentesis or chest tubes may be required for hydrothorax.
4. Partial exchange transfusion may be necessary if the hematocrit is less than 30%.
5. A complete head-to-toe neonatal assessment should be performed to determine the etiology of the hydrops if it is unknown (including echocardiogram, ultrasound of GI and renal systems).
6. Phototherapy when indicated.

Acknowledgment

The author would like to express her thanks to Dr. Jack H.T. Chang for his help in reviewing this chapter.

STUDY QUESTIONS

1. At the time of delivery, an infant with a gastroschisis or omphalocele should have the defect covered with:
  a. A light silicone bag.
  b. Betadine.
  c. Warm, moist dressings.

2. Prune-belly syndrome refers to:
  a. An extremely wrinkled abdomen caused by oligohydramnios.
  b. Congenital absence of abdominal muscles.
  c. The herniation of bowel through the umbilical ring.

3. The incidence of associated anomalies in infants with tracheoesophageal fistula is:
  a. 10–15%.
  b. 30–40%.
  c. Greater than 55%.

4. Clinical presentation of malrotation/volvulus includes:
  a. Scaphoid abdomen.
  b. Dehydration.
  c. Bilious vomiting.

5. Meconium ileus primarily occurs in:
  a. Children with multiple sclerosis.

b. Children with cystic fibrosis.

c. Children with trisomy 13 fibrosis.

6. Gastric decompression in a baby with diaphragmatic hernia is performed for which reason?
   a. To prevent aspiration pneumonia.
   b. To prepare the infant for surgery.
   c. To prevent the stomach and bowel from enlarging secondary to swallowed air.

7. Necrotizing enterocolitis may be associated with:
   a. Birth trauma.
   b. $MgSO_4$ use in the mother during labor.
   c. Umbilical line placement.

8. Most newborns appear jaundiced at bilirubin levels:

a. Greater than 7 mg/dl.

b. Greater than 13 mg/dl.

c. Greater than 17 mg/dl.

9. Phenobarbital is sometimes given to decrease bilirubin because:
   a. It keeps the baby quieter, so that phototherapy is more effective.
   b. It converts unconjugated bilirubin into water-soluble bilirubin, so that it is more easily excreted.
   c. It increases the concentration of ligandin.

10. Breast milk jaundice is found in approximately:
    a. 1% of breast-fed infants.
    b. 10% of breast-fed infants.
    c. 40% of breast-fed infants.

Answers to Study Questions

1. c	5. c	8. a
2. b	6. c	9. c
3. b	7. c	10. a
4. c		

BIBLIOGRAPHY

Cloherty, J.P.: Neonatal hyperbilirubinemia. *In* Cloherty, J.P., and Stark, A. (eds.): Manual of Neonatal Care, 3rd ed. Boston, Little, Brown, 1991, pp. 298–335.

Fanaroff, A., and Martin, R.: Bilirubin and the Laboratory: Advances in the 1980s, Considerations for the 1990s. *In* Neonatal-Perinatal Medicine, 4th ed. St. Louis, C.V. Mosby, 1987.

Frank, G., Turner, B., and Merenstein, G.: Jaundice. *In* Merenstein, G., and Gardner, S. (eds.): Handbook of Neonatal Intensive Care. St. Louis, C.V. Mosby, 1989, pp. 318–335.

Kenner, C., Harjo, J., and Bruggemeyer, A.: Neonatal Surgery: A Nursing Perspective. Orlando, Grune & Stratton, 1988.

Mosijczuk, A., and Vaiani-Ellis, C.: Hematologic disease. *In* Merenstein, G., and Gardner, S. (eds.): Handbook of Neonatal Intensive Care. St. Louis, C.V. Mosby, 1989, pp. 287–318.

Newman, T., and Maisels, M.K.: Neonatal jaundice. Clin. Perinatol., 17:2, 1990.

Romero, R., Pilu, G., Jeanty, P., et al.: Prenatal Diagnosis of Congenital Anomalies. Norwalk, CT, Appleton & Lange, 1988.

Ruttledge, J.C., and Nan-Ou, C.: Selected topics in pediatric pathology. Pediatr. Clin. North Am., 36(2):189, 1989.

Streeter, N.: High Risk Neonatal Care. Aspen Publications, 1986.

Van de Bor, M., et al.: Hyperbilirubinemia in very preterm infants and neurodevelopmental outcome at 2 years of age: Results of a National Collaborative Survey. Pediatrics, 83:915–920, 1989.

Vestal, K., and McKenzie, C.: AACN High Risk Perinatal Nursing. Philadelphia, W.B. Saunders Co., 1983.

REFERENCES

Gryboski, J., and Walker, A.: Gastrointestinal Problems in the Infant, 2nd ed. Philadelphia, W.B. Saunders Co., 1983.

Hayme, H.E., Higginbottom, M.C., and Jones, K.L.: The vascular pathogenis of gastroschisis: Intrauterine interruption of the omphalomesenteric artery. J. Pediatr., 98(2), Feb. 1981.

Maisels, M.J., and Newman, T.B.: Jaundice in the healthy term infant: Time for reevaluation. *In* Yearbook of Neonatal and Perinatal Medicine. New York, Mosby Yearbook, 1990.

Elizabeth A. Estrada
Margaret Brennan-Behm

CHAPTER

14

Neonatal Nutrition

Objectives

1. Describe the general physiology of digestion and absorption of the pre-term infant's gastrointestinal tract.

2. Identify the nutritional store deficiencies most common in pre-term and term infants.

3. Describe the standards used to assess growth in pre-term infants.

4. Describe the basic nutritional requirements for pre-term infants and the factors that influence these requirements.

5. Identify the appropriate uses, routes of delivery, components, complications, and nursing care routines for parenteral nutrition.

6. Compare and contrast the advantages and disadvantages of human milk and commercial formula.

7. Describe the methods used to assess an infant's readiness for enteral nutrition.

8. Describe the various methods for enteral feedings and the advantages and disadvantages of each method.

9. Describe the measures used to assess an infant's nutritional status as well as the causes and treatments for states of malnutrition and feeding intolerances.

The high-risk neonate presents many challenges to the neonatal nurse in providing adequate nutrition to meet basic requirements and support growth. It is important for nurses to become involved in evaluating the neonate's nutritional needs and capabilities from the first minutes to hours of life. An understanding of the gastrointestinal limitations of pre-term infants and the special nutritional needs of high-risk infants is necessary to provide optimal nutrition and prevent complications of malnutrition.

Nurses play a key role in collecting and analyzing data and collaborating with members of the health care team to provide appropriate nutritional management of high-risk infants. Providing nutrition to high-risk neonates, who comprise a wide range of diagnoses and disease processes, is a complex and difficult challenge. This chapter provides a comprehensive review of the nutritional needs of the pre-term and high-risk infant and discusses methods for meeting those needs.

Anatomy and Physiology of the Pre-term Infant's GI Tract

A. Anatomical and physiological characteristics of the pre-term infant's (<33–34 weeks' gestation) **GI tract** (LeFrak, 1987).
1. Anatomical limitations and characteristics.
   a. Lack of suck-swallow coordination.
   b. Absent or weak cough and gag reflexes.
   c. Incompetent gastroesophageal sphincter.
   d. Delayed gastric emptying time.
   e. Decreased small bowel motility.
   f. Incompetent ileocecal valve.
   g. Impaired rectosphincteric reflex.
2. Physiological limitations and characteristics.
   a. Decreased bile salts (fat malabsorption).
   b. Decreased pancreatic lipase (fat malabsorption).
   c. Decreased lactase (lactose malabsorption).
   d. Low enzyme levels (incomplete protein digestion).
   e. Loss of protein and calories in stool.

B. **Feeding-induced hormones** (Uvnas-Moberg et al, 1987).
1. The pre-term infant lacks adequate gut hormone secretion.
2. These hormones are thought to have several important roles in the development and function of the GI tract, including the following:
   a. Digestion of nutrients.
   b. Maturation of gut motility.
   c. Control of exocrine and endocrine pancreatic secretion.
   d. Hepatic function.
   e. Energy metabolism.
3. Failure to stimulate gut hormone secretion has implications for GI mucosal development and gut maturation and function.
4. Stimulus for secretion of gut hormones is bypassed during parenteral nutrition and some methods of enteral feeding.

C. **GI function** (Erdman, 1991).
1. Gut is structurally and functionally mature by 33–34 weeks' gestation for adequate absorption and utilization of nutrients to support growth on enteral feeding.
2. Prior to 33–34 weeks, enzymatic activity necessary for absorption is present in very limited quantities.

D. **Nutrient store deficiencies of the pre-term infant.**
1. Energy.
   a. Fat is utilized as a major energy source by the newborn.
      (1) Sources of fat for the newborn are as follows:
         (a) Release of free fatty acids (FFA) from adipose tissue.
         (b) Ingestion of milk (a diet rich in fat).
         (c) Intravenous intralipids.
      (2) Mobilization of FFA in the pre-term infant is limited due to low adipose tissue stores at birth.
   b. The normal full-term infant has sufficient energy stores (in the form of glycogen and fat) to be utilized during the relative starvation state that normally occurs in the first few days of life.
   c. The pre-term infant has limited stores of fat and glycogen and will quickly exhaust endogenous sources of energy if sufficient exogenous energy is not provided.

2. Vitamins and minerals.
    a. Nutrients, such as vitamins A and E, and minerals and trace elements, such as calcium, phosphorus, iron, copper, zinc, and selenium, which normally accumulate at an appreciable rate predominately in the last trimester of pregnancy, are in low reserve in the pre-term infant.
    b. These nutrients play an essential role in promoting normal tissue growth and repairing injured tissue.
3. Providing adequate quantities of many essential nutrients to prevent further depletion of reserves and to achieve comparable intrauterine accretion rates is difficult and complex.
4. Inadequate nutrition affects the growth and development of all organ systems.

Standards for Adequate Growth

A. Intrauterine growth curves.
1. Widely accepted.
2. Standard for adequate growth is a normal fetus in utero at a post-conceptional age similar to the premature infant ex utero.
3. May be an inappropriate standard for adequate growth for pre-term infants for the following reasons:
    a. Due to immature organ systems of the pre-term infant, it is impossible, even with total parenteral nutrition and commercially prepared premature formulas, to reproduce the transplacental provision of nutrients.
    b. As gestational age decreases, extrauterine provision of comparable nutrients becomes increasingly difficult and may be undesirable in very low birth-weight (VLBW) or critically ill infants.
    c. Severe disease inhibits utilization of nutrients.
    d. Overly aggressive attempts to attain comparable intrauterine growth often result in the following:
        (1) Acidosis.
        (2) Fluid overload.
        (3) Promotion of patent ductus arteriosus (PDA).
        (4) Increased risk of bronchopulmonary dysplasia (BPD) secondary to PDA.

B. Post-natal growth curves for pre-term infants.
1. Weight and head circumference are based on birthweight.
2. Attempt to account for early post-natal water weight loss.
3. Reflect a slower growth velocity than is seen with intrauterine growth curves.

C. Clinicians must bear in mind that definitive criteria for adequate growth remains a controversial issue.

D. Anthropometric measurements and standardized growth curves are necessary tools for assessing growth and nutrition.

E. Whether based on intrauterine or post-natal criteria, a standardized curve that is reflective of a comparable population with respect to geographic location/climate, ethnic, and socioeconomic variables must be selected or developed by each institution.

Nutritional Requirements and Feeding for Full-Term Infants

A. Caloric and fluid requirements.
1. Healthy newborns require approximately 100–120 kcal/kg/day for adequate growth and development.
2. Adequate caloric intake is generally achieved by intake of 150–180 cc/kg/day when 20 kcal/ounce formula or human milk is used.

B. **Protein, fat, and carbohydrate.**
1. Total caloric intake should be represented by the following:
   a. Protein — 7–12%.
   b. Fat — 35–55%.
   c. Carbohydrate — 35–55%.
2. Human milk and commercial infant formulas supply these nutrients within acceptable ratios.
3. Vitamins, minerals, and trace elements.
   a. Vitamin deficiency in healthy, full-term infants is rare.
   b. Human milk and formulas provide adequate amounts of vitamins to meet the needs of most infants. However, supplements of vitamin D, fluoride, and iron are often recommended, especially with breast-fed infants.
   c. Recommended daily requirements and intakes are described in detail elsewhere (Avery and Fletcher, 1987).
4. Human milk and term-infant formulas.
   a. Human milk is the optimal food for most full-term infants. All healthy mothers should be encouraged to breast-feed their infants.
      (1) Human milk may be deficient in vitamin D, especially for dark-skinned infants who are not exposed to adequate amounts of sunlight. Although controversial, vitamin D supplements are generally recommended for all breast-fed infants.
      (2) The unique absorption of iron and zinc from human milk results in rare deficiencies of these minerals, despite their low content in human milk. However, the addition of any other feeding (i.e., formula, cereal, fruit) decreases iron and zinc utilization from human milk).
   b. Commercial formulas for full-term infants are cow milk or soy based. Although both support adequate weight gain for full-term infants, soy-based formulas are not recommended unless the infant exhibits signs/symptoms of lactose intolerance.
5. Supplements. Controversy exists regarding supplementation of human milk or formulas with additional vitamins and minerals. Nonetheless, some recommendations for supplementation are as follows:
   a. Iron.
      (1) The Committee on Nutrition (CON) of the American Academy of Pediatrics (AAP, 1980) recommends iron supplementation of 1 mg/kg/day to all full-term bottle- and breast-fed infants by at least 6 months of age.
      (2) Iron supplements may be given in the form of ferrous sulfate, iron-fortified formula, or iron-fortified cereal.
   b. Vitamin D.
      (1) Adequate amounts supplied in formula.
      (2) Supplementation controversial in breast-fed infants. May require 400 IU/day in the form of multivitamins.
   c. Fluoride.
      (1) The CON of the American Academy of Pediatrics (AAP, 1986) recommends fluoride supplementation in the absence of an adequately fluoridated water supply (0.7–1.0 ppm).
      (2) Supplementation should begin at approximately 2 weeks of age.
      (3) If local water supply contains <0.3 ppm of fluoride, the supplementation recommendation is 0.25 mg/day.
      (4) If local water supply contains ≥0.3 ppm, no supplementation is recommended.

Nutritional Requirements for Pre-term Infants

A. **General considerations.**
1. Recommendations for nutritional requirements and advisable intakes must be utilized as guidelines for meeting nutritional requirements.

2. Individual attention must be given to each infant because nutrient needs can be highly variable.
3. Gestational age and birthweight influence nutrient body stores at birth as well as digestive, absorptive, and metabolic capabilities.
4. The day-to-day clinical status of the infant will heavily influence nutrient requirements.
5. Estimated enteral energy and nutrient requirements and advisable intakes are presented in Table 14–1. These data reflect the most recent recommendations of the AAP (1985).

B. Specific recommendations.
1. Water.
    a. Requirement = amount of water lost from insensible water loss + fecal and urine water + amount retained in newly synthesized tissue.
    b. Actual requirements are highly variable and are dependent on the clinical status of the infant.
    c. Minimum requirement is approximately 150 cc/kg/day for a growing premature infant receiving 120 kcal/kg/day with enteral feedings or 100–150 cc/kg/day for an infant receiving parenteral fluids.
    d. Factors that increase fluid requirements are as follows:
        (1) Abnormal fluid losses (ileostomy, colostomy, chest tubes).
        (2) Diarrhea, vomiting.
        (3) Increase in activity level.
        (4) Labile body temperature, fever, cold stress.
        (5) Low humidity.
        (6) Phototherapy.
        (7) Prematurity.

Table 14–1
ESTIMATED REQUIREMENTS AND RECOMMENDED INTAKES OF ENERGY AND NUTRIENTS FOR PREMATURE INFANTS

	Estimated Requirements Per Day	Advisable Intakes		
		Per Day	*Per kg**	*Per 100 kcal†*
Body Weight 800–1200 g (26–28 wks' gestation)				
Energy (kcal/kg)	120	130		
Protein (g)	3.64	4.0	4.0	3.1
Sodium (mEq)	3.22	3.5	3.5	2.7
Chloride (mEq)	2.79	3.1	3.1	2.4
Potassium (mEq)	2.52	2.5	2.5	1.9
Calcium (mg)	188	210	210	160
Phosphorus (mg)	126	140	140	108
Magnesium (mg)	8.7	10.0	10.0	7.5
Body Weight 1200–1800 g (29–31 wks' gestation)				
Energy (kcal/kg)	120	130		
Protein (g)	4.78	5.2	3.5	2.7
Sodium (mEq)	4.08	4.5	3.0	2.3
Chloride (mEq)	3.47	3.8	2.5	2.0
Potassium (mEq)	3.45	3.4	2.3	1.8
Calcium (mg)	251	280	185	140
Phosphorus (mg)	171	185	123	95
Magnesium (mg)	11.7	13.0	8.5	6.5

*Assuming body weight of 1000 and 1500 g, respectively, for 800–1200 g infants and 1200–1800 g infants.
†Assuming caloric intake of 130 kcal/kg/day.
Adapted from Ziegler, E.E., Biga, R.L., and Foman, S.J.: Nutritional requirements of the premature infant. *In* Suskind, R.M. (ed.): Textbook of Pediatric Nutrition. New York, Raven Press, 1981, p. 32.

(8) Radiant warmers.

(9) Renal dysfunction (glycosuria, acute tubular necrosis).

(10) Third spacing.

e. Factors that restrict fluid requirements are as follows:

(1) Birth asphyxia.

(2) Bronchopulmonary dysplasia (BPD).

(3) Patent ductus arteriosus.

(4) Postoperative status.

(5) Congestive heart failure.

(6) Meningitis.

(7) Renal failure.

2. Calories

a. Energy intake = energy stored + energy expended + energy excreted.

b. Generally, an intake of 120 kcal/kg/day of either human milk or formula will meet the requirements of low birthweight (LBW) infants under normal circumstances (Table 14–2). Some infants may require as much as 150–165 kcal/kg/day for catch-up growth.

c. Parenteral requirements are about 20% less than enteral requirements, or about 70–100 kcal/kg/day.

d. Adequate caloric intake should be assessed based on appropriate daily weight gain or 12 g/kg/day for pre-term infants (LeFrak-Okikawa, 1988).

e. Factors that increase caloric requirements are as follows:

(1) Acute or chronic respiratory disease.

(2) Fluctuations of ambient temperature outside the limits of neutral thermal range.

(3) Hypothermia.

(4) Increased cardiac output; left-to-right shunting.

(5) Increased muscular activity.

(6) Infection.

(7) Malabsorption of prematurity.

(8) Short gut syndrome or other malabsorption syndromes.

(9) Small for gestational age (SGA).

3. Protein.

a. Necessary for cell growth and synthesis of enzymes and hormones.

b. Requirement = growth needs + losses through skin, urine, and feces.

c. Precise requirements are not available; both low-protein (<2 g/kg/day) and high-protein diets (>6 g/kg/day) have been shown to be detrimental to pre-term infants.

d. A protein intake of 2.5–4 g/kg/day with protein intake being 7–12% of total caloric intake is generally recommended.

e. 24–32 non-protein kilocalories must be delivered for each gram of protein administered for proper protein utilization.

f. Must consider amino acid constituents.

(1) In addition to the nine essential amino acids that are necessary for cell

Table 14–2

ENTERAL CALORIC REQUIREMENTS FOR THE PRE-TERM INFANT (kcal/kg/day)

Basal requirements	40–50
Activity	5–15
Cold stress	0–10
Fecal losses	10–15
Specific dynamic action (energy cost of digestion and metabolism)	10
Growth	20–30
Total	85–130

From Kerner, J.A. (ed.): Manual of Pediatric Parenteral Nutrition. New York, John Wiley & Sons, 1983.

growth, pre-term infants require four additional amino acids not essential for full-term infants (histidine, tyrosine, taurine, and cystine).

(2) These are present in adequate amounts in human milk and have recently been added to all premature infant formulas.

g. Whey-predominant formulas appear to be advantageous metabolically to pre-term infants and are provided in pre-term infant formulas. Whey : casein ratio of human milk is 60 : 40; whey : casein ratio of cow milk is 18 : 82.

h. Adequate protein intake may not be achievable with unfortified human milk, especially if the infant is fluid restricted or very small (<1200 g).

4. Fat
  a. Major source of energy for growing pre-term infants and necessary for transport of fat-soluble vitamins.
  b. Guidelines for fat intake are as follows:
    (1) Infants who are <1500 g, pre-term, or SGA require 3 g/kg/day.
    (2) Infants who are >1500 g tolerate 4 g/kg/day.
    (3) Intake should be approximately 35–55% of total caloric intake.
  c. Good source of energy because of high-caloric content and lack of osmolality; however, not all fats are well absorbed by pre-term infants.
  d. Human milk provides about 50% of energy from fat; commercial formulas provide 40–50%.
  e. Because of fatty acid composition and lipase present in human milk, the fat of human milk is more easily digested and absorbed by LBW infants than is the fat derived from cow's milk.
  f. Medium-chain triglycerides (MCTs) are more easily absorbed than long-chain fatty acids in pre-term infants; MCTs are absorbed by passive diffusion and do not require bile salts.
  g. Premature infant formulas use a combination of MCTs and shorter-chain vegetable fatty acids from vegetable oil.
  h. Linoleic acid is an essential fatty acid and should account for at least 3% of total calories (0.5 g/100 kcal). This amount is easily achieved with adequate intakes of human milk and commercial premature formulas. Linolenic acid may also be essential for infants.

5. Carbohydrates.
  a. Glucose is essential for brain function.
  b. Because glucose can be manufactured from other carbohydrates, protein, and fats, there is no absolute requirement for intake. However, pre-term infants rapidly become hypoglycemic without glucose intake.
  c. Carbohydrate intake should provide 35–55% of total calories. Lactose, or a combination of lactose and other sugars, is the preferable carbohydrate for enteral nutrition.
  d. Lactose is the carbohydrate in human milk and is the predominant carbohydrate in most milk-based formulas for full-term infants. The lactose content of human colostrum is significantly lower than mature milk.
  e. Low intestinal mucosal lactase activity of LBW infants may impair digestion of lactose.
  f. The addition of some glucose polymers (e.g., Polycose) may be better tolerated by LBW infants than 100% lactose and provides less osmotic activity per unit weight.
  g. A combination of glucose polymers and lactose is used as the carbohydrate source in many premature formulas.

6. Electrolytes.
  a. Sodium, potassium, and chloride are necessary for growth and play a significant role in water and acid-base balance.
  b. LBW infants have increased sodium needs in the first weeks of life due to underdeveloped renal sodium conservatory mechanisms.
  c. VLBW (<1500 g) infants may require 4–8 mEq/kg/day of sodium to prevent hyponatremia.
  d. Factors that influence electrolyte balance include the following:

      (1) Congenital or post-natal renal failure.

      (2) Diuretic therapy.

      (3) Extent of lung disease.

      (4) Gestational age.

      (5) Sepsis.

  e. Pre-term infant formulas provide higher amounts of sodium, potassium, and chloride than term infant formulas and are generally sufficient for most healthy, growing pre-term infants.

  f. Although pre-term human milk has been found to have higher sodium and chloride levels than term human milk, levels may still be insufficient for the growing pre-term infant.

7. Vitamins and minerals.

  a. Exact requirements of vitamins and trace minerals for pre-term infants have not been established.

  b. Pre-term infants require more of some vitamins and minerals than full-term infants, because their nutrient stores are diminished at birth, and growth often occurs rapidly once the infant is stable and well.

  c. Tables 14–3 and 14–4 provide advisable enteral intakes of vitamins and minerals, respectively, for growing pre-term infants. These data represent the most recent recommendations of the AAP (1985).

  d. Vitamin A (fat soluble).

      (1) Precursor of photosensitive pigments.

      (2) Plays a role in the following:

        (a) Synthesis of mucopolysaccharides.

        (b) Differentiation of mucous membranes.

        (c) Maintenance of the adrenal cortex.

        (d) Remodeling of bone.

        (e) Tissue healing.

      (3) Body content of retinol is generally low in pre-term infants because of low hepatic reserves.

      (4) Low vitamin A levels have been found in infants with BPD.

      (5) Absorption is decreased when fat intake is inadequate or when direct bilirubin is high.

      (6) Vitamin A levels need to be assessed.

        (a) <10 μg/dl = vitamin A deficiency (normal = $30-60$ μg/dl).

        (b) Levels should be obtained and supplements given if necessary.

      (7) Deficiency may lead to the following:

        (a) Apathy.

Table 14–3
RECOMMENDED MINIMUM ENTERAL INTAKE OF VITAMINS FOR PREMATURE INFANTS

Vitamin	Recommended Intake
A	250 IU/100 kcal
D	at least 500 IU/day
E	0.7 IU/100 kcal and at least 1.0 IU/g of linoleic acid
K	4 μg/100 kcal (in addition to 1 mg at birth)
Thiamine	40 μg/100 kcal
Riboflavin	60 μg/100 kcal
Niacin	250 μg/100 kcal
C	8 mg/100 kcal
B_6	35 μg/100 kcal or a minimum of 15 μg per gram of protein
B_{12}	0.15 μg/100 kcal or 0.3–0.5 μg/day
Folic acid	20–50 μg/day
Pantothenic acid	300 μg/100 kcal
Biotin	1.5 μg/100 kcal

Data from American Academy of Pediatrics, Committee on Nutrition: Pediatrics, *60*:519, 1977; and American Academy of Pediatrics, Committee on Nutrition: Pediatrics, *75*:976, 1985.

Table 14-4
RECOMMENDED MINIMUM ENTERAL INTAKE OF MINERALS FOR PREMATURE INFANTS

Mineral	Recommended Intake
Copper	90 μg/100 kcal
Iodine	5 μg/100 kcal
Manganese	5 μg/100 kcal
Zinc	0.5 mg/100 kcal
Iron	2-3 mg/kg/day*

*When infant is 2 months of age and when full feedings are tolerated, iron supplements are recommended. If iron supplements are started prior to 2 months of age, vitamin E supplements should also be given. When infant is >2000 g or when at home, 2-3 mg/kg/day is recommended supplement for breast-fed infants but usually not necessary if iron-fortified formula is used.

Data from American Academy of Pediatrics, Committee on Nutrition: Pediatrics, *75*:976, 1985.

       (b) Decreased resistance to infection.
       (c) Keratinization of mucous membranes.
       (d) Night blindness.
       (e) Poor growth.
       (f) Xerophthalmia.
    (8) Excess may lead to the following:
       (a) Brittle bones.
       (b) Dry skin.
       (c) Loss of hair.
       (d) Increased intracranial pressure.
       (e) Irritability.
  e. Vitamin D (fat soluble).
    (1) Increases intestinal absorption of calcium and phosphorus.
    (2) Promotes reabsorption of calcium and phosphorus in the kidney.
    (3) Facilitates both bone mineralization and calcium and phosphorus mobilization from bone.
    (4) Deficiency may result in clinical rickets or tetany.
  f. Vitamin E (fat soluble).
    (1) Contributes to stability of cell membranes by retarding oxidation of unsaturated fatty acids.
    (2) Poorly absorbed by infants <32 weeks secondary to fat malabsorption.
    (3) Iron supplementation and high intake of polysaturated fatty acids interferes with vitamin E absorption and activity.
    (4) Supplementation may be used to treat hemolytic anemia associated with prematurity.
    (5) Supplementation may be associated with an increased incidence of necrotizing enterocolitis (NEC), intraventricular hemorrhage (IVH), and sepsis.
    (6) Blood levels should be in the range of 1-3 mg/dl.
  g. Vitamin K (fat soluble).
    (1) Necessary for manufacturing several clotting factors (e.g., prothrombin and Factor VII).
    (2) All newborns, full-term and pre-term, require 0.5-1.0 mg IM at birth.
    (3) Deficiency may result in hemorrhagic disease of the newborn (refer to Chapter 3).
    (4) Excess may lead to the following:
       (a) Hemolytic anemia.
       (b) Impaired binding of bilirubin to albumin.
  h. Calcium, phosphorus, and magnesium.
    (1) Necessary for bone mineralization.
    (2) Low stores at birth make the pre-term infant very susceptible to rickets if adequate intakes are not provided during growth.

(3) Calcium and phosphorus retention and absorption are interdependent.

(4) Whether calcium absorption is vitamin D dependent is controversial; phosphorus absorption appears to be independent of vitamin D supplementation.

(5) Alkaline phosphatase levels >300 mg/dl or radiological evidence of rickets indicate a need to increase calcium and phosphorus intake.

(6) Alkaline phosphatase levels should be checked bi-weekly to assess bone mineralization status (normal levels should be <300 mg/dl).

(7) Human milk and term infant formulas are deficient in adequate amounts of calcium and phosphorus for growing pre-term infants.

(8) Human milk fortifiers (Enfamil Human Milk Fortifier and Similac Natural Care) can be added to human milk to supply adequate amounts of calcium and phosphorus to meet pre-term infant needs.

(9) Premature infant formulas (Similac Special Care and Enfamil Premature) have increased amounts of calcium, phosphorus, and magnesium and appear to be adequate for most pre-term infants.

(10) Hypophosphatemia (serum concentration <4 mg/dl) is common in premature infants fed human milk and should be considered an early warning sign of decreased bone mineralization.

i. Iron.

(1) Important for synthesis of hemoglobin, myoglobin, and iron-containing enzymes.

(2) Difficult to provide extrauterine iron to achieve fetal accretion rates because of poor enteral absorption and interference with vitamin E absorption.

(3) Early physiological anemia of prematurity is not benefited by iron therapy.

(a) Maintenance of hematocrit >40% by transfusion of packed red blood cells is indicated by:

i. Presence of clinical symptoms of anemia (i.e., tachycardia, apnea, and bradycardia; fatigue leading to inability to nipple feed).

ii. Chronic oxygen requirements.

iii. Patent ductus arteriosus.

(4) Iron supplementation.

(a) Oral supplementation for premature infants of 2–3 mg/kg/day starting at 2 months of age (and once infant is on full feedings) appears to be well accepted.

(b) Vitamin E supplementation may be needed for premature infants receiving iron supplementation.

j. Zinc.

(1) Plays a role in protein synthesis and is a co-factor of insulin and at least 40 enzymes.

(2) Body stores are limited in the pre-term infant.

(3) Zinc requirements may increase two to four times above the normal requirements for infants with diarrhea, short bowel syndrome, or loss of intestinal fluid.

(4) Deficiency causes the following:

(a) Acrodermatitis enteropathica (diarrhea, dermatitis, alopecia, and apathy).

(b) Anorexia.

(c) Decreased growth hormone.

(d) Decreased wound healing.

(e) Esophagitis.

(f) Growth failure.

(g) Hepatosplenomegaly.

(h) Irritability.

(i) Retarded bone age.

(5) Zinc levels should be monitored; levels <40 μg/dl should be considered low.

Parenteral Nutrition

Total parenteral nutrition (TPN) can provide nutritional support to neonates, but may also be used in conjunction with enteral nutrition to provide partial daily requirements for certain infants.

A. Indications for TPN in the neonatal period (Kerner, 1983).
1. Surgical gastrointestinal disorders (e.g., gastroschisis, tracheoesophageal fistula, malrotation, etc.).
2. Intractable diarrhea of infancy.
3. Short bowel syndrome.
4. Serious acute alimentary diseases, e.g., necrotizing enterocolitis (NEC).
5. Chronic idiopathic intestinal pseudo-obstruction syndrome.
6. Gastrointestinal fistulas.
7. Hypermetabolic states.
8. Renal failure.
9. Intensive care of LBW infants.
10. Special circumstances (e.g., cystic fibrosis, cardiac cachexia, hepatic failure, sepsis).

B. TPN administration.
1. Peripheral route.
   a. Peripheral TPN should be used to achieve adequate nutritional intake when enteral intake is not possible or does not provide sufficient caloric requirements.
   b. Peripheral administration is less invasive than central administration, but IV access may become problematic if parenteral therapy is required for several weeks or more.
   c. Dextrose concentrations may be limited to <12.5% to prevent irritation of small peripheral vessels.
   d. Adequate kilocalorie needs may be met with lipid administration.
2. Central route.
   a. Dextrose concentrations are not restricted as compared to the peripheral route; therefore, complete nutritional management may be more easily achieved, especially when fluids are restricted.
   b. Increased risk of the following:
      (1) Mechanical complications.
      (2) Sepsis.
      (3) Thrombosis of large vessels.
   c. Percutaneous central venous catheters (PCVCs) are being used with increasing frequency in NICUs. They provide long-term venous access and may be put in at the bedside by skilled nursing or medical staff.
   d. Surgically placed central venous catheters (i.e., Broviac or Hickman) provide long-term venous access but have risks of surgery and anesthesia; they may be more stable than PCVCs, owing to sutured cuff.
3. General considerations for TPN.
   a. Due to the malabsorptive problems of the pre-term infant's GI tract and the efficiency of IV nutrient delivery, the suggested nutrient intakes for TPN are slightly different than those for enteral nutrition.
   b. Assessment of nutritional status and complications related to TPN differ from those associated with enteral nutrition. Table 14–5 provides a suggested nutritional assessment monitoring schedule for infants receiving TPN.

C. Guidelines for determining appropriate intake, compositions of available preparations, and guidelines for IV administration are listed below for several important nutritional components.

Table 14-5
SUGGESTED MONITORING SCHEDULE FOR INFANTS RECEIVING TPN

Parameter	Frequency*	Purpose/Comments
Weight	Daily	Indicator of fluid retention and adequacy of kilocalorie intake
Length	Weekly	Assess adequacy of growth
Serum glucose	†	Glucose tolerance; can use Chemstrip
Urine glucose	2-6 times per day	Assess glucose tolerance
Electrolytes	Daily until stable, then 2/wk	Determines appropriateness of levels in TPN
BUN and creatinine	Weekly*	Assess renal function; detect deficient or excessive protein intake (BUN and creatinine >17:1)
Hematocrit	Weekly	Detect anemia (possibly due to lack of iron or vitamins)
Iron, total iron binding capacity, reticulocyte count	As indicated	To determine cause of anemia, and evaluate response to therapy
White blood count	As indicated	If signs of infection appear
Triglycerides	Daily during first 5-7 days; after any rate increase	Assess tolerance of lipids (determine that they are being cleared from the serum)
Serum calcium, phosphate, magnesium	Weekly	Assess adequacy of intake
Alkaline phosphatase	Weekly	Detect early rickets
Bilirubin (fractional)	Weekly*	Assess liver function (detect cholestasis)
Y-GT	Weekly	Assess liver function
Ammonia	As indicated*	Performed if symptoms of hyperammonemia (unexplained lethargy, vomiting, or coma) occur
Prealbumin, transferrin, albumin	Weekly*	Indicators of protein nutrition; prealbumin has half-life of 3-4 days making it a good choice for monitoring nutritional improvement; transferrin is not reliable in iron-deficient patients; albumin has a long half-life (14-18 days), making it slow to respond to nutritional therapy
Vitamin A	Monthly	Assess adequacy of intake
Zinc, copper	Monthly	Assess adequacy of intake

* Before starting TPN and lipids, obtain baseline values for weight, length, serum glucose, electrolytes, renal and liver function tests, CBC, and triglycerides.
† Monitor closely while initiating TPN and during glucosuria and evaluate during any interruption of TPN and for at least 24 hours following cessation of TPN.
Data from Kerner, J.A. (ed.): Manual of Pediatric Parenteral Nutrition. New York, John Wiley, 1983; and Moore, M.C.: Neonatal Network, *6*:33, 1987.

1. Calories: Parenteral requirements are about 20% less than enteral intake, or about 70-100 kcal/kg/day.
   a. Caloric values must be adjusted to meet activity levels, body temperature, and degree of stress.
   b. Activity and catabolic states can cause a 25-75% increase in metabolic demands.
2. Water.
   a. Minimum requirement approximately 100-150 cc/kg/day.
   b. Water requirement varies with gestational and post-natal age and environmental conditions, such as incubator versus radiant heat source and phototherapy.
3. Nutrient considerations (Table 14-6).
   a. Protein.
      (1) Available preparations.

Table 14–6
RECOMMENDED CALORIE, CARBOHYDRATE, FAT, FLUID, AND PROTEIN INTAKE FOR TPN

Component Weight	% of Total Calories	Equivalent Calculation Based On
Carbodydrates	35–55	
Fat	35–55	3–4 g/kg/day
Protein	7–12	2–3 g/kg/day
Kcal		70–100 kcal/kg/day
Fluid		100–150 cc/kg/day

Data from Kerner, J.A. (ed.): Manual of Pediatric Parenteral Nutrition. New York, John Wiley, 1983.

  (a) Pediatric crystalline amino acid solutions.
    i. Require no further metabolism prior to protein utilization.
    ii. Improved nitrogen balance and weight gain when compared with infants receiving standard adult hyperalimentation fluids.
  (b) Amino acids contain 4 kcal/g.
  (2) To calculate amount of protein infant is receiving, use the following formula: protein dose = weight (kg) × % amino acid/100 cc IV fluid × number of 100 cc increments of IV fluid received (LeFrak-Okikawa, 1988).
 b. Fat.
  (1) Available preparations.
    (a) Supplied by soy and/or safflower oil preparations, which provide essential fatty acids (EFAs).
    (b) 10% lipid preparations = 1.1 kcal/cc.
    (c) 20% lipid preparations = 2.2 kcal/cc.
  (2) Guidelines for fat administration during TPN.
    (a) To calculate amount of fat infant is receiving, use the following formula: lipid dose = cc of fat/day ÷ 10 or 5 ÷ weight in kg (divide by 10 if 10% preparation is used; divide by 5 if 20% preparation is used) (LeFrak-Okikawa, 1988).
    (b) 10% preparations may be used when initiating IV fat administration, especially for VLBW infants. Rates of 0.15–0.2 g/kg/hour are suggested to prevent the complications associated with rapid infusion rates.
    (c) 20% preparations are commonly used and are generally well tolerated. They are especially useful for infants requiring a great caloric intake yet are fluid restricted (e.g., infants with BPD).
 c. Carbohydrates (CHO).
  (1) CHO source is glucose monohydrate (dextrose), 3.4 kcal/g.
    (a) Dextrose preparations are made according to the infant's tolerance.
    (b) Standard dextrose concentrations are available in 5% or 10% solutions (per cent = grams of dextrose per deciliter of solution). Other concentrations may be custom made to the individual needs of the infant.
  (2) Guidelines for carbohydrate administration.
    (a) Glucose infusion rates of 5–6 g/kg/day are necessary for minimal caloric intake, protein metabolism, and growth.
    (b) Dextrose concentrations may be increased by 1–2 mg/kg/min each day (until the maximum percentage is obtained for the route being used) as long as serum glucose remains <150 mg/dl and glycosuria <0.5%.
    (c) Insulin may be added to TPN to attain appropriate glucose delivery in infants exhibiting hyperglycemia. The infant's glucose status must

then be monitored very closely (as often as every 15 minutes) until stable and whenever changes in dextrose concentrations or insulin rates are made (LeFrak-Okikawa, 1988).

   d. Calcium and phosphorus.

     (1) Hyperalimentation preparations for infants should contain at least 3–4 mEq (60–80 mg) of calcium and 1.4 mmol (43 mg) of phosphorus per kilogram per day.

     (2) Difficult to supply the small, premature infant with adequate amounts of parenteral calcium and phosphorus to meet in utero fetal accretion rates due to precipitation of minerals in parenteral fluids.

     (3) The use of Trophamine, with additional cystine (Kendall McGaw), as the amino acid solution increases the solubility of these minerals and prevents precipitation when mixed at high concentrations.

   e. Vitamins and minerals (Tables 14–7 and 14–8).

D. **Complications associated with TPN administration.**

1. Potential complications associated with protein administration.

   a. Excessive protein intake is associated with metabolic disturbances (hyperammonemia, metabolic acidosis, azotemia, and hyperaminoacidemia).

   b. Cholestatic jaundice (direct bilirubin >1.5 mg/dl) may occur as a result of excessive protein intake or long-term TPN.

     (1) Occurs in 7–10% of all infants receiving TPN (Moore, 1987).

     (2) Factors that have been correlated with an increased incidence of cholestatic jaundice are as follows:

       (a) GI surgery.

       (b) Hepatitis.

       (c) IVH.

       (d) Patent ductus arteriosus.

       (e) Prolonged ileus.

       (f) Prolonged periods without enteral feeding.

       (g) Sepsis (contributes to the ineffective utilization and metabolism of protein).

       (h) Viral infections (e.g., cytomegalovirus).

2. Potential complications associated with fat administration.

   a. Inadequate fat intake may lead to essential fatty acid (EFA) deficiency and may be evidenced by the following:

     (1) Dry, scaly skin.

     (2) Poor growth.

Table 14–7
SUGGESTED VITAMIN DOSAGES FOR INFANTS RECEIVING TPN

	Infant Weight		
Vitamin	<1 kg	1–3 kg	>3 kg
C (mg)	24	52	80
A (mg)	0.21 (690 units)	0.45 (1495 units)	0.7 (2300 units)
D (μg)	3.00 (120 units)	6.50 (260 units)	10.0 (400 units)
B$_1$ (mg)	0.36	0.78	1.2
B$_2$ (mg)	0.42	0.91	1.4
B$_6$ (mg)	0.30	0.65	1.0
Niacin (mg)	5.10	11.10	17.0
Pantothenic acid (mg)	1.50	3.25	5.0
E (mg)	2.10	4.60	7.0
Biotin (μg)	6.00	13.00	20.0
Folic acid (μg)	42.00	91.00	140.0
B$_{12}$ (μg)	0.30	0.65	1.0
K (μg)	60.00	130.00	200.0

From Moore, M.C.: Neonatal Network, *6*(2):33–40, 1987.

Table 14-8
SUGGESTED MINERAL INTAKE (per kg) FOR INFANTS RECEIVING TPN

Mineral	Amount
Sodium	2.0-3.0 mEq
Potassium	2.0-3.0 mEq
Calcium	3.0 mEq
Phosphate	2.0 mmol
Magnesium	0.25-0.5 mEq
Zinc	300.0 μg (<3 kg)
	100.0 μg (>3 kg)
Copper	20.0 μg
Manganese	2-10.0 μg
Chromium	0.14-0.2 μg
Selenium	3.0 μg

From Moore, M.C.: Neonatal Network, 6(2):33-40, 1987.

(3) Poor platelet aggregation.

(4) Thrombocytopenia.

b. Hyperlipidemia interferes with oxygenation by coating red blood cells, inhibiting carbon dioxide/oxygen exchange, and diminishing pulmonary membrane diffusion capacity. Lipid administration may be contraindicated in infants requiring >60% F_{IO_2} (Pereira et al, 1980).

c. Intravenous lipids may be contraindicated in septic infants due to their interference with leukocyte function (Chen, 1986; Nordenstrom et al, 1979).

d. Intravenous lipids may be contraindicated for infants with severe hyperbilirubinemia because fatty acids compete with bilirubin for binding sites on plasma albumin.

e. Frequent assessment of triglyceride levels is necessary for all jaundiced infants receiving intravenous lipids.

3. Potential complications associated with CHO administration.

a. Hyperosmolarity.

b. Hyperglycemia (serum glucose >150 mg/dl) or glycosuria (>0.5%); frequently seen in VLBW and/or septic infants.

c. Hypoglycemia secondary to insufficient glucose administration or excessive insulin administration.

4. Additional complications associated with TPN.

a. Dehydration secondary to hyperglycemia.

b. Vitamin imbalance.

(1) Vitamin A.

(a) Adheres to infusion pump tubing, resulting in a vitamin A dose that is one-third or less of the amount originally placed in solution (Greene et al, 1986; Riggle and Brandt, 1986).

(b) May also be further destroyed by exposure to light.

(2) Riboflavin.

(a) Destroyed by exposure to light; one-half may be lost in a 24-hour period, with greater loss during phototherapy.

c. Inadequate calcium and phosphorus intake, leading to increased risk for rickets.

d. Trace element deficiency.

e. Extravasation of IV site.

f. Infection.

(1) Contributing factors.

(a) Indwelling venous catheters.

(b) Pre-term infant's limited immunological response to infection.

(c) Lipid preparations provide an excellent medium for bacterial and fungal growth.

5. Measures to prevent/minimize complications associated with TPN.
  a. Double-check all TPN calculations and solutions prior to patient administration.
  b. Utilize a volumetric chamber for 4-hour aliquots of TPN to avoid overhydration in the event of infusion pump malfunction.
  c. Hourly intake recording and IV site assessment.
  d. Readjust fluid volume, dextrose concentration, protein and/or fat intake, and insulin supplementation as soon as problems are identified.
  e. If possible, TPN should be decreased and enteral feedings initiated to stimulate bile production if cholestatic jaundice occurs.
  f. Pharmacy preparation of TPN under laminar air flow hood.
  g. Filtering central TPN with a 0.22 μ in-line filter.
  h. Scrupulous handwashing prior to handling any TPN tubing or IV sites.
  i. Aseptic technique for all dressing or tubing changes.
  j. Opaque coverings for TPN bottles and/or tubing to reduce vitamin A and riboflavin loss.
  k. If alkaline phosphatase levels exceed 300 mg/dl:
    (1) May need to further increase doses of calcium and phosphorus in TPN.
    (2) Adding cysteine hydrochloride to the solution will lower the pH and increase the calcium and phosphorus solubility.
    (3) If calcium and phosphorus doses are maximized, supplementation of calcium and phosphorus via a separate infusion site may be necessary to supply adequate amounts of these minerals while avoiding the risk of precipitation in the TPN solution.

Enteral Feedings: Human Milk and Commercial Formulas

A. Human milk.
1. Full-term infants.
  a. Human milk is the ideal food for most full-term infants.
  b. Pooled human milk may be suitable for healthy, full-term infants, although efficacy has recently been questioned due to possible transmission of human immunodeficiency virus (HIV).
2. Pre-term infants.
  a. Nutritional adequacy of human milk for pre-term infants is controversial.
    (1) Pooled human milk is not recommended.
    (2) Human milk, both term and pre-term, is generally deficient in protein, sodium, calcium, and phosphorus for the growing pre-term infant.
    (3) Although not consistently demonstrated, pre-term human milk has been shown to have higher concentrations of energy, fat, protein, and sodium and lower concentrations of lactose, calcium, and phosphorus than term human milk.
  b. Fortified mother's milk may be the optimal food for pre-term infants.
    (1) Commercially prepared human milk fortifiers (Similac Natural Care or Enfamil Human Milk Fortifier) enhance protein, calorie, vitamin, and mineral content of mother's milk (Table 14–9).
    (2) Premature infant formulas can also be mixed with human milk as a means of nutrient fortification.
3. Advantages of human milk to formula.
  a. Host resistance factors and anti-infective properties.
  b. Easier fat and amino acid absorption and digestion relative to cow's milk formula.
  c. Increased absorption of zinc and iron.
  d. Low renal solute load.
  e. Optimal distribution of calories for full-term infants: 7% provided as protein, 55% as fat, and 38% as carbohydrate.
  f. Presence of thyroid hormones that may delay onset of hypothyroidism.
  g. Maternal involvement in care of her infant.

Table 14-9
COMMONLY USED COMMERCIAL INFANT FORMULAS

Product/Calories Per Ounce	Manufacturer	Comments
Milk-based Formulas for Full-Term Infants		
Enfamil with iron, 20	Mead Johnson	Routine feeding for infants >2000 g.
Similac with iron, 20	Ross	Available without added iron.
Similac PM 60/40, 20	Ross	Decreased potassium and phosphorus content. Not available with added iron.
SMA with iron, 20	Wyeth	Routine feeding for infants >2000 g. Available without added iron. Lower in potassium and phosphorus content than routine formula.
Enfamil with iron, 24	Mead Johnson	Increased nutritional density feeding. Available
Similac with iron, 24	Ross	without added iron.
Milk-based Formulas for Pre-term Infants		
Enfamil Premature Formula with iron, 24	Mead Johnson	Growing LBW infant (<2000 g) feeding.
Similac Special Care with iron, 24	Ross	Increased energy, protein, vitamin, and
SMA "Preemie," 24	Wyeth	mineral content. Available without added iron.
Enfamil Human Milk Fortifier	Mead Johnson	Powder human milk fortifier. Increases caloric, protein, and mineral content. Usual dilution: 1 package fortifier per 25 cc expressed mother's milk.
Similac Natural Care	Ross	A liquid human milk fortifier. Increases caloric, protein, and mineral content. Designed to be mixed with expressed mother's milk or fed alternatively with breast milk.
Soy-based Formulas		
Isomil, 20	Ross	Commonly used for infants who are allergic to
Prosobee, 20	Mead Johnson	cow's milk protein, for those who cannot
Nursoy, 20	Wyeth	tolerate lactose, and those with galactosemia or gluten sensitivity. Has been demonstrated to be nutritionally equivalent to milk-base formulas in supporting weight gain.
Elemental or Therapeutic Formulas		
Pregestimil, 20	Mead Johnson	Ideal elemental formula for full-term infants. Protein, fat, and carbohydrate modified. Iron fortified. Available in powder for easy caloric concentration or as ready to feed.
Alimentum, 20	Ross	Complete elemental formula for infants. Protein, fat, and carbohydrate modified (See Pregestimil).
Nutramigen, 20	Mead Johnson	Protein-modified, lactose-free formula. Indicated for protein allergy or sensitivity, severe or persistent diarrhea. Iron fortified. Available in powder or as ready to feed. Generally not used for pre-term infants.

Data from Clinical Dietetics Staff, Clinical Nutrition Group, and Nutrition Committee (eds.): Infant formulas. *In* Nutrition and Diet Manual. Washington, DC, Children's Hospital National Medical Center, 1989; and Nichols, B.L.: Infant feeding practice: *In* Tsang, R.C., and Nichols, B.L. (eds.): Nutrition During Infancy. Philadelphia, Hanley & Belfus, 1988.

4. Disadvantages of human milk to formula.
   a. Difficult and costly to determine exact nutrient quantities for each mother.
   b. Most likely deficient in protein, calcium, phosphorus, and some vitamins for the growing premature infant.
   c. Artificial expression, collection, and storage of milk may lead to higher risk of contamination by pathogenic bacteria.
      (1) Expressed breast milk is not sterile and is frequently contaminated with many organisms.

      (2) For extremely LBW or other immunocompromised infants, culturing of human milk before it is fed may be indicated (McCoy et al, 1988; Meier and Wilks, 1987).

5. Establishing and maintaining an adequate milk supply.
   a. Most mothers of pre-term or acutely ill infants must establish lactation by expressing milk with a breast pump for several weeks to several months before their infants are allowed to feed at breast.
   b. Nurses can play a key role in helping mothers successfully initiate and maintain an adequate supply of milk for their infants.
      (1) A lactation specialist or a breast-feeding support and education group, composed of nurses, physicians, and dieticians, can provide consistent, up-to-date educational and clinical information to staff and families.
      (2) Mothers often need help with obtaining an electric pump for home use, learning how to use the pump, and learning how to collect and store the breast milk. Additionally, mothers need a great deal of ongoing emotional support and follow-up.
      (3) Institutional standards of care for all mothers who wish to breast feed need to be established.

B. **Commercially prepared formulas** (Table 14–9).
1. Recommendations and standards for commercially prepared formulas were first developed in the 1940s by the U.S. Food and Drug Administration.
2. The Committee on Nutrition (CON) of the American Academy of Pediatrics (AAP) has developed updated recommendations for standards for infant formulas.
3. In 1980, the U.S. Congress passed the Infant Formula Act, which codified the recommendations of the CON and required that all commercially prepared infant formulas meet these standards.
4. Formulas can be classified as milk based, soy based, or elemental (i.e., protein, fat, or carbohydrate modified).
   a. Milk-based formulas.
      (1) Appropriate for most infants.
      (2) Full-term infant formulas are designed to approximate the micronutrient content of human milk.
      (3) Have been demonstrated to be equal to human milk in promoting rapid growth during the first 6 months of life.
      (4) Pre-term infant formulas.
         (a) Provide added calories, protein, vitamins, and minerals to meet the needs of growing LBW infants.
         (b) Modifications in fat, protein, and carbohydrate sources enhance the digestibility and absorption of nutrients for infants with immature GI function.
   b. Soy-based formulas.
      (1) Lactose free.
      (2) Appropriate for infants with:
         (a) Lactose intolerance.
         (b) Galactosemia.
   c. Elemental formulas.
      (1) Appropriate for infants with:
         (a) Protein (cow and soy) allergy/intolerance.
         (b) Fat malabsorption.

Enteral Feeding Methods

A. **Enteral provision of nutrients** (prior to 2 weeks of age) has significant long-term advantages for pre-term infants.
1. Promotion of gut mucosal development.

2. Potential protection against NEC.
3. Improvement in metabolic status.
4. Reduction in the liver enzyme abnormalities that are associated with parenteral nutrition methods.

B. **When to initiate feedings and what method to use are controversial issues.** Several criteria that are applied in making feeding decisions are as follows:

1. Although an infant receiving oxygen and/or mechanical ventilation is not excluded from enteral nutrition, feedings should be postponed until the infant's physiological status is stable (e.g., not requiring resuscitation or demonstrating signs/symptoms of shock).
2. Apnea/bradycardia episodes are not necessarily contraindications for enteral feedings, but feedings may need to be postponed or withheld if apnea/brady-cardia and/or desaturation episodes become acutely severe or frequent.
3. GI peristalsis must be confirmed and assessed by auscultating bowel sounds, monitoring stooling patterns, and measuring abdominal girth.
4. GI perfusion is decreased with patent ductus arteriosus (PDA). Feedings may be postponed until PDA is closed.

C. **Oral feeding.**
1. Indications for oral feedings.
   a. Infant should be free from signs/symptoms of respiratory distress (e.g., respiratory rate <60 breaths/minute; blood gas values within normal limits); clinicians may modify these criteria for infants with chronic lung disease.
   b. Infant demonstrates suck-swallow-breathe coordination (this occurs at approximately 32–34 weeks' gestation for most infants; all infants need to be individually assessed).
   c. Infant's oxygen requirements do not exceed 50% FIO_2 during feedings (Moyer-Mileur, 1986).
   d. For infants who are in transition from gavage feedings, minimal residuals (3 cc/kg) should be obtained (Moyer-Mileur, 1986).
2. Oral feeding routine.
   a. Oral feedings are the feeding method of choice for most infants >34 weeks' gestation.
   b. A healthy infant born at >34 weeks' gestation may have feedings initiated as soon after birth as indicated. Factors to be considered include infant behavior, maternal preference for breast or bottle feeding, and results of hypoglycemia screening for SGA, large for gestational age (LGA), or infants of diabetic mothers (IDM).
   c. For infants 32–34 weeks' gestation and/or infants who are in transition from gavage feeding:
      (1) Feedings should be offered as oral feedings in a progressive fashion; initially, one to three oral feedings per day (the remainder by gavage) with a slow progression, as tolerated by the infant.
      (2) Careful monitoring must take place during feedings to ensure safe intake without complications of aspiration, desaturation (or increased FIO_2 requirements), apnea, and bradycardia. Such complications have been reported to occur less frequently during breast feeding than bottle feeding (Meier and Pugh, 1985).
3. Advantages of oral feeding.
   a. Facilitates the infant's total digestive capacity.
   b. Allows the infant to self-regulate his or her feeding.
   c. Social behavior states of infants are encouraged, especially when there is parental involvement.
   d. Complications of indwelling feeding tubes are avoided (e.g., bacterial inoculation, perforation, etc.).
   e. Does not force parents to adapt to an invasive care routine in the home setting.
4. Disadvantages of oral feeding.

a. May be associated with an exaggerated vagal response in pre-term infants who are in transition from gavage to bottle feedings.

b. Increased risk of aspiration in infants who do not coordinate sucking, swallowing, and breathing during oral feeding.

5. Bottle feeding has been associated with a greater decrease in infant oxygenation during and after feeding as compared with breast feeding (Meier, 1988; Meier and Anderson, 1987).

6. Putting pre-term infants to breast.

a. Recent studies have questioned the practice of postponing breast feeding until bottle feeding is well established (Meier, 1988; Meier and Anderson, 1987; Meier and Pugh, 1985).

  (1) Pre-term infants have been able to breast feed successfully as early as 32 weeks' gestation and may establish mature suck-swallow-breathe coordination earlier with breast feeding as compared with bottle feeding (Meier, 1991).

  (2) Breast feeding may be less physiologically stressful to pre-term infants than bottle feeding (Meier, 1988; Meier and Anderson, 1987).

b. Test-weighing infants (prior to and after breast feeding) using an electronic scale has been shown to be a reliable method of determining infant intake at breast (Meier et al, 1990).

D. Gavage feedings.

1. Provide enteral feeding to infants <32 weeks' gestation and/or infants who are unable to safely feed orally.

2. Non-intubated infants who are exhibiting mild respiratory distress should be fed via an orogastric (OG) feeding tube rather than a nasogastric (NG) feeding tube because infants are mainly obligatory nose breathers (Van Someren et al, 1984). However, the nasal route is easier to secure, which may decrease the risk of tube displacement and potential for aspiration.

3. Parenteral nutrition may be required to supplement enteral intake when feedings are being initiated.

4. Intermittent gavage feeding routine.

a. A 3.5–8.0 Fr feeding tube is inserted using a standard measuring technique: from the nose to the ear to the lower end of the sternum and adding 1 cm, or from the ear to the nose to a point midway between the xiphoid process and the umbilicus (Weibley et al, 1987).

b. The tube should be secured into place with tape.

c. Proper placement should be assessed after insertion and prior to each feeding by:

  (1) Aspirating stomach contents.

  (2) Slowly injecting 0.5–1 cc of air into the feeding tube while auscultating the stomach with a stethoscope.

d. Polyvinylchloride tubes may be indwelling for 1–3 days or may be removed following each feeding, depending on clinical preferences. (Frequent insertion of tubes may cause mucosal trauma and is stressful for infants; therefore, indwelling tubes are recommended.) Silastic or polyurethane tubes do not harden over time and may be left in place for several weeks to months, but they are slightly harder to secure with tape because the outer surface is slippery.

e. Administer feedings by gravity over 15–30 minutes; gravity allows for a natural "burp" through the tube and avoids direct, forceful pressure into the GI tract.

f. During the feeding, the infant should be closely observed for intolerance and complications (e.g., emesis, bradycardia, apnea).

g. Following the feeding, the tube should be cleared with air and the tube capped off to air. If the tube is to be removed following each feeding, remove tube by pinching it off and withdrawing it quickly.

h. Following the feeding, the infant should be burped and positioned on his or her right side or abdomen with the head of the bed elevated at a 30 degree angle.

5. Indications for continuous gavage feedings.
   a. VLBW infants whose gastric capacity is limited, and infants who require a steady influx of glucose (e.g., IDM with severe hypoglycemia).
   b. Infants with malabsorptive syndromes (e.g., short bowel syndrome, post-NEC, neonatal abstinence syndrome).
   c. Intractable gastroesophageal reflux.
6. Continuous gavage feeding routine.
   a. See previous discussion under Intermittent gavage feeding routine, Sections a. through d. and f.
   b. A 4-hour feeding volume should be aseptically prepared and purged through the appropriate infusion pump tubing. (Syringe infusion pumps are recommended due to their low priming volume and inexpensive cost.)
   c. For human milk feedings, infusion pump tubing should be changed every 4 hours (i.e., with each 4-hour feeding volume set-up) to eliminate exponential bacterial growth in expressed mother's milk (Lemons et al, 1983).
   d. Following insertion, taping, and assessment for proper placement, the infant's feeding tube is connected to the infusion pump tubing.
   e. The infusion pump is programmed to deliver the appropriate rate and volume to the infant.
   f. Hourly enteral feeding intake should be recorded.
   g. Assess every 2–4 hours:
      (1) Gastric residuals (up to 2–3 hours of infusion volume may be normal, with no other signs of feeding intolerance).
      (2) Abdominal girth.
7. Advantages of gavage feedings.
   a. Allow infants who are unable to safely feed orally the benefits of enteral nutrition (e.g., stimulation of bile flow and feeding-induced hormones, improved weight gain patterns).
8. Disadvantages of gavage feedings.
   a. Provide source for bacterial inoculation of the GI tract via feeding tube and milk.
   b. Potential risks associated with improper placement of feeding tube.
   c. Enteric gut hormone secretion is altered.
   d. Do not allow the infant to self-regulate feeding.
   e. Require skilled nursing personnel.
   f. Parental involvement with this feeding method is limited in many nursery settings.
9. Advantages of continuous versus intermittent gavage feeding.
   a. Allows for a more controlled fluid and caloric administration.
   b. May be better tolerated than intermittent feedings for VLBW infants or infants who have suffered GI injury or surgery.
10. Disadvantages of continuous versus intermittent gavage feeding.
   a. Higher risk of aspiration when infant is unattended.
   b. Does not promote gastric readiness for bolus feedings (i.e., stomach capacity remains small).
   c. Intermittent gavage feedings have been associated with the following:
      (1) Decreased oxygenation during feeding (Herrell et al., 1980).
      (2) Impaired pulmonary function after feeding (Patel et al., 1977; Yu, 1976; Yu and Rolfe, 1976).
      (3) Decreased peripheral circulatory responses during feeding (Yao et al., 1971).

E. Transpyloric feedings.
1. Indications for transpyloric feedings.
   a. Infants who are at great risk for aspiration (e.g., gastroesophageal reflux, receiving nasal continuous positive airway pressure); risk is minimized because the end of the tube is located beyond the pyloric sphincter.

2. Transpyloric feeding routine.
   a. A Silastic or polyurethane nasojejunal tube is inserted, using a standard measuring technique (i.e., from the tip of the infant's nose to the knee).
   b. Placement is assessed by checking pH of aspirated fluid (pH of 5–7 indicates transpyloric placement); x-ray confirmation is also usually indicated.
   c. An OG feeding tube is inserted prior to feeding for assessment of gastric residuals.
   d. Infusion pump and tubing should be prepared and connected to the feeding tube as outlined in the section on continuous gavage feedings.
3. Advantages of transpyloric feeds versus gastric feeds.
   a. Less chance of aspiration because feedings are administered below the pyloric sphincter.
4. Disadvantages of transpyloric feedings versus gastric feedings.
   a. Increased risk of intestinal perforation.
   b. Require tube verification by x-ray, as well as increased nursing time to place tube; both are costly.
   c. May induce symptoms of malabsorption (i.e., frequent stooling and increased excretion of fat and potassium) because the stomach is not able to aid in the digestive process.

F. Gastrostomy feedings.
1. Indications for gastrostomy feeding.
   a. Congenital anomalies of the GI tract requiring surgical intervention.
   b. Severely asphyxiated infants who are unable to suck and swallow.
   c. Other infants requiring long-term gavage feedings.
2. Gastrostomy feeding routine.
   a. Residuals are assessed prior to each feeding by unclamping and lowering the gastrostomy tube or by aspirating gastric contents.
   b. Feedings are administered by gravity over 15–30 minutes or may be delivered by continuous drip.
   c. The tube should be cleared with water or air after feeding is finished.
   d. The tube may be left unclamped after feedings at a level of 10–12 cm above the patient for "burping" or clamped after feeding, depending on infant tolerance and comfort.
   e. Tube migration should be evaluated with any sign of feeding intolerance.
3. Advantages of gastrostomy feedings.
   a. Allows for enteral feedings if oral or gavage routes are not feasible (e.g., esophageal atresia).
   b. More comfortable feeding method than gavage feedings for infants with long-term oral feeding problems.
4. Disadvantages of gastrostomy feeding method.
   a. Infant may not be provided with the opportunity to develop suck-swallow-breathe coordination. Sham feedings and non-nutritive sucking may provide a solution to this disadvantage (DeBear, 1986). Sham feedings are non-nutritive oral feedings that allow fluids to drain via a mucous fistula, thereby avoiding the lower esophagus.
   b. See previous discussion under Disadvantages of gavage feedings, Sections a. through f.

Nutritional Assessment

A. Anthropometric.
1. Anthropometric measurements should be monitored at the following intervals:
   a. Weights—daily.
   b. Length and head circumference—weekly.
2. Weight, head circumference, and length should be plotted on growth curves weekly.

3. Intake.
   a. Fluid, protein, and calorie intake should be calculated daily.
   b. Need for vitamin/mineral supplements should be assessed at least weekly.
   c. Laboratory.
      (1) Laboratory values should be monitored at regular intervals (Merenstein and Gardner, 1989). Growing pre-term infants may require
         (a) Weekly—electrolytes, calcium, phosphorus, total protein, albumin, hemoglobin
         (b) Twice monthly—alkaline phosphatase.
      (2) See Table 14–5 for suggested laboratory monitoring while the infant is receiving TPN.

B. **Feeding tolerance.**
1. Premature infants are at risk for a variety of problems related to enteral feedings secondary to physiological limitations of the pre-term infant's GI tract (see page 255).
2. During the initiation of feedings and until full feedings are maintained and well tolerated, the nurse should assess the following prior to each feeding or every 2–4 hours during continuous feedings:
   a. Presence of bowel sounds.
   b. Correct placement of gastric or transpyloric tube, if present (see sections on gavage and transpyloric feeding methods).
   c. Gastric residual.
   d. Abdominal girth measurement—compare with previous measurements.
   e. Observation of distended bowel loops on abdominal surface.
3. Frequency, amount, and consistency of stools must be noted with each stool and documented.
   a. Slow GI motility may lead to constipation and result in gastric distention, gastric residuals, and possibly vomiting.
   b. Glycerine suppositories may be needed to facilitate stooling.
4. All stools should be checked for occult blood and reducing substance once feedings are started.
   a. If Hemetest is positive, further evaluation is needed.
   b. Occult blood may be present if maternal blood was swallowed, if meconium stools are still being passed, following esophageal or gastric irritation from feeding tubes, and from rectal fissures.
   c. Reducing substance in stools may signify carbohydrate malabsorption but may also be a normal finding in infants who are breast fed.
      (1) Results from reducing substance testing are accurate only when done on fresh stool because bacteria in stool decreases the sugar content within minutes.
      (2) Carbohydrate malabsorption has been detected in infants with NEC and may represent an early predictor of the risk for development of NEC.
         (a) Greater than 0.5% (500 mg/dl) of sugar in the stool indicates abnormal amounts of sugar (Krom and Frank, 1989) and warrants further observation for clinical features of NEC.
         (b) In the absence of significant indicators of NEC, a reduction in the concentration of carbohydrate or volume of feedings may alleviate the problem until GI function matures.

Nursing Interventions to Facilitate Tolerance of Enteral Feedings

A. **Non-nutritive sucking during gavage feedings.**
1. Accelerates maturation of the sucking reflex.
2. Improves weight gain.
3. Decreases oxygen consumption.

4. Facilitates earlier advancement to full oral feedings and earlier discharge to home.

B. Prone or side-lying position during or after feedings.
1. Improves gastric emptying time.
2. Decreases the chance of regurgitation and aspiration.

C. Holding in flexed, semi-upright position during oral or gavage feedings.
1. Promotes flexed posture.
2. Encourages social interaction.
3. Decreases the chance of regurgitation and aspiration.

D. Reduction in stress and stimulation prior to or during feedings.
1. Reduces fluctuations in oxygenation that may interfere with GI perfusion and function.
2. Promotes an infant behavioral state that is conducive to social interactiveness.

STUDY QUESTIONS

1. Which one of the following is true regarding post-natal growth curves?
   a. Attempt to account for early post-natal water weight loss.
   b. Growth velocity is faster than is seen with intrauterine growth curves.
   c. Standard for adequate growth is a normal fetus in utero.

2. The recommended protein intake for premature infants is:
   a. 0.5–2.0 g/kg/day
   b. 2.5–4.0 g/kg/day
   c. 4.5–6 g/kg/day

3. Which one of the following is an indication for starting TPN?
   a. Inability to bottle feed successfully
   b. SGA infant
   c. Surgical GI disorder

4. Centrally administered TPN is advantageous to peripheral TPN because:
   a. Central lines have fewer complications than peripheral lines.
   b. Dextrose, calorie, and protein contents can be higher.
   c. Surgically placed lines are easy to place and carry few risks to LBW infants.

5. Suck-swallow-breathe coordination is thought to occur when an infant reaches:

   a. 29–31 weeks' gestation
   b. 32–34 weeks' gestation
   c. 35–37 weeks' gestation

6. Which one of the following is true regarding human milk?
   a. Expressed human milk is sterile.
   b. Fat and amino acids are more easily digested as compared with formula.
   c. Pooled human milk is nutritionally adequate for pre-term infants.

7. Pre-term infant formulas contain:
   a. Less calories and protein than term infant formulas.
   b. More calories and protein than term infant formulas.
   c. No lactose.

8. Reducing substance in stools of $> 0.5\%$ may signify:
   a. Carbohydrate malabsorption.
   b. Protein intolerance.
   c. Zinc deficiencies.

9. Non-nutritive sucking during gavage feeding:
   a. Accelerates maturation of the sucking reflex.
   b. Increases oxygen consumption.
   c. Interferes with weight gain.

Answers to Study Questions

1. a   4. b   7. b
2. b   5. b   8. a
3. c   6. b   9. a

REFERENCES

American Academy of Pediatrics, Committee on Nutrition: Nutritional needs of low-birth weight infants. Pediatrics, 60:519–530, 1977.

American Academy of Pediatrics, Committee on Nutrition: Vitamin and mineral supplement needs in normal children in the United States. Pediatrics, 66:1015–1012, 1980.

American Academy of Pediatrics, Committee on Nutrition: Nutritional needs of low-birth-weight infants. Pediatrics, 75:976–986, 1985.

American Academy of Pediatrics, Committee on Nutrition: Fluoride Supplementation. Pediatrics, 77:758–761, 1986.

Avery, G.B., and Fletcher, A.B.: Nutrition. In Avery, G.B. (ed.): Neonatology: Pathophysiology and Management of the Newborn, 3rd ed. Philadelphia, J.B. Lippincott, 1987, pp. 1173–1229.

Chen, W.J.: Utilization of intralipid in septic rats: Effects of sepsis on the clearance of exogenous fat emulsion from various organs. J. Parenter. Enter. Nutr., 10:482–486, 1986.

Clinical Dietetics Staff, Clinical Nutrition Group, and Nutrition Committee (eds.): Infant formulas. In Nutrition and Diet Manual. Washington, DC, The Children's Hospital National Medical Center, 1989.

DeBear, K.: Sham feeding: Another kind of nourishment. Am. J. Nurs., 10:1142–1143, 1986.

Erdman, S.: Development and growth of the newborn gut. Clinical Update '91: Gastrointestinal Dysfunction. Denver, Conference of the National Association of Neonatal Nurses, 1991.

Greene, H.L., Courtney-Moore, M.E., Phillips, B., et al: Evaluation of a pediatric multiple vitamin preparation for total parenteral nutrition: II. Blood levels of vitamins A, D, and E. Pediatrics, 77:539–547, 1986.

Herrell, N., Martin, R.J., and Fanaroff, A.: Arterial oxygen tension during nasogastric feeding in the preterm infant. J. Pediatr., 96:914–916, 1980.

Kerner, J.A. (ed.): Manual of Pediatric Parenteral Nutrition. New York, John Wiley, 1983.

Krom, F.A., and Frank, C.G.: Clinitesting neonatal stools. Neonatal Network, 8(2):37–40, 1989.

Lefrak, L.: Feeding Problems of the VLBW Infant. Chicago, The National Conference of Neonatal Nursing, Contemporary Forums, 1987.

Lefrak-Okikawa, L.: Nutritional management of the very low birth weight infant. J. Perinat. Neonat. Nurs., 2(1):66–77, 1988.

Lemons, P.M., Miller, K., Eitzen, H., et al: Bacterial growth in human milk during continuous feeding. Am. J. Perinatol., 1:76–80, 1983.

McCoy, R., Kadowaki, C., Wilks, S., et al: Nursing management of breast feeding preterm infants. J. Perinat. Neonat. Nurs. 2(1):42–55, 1988.

Meier, P.: Breast feeding the premature infant. Clinical Update '91: Gastrointestinal Dysfunction. Denver, Conference of the National Association of Neonatal Nurses, 1991.

Meier, P.P.: Bottle and breast feeding: Effects on transcutaneous oxygen pressure and temperature in preterm infants. Nurs. Res., 37:36–41, 1988.

Meier, P., and Anderson, G.C.: Responses to bottle and breast feeding in small preterm infants: A report of five cases. Am. J. Maternal-Child Nurs., 12:97–105, 1987.

Meier, P.P., Lysakowski, T.Y., Engstrom, J.L., et al: The accuracy of test-weighing for preterm infants. J. Pediatr. Gastroenterol. Nutr. 10:62–65, 1990.

Meier, P., and Pugh, E.J.: Breastfeeding behavior of small preterm infants. Am. J. Maternal-Child Nurs., 10:396–401, 1985.

Meier, P., and Wilks, S.: The bacteria in expressed mother's milk. Am. J. Maternal-Child Nurs., 12:420–423, 1987.

Merenstein, G., and Gardner, S.: Neonatal nutrition. In Handbook of Neonatal Intensive Care, 2nd ed. St. Louis, C.V. Mosby, 1989, p. 182.

Moore, M.C.: Total parenteral nutrition for infants. Neonatal Network, 6(2):33–40, 1987.

Moyer-Mileur, L.J.: Nutrition. In Streeter, N.S. (ed.): High-risk Neonatal Care. Rockville, MD, Aspen, 1986, pp. 263–296.

Nichols, B.L.: Infant feeding practice. In Tsang, R.C., and Nichols, B.L. (eds.): Nutrition During Infancy. Philadelphia, Hanley & Belfus, 1988, pp. 367–377.

Nordenstrom, J., Jarstrand, C., and Wiernik, A.: Decreased chemotactic and random migration of leukocytes during intralipid infusion. Am. J. Clin. Nutr., 32:2416–2422, 1979.

Patel, B.D., Dinwiddie, R., Kumar, S.P., and Fox, W.W.: The effects of feeding on arterial blood gas and lung mechanics in newborn infants recovering from respiratory disease. J. Pediatr., 90,435–438, 1977.

Pereira, G.R., Fox, W.W., Stanley, C.A., et al: Decreased oxygenation and hyperlipemia during intravenous fat infusions in premature infants. Pediatrics, 66:26–30, 1980.

Riggle, M.A., and Brandt, R.B.: Decrease of available vitamin A in parenteral nutrition solutions. J. Parenter. Enter. Nutr., 10:388–392, 1986.

Uvnas-Moberg, K., Widstrom, A.M., Marchini, G., et al: Release of GI hormone in mother and infant by sensory stimulation. Acta Pediatr. Scand., 76:851–860, 1987.

Van Someren, V., Linnett, S., Stothers, J., et al: An investigation into the benefits of resisting nasoenteric feeding tubes. Pediatrics, 74:379–383, 1984.

Weibley, T.T., Adamson, M., Clinkscales, N., et al: Gavage tube insertion in the premature infant. Am. J. Maternal-Child Nurs., 12:24–27, 1987.

Yao, A.C., Wallgren, C.G., Sinha, S.N., and Lind, J.: Peripheral circulatory response to feeding in the newborn infant. Pediatrics, 47(2):378–383, 1971.

Yu, V.Y.: Cardiorespiratory response to feeding in newborn infants. Arch. Dis. Child., *51*:305–309, 1976.

Yu, V.Y., and Rolfe, P.: Effect of feeding on ventilation and respiratory mechanics in newborn infants. Arch. Dis. Child., *51*:310–313, 1976.

Ziegler, E.E., Biga, R.L., and Foman, S.J.: Nutritional requirements of the premature infant. *In* Suskind, R.M. (ed.): Textbook of Pediatric Nutrition. New York, Raven Press, 1981, pp. 29–39.

BIBLIOGRAPHY

American Academy of Pediatrics, Committee on Nutrition: Commentary on breast-feeding and infant formulas, including proposed standards for formulas. Pediatrics, *57*:278–285, 1976.

American Academy of Pediatrics, Committee on Nutrition: Special diets for infants with inborn errors of amino acid metabolism. Pediatrics, *57*:783–791, 1976.

Anderson, G.H. Atkinson, S.A., and Bryan, M.H.: Energy and macronutrient content of human milk during early lactation from mothers giving birth prematurely and at term. Am. J. Clin. Nutr., *34*:258–265, 1981.

Atkinson, S.A., Bryan, M.H., and Anderson, G.H.: Human milk feeding in premature infants: Protein, fat, and carbohydrate balances in the first two weeks of life. J. Pediatr., *99*:617–624, 1981.

Avery, G.B., and Fletcher, A.B.: Nutrition. *In* Avery, G.B. (ed.): Neonatology: Pathophysiology and Management of the Newborn, 3rd ed. Philadelphia, J.B. Lippincott, 1987, pp. 1173–1229.

Aynsley-Green, A., Adrian, T.E., and Bloom, S.R.: Feeding and the development of enteroinsular hormone secretion in the preterm infant: Effects of continuous gastric infusions of human milk compared with intermittent boluses. Acta Paediatr. Scand., *71*:379–383, 1983.

Bernbaum, J.C., Pereira, G.R., Watkins, J.B., et al: Nonnutritive sucking during gavage feeding enhances growth and maturation in preterm infants. Pediatrics, *71*:41–45, 1983.

Bhatia, J., and Foman, S.J.: Formulas for premature infants: Fate of the calcium and phosphorus. Pediatrics, *72*:37–40, 1983.

Bodefeld, E., Schachinger, H., Huch, A., et al: Continuous TCP_{O_2} monitoring in healthy and sick newborn infants during and after feeding. Birth Defects: Original Article Series, *15*:503–508, 1979.

Brosius, K.K., Ritter, D.A., and Kenney, J.D.: Postnatal growth curve of the infant with extremely low birth weight who was fed enterally. Pediatrics, *74*:778–782, 1984.

Chatas, M.K.: Percutaneous central venous catheters in neonates. J. Obstet. Gynecol. Neonatal Nurs., *15*:324–329, 1986.

Churella, H.R., Bachhuber, W.L., and MacLean, W.C.: Survey: Methods of feeding low-birth-weight infants. Pediatrics, *76*:243–249, 1985.

Cook, D.A., and Sarett, H.P.: Design of infant formulas for meeting normal and special needs. *In* Lifshitz, F. (ed.): Pediatric Nutrition: Infant Feedings—Deficiencies—Diseases. New York, Marcel Dekker, 1982, pp. 71–85.

Fanaroff, A.A., and Klaus, M.H.: Feeding and selected disorders of the gastrointestinal tract. *In* Klaus, M.H., and Fanaroff, A.A. (eds.): Care of the High-risk Neonate, 3rd ed. Philadelphia, W.B. Saunders Co., 1986, pp. 113–146.

Fletcher, A.B., and Avery, G.B.: Nutrition for full-term and preterm infants. Infant Nutr., *75*(1):113–122, 1984.

Foman, S.J., Ziegler, E.E., and Vazquez, H.D.: Human milk and the small premature infant. Am. J. Dis. Child., *131*:463–467, 1977.

Frank, L., and Sosenko, R.S.: Undernutrition as a major contributing factor in the pathogenesis of bronchopulmonary dysplasia. Am. Rev. Respir. Dis., *138*:725–729, 1988.

Georgieff, M.K., and Sasanow, S.R.: Nutritional assessment of the neonate. Clin. Perinatol., *13*:73–89, 1986.

Greer, F.R., McCormick, A, and Loker, J.: Changes in fat concentration of human milk during delivery by intermittent bolus and continuous mechanical pump infusion. J. Pediatr., *105*:745–749, 1984.

Guss, E.: Breast-feeding. *In* Streeter, N.S. (ed.): High-risk Neonatal Care. Rockville, MD, Aspen, 1986.

Gutman, L.T., Idriss, Z.H., Gehlbach, S., et al: Neonatal staphylococcal enterocolitis: Association with indwelling feeding catheters and *S. aureus* colonization. J. Pediatr. *88*:836–839, 1976.

Heird, W.C., Okamoto, E., and Anderson, T.L.: Nutrition, body fluids, and acid-base homeostasis. *In* Fanaroff, A.A., & Martin, R.J. (eds.): Behrman's Neonatal-Perinatal Medicine: Diseases of the Fetus and Infant, 3rd ed. St. Louis, C.V. Mosby, 1983, pp. 302–308.

Helms, R.A.: Comparison of a pediatric versus standard amino acid formulation in preterm neonates requiring parenteral nutrition. J. Pediatr., *110*:466–470, 1987.

Kerner, J.A. (ed.): Manual of Pediatric Parenteral Nutrition. New York, John Wiley, 1983.

Lemons, P., Stuart, M., and Lemons, J.A.: Breast-feeding the premature infant. Clin. Perinatal Neonatal Nurs., *13*(1):111–122, 1986.

Measel, C.P., and Anderson, G.C.: Nonnutritive sucking during tube feedings: Effect on clinical course in premature infants. J. Obstet. Gynecol. Neonatal Nurs., *8*:265–272, 1979.

Merenstein, G., and Gardner, S.: Total parenteral nutrition. *In* Handbook of Neonatal Intensive Care, 2nd ed. St. Louis, C.V. Mosby, 1989, pp. 261–283.

Myant, N.B.: Lipid metabolism. *In* Phillipp, E.E., Barnes, J., and Newton, M. (eds.): Scientific Foundations of Obstetrics and Gynecology. Chicago, Heineman, 1986, pp. 403–417.

Ohio Neonatal Nutritionists: Nutritional Care for High Risk Newborns. Philadelphia, George Stickley, 1985.

Ostertag, S.G., LaGamma, E.F., Reisen, C.E., et al: Early enteral feeding does not affect the incidence of necrotizing enterocolitis. Pediatrics, 77:275–280, 1986.

Shenai, J.P., Chytil, F., and Stahlman, M.T.: Vitamin A status in neonates with bronchopulmonary dysplasia. Pediatr. Res., 19:185–189, 1985.

Steichen, J.J., Krieg-Wispe, S., and Tsang, R.C.: Breastfeeding the low birth preterm infant. Clin. Perinatol., 14:131–171, 1987.

Szabo, J.S., Hillemier, C., and Oh, W.: Effect of non-nutritive and nutritive suck on gastric emptying in premature infants. J. Pediatr. Gastroenterol. Nutr., 4:348–351, 1985.

Tsang, R.C., and Nichols, B.L. (eds.): Nutrition During Infancy. Philadelphia, Hanley & Belfus, 1988.

Wharton, B.A., Bremer, H.J., Orzalesi, M., et al: (Committee on Nutrition of the Preterm infant, European Society of Paediatric Gastroenterology and Nutrition): Nutrition and Feeding of Preterm Infants. Oxford, Blackwell Scientific Publications, 1987.

Wilks, S., and Meier, P.: Helping mothers express milk suitable for preterm and high-risk infant feeding. Am. J. Maternal-Child Nurs., 13:121–123, 1988.

Ziegler, E.E., O'Donnell, A.M., Nelson, S.E., et al: Body composition of the reference fetus. Growth, 40,329–341, 1976.

Laura Campbell Stokowski

Metabolic Disorders

Objectives

1. Describe mechanisms of glucose homeostasis in the fetus and neonate.

2. Identify key features and usual management of common problems of glucose regulation in the neonatal period.

3. Describe the physiology of fluid and electrolyte (sodium, potassium, calcium, and magnesium) regulation in the newborn.

4. Identify etiologies of fluid and electrolyte imbalances in the newborn.

5. Delineate common approaches to maintaining fluid and electrolyte balance in the premature and sick neonate.

6. Describe the normal maintenance of acid-base equilibrium in the neonate, including metabolic acidosis and alkalosis.

7. Identify inborn errors of metabolism that may present in the neonatal period.

8. Outline the evaluation and initial management of an infant with a possible inborn error of metabolism.

9. Describe the long-term consequences of untreated metabolic disorders.

An essential part of successful transition to extrauterine life is the achievement of metabolic control. Because mature control of metabolic processes may not occur for many months after birth, premature and other stressed neonates can experience transient disturbances of glucose, fluid, electrolyte, and acid-base balance. Permanent metabolic disorders, such as those caused by inborn errors of metabolism, may also manifest in the neonatal period. Both transient and permanent metabolic derangements can be life threatening, so astute caretakers monitor metabolic functions closely in their neonatal patients.

Glucose Metabolism and Disorders

GLUCOSE HOMEOSTASIS

A. **Physiology.** Glucose is vital for normal cellular metabolism throughout the body and is the main energy substrate for the brain. Blood glucose concentration at any given time is determined by the balance between availability and utilization of glucose. Key concepts in glucose regulation include the following:

1. Glycolysis, the process of glucose utilization, can occur with oxygen (aerobic) or without oxygen (anaerobic). The anaerobic pathway requires significantly more fuel than aerobic metabolism.
2. Exogenous glucose not required for immediate energy needs is stored as glycogen in the liver, heart, and skeletal muscles. During starvation, glycogen is released into the bloodstream by a process called *glycogenolysis.*
3. Because hepatic glycogen is limited, another source of endogenous glucose is gluconeogenesis: the production of glucose from non-glucose substrates resulting from the breakdown of body fat and protein such as glycerol, lactate, pyruvate, and amino acids.

B. **Fetal glucose homeostasis.** A supply of glucose diffuses across the placenta. Glycogen storage for post-natal energy needs begins early in gestation, with most accumulating during the third trimester. Insulin, necessary for fetal growth, is detectable early in gestation, but the insulin response to a glucose load remains immature even at term.

C. **Neonatal glucose homeostasis.** At birth, metabolic adjustments must be made to achieve normoglycemia in spite of sudden withdrawal of placental glucose.

1. At birth the newborn's blood glucose is 70–80% of the maternal level.
2. The newborn's blood glucose level falls, reaching a nadir at 1–3 hours of age.
3. To meet high metabolic demands for glucose during this post-birth period of "starvation," plasma glucagon rises and, with other hormonal changes, triggers the endogenous production of glucose by releasing hepatic glycogen, activating lipolysis, and initiating gluconeogenesis. Liver glycogen is 90% diminished by 3 hours of age.
4. The newborn's basal blood glucose level rises progressively during the first days of life.

DISORDERS OF GLUCOSE METABOLISM

A. **Hypoglycemia.**

1. Pathophysiology of hypoglycemia.
   a. The normal post-natal drop in blood glucose can be magnified by increased glucose need, low glycogen or fat stores, and/or immature hormonal regulation of glucose.
   b. Due to the high glucose demand of the relatively large neonatal brain, the most devastating effect of low circulating glucose is neuronal damage. It is not known to what degree protective effects of alternate fuels for brain metabolism may be operating during hypoglycemia.
2. Etiologies of hypoglycemia.
   a. Inadequate production of glucose.
      (1) Pre-term infants—born before late pregnancy storage of glycogen.
      (2) Intrauterine growth retardation (IUGR)—low glycogen and fat stores, impaired gluconeogenesis.
      (3) Post-term infants—glycogen depletion from placental insufficiency.
      (4) Delayed feedings or conditions causing vomiting or malabsorption.
   b. Increased utilization of glucose.
      (1) Birth asphyxia/anoxia; respiratory distress—increased energy needs.
      (2) Cold stress—rapid depletion of glycogen.

(3) Polycythemia—increased utilization of glucose by red blood cells.
  c. Increased uptake of glucose related to hyperinsulinism.
    (1) Infant of diabetic mother (IDM).
    (2) Erythroblastosis fetalis.
    (3) Beckwith-Wiedemann syndrome.
    (4) Pancreatic islet cell adenoma/nesidioblastosis.
    (5) High glucose infusion or tocolytics used prior to delivery.
  d. Other etiologies.
    (1) Inborn errors of metabolism (e.g., galactosemia).
    (2) Endocrine disorders.
    (3) Iatrogenic: umbilical artery catheter (UAC) tip position near the pancreas.
3. Clinical presentation and assessment.
  a. Onset of hypoglycemia is usually in the first 6 hours of life.
  b. Many neonates are asymptomatic, especially pre-term infants.
  c. Symptoms most often described:
    (1) Tremors; jitteriness.
    (2) Abnormal cry (high pitched or weak).
    (3) Apnea, irregular respirations, cyanosis.
    (4) Lethargy, apathy, refusal to feed.
    (5) Hypotonia.
    (6) Eye rolling; seizures.
  d. Differentiation between jitteriness and seizures:
    (1) Jitteriness is fine, rhythmic tremulousness, usually in response to a stimulus; ceases with gentle flexion of the limb.
    (2) Seizures are clonic jerking movements that are not stimulus sensitive; can still be felt with passive flexion and may be associated with abnormal gaze/eye movement.
  e. Assessment of gestational age and measurement of body weight, length, and head circumference to determine if size is appropriate for gestational age due to increased risk of hypoglycemia in small (SGA) or large for gestational age (LGA) infants.
4. Diagnostic studies in hypoglycemia.
  a. Hypoglycemia. The lowest acceptable limit for blood glucose concentration in the newborn is controversial. Several approaches have been taken to define hypoglycemia:
    (1) Values of *plasma* glucose based on normative data (Cornblath and Schwartz, 1991).
      (a) Pre-term: <25 mg/dl.
      (b) Full-term: <72 hours of age—<35 mg/dl; ≥72 hours of age—<45 mg/dl.
    (2) Other widely used clinical definition: plasma glucose <40 mg/dl regardless of size or gestational age, based on the assumption that the pre-term or SGA infant's brain is no more tolerant to hypoglycemia than the full-term infant's brain. A level of 40 mg/dl (45 mg/dl after 24 hours of age) is thought to provide a safe margin for error.
    (3) Whatever glucose level produces symptoms in the infant, indicating true cellular glucose insufficiency.
  b. Blood glucose screening. Common rapid bedside methods utilize whole blood, an enzymatic reagent strip, and a color chart or a reflectance meter to read results. Limitations of these techniques include the following:
    (1) Underestimation of actual glucose level when whole blood is used, as glucose is primarily in plasma. Red blood cells are low in glucose, causing the test result to be approximately 10–15% lower than plasma values. The discrepancy is even greater in the presence of polycythemia.
    (2) Technical variables can drastically alter results, including timing of reaction, pressure applied during blotting or wiping, size and distribution of blood droplet on reagent strip, water temperature or strength of stream,

and difficulty using color comparison charts. Electronic devices remove some but not all of these variables.

c. Laboratory confirmation of test strip value—blood sample should be drawn from a warmed heel and placed on ice until analyzed. Concentration of glucose in the plasma, rather than whole blood, is measured, allowing a more accurate diagnosis of hypoglycemia.

5. Patient care management.
   a. Anticipate hypoglycemia in infants at risk; obtain good antenatal history and screen at increased frequency in the early hours of life until normoglycemic:
      (1) Begin at ½–1 hour of age; continue hourly for at least 4–6 hours.
      (2) Once stable, screen every 2–4 hours or before feedings for 24–48 hours.
   b. Provide glucose substrate through early enteral feeding of formula or breast milk or IV glucose at 4–8 mg/kg/min.
   c. If infant is symptomatic or does not respond to initial infusion of glucose, "mini-boluses" of $D_{10}W$ may be given (generally 2 ml/kg) and followed with a constant infusion.
   d. Infants with refractory hypoglycemia may require:
      (1) High concentrations of IV glucose; a central line should be used to administer concentrations >12.5%.
      (2) Hydrocortisone (reduces glucose utilization, promotes gluconeogenesis).
      (3) Glucagon (releases glycogen; used only in infants with adequate hepatic stores).

6. Complications.
   a. Rebound hypoglycemia—a result of transient hyperinsulinemia in response to a bolus of glucose.
   b. Skin/tissue necrosis from extravasation of high glucose concentrations in peripheral IV solutions—elevation of the affected area and subcutaneous injections of hyaluronidase may be helpful in limiting damage (Raszka et al., 1990).

7. Outcome.
   a. Neurological impairment is a long-term consequence of severe symptomatic hypoglycemia. Seizures are associated with increased CNS morbidity.
   b. Controversy exists as to whether asymptomatic hypoglycemia is a normal physiological phenomenon or can result in permanent CNS damage.

B. **Infant of the diabetic mother (IDM).**

1. Pathophysiology.
   a. Under conditions of maternal hyperglycemia, high glucose concentrations cross the placenta freely, but insulin does not.
   b. The fetal pancreas undergoes islet cell hypertrophy, producing insulin in response to the excessive glucose. This causes a high rate of fetal growth and, because of rapid glucose disposition, an exaggerated and sometimes persistent post-natal hypoglycemia.
   c. Severity of neonate's problems is related to the degree of maternal diabetic control during pregnancy.

2. Clinical presentation and assessment.
   a. Hypoglycemia may occur immediately after birth without symptoms.
   b. Typical IDMs are macrosomic/LGA. Evidence of birth injury may be present in these infants due to their large size. Some IDMs are small for gestational age due to placental insufficiency in advanced stages of diabetes.
   c. Prematurity.
   d. Respiratory distress syndrome. Fetal hyperinsulinemia may inhibit surfactant production, delaying lung maturation.
   e. Polycythemia: venous hematocrit >65%; plethoric appearance.
   f. Jaundice.
   g. Ruddy complexion, cherubic face.
   h. Congenital malformations (sacral dysgenesis, situs inversus, ureter duplex, renal agenesis, cardiac anomalies, anencephalus, holoprosencephaly, small

left colon syndrome) are two to three times more likely if mother has insulin-dependent diabetes during organogenesis. Precise etiology (teratogenic factors or genetic predisposition) is unknown.

3. Laboratory and diagnostic studies.
   a. Blood glucose screen with laboratory confirmation of plasma glucose.
   b. Calcium and magnesium levels due to risk of hypocalcemia or hypomagnesemia.
   c. Venous hematocrit to anticipate problems related to polycythemia.
   d. X-rays to rule out fractures resulting from traumatic delivery.
   e. Gastric aspirate and/or tracheal aspirate for analysis of phospholipids to rule out the risk of respiratory distress syndrome in symptomatic infants.
   f. Other tests to detect and diagnose congenital anomalies.
4. Patient care management.
   a. Anticipate problems of IDM prior to delivery. Obtain maternal and cord blood glucose concentrations at delivery, if possible.
   b. Monitor neonatal blood glucose immediately after birth and every 30 minutes for several hours.
   c. Provide early feeding (if indicated) and/or IV glucose. High glucose concentrations may be required.
   d. Monitor glucose levels prior to feedings when IV glucose is weaned.
5. Complications, in addition to those of hypoglycemia, include the following:
   a. Shoulder dystocia — occurs in macrosomic infants, particularly when mid-forceps delivery or vacuum extraction required; may result in brachial plexus injury (Erb's palsy) or fractures.
   b. Renal vein thrombosis — secondary to polycythemia/hyperviscosity.
6. Outcome.
   a. Perinatal mortality of the IDM has improved dramatically but continues to be approximately twice that of the normal population.
   b. Morbidities associated with IDM include neurological abnormalities, developmental delay, behavioral differences, obesity, and diabetes.
   c. Improved outcomes have been seen in infants of well-managed diabetics.

C. **Hyperglycemia.**
1. Pathophysiology. The extremely premature infant is often unable to tolerate full enteral feedings early in life and must be nourished by parenteral glucose infusions for long periods. Unable to suppress endogenous glucose production even if receiving an exogenous supply, and lacking mature insulin and glucagon control of glucose, these infants may not be able to tolerate glucose loads as low as 4 mg/kg/minute.
2. Etiologies of hyperglycemia (in addition to glucose intolerance).
   a. IUGR (may also have decreased insulin responsiveness to glucose).
   b. Excessive glucose load (>6–8 mg/kg/minute, exceeding the normal rate of glucose production of the liver).
   c. Medications, e.g., methylxanthines, corticosteroids, Intralipid infusions.
   d. Iatrogenic — related to infusion of glucose via UAC. Higher blood glucose values may be obtained from the heel on the same side as the iliac vessel used for cannulation (Jacob and Davis, 1988).
3. Clinical presentation and assessment of hyperglycemia.
   a. Onset as early as 24 hours, usually before 3 days of life.
   b. Often asymptomatic. Neurological signs may be secondary to CNS damage.
4. Laboratory and diagnostic studies.
   a. Definition of hyperglycemia: plasma glucose >150 mg/dl.
   b. Hyperglycemia may not be detected by whole blood screening alone.
   c. Urine glucose test. Very low birthweight (VLBW) infants have low renal threshold for glucose and may spill sugar at blood glucose levels as low as 80–100 mg/dl.
5. Differential diagnosis.
   a. Sepsis and infection.

      b. Transient neonatal diabetes.
6. Patient care management.
      a. Screen infants at risk for hyperglycemia, particularly VLBW infants.
      b. Decrease glucose load. Insulin may be used to normalize blood glucose without reducing caloric intake, thus promoting weight gain.
      c. Enteral feeding, if feasible, to promote tolerance of higher glucose load.
7. Complications.
      a. Hyperglycemia increases serum osmolality. If sustained, this may directly damage brain cells and contribute to intraventricular hemorrhage (IVH). High blood glucose levels do not guarantee adequate glucose uptake by the brain.
      b. Hyperglycemia can disrupt fluid and nutritional balance by causing osmotic free water loss, dehydration, and weight loss.
      c. Insulin management may be difficult in the extremely pre-term infant; blood sugar levels can fluctuate widely. A precisely controlled continuous infusion pump is essential.

Fluid Balance and Disorders

A. **Fluid balance in the newborn.**
1. Physiologic factors affecting fluid balance.
      a. Body water composition. Water, the most abundant component of the body, is distributed in two main compartments: intracellular fluid (ICF) and extracellular fluid (ECF), the latter being composed of intravascular and interstitial spaces. As gestation progresses, fetus undergoes a change in total body water (TBW) distribution:
        (1) At 24 weeks, TBW percentage is high; the majority is in ECF compartments.
        (2) By term, TBW is lower, and a greater percentage of fluid has shifted from ECF to ICF compartments. These changes are largely due to increases in body fat content with increasing gestation.
        (3) After birth, an acute increase in intravascular volume occurs, which can be influenced by the timing of cord clamping. Then all infants, regardless of gestational age, experience a contraction of ECF volume manifested by diuresis in the first week of life. This is considered physiological and is reflected in the usual post-natal weight loss of 5–10% in full-term and up to 20% in pre-term infant.
2. Renal function.
      a. Fetal kidneys produce urine as early as 5 weeks' gestation; volume increases with advancing gestation. The function of the kidneys in utero is to maintain amniotic fluid volume, whereas water and electrolyte balance is regulated by the placenta. Fetal nephrons are functional but immature until 34 weeks; renal blood flow, renal tubular function, and glomerular filtration rate (GFR) are all immature in the fetus and extremely pre-term infant.
      b. After birth, renal blood flow increases as renal vascular resistance falls. Improved renal function in the days after birth from increased GFR is more pronounced in the full-term than the pre-term infant.
      c. Both full-term and pre-term infants can dilute urine; however, when faced with a rapid fluid load, the pre-term infant may have a delayed response, resulting in fluid retention.
      d. Because of decreased responsiveness to antidiuretic hormone (ADH), neonates can not efficiently concentrate urine in response to fluid deprivation. Maximum concentrating ability of 600–800 mOsm/liter is about half that of the adult.
      e. The ability of the kidneys to reabsorb sodium, bicarbonate, and glucose is also limited in the newborn, particularly in the pre-term infant.

B. **Maintenance of fluid homeostasis.**

1. Post-natal influences on fluid balance. Fluid losses in the newborn period come from renal and extrarenal sources, which include the unquantifiable insensible water losses (IWL) of the skin and respiratory tract. A number of factors have been identified that may increase or decrease IWL in the neonatal period (Table 15–1). The thermal environment is particularly important to fluid balance.

   a. Renal losses. Urine output ranges from 1 to 4 ml/kg/hour; highest flow rates occur during the physiological reduction in ECF.

   b. Transepidermal water loss (TEWL). A function of immaturity, TEWL occurs as body water diffuses through the epidermis and is lost to the atmosphere. Because the epidermis is a poor barrier in the pre-term infant, TEWL can be as high as 40–150 ml/kg/day, compared with 10–15 ml/kg/day in the term infant. Other features of the skin that predispose to high evaporative losses are high skin water content, low subcutaneous fat, high surface area, and high skin vascularity. Barrier function of the skin improves by 2 weeks' post-natal age.

   c. Respiratory losses—estimated to be 0–10 ml/kg/day; related to temperature and humidity of inspired gases and minute ventilation.

   d. Stool losses—if stooling, losses estimated to be 5 ml/kg/day in the first week of life, increasing to 10 ml/kg/day thereafter.

   e. Other losses include gastric drainage, ostomies, surgical wounds.

2. Fluid requirements of the newborn. The goal of fluid therapy is to achieve normal hydration (normal electrolytes, osmolality, glucose, acid-base balance, and adequate blood volume) without placing undue demands on the body's immature organ systems. Generally, this means replacing urine volume plus an estimate of IWL to maintain body weight of at least 85–90% of birthweight.

   a. Fluid administration to premature and sick infants. The usual approach is as follows:

      (1) First day of life: relative fluid restriction of 60–100 ml/kg, depending on degree of control over evaporative and other fluid losses. Extremely pre-term infants may require more fluid relative to body weight because of high insensible losses.

      (2) On day 2 to 3, fluids may be increased slightly depending on renal response and body weight. Fluid restriction is maintained longer for infants with severe cardiorespiratory and other problems such as renal failure and perinatal asphyxia.

      (3) Thereafter, fluids are usually liberalized if indicated by adequate renal function, weight loss, and general improvement. Fluids are gradually increased to about 120–200 ml/kg/day by the end of first week.

   b. Fluid needs for growth of new tissue (after the initial weight loss): 6–15 ml/kg/day.

Table 15–1
ENVIRONMENTAL INFLUENCES ON IWL*

Factors that May Increase IWL	Factors that May Decrease IWL
Extreme prematurity	Increasing body weight/gestation
Post-natal age <1 week	Increasing post-natal age
Radiant warmer	Plastic film blanket on radiant warmer
Convection; drafts	Heat shield within incubator
High ambient temperature	Neutral thermal environment
Low humidity	High relative humidity; mist tent
Hyperthermia	Transparent dressings on skin
Ventilation with dry gases	Humidification of inspired gases
Phototherapy	Clothing
Activity	

*IWL, insensible water loss.

3. Assessment of fluid balance. Because calculations of fluid requirements may involve guesswork, close monitoring of hydration status is necessary to achieve the goals of fluid therapy.
   a. Measurement of body weight. Weight may change with alterations in fluid balance only if there is a change in total body water. Internal shifts of body fluid may not be detected by weight alone. Weighing small infants with accuracy is difficult because small errors (such as failure to subtract weight of an armboard) can have significant consequences if therapeutic decisions are based on body weight. Bed scales may improve accuracy by making the weighing procedure easier.
   b. Measurement of urine volume. Neonates, particularly premature infants, tend to void frequently in small amounts. If urine is collected onto diapers lying under radiant warmers, these volumes are subject to evaporation between the time of voiding and the time of weighing for determination of output. The smaller the voided volume, the higher rate of evaporation (Cooke et al., 1989).
   c. Urine specific gravity—an indirect measure of urine osmolality; if normal (1.002–1.012), specific gravity reflects a normal urine osmolarity (100–300 mOsm/liter). Unreliable if glucose, blood, or protein are in the urine.
   d. Assessment parameters—quality of skin turgor and mucous membranes, presence of edema, appearance of eyes, level of anterior fontanel. Hemodynamic assessment includes pulse quality, blood pressure, and perfusion (capillary refill time, temperature, acid-base balance).

DISORDERS OF FLUID BALANCE

A. **Fluid depletion (dehydration).**
1. Etiologies and precipitating factors.
   a. Extreme prematurity (<28 weeks, <800 g)—during first week of life can manifest a syndrome known as "hyperosmolar hypernatremic dehydration." With large TEWL, the ECF reservoir contracts rapidly, resulting in a sodium excess that cannot be excreted efficiently by the kidneys.
   b. Glycosuria with osmotic diuresis.
   c. Diarrhea.
   d. Diabetes insipidus—pure renal water loss related to failure to secrete or respond to ADH.
   e. Abdominal or pleural cavity exposure during surgery.
   f. Miscalculation of fluid losses; inadequate fluid intake.
2. Clinical presentation and assessment.
   a. Weight loss occurs if there is a reduction in TBW.
   b. Low urine output (<0.5 ml/kg/hour); specific gravity may be high. Urine output may be normal or high in the extremely low birthweight infant.
   c. Poor skin turgor (gently pinched skin is slow to retract), dry skin and mucous membranes; in severe cases, sunken fontanel or eyeballs.
   d. Hemodynamic changes may include tachycardia and/or increased pulses with peripheral vasoconstriction (pale, cool, mottled skin with prolonged capillary filling time); central blood pressure may be normal.
3. Laboratory and diagnostic tests.
   a. Serum sodium can be low, normal, or high depending on cause of dehydration.
   b. In hyperosmolar hypernatremic dehydration there may be several abnormalities: elevated serum sodium, potassium, and glucose; and glycosuria.
   c. Hematocrit may increase due to hemoconcentration.
   d. Tests of renal function (BUN, creatinine).
4. Differential diagnosis.
   a. Shock, hypovolemia.
   b. Renal failure.

5. Patient care management. Prevention is the most important aspect of managing hyperosmolar dehydration:
   a. Minimize TEWL from birth. Methods that have been successfully used to decrease TEWL include use of incubators, heat shields, plastic film "blankets," and supplemental humidity. Application of a semi-permeable polyurethane dressing directly to the skin of VLBW infants has been shown to reduce TEWL without affecting skin maturation (Knauth et al., 1989).
   b. Reduce respiratory water losses to zero by using only humidified gas mixtures for respiratory support.
   c. Fluid need is approximately 80–100 ml/kg/day with sodium restriction unless hyponatremic. Sodium is added gradually when serum sodium level decreases.
   d. Monitor hydration closely; weigh every 8–12 hours. Weight loss up to 20% is often tolerated if other parameters indicate adequate hydration.
   e. Giving too much fluid in response to hypernatremic dehydration can worsen the problem by aggravating hyperglycemia and increasing risk of heart failure, pulmonary edema, and CNS injury.
6. Complications.
   a. Excessive weight loss contributing to morbidity and mortality.
   b. Hypotension; tissue damage from hypoperfusion.
   c. Impaired excretion of drugs when urine output is minimal.
   d. Inadequate excretion of daily solute load, aggravating electrolyte imbalances.

B. Fluid overload.
1. Etiologies and precipitating factors.
   a. Poor cardiac function; congestive heart failure (CHF); patent ductus arteriosus (PDA).
   b. Bronchopulmonary dysplasia.
   c. Renal failure; hypoperfusion.
   d. Miscalculation of fluid needs; provision of too much fluid (may be due to failure to account for all sources of fluid such as flush solutions, medications, colloid).
   e. Syndrome of inappropriate antidiuretic hormone (SIADH)—most commonly encountered in infants with CNS infection or injury, but also seen in sick, stressed premature infants. ADH is secreted continuously or intermittently, inappropriate to usual osmotic and volume stimuli. The result is fluid retention with a low serum osmolality and low urine output.
2. Clinical presentation and assessment—varies with underlying cause of fluid overload.
   a. Weight gain (if there is a net increase in TBW).
   b. Urine output can be increased if kidneys are handling the fluid load normally; with renal failure and CHF, urine output is decreased.
   c. Peripheral edema (dorsum of hands, feet; pretibial; presacral; facial).
   d. Pulmonary edema, rales.
   e. Hemodynamic changes—may be a symptomatic PDA, tachycardia, increased pulses or blood pressure; with CHF, venous filling pressure is high.
3. Laboratory and diagnostic tests.
   a. Plasma osmolality is low (<280 mOsm/liter); urine osmolality is normal.
   b. In SIADH, osmolalities and sodium levels of urine and plasma are diagnostic: urine output is low with high specific gravity and sodium levels; serum sodium and osmolality are low.
   c. In CHF, sodium retention may be present.
   d. Tests of renal function may be ordered.
4. Patient care management.
   a. Cautious fluid management with consideration of renal function. Calculations of daily intake must take into account fluids given to administer medications and flush intravascular catheters.

b. Diuretics may be used in some cases.
c. Infants with severe edema need protective care for skin and joints.
5. Complications.
   a. Hyponatremia.
   b. Edema; cellular water intoxication. Sequestration of fluid in body tissues ("third spacing") can occur with a loss of effective intravascular volume.
   c. Excessive fluid administration early in life has been associated with worsening of respiratory distress syndrome, predisposition to the development of bronchopulmonary dysplasia, symptomatic PDA, and necrotizing enterocolitis.

Electrolyte Balance and Disorders

SODIUM

A. Sodium homeostasis.
1. Functions of sodium (Na). Na, the major extracellular cation, is closely involved in water balance. Na and other electrolytes are found in varying concentrations in all body fluid compartments; they determine the tonicity of the fluid compartment and influence the passage of water through vascular and cell membranes. In this way, electrolytes control the osmotic equilibrium between compartments. When serum Na is elevated, blood becomes hypertonic, causing a shift of fluid from intracellular to extracellular spaces, resulting in cellular dehydration. A low serum Na causes hypotonicity and a shift into intracellular spaces.
2. Regulation of Na. Na balance is influenced by aldosterone, a potent inhibitor of Na excretion. Normally, the kidneys filter Na, reabsorb most of it, and excrete a small amount. The pre-term infant's tendency to excrete too much Na is due to a decreased responsiveness to aldosterone and renin and often leads to negative Na balance. Paradoxically, due to a low GFR and renal blood flow, the extremely pre-term infant may be unable to excrete an Na load effectively. Thus, the pre-term infant is susceptible to both salt wasting and salt retention.

B. Disorders of sodium.
1. Hyponatremia.
   a. Pathophysiology. Na depletion can be associated with both dehydration and fluid overload. Excess excretion of Na can cause a proportionate loss of water (isotonic dehydration) with contraction of the ECF volume and renal failure. Without water loss, high Na loss results in hypotonic ECF, causing a shift of water into cells and cellular edema.
   b. Etiologies and precipitating factors.
      (1) Prematurity—renal and hormonal immaturity with tendency toward Na excretion.
      (2) Medications, e.g., indomethacin, furosemide, methylxanthines.
      (3) Water retention due to SIADH.
      (4) Dilutional hyponatremia due to excessive free water intake.
      (5) Inadequate Na intake during period of rapid growth.
   c. Clinical presentation and assessment.
      (1) May be asymptomatic or present with signs if fluid overload (edema) or dehydration.
      (2) Apnea, irritability, twitching, or seizures if Na drops acutely.
   d. Laboratory and diagnostic studies.
      (1) Serum Na low (<130 mEq/liter) and osmolality low (<280 mOsm/liter).
      (2) Urine Na excretion rate to rule out excessive Na^+ losses.
      (3) Glucose level to check for concurrent hyperglycemia.
   e. Differential diagnosis.
      (1) SIADH.
      (2) Congenital adrenal hyperplasia (salt-losing form).

f. Patient care management.
   (1) Na supplementation after post-natal diuresis begins (usually day 2). Maintain adequate Na intake in IV/oral nutrition.
   (2) Monitor weight, urine output, parameters of hydration, and adequacy of intravascular volume.
   (3) SIADH is managed with fluid restriction and monitoring Na, osmolality, and urine output.
g. Complications.
   (1) If SIADH is not recognized and Na is administered for hyponatremia, the problem can be worsened by expanding the ECF volume.
   (2) Hyponatremia reduces plasma osmolality, creating an osmotic gradient at the blood-brain barrier. Fluid moves into the cells of the brain causing cerebral edema. Too rapid correction of low Na may be harmful because the brain cannot adjust quickly enough to the rising osmolality.
   (3) Poor growth due to chronic hyponatremia.
2. Hypernatremia.
   a. Pathophysiology. The extremely premature infant may have an impaired ability to excrete a high Na load. Usually, hypernatremia reflects a deficiency of water relative to total body Na content and is actually a disorder of water balance rather than a disorder of Na balance.
   b. Etiology and precipitating factors.
      (1) Excessive IWL with insufficient fluid intake leading to hypernatremic dehydration.
      (2) High Na intake inadvertently administered to infant: maintenance NaCl, arterial line infusions, $NaHCO_3$, medications.
      (3) Diabetes insipidus—deficiency of pituitary-secreted hormone vasopressin (ADH) causing loss of water in excess of loss of Na.
   c. Clinical presentation and assessment.
      (1) Signs of dehydration.
      (2) Neurological signs of severe hypernatremia: high-pitched cry, listlessness, irritability, apnea. Can progress to seizures and coma.
   d. Laboratory and diagnostic studies.
      (1) Serum Na (>150 mEq/liter) and osmolality (>300 mOsm/liter).
   e. Patient care management.
      (1) Gradual Na restriction to avoid sudden fall in plasma osmolality. If maintenance Na has not been started, it is usually delayed.
      (2) Hypernatremic dehydration is managed as described above.
      (3) In extreme cases, exchange transfusion may be necessary.
   f. Complications. As hypernatremia develops, intracellular water can be depleted, causing cells to shrink. In the brain, this may contribute to CNS injury. IVH may result from a sudden increase in plasma osmolality.

POTASSIUM

A. **Potassium homeostasis.**
1. Functions of potassium (K)—the major cation in ICF; K contributes to intracellular osmotic activity and in part determines ICF volume. K plays a fundamental role along with Na in membrane transport and in the propagation of nerve and muscle action potential.
2. Regulation of potassium. The amount and distribution of K in the body is influenced by renal excretion, GFR, aldosterone, insulin, and acid-base balance.

B. **Disorders of potassium.**
1. Hypokalemia.
   a. Pathophysiology. Because K is 90% intracellular, it is assessed indirectly by measuring the quantity in the serum. A low serum K implies insufficient K within the cells, which may impede cellular function.
   b. Etiology and precipitating factors.
      (1) Excessive renal wasting of K secondary to diuretic therapy.

(2) Increased GI losses from an ostomy or nasogastric tube.
(3) Insulin therapy.
(4) Bicarbonate therapy; metabolic alkalosis.
(5) Inadequate K intake.
c. Clinical presentation and assessment.
   (1) Cardiac effects are common: flattened T waves, prominent U waves, ST depression.
   (2) Muscle weakness; ileus.
d. Laboratory and diagnostic studies.
   (1) Serum K (<3.5 mEq/liter); must be interpreted with acid-base status in mind because alkalosis drives K into cells, resulting in a low serum K.
   (2) EKG to evaluate for myocardial dysfunction.
e. Patient care management.
   (1) Begin K supplementation when urine output is well established, usually on the second to third day of life.
   (2) To correct hypokalemia, increase K gradually, monitoring serum K.
f. Complication. Hypokalemia potentiates digitalis toxicity.

2. Hyperkalemia.
   a. Pathophysiology. Owing to immature tubular function and poor response to aldosterone, the neonatal kidneys may not handle an increased K load.
   b. Etiology and precipitating factors.
      (1) Endogenous release of K from tissue destruction, acidosis, hypoperfusion, hemorrhage, bruising.
      (2) Renal failure.
      (3) Extreme prematurity (non-oliguric hyperkalemia).
      (4) Adrenal insufficiency.
      (5) Spurious value from heel stick sample (due to hemolysis of cells).
      (6) Transfusion with blood >3 days old.
      (7) Metabolic acidosis: low intracellular pH causes K leakage from cells.
   c. Clinical presentation and assessment.
      (1) Muscle weakness.
      (2) Cardiac effects: ventricular tachycardia, peaked T wave, widened QRS. The more rapid the rise in K, the more serious the cardiac toxicity.
   d. Laboratory and diagnostic studies.
      (1) Serum K (>7.0 mEq/liter)—drawn from venipuncture or arterial line. Must consider acid-base status, because acidosis shifts K out of cells.
      (2) Tests of renal function: BUN, creatinine.
      (3) EKG to evaluate for myocardial dysfunction.
   e. Patient care management.
      (1) Restrict K intake; monitor serum K.
      (2) If cardiac changes are evident, other forms of treatment include the following:
         (a) Calcium gluconate—lowers cell membrane threshold transiently, antagonizing the effects on the heart muscle.
         (b) Glucose and insulin—expand ECF volume, increase intracellular uptake of K, and may increase excretion of K. Because overall K content in the body may not decrease with this therapy, strategies to remove K from the body may also be required.
         (c) $NaHCO_3$—decreases serum K by shifting K into cells.
         (d) Cation exchange resin (Kayexalate)—Na is exchanged for K in the intestine to increase excretion of K.
         (e) Exchange transfusion.
         (f) Peritoneal dialysis for severe, intractable hyperkalemia.
   f. Complications.
      (1) Hyperkalemia is life threatening; can lead to cardiac arrest.
      (2) Kayexalate can cause hypocalcemia, hypomagnesemia, hypernatremia.

CALCIUM

A. **Calcium homeostasis.**

1. Functions of calcium (Ca)—plays a central role in many physiological processes: maintains cell membrane permeability; activates enzyme reactions for muscle contraction, nerve transmission, and blood clotting. Ca is vital for normal cardiac function and development of the skeleton, where 99% of the body's Ca is stored.
2. Regulation of calcium—hormonal and non-hormonal influences.
   a. Parathyroid hormone (PTH) increases serum Ca by mobilizing Ca from bone and intestines and reducing renal excretion of Ca. PTH is stimulated by low serum Ca or magnesium (Mg) levels and is suppressed by high Ca and Mg levels.
   b. Vitamin D—acts with PTH to restore Ca to normal levels by increasing absorption of Ca and phosphorus from the intestines and bone.
   c. Calcitonin—a Ca counter-regulatory hormone; lowers Ca levels by antagonizing the Ca mobilizing effects of PTH on bone and intestines.
3. Serum Ca is transported in three forms:
   a. Protein-bound calcium.
   b. Inactivated Ca (complexed with bicarbonate, phosphorus, or citrate).
   c. Free ionized calcium (iCa)—physiologically active form, capable of being transported across the cell membrane. Amount of iCa depends on serum protein content, blood pH, and other factors. Acidosis increases iCa; alkalosis decreases iCa.

B. **Fetal calcium metabolism.** Fetal Ca needs are met by active transport of Ca across the placenta. Ca accretion by the fetus increases during the last trimester because Ca is incorporated into newly forming bones. Because maternal PTH and calcitonin do not cross the placenta, the fetus is relatively hypercalcemic, which suppresses fetal PTH and stimulates fetal calcitonin.

C. **Neonatal calcium metabolism.** When the supply of Ca ceases at birth, the neonate must rely on endogenous stores and dietary Ca to avoid hypocalcemia. After birth, Ca level declines, reaching its physiological nadir at 24 hours, but PTH activity nevertheless remains low. By 48–72 hours of age, PTH and vitamin D levels rise and calcitonin declines, allowing Ca to be mobilized. Serum Ca is thus normalized despite a low Ca intake.

D. **Disorders of calcium metabolism.**

1. Hypocalcemia.
   a. Pathophysiology. Failure to achieve Ca homeostasis after birth can occur from inadequate Ca stores, immature hormonal control, inability to mobilize Ca, or interference with Ca utilization.
   b. Precipitating factors and etiologies of early hypocalcemia.
      (1) Premature infants—miss much of third-trimester stores of Ca and are relatively hypoparathyroid (blunted PTH response to hypocalcemia).
      (2) IDM—prolonged delay in PTH production after birth.
      (3) Placental insufficiency—reduced Ca stores.
      (4) Birth asphyxia and stress—precipitate a surge in calcitonin, which suppresses Ca levels. In addition, tissue damage and glycogen breakdown release phosphorus into the circulation, which decreases Ca uptake.
      (5) Treatment with $NaHCO_3$—shifts Ca from ionized to protein-bound form, decreasing its effectiveness.
      (6) Low dietary intake—fasting, insufficient maintenance Ca.
      (7) Iatrogenic—exchange transfusion can cause hypocalcemia because the Ca ions complex to citrate in citrate-preserved blood.
   c. Late hypocalcemia may be caused by:
      (1) Maternal hyperparathyroidism (fetal/neonatal hypoparathyroidism).

(2) High phosphate formula—newborn kidney has difficulty excreting the excess phosphate, causing hyperphosphatemia, which suppresses Ca.

(3) Intestinal malabsorption.

(4) Hypomagnesemia.

(5) DiGeorge syndrome—absence of thymus and parathyroid glands.

(6) Furosemide therapy.

d. Clinical presentation and assessment.

(1) Mild hypocalcemia is usually asymptomatic; signs of neuromuscular hyperactivity (jitteriness, twitching, high-pitched cry) may be observed.

(2) Severe, symptomatic hypocalcemia (neonatal tetany) is rare—presents with extreme jitteriness, seizures, laryngospasm, stridor, prolonged QT interval; associated with hypomagnesemia.

e. Laboratory and diagnostic studies.

(1) Serum total calcium (<7 mg/dl); ionized Ca if testing is available. Proportion of iCa cannot be reliably predicted from the total serum Ca.

(2) Magnesium, phosphorus levels and determination of acid-base balance.

f. Patient care management.

(1) Monitor serum Ca of infants at risk (premature, SGA, asphyxiated, IDM). Prophylactic supplemental Ca is often given to infants at risk for hypocalcemia.

(2) Early, mild hypocalcemia often resolves without treatment.

(3) Severe hypocalcemia treated with boluses and/or maintenance infusion of calcium gluconate; continuous infusion usually preferred over boluses.

(4) Treatment of late hypocalcemia depends on the underlying cause.

g. Complications.

(1) Rapid infusions of parenteral Ca can cause bradycardia or cardiac arrest. Boluses, if required, should be administered slowly while monitoring heart rate. Infusing parenteral Ca over 20–30 minutes by syringe pump effectively prevents this complication.

(2) Tissue necrosis and calcifications from extravasated Ca. Peripheral infiltrations respond to treatment with subcutaneous hyaluronidase.

(3) Intestinal and liver necrosis have been reported with Ca infusion given via umbilical catheters.

(4) Rickets can be a long-term complication of problematic Ca homeostasis. Demineralization of the bone may occur despite adequate intake.

2. Hypercalcemia.

a. Pathophysiology. A rise in serum Ca level can rapidly overwhelm the infant's compensatory mechanisms for Ca equilibrium. An excess supply of Ca has multiple effects and is potentially lethal.

b. Etiology and precipitating factors.

(1) Hyperparathyroidism—primary neonatal disorder or secondary to maternal hypoparathyroidism with chronic stimulation of the fetal parathyroid gland.

(2) Phosphate depletion—low dietary intake; may be associated with low phosphate content in human milk.

(3) Subcutaneous fat necrosis—precedes hypocalcemia; pathogenic mechanism unknown.

(4) Idiopathic infantile hypercalcemia—abnormal vitamin D metabolism.

(5) Iatrogenic—overtreatment with calcium infusion.

c. Clinical presentation and assessment.

(1) Hypotonia, weakness, irritability and poor feeding (neurological signs and symptoms due to a direct effect of Ca on the CNS).

(2) Hypertension.

(3) Weight loss, vomiting.

(4) Constipation.

(5) Polyuria/dehydration—due to interference with action of ADH.

(6) Fat necrosis — found over back and limbs; associated with difficult delivery, hypothermia, IDM.
d. Laboratory and diagnostic tests.
  (1) Serum Ca (>11 mg/dl).
  (2) In hyperparathyroidism, serum phosphate levels may be low, urine Ca and phosphate excretion high.
  (3) EKG — cardiac effects include shortened QT interval and arrhythmias.
  (4) Radiological evidence of skeletal demineralization.
e. Patient care management.
  (1) Correct the primary cause, if possible. Hyperparathyroidism may require subtotal parathyroidectomy.
  (2) Promote excretion of Ca — furosemide has calciuretic effect.
  (3) Restrict dietary Ca intake; increase intake of phosphate if needed.
  (4) Glucocorticoids decrease intestinal absorption of Ca.
  (5) Calcitonin infusion may be given to oppose the effects of PTH.
f. Complications.
  (1) Nephrocalcinosis; renal failure; renal tubular acidosis.
  (2) Metastatic calcification of damaged cells/tissues throughout body, including the brain.
  (3) Hypertensive encephalopathy.

MAGNESIUM

A. Magnesium homeostasis.
1. Functions of magnesium (Mg). Mg is a catalyst for many intracellular enzyme reactions, including muscle contraction and carbohydrate metabolism. Mg is critical for normal parathyroid function and bone–serum Ca homeostasis.
2. Fetal and neonatal magnesium homeostasis. The fetus receives its supply of Mg by active transport across the placenta. Maternal health and diet can influence the amount of Mg accrued by the fetus. After birth, Mg level normally falls along with Ca level, then rises to normal within 48 hours.

B. Disorders of magnesium.
1. Hypomagnesemia.
  a. Pathophysiology. A low Mg level in a neonate is directly related to the maternal level prior to birth. Although an acute decline in Mg stimulates PTH release, chronic Mg deficiency suppresses PTH and blocks the hormone's actions on the bone and kidneys. Hypocalcemia ensues.
  b. Etiologies and precipitating factors. Hypomagnesemia is associated with the following:
    (1) Hypocalcemia.
    (2) Prematurity.
    (3) Placental insufficiency: IUGR.
    (4) IDM.
    (5) Maternal Mg deficiency or hyperparathyroidism.
    (6) Increased phosphate load.
    (7) Malabsorption, diarrhea, vomiting, nasogastric suction.
    (8) Exchange transfusion — citrate also binds Mg.
    (9) Diuretic therapy — furosemide leads to Mg wasting.
  c. Clinical presentation and assessment. Because the major effect of low Mg is on Ca levels, the infant usually presents with hypocalcemia and may have the associated symptoms: eye rolling, twitching, tetany, muscle weakness, and focal or generalized seizures. Hypomagnesemia should be considered in any infant who does not respond to therapy for hypocalcemia.
  d. Laboratory and diagnostic studies — serum Mg level (<1.5 mg/dl).
  e. Patient care management.
    (1) Treat hypocalcemia.

(2) If severe, administration of magnesium sulfate may be necessary to relieve symptoms until Ca balance is restored.

(3) Seizures are usually unresponsive to anticonvulsants.

f. Complications. Overtreatment with magnesium sulfate can result in hypotonia and respiratory depression, hypotension, and cardiac arrhythmias.

2. Hypermagnesemia.

a. Pathophysiology. An excessive load of Mg, from the mother or an exogenous source, is slow to be excreted by the neonatal kidneys. In the meantime, precipitous Mg levels can cause CNS and neuromuscular depression with a marked decrease in skeletal muscle contractility.

b. Etiology and precipitating factors.

(1) Magnesium sulfate treatment for pre-term labor.

(2) Excessive administration of Mg.

(3) Antacid therapy for gastric irritation and bleeding.

c. Clinical presentation and assessment.

(1) Respiratory depression, apnea.

(2) Neuromuscular depression: lethargy, poor suck, loss of reflexes, muscle weakness, hypotonia.

(3) GI hypomotility, abdominal distention.

(4) Hypotension, cardiac arrhythmias.

(5) Infants may also be asymptomatic.

d. Laboratory and diagnostic studies—high serum Mg (>2.5 mg/dl).

e. Patient care management.

(1) Prepare to resuscitate infants born to mothers receiving large doses of magnesium sulfate.

(2) General supportive care for hypotension, respiratory distress.

(3) Administer calcium gluconate to counteract effects of Mg. Urinary Mg can be increased with administration of furosemide.

(4) If unresponsive to treatment, exchange transfusion may be necessary.

Acid-Base Balance

A. Acid-base physiology.

1. pH. Acid-base balance is normal when the pH of the blood is between 7.35 and 7.45. pH is determined by the hydrogen ion (H^+) concentration in ECF. A complex system of buffers, conservation, and excretion regulates the H^+ concentration, thus keeping the pH in the normal range.

2. Buffering system—first line of defense against excess H^+ concentration. Buffers, including bicarbonate (HCO_3^-), plasma proteins, and hemoglobin, act rapidly to pick up excess H^+. The major buffer, HCO_3^- teams with H^+ to form carbonic acid, which dissociates into water and CO_2 and can be eliminated.

3. Lung regulation. The lungs remove large amounts of carbonic acid from the body in the form of CO_2. The rate of removal can be increased or decreased by altering minute ventilation.

4. Kidney regulation. The kidney acts to maintain the equilibrium between acids and bases in the body by excreting H^+ and other acids, and reabsorbing HCO_3 and other buffers. In this way, the body eliminates the daily load of non-volatile acids produced by normal metabolism.

5. Compensation. When one or more of the body's regulatory systems fails, other systems have a limited ability to maintain the acid-base equilibrium. When the pH is outside of the normal range (<7.35 or >7.45), compensatory mechanisms have failed.

a. An acid-base deviation is termed *respiratory* if it is due to an abnormal P_{CO_2} level and *metabolic* if due to an abnormal level of plasma HCO_3^-.

b. The lungs attempt to compensate for a metabolic aberration, and the kidneys for a respiratory aberration. The result is a change in pH toward normal despite abnormal blood P_{CO_2} or HCO_3^-. The lungs compensate much more quickly than the kidneys; however, neither can totally normalize the pH unless the underlying disorder is corrected.

B. **Disorders of acid-base balance.** Only those classified as primary metabolic problems are discussed here.

1. Metabolic acidosis.
   a. Pathophysiology. A pH below 7.35 can be the result of loss of bicarbonate (buffering capacity) or excess acid production. The normal HCO_3^- level in the neonate is 18–21 mEq/liter, lower than in the adult. Immature or dysfunctional organ systems, including the lungs and kidneys in the premature or sick neonate, contribute to acidosis.
   b. Etiologies and precipitating factors.
      (1) Loss of bicarbonate.
         (a) Failure of the kidney to conserve HCO_3^-. The common acidosis of prematurity is partly due to low renal threshold for HCO_3^-.
         (b) Renal tubular acidosis.
         (c) Severe diarrhea.
         (d) Rapid ECF expansion.
      (2) Excess acid load—ingestion or endogenous production of acid that cannot be handled by the neonate.
         (a) Inborn errors of metabolism (disorders of amino acid, organic acid, and carbohydrate metabolism).
         (b) Conditions resulting in hypoxia or hypoperfusion, leading to anaerobic metabolism and lactic acidosis (respiratory distress, congenital heart disease, PDA, sepsis, asphyxia, hypotension, shock, hypothermia, anemia, hypoglycemia).
         (c) Calorie deprivation—catabolism of protein or fat for energy.
         (d) New bone formation during growth—when Ca is incorporated into bone, H^+ is liberated.
         (e) Intolerance of dietary protein and amino acids.
      (3) Underexcretion of acid—immaturity, damage or hypoperfusion affecting the kidney's ability to excrete acid; can be due to shock or hypoxic renal damage. Pre-term infants have difficulty excreting H^+.
   c. Clinical presentation and assessment.
      (1) Presenting signs depend on underlying cause.
      (2) Lethargy, seizures, or coma reflect CNS acidosis.
      (3) In some infants, there may be evidence of respiratory compensation: increased rate (tachypnea) or depth (hyperpnea) of breathing.
      (4) Laboratory and diagnostic studies.
         (a) Blood pH < 7.35 (acidemia).
         (b) Serum HCO_3^- level (<18 mEq).
         (c) Anion gap to differentiate between excess acid and insufficient HCO_3^- as cause of acidosis: anion gap = (serum $Na^+ + K^+$) − (serum $Cl^- + HCO_3^-$). Usual range is 8–16 mEq. If high (>20 mEq), acidosis is due to excess acid. If normal with elevated serum Cl^-, acidosis is due to loss of HCO_3^-).
         (d) Urine pH >7 with systemic acidosis suggests renal tubular acidosis. If low (<5), kidneys are excreting acid adequately.
         (e) Other blood gases to rule out primary respiratory problem.
   d. Patient care management.
      (1) Treat underlying problem.
      (2) Correction of severe acidosis (pH < 7.2).
         (a) $NaHCO_3$—concentration 0.5 mEq/ml, 1–2 mEq/kg dose. Administer slowly by syringe pump or by continuous drip; rapid increase in osmolality and pH may be dangerous.
         (b) Tromethamine (THAM)—alkali with advantage of not contributing to Na load. Lowers Pco_2; has rapid cellular penetration but 50% less base activity than $NaHCO_3$.

   e. Complications.
      (1) Severe acidosis can depress myocardial contractility and cause arteriolar vasodilatation, hypotension, and pulmonary edema.
      (2) Impaired surfactant production.
      (3) Electrolyte imbalance: decreased ionized calcium; hyperkalemia.
      (4) Adverse effects of $NaHCO_3$ include cerebral hemorrhage or edema related to wide swings in plasma osmolity. $NaHCO_3$ can also worsen acidosis by rapidly increasing CO_2 if lung disease is present and ventilation is inadequate. $NaHCO_3$ can aggravate hyponatremia and cause tissue injury if extravasated.
2. Metabolic alkalosis.
   a. Pathophysiology—an increase in extracellular HCO_3^-; may be due to abnormally low H^+ concentration.
   b. Etiologies and precipitating factors.
      (1) Gain of HCO_3^-—alkali therapy; exchange transfusion.
      (2) Loss of H^+—vomiting, nasogastric suction, furosemide therapy (promotes excretion of K^+ and H^+).
      (3) Compensation for chronic respiratory acidosis.
      (4) Rapid ECF reduction.
   c. Clinical presentation and assessment. Presenting signs depend on underlying cause or primary disorder.
   d. Laboratory and diagnostic studies.
      (1) Blood pH > 7.45 (alkalemia).
      (2) Serum HCO_3^- increased (>26 mEq/liter).
   e. Patient care management.
      (1) Decrease HCO_3 intake if alkali therapy is cause of alkalosis.
      (2) Restoring fluid and electrolyte balance is critical.
   f. Complications. Severe alkalosis can cause:
      (1) Tissue hypoxia, neurological damage, seizures.
      (2) Electrolyte disturbances: increased ionized calcium, hypokalemia.
      (3) Impairment of tissue oxygen delivery.

Inborn Errors of Metabolism

A. **Common features.** Occasionally, a very ill neonate is admitted to the neonatal intensive care unit and no cause can be found for derangements such as acidosis, hyperglycemia, and seizures. Some of these infants will have an inborn error of metabolism (IEM), which is an inherited disorder that can lead to irreversible brain damage or even death. There are more than 500 known errors of metabolism. Individually, most are very rare, but collectively they contribute significantly to neonatal morbidity and mortality.
1. Pathophysiology of IEM.
   a. The lesion that disrupts normal metabolism is usually the absence or deficiency of a critical enzyme. When important biochemical reactions are blocked, various precursors and metabolites can accumulate, most of which are toxic to tissues and organs, including the CNS.
   b. The fetus is usually unaffected because the placenta effectively removes toxins; thus, the neonate is generally born at term in good health.
   c. Inheritance pattern of most metabolic disorders is autosomal recessive.
2. Clinical presentation of IEM.
   a. With few exceptions, infants with metabolic disease appear normal at birth. Within hours, days, or weeks, non-specific signs and symptoms may appear that could be attributed to many different disorders in the neonate. Sepsis neonatorum and CNS pathology may at first be suspected. A metabolic cause should be considered in any sick neonate, because many of the disorders can be treated only if detected early.

b. Clues that point to the possibility of an IEM include the following:
   (1) Failure of a sick neonate to respond to usual therapies.
   (2) Unusual severity and intractability of problems such as metabolic acidosis.
   (3) Acute onset: rapid progression of symptoms.
   (4) A full-term neonate with onset of symptoms after an interval of apparent normal health after birth, or symptoms that correspond with introduction of milk feedings.
   (5) A history of previous unexplained neonatal death in the family or parental consanguinity.
c. Clinical assessment may reveal all or some of the following:
   (1) Neurological signs, ranging from lethargy, irritability, and weak suck to tremors, seizures, flaccidity, or rigidity and coma.
   (2) Respiratory distress secondary to neurological depression or compensatory hyperpnea or tachypnea from severe metabolic acidosis.
   (3) GI symptoms — vomiting, diarrhea, poor feeding, failure to gain weight.
   (4) Unusual odor or color of the urine, suggesting certain metabolic errors.
d. Laboratory findings — vary with individual disorders.
3. Diagnosis of IEM.
   a. Prenatal diagnosis: amniocentesis or chorionic biopsy and DNA analysis.
   b. Newborn screening.
      (1) Tests available for a wide array of inborn errors. The battery used for routine screening in each U.S. state varies; many test for phenylketonuria (PKU), galactosemia, maple syrup urine disease, tyrosinemia, and homocystinuria. PKU testing is mandated by law throughout Canada.
      (2) Newborn screening alone cannot be relied on to detect all inborn errors because in some instances (e.g., maple syrup urine disease) irreversible damage occurs before results of newborn screening are known. A small percentage of infants with hypothyroidism or homocystinuria will not be picked up on the newborn screen.
      (3) Infants discharged before 24 hours of age should have a PKU repeated at 2–3 weeks of age; infants who expire should be screened also. Some states repeat the entire genetic screen at 2–3 weeks of age.
   c. Neonatal diagnosis: several levels of investigation.
      (1) For suspicion of an IEM, general tests such as blood gases, plasma NH_4, blood glucose, urinary ketones, and urine-reducing substances help to classify the disorder for purposes of immediate management.
      (2) A metabolic screen of blood or urine is performed to determine the type of disorder (e.g., urea cycle defect).
      (3) Enzyme analysis of blood, urine, cerebrospinal fluid, and skin or other tissues will establish a definitive diagnosis.
   d. Post-mortem diagnosis: if a neonate dies before a diagnosis has been established, the following should be collected for analysis: blood, urine, biopsies of skin and liver. Only when an exact diagnosis is found can prenatal testing be offered for subsequent pregnancies.
4. Patient care management.
   a. General supportive care: respiratory support; antibiotics; fluids; correct electrolyte imbalances; attempt to correct acidosis.
   b. Nutrition. In the absence of a specific diagnosis, the goal is to induce an anabolic state. If organic acid or urea cycle defects are suspected, protein intake should be stopped. A high-calorie intake with glucose and fat (and insulin if necessary) will suppress catabolism and production of toxic metabolites and encourage anabolism of endogenous protein. A central venous line may be required to maintain high-calorie infusions.
   c. Megavitamins in pharmacological doses may benefit infants with certain disorders. Vitamin B_{12}, biotin, riboflavin, nicotinamide, and thiamine have all been used alone or in combination; pyridoxine is life saving in pyridoxine-dependent seizures.

d. Hemodialysis—most rapid and efficient way to remove toxic substances distributed throughout the body.
e. Peritoneal dialysis—less effective then hemodialysis.
f. Exchange transfusion—may transiently improve infant's condition. Removes only metabolites bound to plasma, thus is ineffective in removing metabolites distributed in the total body water.
g. Long-term therapy is dietary and varies depending on specific disorder.

Specific Disorders of Metabolism

The most common disorders presenting in the neonatal period are listed in Table 15–2.

A. Disorders of amino acid metabolism.
1. Phenylketonuria (PKU)—deficiency of the liver enzyme needed for conversion of phenylalanine to tyrosine. Phenylalanine is normally produced in the breakdown of tissue protein and from digestion of dietary protein. When its conversion to tyrosine is blocked, phenylalanine accumulates in body fluids and causes CNS damage.
   a. Incidence: 1:15,000.

Table 15–2
INBORN ERRORS OF METABOLISM WITH NEONATAL ONSET

Amino Acid Disorders
Phenylketonuria*
Maple syrup urine disease*
Non-ketotic hyperglycinemia
Hereditary tyrosinemia*

Organic Acid Disorders
Isovaleric acidemia
Propionic acidemia
Glutaric acidemia type II
Methylmalonic acidemia
Biotinidase/multiple carboxylase deficiency*

Urea Cycle Defects/Hyperammonemia
Carbamyl phosphate synthetase deficiency
Ornithine transcarbamylase deficiency
Citrullinemia
Argininosuccinic aciduria
Arginase deficiency
Transient hyperammonemia of the newborn

Disorders of Carbohydrate Metabolism
Galactosemia*
Hereditary fructose intolerance
Fructose-1,-6-diphosphatase deficiency
Pyruvate dehydrogenase deficiency
Pyruvate carboxylase deficiency
Glycogen storage disease

Other
Lysosomal storage disorders
Congenital adrenal hyperplasia*
Cystic fibrosis*
α_1-Antitrypsin deficiency
G6PD deficiency
Pyridoxine deficiency

   *Newborn screening test available.

b. Presentation: effects begin after birth; symptoms usually appear after 3 months of age. Early symptoms include vomiting, feeding difficulties, irritability, overactivity, infantile eczema, hypopigmented skin and hair, and "musty" smelling urine (due to phenylacetic acid).

c. Management: dietary restriction of phenylalanine. Treatment should begin as early as possible.

d. Outcome: mental retardation results from untreated PKU; 95% will have IQ <50. With diet, intelligence can be in the normal range. As more patients with PKU survive, effects of maternal untreated PKU on the fetus are becoming known: microcephaly, mental retardation, and congenital heart disease can occur even in infants without PKU.

2. Maple syrup urine disease (MSUD)—absence of enzymes required for a step in the degradation of three branched-chain amino acids: leucine, isoleucine, and valine. These amino acids are converted to highly toxic ketoacids that cannot be oxidized and therefore accumulate in the blood.

a. Incidence: 1:250,000 to 1:300,000.

b. Presentation: infants appear normal at birth but by first 48–72 hours present with vomiting, rapid shallow respirations, high-pitched cry, hypotonicity alternating with hypertonicity, followed by seizures and coma. Severe acidosis and hypoglycemia are common. Urine may have characteristic sweet maple syrup odor.

c. Management: peritoneal dialysis to clear ketoacids and amino acids; thiamine administration may benefit some infants.

d. Outcome: neonates die very quickly if untreated. Mental retardation is not avoidable if symptoms occur prior to treatment.

B. Disorders of organic acid metabolism.

1. Pathophysiology. Organic acids are intermediate metabolites of amino acid metabolism. When an enzyme defect prevents its metabolism, the affected organic acid accumulates, causing CNS damage and placing a significant burden on the immature kidneys. The most common disorder is methylmalonic acidemia.

2. Presentation—metabolic acidosis with compensatory hyperpnea, feeding difficulties and vomiting, CNS depression, seizures, hypoglycemia, electrolyte disturbances, leukopenia, thrombocytopenia, and hyperammonemia. A hallmark is an elevated anion gap. Isovaleric acidemia produces an odor reminiscent of "sweaty feet."

3. Management. In addition to protein restriction, dialysis, and megavitamin, carnitine and glycine have been administered in some organic acidemias to provide an alternative pathway for excretion of toxic compounds.

C. Disorders of urea cycle/hyperammonemia.

1. Pathophysiology. The urea cycle is the major pathway for detoxification of ammonia, a by-product of nitrogen degradation. A defect can occur at any of the five steps in the cycle, resulting in accumulation of ammonia and profound encephalopathy.

2. Presentation. Progressive illness begins with poor feeding, vomiting, and dehydration. Drowsiness is followed by seizures, coma, cardiovascular collapse, and death. A clue from the history is recent weaning from breast milk (relatively low in protein) to higher protein milk feedings. Pre-term infants can exhibit transient hyperammonemia while on parenteral nutrition.

3. Diagnostic studies—blood NH_4 levels often >1000 μM/liter. If diagnostic tests do not identify a cause, the infant may have transient hyperammonemia of the newborn.

4. Management—stop protein intake, institute dialysis as soon as possible to reduce ammonia levels. Sodium benzoate is used to achieve an alternate route for elimination of nitrogen.

5. Outcome—neurological improvement is seen as NH_4 level declines. Degree of

permanent damage depends on duration of hyperammonemic coma. Mortality is 50% from urea cycle defects, 30% from transient hyperammonemia.

D. **Disorders of carbohydrate metabolism.** The most common disorder in this category with onset in the neonatal period is galactosemia.

1. Pathophysiology. Lactose is a disaccharide composed of glucose and galactose. In galactosemia, the enzyme that mediates the conversion of galactose to glucose is absent; thus, infants cannot digest lactose. The partially metabolized galactose is extremely toxic to the brain, liver, and kidneys.
2. Incidence: 1 : 60,000 to 1 : 80,000.
3. Presentation.
   a. Infants may be SGA and fail to gain weight. Vomiting and diarrhea correspond with introduction of lactose feedings.
   b. Liver damage soon follows, with jaundice, hepatomegaly, and cirrhosis.
   c. Hypoglycemia and anemia may be present.
   d. Cataracts begin to develop early in life.
   e. Often present with fulminant gram-negative sepsis due to damage to intestinal mucosa by galactose-1-phosphate, allowing invasion by *Escherichia coli*.
4. Diagnostic studies — blood enzyme level; urine-reducing substances (urine "dip-stick" tests detect only glucose and will be negative).
5. Management — withhold lactose from the diet; substitute lactose-free formula. Sepsis must be aggressively treated.
6. Outcome — if untreated, mental retardation and cerebral palsy can result. Mortality is 20%. Early treatment helps to preserve intellect. With treatment, cataracts and liver damage are reversible.

E. **Other inborn errors of metabolism.**

1. Glucose-6-phosphate dehydrogenase (G6PD) deficiency.
   a. Pathophysiology. G6PD deficiency is an inherited disorder of red blood cell metabolism. Using the enzyme G6PD, the normal red blood cell (RBC) produces glutathione, which protects its membrane from oxidation. Without glutathione, hydrogen peroxide accumulates within the RBC, damaging and eventually lysing the cell. The RBC is also vulnerable to damage by other oxidants such as chemicals and certain drugs (sulfonamides, aspirin).
   b. Incidence: 100 million affected worldwide, especially prevalent in Mediterranean, Asian, and Middle East populations. A mild variant is found in 13% of American blacks.
   c. Clinical presentation and assessment. Although more than 100 variants exist, two basic forms of clinical expressions have been described:
      (1) Spontaneous chronic hemolytic anemia — neonates may be jaundiced (especially if premature) and anemic. Coombs' test is negative.
      (2) Episodic hemolysis — induced by exposure to infection or oxidant substances. These neonates may be asymptomatic at birth. Onset of symptoms occurs at 48–96 hours after ingestion of the substance.
   d. Diagnostic studies.
      (1) Test of erythrocyte G6PD activity.
      (2) Serum bilirubin.
      (3) Hemoglobin and hematocrit; reticulocyte count to evaluate anemia.
   e. Patient care management. No cure is available; management is supportive and preventive.
      (1) Treat hyperbilirubinemia: phototherapy, exchange transfusion.
      (2) Correct anemia.
      (3) Treat infection if present; minimize exposure to oxidants.
      (4) Vitamin E has been used for its antioxidant properties.
      (5) Parent education regarding avoidance of oxidant substances and drugs; these should also be avoided by a breast-feeding mother of an affected infant.
   f. Complications.

(1) Acute hemolysis triggered by oxidants; can be fatal.

(2) Bilirubin encephalopathy.

2. Cystic fibrosis (CF).

a. Pathophysiology. CF is a multisystem disorder characterized by generalized dysfunction of exocrine glands. The affected organs are those that secrete mucus: the lungs, pancreas, intestinal tract, salivary glands, biliary tract, and genitourinary tract. Mucus secretions are viscous and may plug glands and ducts, causing dysfunction and tissue damage. Although the gene marker for CF has been located, the underlying error of metabolism remains unknown.

b. Incidence—1:2000 white (average); 1:13,000 blacks.

c. Clinical presentation and assessment. Neonates are usually asymptomatic unless there is a meconium ileus, which occurs in 10% of cases.

(1) Meconium ileus: meconium cannot pass through the distal ileum, causing distention, bowel loops, vomiting, failure to pass meconium.

(2) Other signs: failure to thrive (FTT), bulky and fatty stools, prolonged jaundice, early respiratory infection.

d. Diagnostic studies.

(1) Neonatal and prenatal screening tests for CF are available.

(2) Sweat test—analysis of sodium and chloride; may be difficult to collect enough sweat in the newborn.

(3) Abdominal x-ray and meglumine diatrizoate (Gastrografin) enema to evaluate bowel obstruction—typical findings are dilated proximal bowel and microcolon.

e. Patient care management. Because the neonate is usually asymptomatic, treatment for CF is aimed at prevention of complications.

(1) Optimal nutrition; monitor growth and development.

(2) Monitor for and treat respiratory infection.

(3) Treatment of meconium ileus.

(a) Gastrografin enema may relieve obstruction (substance is hypertonic and irritating; may stimulate bowel activity).

(b) Surgical resection of dilated bowel may be necessary.

f. Complications.

(1) Volvulus; perforation (can occur in utero) with meconium peritonitis.

(2) Chronic obstructive pulmonary disease; frequent lung infection.

(3) Digestive difficulties; biliary cirrhosis.

(4) FTT; delayed growth and development.

(5) Sterility in males.

g. Outcome.

(1) Infant mortality 13% due to malnutrition and malabsorption.

(2) Mean survival 22 years; some improvement with early therapy.

STUDY QUESTIONS

1. Hypoglycemia in the infant of a diabetic mother is thought to be caused by:
   a. Decreased glucose uptake.
   b. Hyperinsulinism.
   c. Low glycogen stores.

2. The most serious effect of low circulating glucose is:
   a. CNS injury.
   b. Osmotic diuresis.
   c. Weight loss.

3. What is the primary reason for the typical loss of weight in the first week of life?

   a. Inadequate fluid intake.
   b. Metabolism of tissue protein for energy.
   c. Reduction of the extracellular fluid reservoir.

4. Transepidermal water loss may be decreased by:
   a. High ambient temperature.
   b. Use of a plastic film "blanket."
   c. Use of a radiant warmer.

5. The presumed mechanism of hypernatremic dehydration in a VLBW infant is:

a. Diabetes insipidus.
b. Postnatal extracellular fluid loss.
c. SIADH.

6. A cause of hypocalcemia that may be overlooked is:
   a. Fat necrosis.
   b. Hypomagnesemia.
   c. Metabolic acidosis.

7. The neonate born to a mother who received large doses of magnesium sulfate prior to delivery may present with:
   a. Apnea.
   b. Hypertension.
   c. Hypertonicity.

8. Which of the following signs/symptoms might be seen in hyperkalemia?
   a. Bradycardia.
   b. Muscle weakness.
   c. Peaked T waves.

9. Hypoxia and hypoperfusion can result in which of the following acid-base disturbances?
   a. Metabolic acidosis.
   b. Metabolic alkalosis.
   c. Respiratory acidosis.

10. A 3-day-old neonate presents with hyperammonemia and dehydration. Which of the following disorders is a likely cause?
    a. G6PD deficiency.
    b. PKU.
    c. Urea cycle defect.

11. What is the most frequent outcome of untreated inherited metabolic disease?
    a. Chronic metabolic acidosis.
    b. Mental retardation.
    c. Sterility.

Answers to Study Questions

1. b	5. b	9. a
2. a	6. b	10. c
3. c	7. a	11. b
4. b	8. c	

REFERENCES

Cooke, R.J., Werkman, S., and Watson, D.: Urine output measurements in premature infants. Pediatrics, *83*(1):116–118, 1989.

Cornblath, M., and Schwartz, R.: Disorders of Carbohydrate Metabolism in Infants, 3rd ed. Boston, Blackwell Scientific Publications, 1991, pp. 91–92.

Jacob, J., and Davis, R.F.: Differences in serum glucose determinations in infants with umbilical artery catheters. J. Perinatol., *8*(1):40–42, 1988.

Knauth, A., Gordin, M., McNelis, W., et al.: Semipermeable polyurethane membrane as an artificial skin for the premature neonate. Pediatrics, *83*(6):945–950, 1989.

Raszka, W.V., Thomas, K.K., Franklin, F.R., et al.: The use of hyaluronidase in the treatment of intravenous extravasation injuries. J. Perinatol., *10*(2):146–149, 1990.

BIBLIOGRAPHY

American Academy of Pediatrics, Committee on Genetics: Newborn screening fact sheets. Pediatrics, *83*(3):449–464, 1989.

Anast, C.S.: Disorders of mineral and bone metabolism. *In* Avery, M.E., and Taeusch, H.W. (eds.): Schaffer's Diseases of the Newborn, 6th ed. Philadelphia, W.B. Saunders Co., 1991.

Aynsley-Green, A., and Soltesz, G.: Disorders of blood glucose homeostasis in the neonate. *In* Robertson, N.R.C. (ed.): Textbook of Neonatology. Edinburgh, Churchill Livingstone, 1986.

Brem, A.: Disorders of potassium homeostasis. Pediatr. Clin. North Am., *37*(2):419–428, 1990.

Brewer, E.D.: Disorders of acid-base balance. Pediatr. Clin. North Am., *37*(2):429–448, 1990.

Burton, B.K.: Inborn errors of metabolism: The clinical diagnosis in early infancy. Pediatrics, *79*(3):359–369, 1987.

Collins, J.: A practical approach to the diagnosis of metabolic disease in the neonate. Dev. Med. Child Neurol., *32*:70–86, 1990.

Cornblath, M., Schwartz, R., Aynsley-Green, A., et al.: Hypoglycemia in infancy: The need for a rational definition. Pediatrics, *85*(5):834–837, 1990.

Costarino, A., and Baumgart. S.: Modern fluid and electrolyte management of the critically ill premature infant. Pediatr. Clin. North Am., *33*(1):153–178, 1986.

Gabble, S.G., and Oh, W.: The Infant of the Diabetic Mother: Report of the 93rd Ross Conference on Pediatric Research. Columbus, OH, Ross Laboratories, 1987.

Modi, N.: Development of renal function. Br. Med. Bull., 44(4):935–956, 1988.

Ogata, E.S.: Carbohydrate metabolism in the fetus and neonate and altered neonatal glucoregulation. Pediatr. Clin. North Am., 33(1):25–46, 1986.

Samie, S.E., and Chevalier, R.: Special needs of the newborn infant in fluid therapy. Pediatr. Clin. North Am., 37(2):323–336, 1990.

Schmidt, K.: A primer to the inborn errors of metabolism for perinatal and neonatal nurses. J. Perinat. Neonat. Nurs., 2(4):60–71, 1989.

Wraith, J.E.: Diagnosis and management of inborn errors of metabolism. Arch. Dis. Child., 64:1410–1415, 1989.

Laura Campbell Stokowski

Endocrine Disorders

Objectives

1. Outline the basic ontogenesis of endocrine systems in the fetus, including the thyroid gland, adrenal cortex, and reproductive organs.

2. Describe the function and regulation of endocrine systems at birth.

3. Identify causes and manifestations of endocrine dysfunction in the neonate, including hypothyroidism, hyperthyroidism, congenital adrenal hyperplasia, and disorders of sexual development.

4. Describe the approach to patient management and specific hormonal therapies of endocrine disorders presenting in the neonatal period.

5. List the elements of effective screening for congenital endocrine disorders, including hypothyroidism and 21-hydroxylase deficiency.

6. Outline the evaluation of the infant with ambiguous or abnormal features of the genitalia, including physical examination and diagnostic tests.

7. Discuss the nursing care of parents of infants born with permanent endocrine disorders.

Endocrine disorders in the newborn are not nearly as common as those of the respiratory, cardiac, or neurological systems. Yet, a knowledge of endocrine function and dysfunction in the neonate is essential, because although rare, endocrine disease is easily missed, usually treatable, and if untreated, can lead to significant morbidity and other unfortunate consequences for the child and family. Although a wide range of endocrine dysfunction is possible, the most common disorders likely to be encountered in the neonate are those of the thyroid, adrenal cortex, and developing sexual organs.

The Endocrine System

A. **Endocrine glands**—the pituitary, the pineal, the thyroid, the parathyroid, the thymus, and pancreatic islet cells, the adrenals, and the gonads.

B. **Endocrine hormones**.

1. Hormone production.

a. Hypothalamus functions as control center for the endocrine system by producing hormone release factors. These trigger the pituitary to secrete tropic hormones, which in turn stimulate the target glands or tissues to produce hormones.

b. Pituitary tropic (stimulating) hormones include adrenocorticotropic hormone (ACTH), growth hormone (GH), thyroid-stimulating hormone (TSH), follicle-stimulating hormone (FSH), luteinizing hormone (LH), and prolactin (PRL).

2. Hormone function.
   a. Hormones control and integrate body functions such as energy production and metabolism, water and electrolyte balance, growth and development, and reproductive processes.
   b. Hormones circulate in the blood in free form and bound to protein. Free-form hormones are the active fraction available to the target tissues; protein-bound hormones represent the hormone reserve in the plasma.

3. Hormone regulation. Hormone levels are regulated by a negative feedback system. Glands secrete hormones until physiological blood levels are reached. A message is then sent back to glands or high control center, which inhibits further hormone synthesis.

Thyroid Gland Disorders

A. Anatomy and physiology.
1. Functions of thyroid gland—concentrate and store iodide; synthesize and release thyroid hormones and thyroid binding globulins.
2. Thyroid hormones—T_4 (thyroxine) and T_3 (tri-iodothyronine) influence metabolism, oxygen consumption, heat production, cardiac output, and development of bones, the central nervous system, and the lungs.
3. Fetal thyroid development.
   a. Fetal thyroid gland begins to function by the 8th week of gestation; thyroid hormones are measurable by the 12th week.
   b. Maternal thyroid hormones do not cross the placenta; the fetus is dependent on its own thyroid production in utero.
4. Physiology of the thyroid at birth.
   a. Shortly after birth, in response to stress of delivery, serum TSH rises sharply. TSH peaks at 30 minutes of age then falls to normal levels over the first week of life.
   b. TSH surge causes T_3 and T_4 to rise also, peaking at 48 hours, then decreasing to normal levels. Post-natal changes occur in the pre-term infant as well but are quantitatively lower.
   c. Thyroid system control (normal T_4 to TSH ratio) matures by 1 month post-natal life in the term infant and at the equivalent post-conceptional age in the pre-term infant.

B. Hypothyroid states.
1. Congenital hypothyroidism—etiologies.
   a. Defects in morphogenesis.
      (1) Thyroid dysgenesis—absent, partial, or ectopic gland (primary hypothyroidism); most common cause of congenital hypothyroidism.
      (2) Defects of the pituitary gland (secondary hypothyroidism).
      (3) Defects of the hypothalamus (tertiary hypothyroidism).
   b. Defects in thyroid hormone biosynthesis—failure of one of the steps in formation of thyroid hormones.
   c. Maternal factors causing neonatal hypothyroidism.
      (1) Treatment with radioactive iodine (crosses the placenta and destroys the fetal thyroid); anti-thyroid drugs; maternal ingestion of iodide or intravaginal use of iodinated solutions (povidone-iodine) prior to delivery.
      (2) Deficient supply of dietary iodide (endemic cretinism).

2. Acquired or transient hypothyroidism.
   a. Transient inhibition of thyroid hormone production, particularly in pre-term infants, from the use of iodine-containing topical disinfectants, ointments, or intravenous contrast media.
   b. Transient hypothyroxinemia (low T_4): immaturity of the hypothalamic-pituitary-thyroid axis and reduced T_4 to T_3 conversion occurs in 50% of infants born before 30 weeks' gestation. This relative hypothyroxinemia corrects spontaneously in 4–8 weeks without treatment.
   c. "Low T_3 syndrome": the effects of nonthyroidal illness (e.g., respiratory distress syndrome) on thyroid metabolism. May be a protective mechanism reducing the metabolic rate during illness; there is no thyroid abnormality per se.
3. Diagnosis of hypothyroid states.
   a. Maternal prenatal history—exposure to radioactive iodine, anti-thyroid drugs, goitrogenic drugs (e.g., lithium).
   b. Newborn screening for hypothyroidism—United States uses two-tiered test:
      (1) Thyroxine (T_4) is measured first. If low, TSH is measured. A low T_4 with high TSH is presumptive primary hypothyroidism. A low T_4 and low TSH require further evaluation to rule out secondary or tertiary hypothyroidism.
      (2) Most false-positive results from screening are premature infants with low T_4 and normal TSH levels.
      (3) Some infants with primary hypothyroidism are missed because T_4 is normal at the time of screening; this can occur if the newborn's blood is sampled too early.
      (4) Incidence of congenital hypothyroidism by screening programs: $1:3500$ to $1:4500$.
      (5) Ideal screening procedures.
         (a) Sample drawn on days 3–6 of life (repeated if drawn earlier).
         (b) Good-quality blood spot on filter paper (fully saturated circles) and dried at room temperature without handling or contamination.
   c. Common thyroid function tests—gestational age, post-natal age, and clinical condition must be taken into account when interpreting results (Table 16–1).

Table 16–1
THYROID FUNCTION TESTS IN HYPOTHYROID STATES

	T_4	Free T_4	T_3	TSH	TRH Stimulation
Primary hypothyroidism; transient hypothyroidism	Low	Low	Normal	High or low	Exaggerated
Secondary hypothyroidism (pituitary)	Low	Low	Normal or low	Low	No response
Tertiary hypothyroidism (hypothalamic)	Low	Low	Low	Normal or high	Delayed; prolonged
Hypothyroxinemia (premature infant)	Low	Low	Low	Normal or low	Normal
Low T_3 syndrome (non-thyroidal)	Normal or low	Normal or low	Low	Normal	Normal

      (1) Radioimmunoassay of total and free T_4 and T_3; and TSH.

      (2) Thyroid binding globulin (TBG) level—reveals the binding capacity of T_4.

4. Clinical presentation of hypothyroid states in neonatal period depends on the amount of functioning thyroid tissue.

  a. Most neonates (95%) have few or no signs of hypothyroidism at birth.

  b. Classic findings (may be present in neonates born with no thyroid gland) include the following:

    (1) Typical facies—wide-set eyes; short nose with flattened bridge; enlarged, protruding tongue; and large fontanelles.

    (2) Umbilical hernia.

    (3) Delayed stooling (>20 hours after birth); constipation.

    (4) Gestation >42 weeks; birthweight >4 kg.

    (5) Poor feeding, weak suck, distention, vomiting.

    (6) Hypothermia; cool, mottled, dry skin.

    (7) Hypoactivity, hypotonia, lethargy, slow reflexes, hoarse cry.

    (8) Jaundice.

    (9) Slow pulse rate.

  c. Subtle, non-specific findings such as temperature instability and slow gut motility may be present in very low birthweight (VLBW) infants with transient hypothyroxinemia.

  d. Neonatal hypothyroid goiter—hypertrophied thyroid gland due to maternal ingestion of goitrogens or an inborn error of thyroid hormone biosynthesis.

    (1) A small goiter may be unnoticed due to shortness of newborn neck; can also be large, asymmetrical, and mistaken for a hygroma.

    (2) Hypertrophy occurs in the posterior lobes; can compress the trachea and cause respiratory distress.

5. Patient care management.

  a. Congenital hypothyroidism.

    (1) Thyroid replacement with synthetic T_4; goal is to maintain normal serum thyroxine level for age, not necessarily to suppress TSH to normal levels.

    (2) Close monitoring is necessary to prevent overtreatment or undertreatment.

      (a) Overtreatment can result in advanced bone age, craniosynostosis, thyrotoxicosis. Early signs of toxicity with L-thyroxine are irritability, hyperactivity, loose stools. Can occur even after periods of apparent stability on replacement therapy.

      (b) Undertreatment leads to clinical hypothyroidism, delayed bone maturation, and neurological damage.

    (3) Treatment may have to begin before the specific diagnosis is known, waiting until child is older to determine the underlying cause.

  b. Transient hypothyroid states.

    (1) Controversy exists regarding need for replacement therapy.

    (2) Infants with persistently elevated TSH need replacement therapy.

    (3) If transient hypothyroidism is untreated, serial thyroid function tests should be followed.

6. Complications.

  a. Hypothyroid goiter with respiratory compromise

    (1) Thyroid replacement with parenteral T_4 is imperative.

    (2) Intubation and assisted ventilation may be necessary.

    (3) Surgery may also be required.

  b. Iodine intoxication with exacerbation of hypothyroid states can occur in sick and well premature infants, although serum TSH may not rise for 7–14 days. Urinary iodine levels can be measured to give an indication of undesired iodine absorption.

7. Outcome.

  a. Congenital hypothyroidism.

    (1) One of the most preventable causes of mental retardation. The earlier

the origin (e.g., intrauterine onset as with thyroid agenesis), the poorer the neurological outcome.

    (2) Life-long thyroid replacement is necessary to prevent neurophysiological disorders and mental retardation. Early treatment improves prognosis — IQ is higher in infants diagnosed and treated prior to 3 months of age.

  b. Transient hypothyroidism — long-term effects on growth and development are unknown. Treatment with L-thyroxine does not appear to alter growth and development of pre-term infant with transient hypothyroxinemia (Chowdhry et al, 1984).

C. Hyperthyroid states.

1. Graves' disease — a thyroid autoimmune condition in which there is production of thyroid-stimulating immunoglobulin (TSI) of the IgG class.

  a. Untreated maternal Graves' — TSIs cross the placenta and stimulate fetal thyroid production. The resultant neonatal hyperthyroidism is transient; improvement is seen as TSI levels fall after birth.

  b. Treated maternal Graves' — iodine and/or anti-thyroid drugs cross the placenta, inducing a fetal goiter. After birth, the infant's thyroid is stimulated by residual TSI and releases large quantities of T_4 into the circulation. The neonate becomes thyrotoxic at 7–10 days of life.

  c. True neonatal Graves' disease — permanent disorder. The infant produces its own antibodies that stimulate the thyroid gland, causing hyperthyroidism.

2. Diagnosis.

  a. Cord blood thyroid levels.

    (1) Total and free T_4 and T_3 elevated (may initially be normal in infants born to mothers with treated Graves'). Repeated hormone levels on infant's serum are needed.

    (2) TSH low due to suppression.

  b. TSI levels in the mother and infant.

3. Clinical presentation of hyperthyroidism.

  a. Serious signs may become apparent in first 24 hours.

  b. Signs associated with hyperthyroidism/thyrotoxicosis are as follows:

    (1) Premature birth of an intrauterine growth-retarded (IUGR) infant.

    (2) Vomiting, diarrhea.

    (3) Exophthalmos.

    (4) Hyperactivity, hyperirritability, tremors.

    (5) Excessive sweating, hyperthermia.

    (6) Often associated with congenital anomalies.

  c. Hyperthyroid goiter — present in 50% of infants; may increase in size during the neonatal period.

  d. Sympathetic stimulation.

    (1) Tachycardia (>200 beats/minute).

    (2) Cardiovascular failure, cardiomegaly, hepatosplenomegaly.

  e. Advanced bone age — craniosynostosis and frontal bossing may be present.

4. Patient care management.

  a. Drug therapy for severe cases.

    (1) Antithyroid drugs, (propylthiouracil) to block formation of thyroid hormones. Replacement therapy with thyroxine may be necessary.

    (2) Lugol's iodine inhibits release of T_4 from the thyroid.

    (3) Propranolol is used to reduce sympathetic overstimulation.

    (4) Digitalis may be administered to neonates with congestive heart failure (CHF).

    (5) Glucocorticoids are helpful as they acutely inhibit thyroid secretion.

    (6) Sedation is often given for neurological symptoms.

5. Complications.

  a. Unrecognized thyrotoxicosis can lead to severe asphyxia or death from tracheal compression by a goiter.

b. Other complications are CHF, thrombocytopenia, hypothyroidism, premature craniosynostosis, and thyroid storm (severe thyrotoxicosis precipitated by stress that results in coma and death if untreated).
6. Outcome.
   a. Hyperthyroidism can be transient (1–3 months in 30%) or can persist into infancy or childhood. Persistent hyperthyroidism may actually be true Graves' disease with neonatal onset rather than effects of maternal Graves' disease.
   b. Growth retardation can be a long-term result.
   c. Mortality rate of neonatal thyrotoxicosis is 15–20%.

Adrenal Gland Disorders

A. **The adrenal gland**—highly vascular organ comprised of two distinct endocrine organs: an inner portion (adrenal medulla) and an outer layer (adrenal cortex), which are functionally independent although enclosed within a common capsule.
1. The adrenal medulla produces catecholamines (epinephrine, norepinephrine, dopamine).
2. The adrenal cortex provides steroid compounds derived from cholesterol that have diverse effects throughout the body.

B. **Adrenal hormones and their actions.**
1. Glucocorticoids (primarily cortisol) play a key role in homeostasis of glucose and in the body's reaction to stress. Fetal glucocorticoids are involved in histological and biochemical maturation of the lung.
2. Mineralocorticoids (primarily aldosterone) maintain sodium homeostasis by stimulating active sodium reabsorption and potassium excretion at the distal tubule of the renal nephron.
3. Androgens (primarily testosterone) are involved in sexual development and maturation.

C. **Physiology of the adrenal glands at birth.**
1. The adrenal glands are capable of producing glucocorticoid regardless of gestational age. Cortisol levels are high at birth but begin to fall as maternal and placental contributions are withdrawn.
2. Cortisol regulation in the neonate is responsive to endogenous stimulation such as stress or severe respiratory disease.
3. The renin-angiotensin system controlling aldosterone production is active at birth but may be immature in the pre-term infant. Plasma renin activity and aldosterone levels are normally high in the newborn.

D. **Adrenal hypofunction**—etiologies in the newborn.
1. Congenital adrenal hyperplasia (see following section).
2. Maternal glucocorticoid therapy—can suppress fetal adrenal glands.
3. Adrenal hemorrhage—related to hemorrhagic diathesis, shock, anoxia, birth trauma.
4. Hypopituitarism—the pituitary fails to produce ACTH, resulting in hypoplasia of the adrenal cortex.

E. **Congenital adrenal hyperplasia (CAH).**
1. Condition resulting from an abnormality in one of the enzymes needed for steroid biosynthesis; autosomal recessive genetic defect that affects males and females equally.
2. Five different enzyme deficiencies can occur, each of which blocks a step in the transformation of cholesterol to cortisol. Most common type (90–95%) is 21-hydroxylase (21-OH) deficiency.
3. Pathophysiology (Fig. 16–1).
   a. Lack of fetal 21-OH prevents conversion of progesterone to its two end products: cortisol and aldosterone.

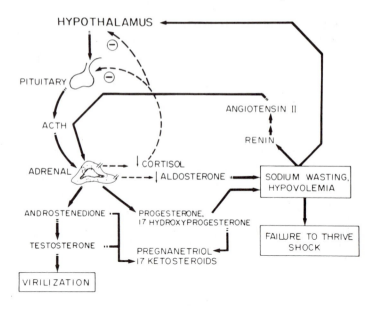

Figure 16-1
Pathophysiology of congenital adrenal hyperplasia caused by 21-hydroxylase deficiency. In the absence of cortisol, ACTH stimulates the adrenal cortex to produce virilizing androgens. Diminished production of aldosterone leads to salt wasting and hypovolemia. (From Danish, R.: Abnormalities of sexual differentiation. *In* Fanaroff, A., and Martin, R. (eds.): Neonatal-Perinatal Medicine, 4th ed. St. Louis, C.V. Mosby Co., 1987.)

  b. The absence of cortisol causes overproduction of ACTH, which stimulates the adrenal cortex, resulting in hyperplasia.
  c. The adrenal cortex responds by producing large amounts of androgens instead of cortisol. At a critical stage in fetal development, these androgens cause virilization of the external genitalia in females.
  d. A precursor to cortisol, 17-hydroxyprogesterone (17-OHP), accumulates in the blood because it cannot undergo the step to convert it to cortisol.
4. Clinical presentations—varies with degree of enzyme deficiency. Although all affected neonates have some glucocorticoid and mineralocorticoid deficiency, it is not always apparent at birth. The following clinical syndromes have been described:
  a. Compensated/non–salt-losing disease (25% of patients).
    (1) An incomplete enzymatic block results in enough aldosterone production to maintain fluid and electrolyte homeostasis, so clinical signs are absent.
    (2) The disease may not be detected until a metabolic emergency occurs, particularly in males, because genitals appear normal.
  b. Uncompensated/salt-losing disease (75% of patients).
    (1) The enzymatic block is complete; both cortisol and aldosterone are deficient. Because aldosterone is necessary for absorption of sodium and water and for excretion of potassium, the aldosterone-deficient infant becomes hyponatremic, hyperkalemic, and dehydrated.
    (2) The neonate has a history of a progressive disorder from birth, beginning with weight loss and mild fluid and electrolyte imbalance and progressing to more serious signs of aldosterone deficiency that result in death if untreated.
    (3) Onset of salt-losing state can be as early as 1 week of age; usually occurs in the first month in untreated disease. Onset is delayed because the newborn normally has a high aldosterone level in the first week from slow hepatic clearance, but as the liver matures, aldosterone is used up and the infant cannot restore it.
5. Assessment and physical examination.
  a. Signs and symptoms that may be seen in the neonatal period include the following:
    (1) Lethargy, poor appetite, weakness.
    (2) Regurgitation, vomiting, diarrhea.

(3) Dehydration (depressed fontanel, dry skin and mucous membranes, recessed eyes).

(4) Hypotension, shock.

(5) Failure to thrive (FTT), weight loss in early life.

(6) Other signs may include apnea, seizures, hypoglycemia.

  b. Appearance of the genitalia.

(1) In girls with 21-OHD (female genotype, 46XX) external genitalia are masculinized.

(2) In boys with 21-OHD (male genotype, 46XY) external genitalia are normal.

6. Diagnosis of 21-OHD CAH.

  a. Index of suspicion—a family history of a sibling with CAH or unexplained death of a male infant. Should also be ruled out in any infant with abnormal genitalia.

  b. Newborn screening for CAH.

(1) 17-OHP level (a cortisol precursor) used to screen for 21-OHD; can be done at same time as routine newborn screening for phenylketonuria and other conditions.

(2) Incidence varies geographically and culturally

  (a) United States in general—1:12,000.

  (b) Yupik Eskimo (of Alaska)—1:684 (salt-losing type).

  (c) Elsewhere, incidence ranges from 1:5000 to 1:23,000.

(3) Some false positives occur in pre-term infants due to normally higher 17-OHP levels.

(4) Optimal timing of sample is 48–72 hours of age.

  c. In symptomatic infants, prompt diagnosis depends on recognition of adrenal insufficiency. Specific tests can then be conducted to determine the exact error of steroid biosynthesis.

  d. Diagnostic tests—common tests and findings in 21-OHD CAH.

(1) Serum levels of steroids and precursors: 17-OHP level is markedly elevated, even more than usually seen in sick, stressed infants. Cortisol levels (baseline and after ACTH administration) are low. Testosterone level is increased.

(2) Plasma renin activity (increased); aldosterone level (can be normal or even elevated).

(3) Serum and urine electrolytes reveal hyponatremia and natriuresis. Hyperkalemia can cause EKG changes such as peaked T wave and prolonged ST segment. In compensated CAH, electrolytes may be normal.

(4) In infants with ambiguous genitalia—blood karyotype to establish the genetic sex (genotype) and radiographic studies and ultrasound to determine the anatomy of internal structures.

7. Differential diagnosis.

  a. Pyloric stenosis is the chief alternative diagnosis in male infants with normal genitalia because of similar time of onset (end of neonatal period) and presentation (FTT, dehydration, projectile vomiting). Pyloric stenosis presents with metabolic (hypochloremic) alkalosis rather than acidosis.

  b. Aldosterone deficiency.

  c. Ambiguous genitalia of different etiology.

  d. Other medical problems, such as inappropriate anti-diuretic hormone, renal disease, or sepsis.

8. Patient care management.

  a. Goals: restore physiologic levels of cortisol, suppress ACTH and androgen overproduction, and maintain fluid and electrolyte homeostasis.

  b. Hormonal therapy: hydrocortisone (glucocorticoid) and, for salt-losing patients, fluorohydrocortisone (mineralocorticoid).

  c. Dietary salt supplementation to prevent hyponatremia.

  d. Monitoring therapy: measurement of plasma cortisol, cortisol precursors,

ACTH, plasma renin activity (PRA), electrolytes, growth and bone maturation; assessment for signs of virilization, hypertension, or other unwanted effects of therapy.
- e. Treatment of salt-losing state/adrenal crisis.
  - (1) Intravenous fluids, glucose, and electrolytes to correct imbalances.
  - (2) Glucocorticoid and mineralocorticoid administration.
  - (3) Treatment of shock; volume replacement.
  - (4) Correction of acidosis.
  - (5) Monitoring for cardiac toxicity due to hyperkalemia.
- f. Genetic counseling (multiple sibling involvement is common).
  - (1) Pre-natal diagnosis is possible with amniotic fluid measurement of 17-OHP or by HLA genotyping of amniotic cells.
  - (2) Intrauterine treatment can prevent virilization of female fetuses. Dexamethasone given to mother crosses the placenta and suppresses fetal ACTH.
- g. Parent education should include:
  - (1) Expectations, prognosis, and future therapy required.
  - (2) Importance of follow-up of growth and development; monitoring of and consequences of discontinuing therapy.
  - (3) Medication administration and stress/illness therapy.

9. Complications.
   - a. Adrenal crisis/collapse under stress.
     - (1) Sudden signs of cortisol insufficiency (shock, hypotension, acidosis, hypoglycemia, seizures) plus sodium depletion.
     - (2) May be precipitated in undiagnosed, untreated, or inadequately treated CAH during episode of illness or stress, such as surgery, in the neonatal period. Can occur in both compensated and uncompensated forms of CAH.
     - (3) Stress therapy (e.g., fever, illness, surgery) requires two to three times the normal dose of hydrocortisone, given IV or IM if the infant is vomiting.
   - b. Poorly controlled CAH can have serious consequences.
     - (1) Failure to suppress ACTH and androgen production can result in signs of virilization and accelerated growth or bone maturation, as well as signs of salt-losing state.
     - (2) Consequences of overtreatment include hypertension, pulmonary edema, CHF, growth failure, adrenal atrophy, and decreased resistance to infection.

10. Outcome.
    - a. Life-long hormonal replacement is necessary, and additional therapy may be required at puberty.
    - b. Untreated disease or delayed diagnosis can result in the following:
      - (1) Sudden deterioration or death in undiagnosed infants.
      - (2) Progressive virilization in both sexes with phallic enlargement, early growth of facial and pubic hair, and so forth.
      - (3) Inappropriate sex assignment, leading to late (traumatic) sex change or permanent infertility if "wrong" sex retained. A virilized female with CAH, misdiagnosed as a male with undescended testes and hypospadias, might be circumcised.
      - (4) Acceleration of growth and bone maturation (may be the first manifestation of undiagnosed CAH). Short stature results from early epiphyseal closure.
    - c. Mortality is 9% from adrenal crisis in the newborn period.

Disorders of Sexual Development

A. **Stages of normal sexual development in the embryo/fetus.**
1. Fertilization—determination of genetic sex based on X or Y chromosome.

2. Primitive gonad development—occurs in first 5 weeks.
   a. Gonads form on genital ridge near kidneys.
   b. Primitive germ cells migrate from yolk sac to genital ridge.
   c. At this state, gonads are indifferent structures—can become either testes or ovaries.
3. Gonadal differentiation—begins at week 6 of gestation.
   a. Tendency of primitive gonad is to become an ovary.
   b. Differentiation to a testis depends on presence of H-Y antigen on the Y chromosome.
   c. Testis begins secreting testosterone; ovary differentiates more slowly, does not secrete hormone.
4. Genital duct differentiation—begins at week 8 of gestation.
   a. Starts with indifferent state; two pairs of ducts form in all embryos: the müllerian ducts and the wolffian ducts.
   b. Tendency is for müllerian ducts to differentiate into female urogenital structures (fallopian tubes, uterus, cervix, vagina) and for wolffian ducts to regress.
   c. Differentiation of wolffian ducts into male urogenital structures depends on presence of anti-müllerian hormone (AMH) and testosterone. These hormones cause the müllerian ducts to regress and wolffian ducts to persist, forming excretory ducts to testes, seminal vesicles, and prostatic glands.
5. External genital differentiation (Fig. 16.–2) begins week 10–12.
   a. Starts with undifferentiated structures: a small genital tubercle, central urogenital slit surrounded by genital folds, and lateral genital swellings.
   b. Tendency is for external genitalia to become feminized: genital tubercle forms the clitoris, genital folds become the labia minora, genital swellings form the labia majora, and the genital sinus remains open to the vagina.

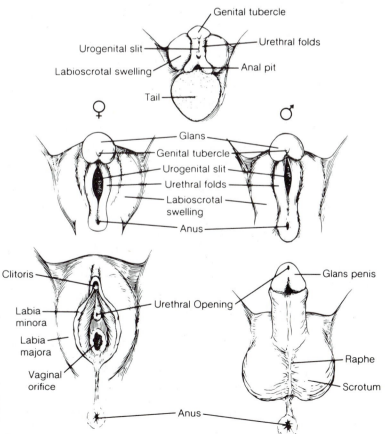

Figure 16–2
Development and differentiation of male and female external genitalia. (From Pelliniemi, L. J., and Dym, M.: In Tulchinsky, D., and Ryan, K. J. (eds.): Maternal-Fetal Endocrinology. Philadelphia, W. B. Saunders Co., 1980, p. 268.)

c. In the presence of testosterone and its metabolite, dihydrotestosterone (DHT), genital structures are masculinized: genital tubercle becomes the glans penis, genital folds form the ventral surface of the urethra and penile shaft, genital swellings become the scrotum, and the genital slit fuses.

B. Abnormalities of sexual differentiation.
1. Disorders of gonadal differentiation.
   a. Turner's syndrome (absent or defective X chromosome; 45X) occurs in 1:2000 to 1:3000 live female infants; manifestations are bilateral "streak gonads" and classic somatic features.
   b. Klinefelter's syndrome (extra X chromosome; 47XXY) occurs in 1:600 live male births; infants have dysgenesis of seminiferous tubules, small testes, and possibly other congenital anomalies.
   c. True hermaphroditism—presence of ovarian and testicular tissue.
2. Disorders of external genital differentiation.
   a. Female pseudohermaphroditism (FPH)—female genotype with male-appearing (virilized) external genitalia. Internal organs (gonads, genital ducts) are normal female structures. Degree of masculinization depends on when during gestation development was influenced by androgens. Etiologies include congenital adrenal hyperplasia (21-OHD), maternal androgen-producing tumors, and maternal hormone therapy during the third month of gestation.
   b. Male pseudohermaphroditism (MPH)—male genotype with feminization or incomplete masculinization of external genitalia. Etiologies include the following:
      (1) Congenital adrenal hyperplasia (several different variants).
      (2) Testicular dysgenesis—complete or partial failure of testicular development; effects depend on the ability of the abnormal testis to produce testosterone and anti-müllerian hormone.
      (3) Defect of androgen biosynthesis—inability to synthesize testosterone.
      (4) Androgen insensitivity (partial or complete)—internal genital ducts and external genital structures do not respond normally to testosterone during differentiation, resulting in testicular feminization. Complete androgen resistance is not recognized in the neonate because external genitalia are those of a normal female infant.
      (5) 5-alpha reductase deficiency—without this enzyme, the external genital organs cannot convert testosterone to dihydrotestosterone, which is needed to complete their development.
      (6) Persistent müllerian duct—uterus and fallopian tubes fail to regress in a phenotypic male due to a defect in synthesis, secretion, or response to anti-müllerian hormone (AMH).
   c. Other structural abnormalities.
      (1) Cryptorchidism—undescended testes. Most common urogenital abnormality, primarily because of high incidence in premature infants. Congenital absence of the testes is known as *anorchia*.
      (2) Hypospadias—incomplete fusion of the penile urethra. The urethral meatus is found proximal to the glans penis, on the ventral surface of the penis or the perineum. Second most common urogenital abnormality, occurring in 1:700 males.
      (3) Microphallus—penile size 2.5 SD below mean for age (<1.9 cm stretched length in a term infant); may be associated with rudimentary (small) testes. Usual cause in 46XY infant is hypogonadotropic hypogonadism.
      (4) Müllerian aplasia and vaginal agenesis—congenital absence of fallopian tubes or vagina; occurs in 1:5000 female births.

C. Clinical presentation. Neonates with disorders of sexual development may present with a wide range of abnormalities:
1. There may be ambiguous or abnormal features of genitalia, asymmetrical genitalia, or a single abnormality such as undescended testes.

2. Many disorders can present with normal-appearing external genitalia.
3. Other presenting signs and symptoms relate to a primary endocrine disorder (adrenal insufficiency, hypopituitarism, growth hormone deficiency, etc.).
4. Genital ambiguity can be associated with malformation syndromes such as trisomy 13.

D. **Clinical assessment and physical examination.**

1. Examination of the genitalia—close scrutiny not only of babies with clearly abnormal genitals but also "females" with inguinal masses, hernias, or slight clitoral enlargement and "males" with unpalpable testes, hypospadias, or unusually small genitalia.
   a. Gonads: presence, location (scrotal sac, inguinal canal, groin), size, symmetry.
   b. Phallus: size (if small, is it a true penis or hypertrophied clitoris?), presence of chordee (downward curvature of the penis).
   c. Urethral meatus: location relative to normal position.
   d. Inguinal canal/groin: testes versus other masses.
   e. Labiosacral folds: degree and location of fusion (partial, complete), true folds versus empty scrotal sac.
   f. Vaginal opening: lift clitoris to examine the sinus.
   g. Pigmentation of external genitalia.
2. Assessment findings—variations that may be expressed include the following:
   a. Female pseudohermaphrodite: degrees of virilization (Fig. 16–3).
      (1) Clitoral hypertrophy—may resemble a phallic urethra.
      (2) Gonads not palpable in labiosacral folds or "scrotum."
      (3) Partial or complete fusion of the posterior genital fold.
      (4) Single urogenital orifice: perineoscrotal hypospadias.
      (5) Mucoid or bloody discharge.
      (6) Hyperpigmentation of labiosacral folds; may be rugated.
   b. Male pseudohermaphrodite: degrees of feminization (Fig. 16–4).
      (1) Absence of testes in scrotum; undescended testes.
      (2) Small phallus; may look like clitoromegaly.
      (3) Single urogenital orifice; may have a small vaginal pouch.
      (4) Incomplete fusion of genital fold; may resemble labia majora.
      (5) Inguinal hernia (persistent müllerian duct).
   c. True hermaphrodite (very rare)—have marked genital ambiguity, with undescended testes or a unilateral gonad, perhaps an inguinal hernia containing a gonad or incomplete fusion of the labiosacral folds.

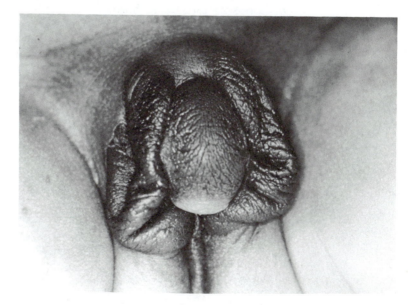

Figure 16–3
Virilization in a 46XX infant with 21-hydroxylase deficiency. Note clitoral hypertrophy and hyperpigmented and rugated labiosacral folds, resembling an empty scrotum. (Courtesy of Michael S. Kappy, M.D., Ph.D.)

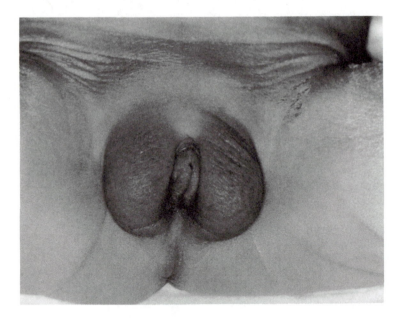

Figure 16–4
46XY infant with ambiguous genitalia due to 5-alpha reductase deficiency. Note absence of a penis and lack of fusion of labiosacral folds, indicating incomplete virilization. (Courtesy of Michael S. Kappy, M.D., Ph.D.)

E. **Diagnosis**—a combination of genetic evaluation, clinical and biochemical findings, and examination of internal structures.
1. Goals of diagnosis.
   a. Determine as quickly as possible the appropriate gender for rearing of the infant—should be considered a psycho-social emergency.
   b. Identify and treat the underlying disorder—anticipate acute medical problems for which the infant may be at risk (e.g., hyponatremia, dehydration).
2. Family history—a similarly affected infant or family member, ingestion of androgens during pregnancy, maternal virilization or uncontrolled CAH.
3. Determination of chromosomal sex—the karyotype (blood, bone marrow) is the definitive method for analyzing sex chromosome constitution. Buccal smear for chromosome analysis is considered inaccurate and is no longer recommended (Pagon, 1987).
4. Diagnosis of underlying endocrine disorder.
   a. Tests for adrenal insufficiency.
   b. Levels of luteinizing hormone, follicle-stimulating hormone, testosterone and DHT.
   c. Human chorionic gonadotropin (HCG) stimulation test measuring testosterone response in males, to see if the target tissues will respond to androgen.
5. Evaluation of internal structures—ultrasound of uterus and fallopian tubes and radiographic studies to view the anatomical connections between the urethra and the genitals.

F. **Patient care management**.
1. Gender assignment.
   a. Defer sex assignment based on external features until the appropriate sex for rearing is known. Recommended sex of rearing is not always the chromosomal sex.
   b. Choice depends on prognosis for functional capacity of the genitals and gender-appropriate reconstruction.
   c. Prognosis for development of secondary sex characteristics may also influence gender choice.
   d. Parental wishes are important; some cultures prohibit gender "reassignment."
2. Usual recommendation for gender assignment.

    a. Female pseudohermaphrodite should be raised as a female—internal structures are normal, fertility is common.

    b. Male pseudohermaphrodite is more complex—decision is based on size and potential for growth of the penis.

        (1) HCG stimulation test: if penis enlarges, may be able to raise as male. Responsiveness does not predict a normal penile size in adulthood.

        (2) In cases of severe microphallus (4 SD below the mean or length <1.5 cm based on term size), it is safer to assign a female sex. This is the case with androgen insensitivity in which there is a vaginal cavity.

    c. Males with 5-alpha reductase deficiency will usually virilize at puberty.

3. Treatment.

    a. Replacement of deficient hormones as required.

        (1) Glucocorticoid/mineralocorticoid for treatment of CAH.

        (2) Testosterone for males with incomplete virilization; must monitor bone age.

        (3) Pituitary hormones for hypopituitarism.

    b. Surgical reconstruction—most recommend that it be done as early as feasible prior to 1 year.

        (1) Surgical repair for FPH involves clitoral recession and repair of the urogenital sinus and vagina (vaginoplasty often deferred until child is older).

        (2) Surgical repair for MPH to be raised as a female involves castration and orchiectomy.

4. Care of the parents.

    a. Initial communication of newborn's gender.

        (1) Do not announce the infant's sex if the genitalia appear abnormal or suggest the baby is neither a boy nor a girl.

        (2) Tell parents the baby's genitals are not completely developed (use "incomplete" rather than "ambiguous"); that the baby will be one sex or the other, but some tests need to be done to determine how best the unfinished organs can be finished.

    b. Ongoing communication regarding diagnostic tests and final diagnosis. The nurse's knowledge of fetal sexual development and of the bipotential nature of developing sexual organs can be used to help parents understand the influences that came to bear on the development of their baby's genitals.

    c. Provide continuous psychological support.

        (1) Anticipate parents' reactions—shock, grief, anger, confusion, disbelief. Frustration with long wait for diagnostic test results may be expressed.

        (2) Share information honestly, particularly when difficult decisions regarding gender assignment must be made.

        (3) When sex of rearing assignment is different from the apparent (genital) sex or the chromosomal sex, assist parents to understand the many facets of an individual's gender identity. This may involve helping them gain a new perspective and discard the traditional view that a person's self-concept as a male or female is determined solely by chromosomes or the appearance of the genitalia.

    d. Recognize impact of parents' feelings and resolution of grief on the child's development—make plans for continuing emotional support, and assist parents to deal with reactions of others who may be aware of the diagnosis. Explore cultural beliefs that may be at the root of parent/family reactions.

    e. Educate parents regarding long-term outlook and therapy (including surgery); emphasize prognosis for normal gender identity with appropriate treatment.

5. Outcome—depends on timing of treatment, adequacy of and compliance with treatment, success of surgical procedures.

    a. Psychosocial adjustment, gender identity, and sexual orientation are not expected to be different if the environment is one that accepts the child's sex of rearing with conviction. In complex cases (staged reconstructive surgery, atypical onset of puberty, infertility), ongoing psychological support for the child and family is essential.

      b. Sexual maturation — hormonal therapy usually required to induce development of gender-appropriate secondary sex characteristics at the desired time.

      c. Reproductive capacity — fertility is possible with some disorders of sexual development, such as FPH, but is rare or impossible in others, such as MPH raised as a female.

  6. Complications.

      a. Inappropriate sex assignment — problem has not been adequately diagnosed in the neonatal period. Some sex reassignments have been made at 2 years of age; not recommended after 18 months.

      b. Gonadal or genital duct malignancy is common; requires surgical removal of internal structures.

STUDY QUESTIONS

1. The most common cause of congenital hypothyroidism is:
   a. Dysgenesis of the thyroid gland.
   b. Maternal Graves' disease.
   c. Prematurity/low birthweight.

2. Which of the following may indicate thyrotoxicosis in a neonate?
   a. Dehydration, hyponatremia, hypotension.
   b. Jaundice, constipation, lethargy.
   c. Tachycardia, irritability, hyperthermia.

3. What is the presumed mechanism for hypothyroidism in well pre-term infants?
   a. Immaturity of the hypothalamus.
   b. Inadequate intake of iodine.
   c. Reduced metabolic rate.

4. A low T_4 and a high thyroid stimulating hormone level are indicative of:
   a. Congenital hypothyroidism.
   b. Thyrotoxicosis.
   c. Transient hypothyroxinemia.

5. Untreated hypothyroidism can result in which of the following?
   a. Mental retardation.
   b. Premature craniosynostosis.
   c. Rapid linear growth.

6. Which of the following may be a life-threatening complication of 21-hydroxylase congenital adrenal hyperplasia?
   a. Hypertension.
   b. Neonatal goiter.
   c. Salt-losing state.

7. The basis for neonatal screening of 21-hydroxylase deficiency is measurement of:
   a. ACTH level.
   b. Cortisol precursors.
   c. Testosterone level.

8. A common cause of virilization in a female infant?
   a. Congenital adrenal hyperplasia.
   b. Maternal estrogen therapy.
   c. Turner's syndrome.

9. Which one of the following is least likely to represent a normal finding in the assessment of the newborn genitalia?
   a. Clitoromegaly.
   b. Partial fusion of labiosacral folds.
   c. Undescended testes.

10. A situation when the sex-of-rearing may be different from the chromosomal sex is:
    a. A 46XX infant with complete virilization due to CAH.
    b. A female with virilization due to a maternal androgen-producing tumor.
    c. A male with severe microphallus unresponsive to exogenous testosterone.

Answers to Study Questions

1. a	5. a	8. a
2. c	6. c	9. b
3. a	7. b	10. c
4. a		

REFERENCES

Chowdhry, P., Scanlon, J., Auerbach, R., et al: Results of controlled double-blind study of thyroid replacement in very low-birth-weight premature infants with hypothyroxinemia. Pediatrics, 73(3):301–305, 1984.

Pagon, R.: Diagnostic approach to the newborn with ambiguous genitalia. Pediatr. Clin. North Am. 34(4):1019–1031, 1987.

BIBLIOGRAPHY

American Acedemy of Pediatrics and American Thyroid Association: Newborn screening for congenital hypothyroidism: recommended guidelines. Pediatrics, 80(5):745–749, 1987.

American Academy of Pediatrics, Committee on Genetics: Newborn screening fact sheet. Pediatrics, 83(3):449–464, 1989.

Brook, C. (ed.): Clinical Paediatric Endocrinology. Oxford, Blackwell Scientific Publications, 1989.

Danish, R.: Abnormalities of sexual differentiation. In Fanaroff, A., and Martin, R. (eds.): Neonatal-Perinatal Medicine, 4th ed. St. Louis, C.V. Mosby, 1987.

Fisher, D.: Euthyroid low thyroxine (T_4) and triiodothyronine (T_3) states in premature and sick neonates. Pediatr. Clin. North Am., 37(6):1297–1312, 1990.

Forest, M.G.: Endocrine disorders in the newborn. In Stern, L., and Vert, P. (eds.): Neonatal Medicine. New York, Masson Publishing, 1987.

Kaplan, S. (ed.): Clinical Pediatric Endocrinology. Philadelphia, W.B. Saunders Co., 1990.

L'Allemand, D., Gruters, A., Beyer, P., et al: Iodine in contrast agents and skin disinfectants is the major cause for hypothyroidism in premature infants. Hormone Res., 28:42–49, 1987.

Mazur, T.: Ambiguous genitalia: Detection and counseling. Pediatr. Nurs., 9(6):417–422, 1983.

McCauley, E.: Disorders of sexual differentiation and development. Pediatr. Clin. North Am., 37(6):1405–1419, 1990.

Mercado, M., Yu, V.Y.H., Francis, I., et al: Thyroid function in very preterm infants. Early Hum. Dev., 16:131–141, 1988.

Smerdely, P., Boyages, S.C., Wu, D., et al: Topical iodine-containing antiseptics and neonatal hypothyroidism in very-low-birth-weight infants. Lancet 2:661–664, 1989.

Sharon M. Glass

CHAPTER

17

Hematological Disorders

Objectives

1. Differentiate the processes of hematopoiesis and erythropoiesis.

2. Recall erythrocyte and leukocyte development from pluripotent stem cells.

3. Relate the consequences of anemia to the management of the infant.

4. Evaluate the clinical presentation of disseminated intravascular coagulation (DIC) in relation to the coagulation consumption and fibrinolysis.

5. Describe the etiological factors of hemorrhagic disease of the newborn.

6. Describe key indicators for nursing assessment of the thrombocytopenic infant.

7. Evaluate the neonatal consequences of maternal immune thrombocytopenic purpura (ITP).

8. Discuss the role of partial exchange transfusion in the treatment of neonatal polycythemia.

9. Describe current recommendations for use of blood components.

10. Analyze the components of the complete blood count (CBC) and describe the usefulness of each in the determination of neonatal sepsis.

This chapter presents an overview of development of blood cells and coagulation factors and includes normal birth values and common diagnostic tests. Blood products and transfusion therapies are discussed with current recommendations for use. Common hematological problems and therapies affecting the newborn are outlined. An evaluation of the CBC components useful for identification of sepsis is included.

Development of Blood Cells (Baehner, 1990; Miller, 1990a, 1990b, 1990c; Oski and Naiman, 1982)

A. Hematopoiesis: formation, production, and maintenance of blood cells.
1. Pluripotent stem cells, from which all blood cells derive, present in yolk sac at 16 days' gestation.
2. Circulation begins by day 22, with primitive cells arising intravascularly from vessel walls.

3. Extravascular liver hematopoiesis begins with migration of pluripotent stem cells from yolk sac, well established by 9 weeks' gestation.
4. Liver hematopoiesis peaks at 4–5 months' gestation, then slowly regresses as medullary (bone marrow) hematopoiesis predominates from 22 weeks' gestation.
5. Sites of extramedullary hematopoiesis (spleen, lymph nodes, thymus, kidneys) aid production of cells during fetal life when long bones are small.
6. Pluripotent cells develop into committed unipotent stem cells (colony-forming units), which evolve into specific cell lines (Figure 17–1).
7. Stress can influence the rate of differentiation of pluripotent cells, yielding different concentrations of committed precursor cells.

B. **Erythropoiesis:** production of erythrocytes (red blood cells).
1. Erythroid precursors develop from a committed unipotent cell that also differentiates to produce granulocytes, monocytes, and platelets.
2. Erythropoiesis and synthesis of hemoglobin are regulated by a hormone, erythropoietin.
3. Erythropoietin is produced post-natally in the kidneys, but during fetal life, extrarenal sites (liver, submandibular glands) predominate.

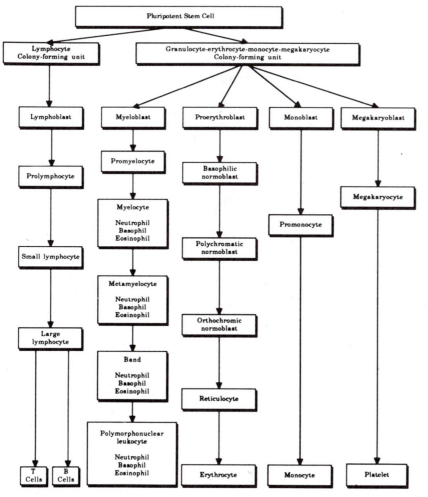

Figure 17–1
Maturation of blood cell components.

4. Erythropoietin production is increased in response to anemia and low oxygen availability to tissues and decreased in response to hypertransfusion.

C. **Hemoglobin:** major iron-containing component of the red blood cell (RBC).
1. Delivers oxygen from lungs to tissue cells through the circulation.
2. By 10 weeks' gestation, fetal hemoglobin (Hb F) is the major component of the RBCs.
3. Transition from predominant production of Hb F to production of adult hemoglobin (Hb A) begins at the end of fetal life.
   a. RBCs contain 70–90% Hb F at birth.
4. Hb F has a greater affinity for oxygen than Hb A, resulting in decreased oxygen release to the tissues.
   a. Hemoglobin binds with 2, 3-diphosphoglycerate (2,3-DPG) to release an oxygen molecule.
   b. Hb F has far less affinity for 2,3-DPG than Hb A.
   c. Levels of 2,3-DPG are directly proportional to gestational age.
5. Normal birth values (Table 17–1).
   a. Values depend on gestational age and volume of placental transfusion (timing of cord clamping).
   b. Peripheral vasoconstriction and stasis yield higher values from capillary samples.

D. **Hematocrit:** percentage of RBCs in a unit volume of blood.
1. Values rise immediately after birth and then decline to cord levels in the first week.
2. Normal birth values (see Table 17–1).
   a. Values depend on gestational age and volume of placental transfusion (timing of cord clamping).
   b. Peripheral vasoconstriction and stasis yield higher values from capillary samples.

E. **Red blood cells.**
1. Erythroid precursors mature in the bone marrow through the normoblast and reticulocyte stages (Figure 17–1).
2. Reticulocytes, in the absence of stress, mature 1–2 days in the bone marrow and then another day in the circulation before maturing to erythrocytes.
   a. Reticulocyte count is inversely proportional to gestational age at birth (see Table 17–1) but falls rapidly to <2% by 7 days.
   b. Persistent reticulocytosis may indicate chronic blood loss or hemolysis.
3. RBC function.
   a. Tissue oxygenation by hemoglobin transport.
   b. Carbon dioxide removal through reaction with carbonic anhydrase.

Table 17–1
NORMAL BLOOD VALUES IN PREMATURE AND TERM INFANTS

Value	Gestational Age (wks) 28	34	Full-Term Cord Blood	Day 1	Day 3	Day 7	Day 14
Hb (gm/dl)	14.5	15.0	16.8	18.4	17.8	17.0	16.8
Hematocrit (%)	45	47	53	58	55	54	52
Red cells (mm³)	4.0	4.4	5.25	5.8	5.6	5.2	5.1
MCV (μ^3)	120	118	107	108	99	98	96
MCH (pg)	40	38	34	35	33	32.5	31.5
MCHC (%)	31	32	31.7	32.5	33	33	33
Reticulocytes (%)	5–10	3–10	3–7	3–7	1–3	0–1	0–1
Platelets (1000s/mm³)			290	192	213	248	252

MCV, mean corpuscular volume; MCH, mean corpuscular hemoglobin; MCHC, mean corpuscular hemoglobin concentration.
From Klaus, M.H., and Fanaroff, A.A.: Care of the High Risk Neonate, 3rd ed. Philadelphia, W.B. Saunders Co., 1986.

   c. Hemoglobin can serve as a buffer to maintain acid-base balance.

4. RBC count.
   a. Number of circulating mature RBCs per cubic millimeter (mm³) (see Table 17–1).
   b. Count equals production minus destruction or loss.
   c. RBC lifespan proportional to gestational age.
      (1) Adult—100–120 days.
      (2) Full-term—60–70 days.
      (3) Premature—35–50 days.
   d. Nucleated RBCs are circulating immature (pre-reticulocyte) red cells.
      (1) Number is inversely proportional to gestational age and declines rapidly in the first week.
      (2) Increase may indicate hemolysis, acute blood loss, hypoxemia, congenital heart disease, or infection.

5. RBC indices: measure of RBC size and hemoglobin content used for designation of anemias (see Table 17–1).
   a. Mean corpuscular volume (MCV): average size and volume of a single RBC.
      (1) MCV decreases as gestation progresses and continues to decrease after birth to adult size by 4–5 years.
      (2) Increased MCV: macrocytes.
      (3) Decreased MCV: microcytes.
   b. Mean corpuscular hemoglobin (MCH): average amount (weight) of hemoglobin per single RBC.
      (1) MCH parallels the MCV decrease.
      (2) Increased MCH: hyperchromic cells.
      (3) Decreased MCH: hypochromic cells.
   c. Mean corpuscular hemoglobin concentration (MCHC): average concentration of hemoglobin per single RBC calculated from the amount of hemoglobin per 100 ml of cells.
      (1) MCHC remains constant, with adult values reached by 6 months.
      (2) Increased MCHC: hyperchromic cells.
      (3) Decreased MCHC: hypochromic cells.

F. White blood cells (WBC).

1. Leukocyte precursors mature in the bone marrow and lymphatic tissues, in the absence of stress, through the promyelocyte, myelocyte, and metamyelocyte stages and enter the circulation at the polymorphonuclear stage (see Figure 17–1).
2. WBCs are carried in the circulation to the extravascular tissues where they function as an important part of the immunologic system in reaction to foreign protein.
3. Granulocytes, lymphocytes, and monocytes are types of WBCs.
   a. Granulocytes—cell lines include basophils, eosinophils, and neutrophils.
      (1) Basophils.
         (a) Important in inflammatory responses.
         (b) Least numerous of the granulocytes: 0.5–1% of total WBC count.
      (2) Eosinophils.
         (a) Perform the same functions as neutrophils but are more sluggish in response.
         (b) Important in allergic and anaphylactic responses and most effective granulocyte for parasitic destruction.
         (c) Benign eosinophilia of prematurity inversely proportional to gestational age may be seen in infants who receive total parenteral nutrition, multiple blood transfusion, and endotracheal intubation, and may be physiological response to foreign antigens (Bhat and Scanlon, 1981).
         (d) Normally comprise 1–3% of total WBC count.
      (3) Neutrophils.

        (a) Function as phagocytes to ingest and destroy small particles, such as bacteria, protozoa, cells and cellular debris, dust, and colloids.

        (b) Stress can increase production and bone marrow release of immature forms.

        (c) Neutrophils are increased at birth but decrease during the first week to reach percentages approximately equal to lymphocytes.

  b. Lymphocytes.

    (1) Thymus-derived (T) lymphocytes.

      (a) Important in graft-versus-host and delayed hypersensitivity reactions.

    (2) Bone marrow–derived (B) lymphocytes.

      (a) Important in production and secretion of immunoglobulins and antibodies.

  c. Monocytes

    (1) Transformed into macrophages in tissues (i.e., lung: alveolar macrophage; liver: Kupffer cell macrophages).

    (2) Responsible for clearance of old blood cells, cellular debris, opsinized bacteria, antigen-antibody complexes, and activated clotting factors from the circulation.

4. WBC count.

  a. Number of circulating WBCs/mm³ (Table 17–2).

  b. WBC count is proportional to gestational age, with the total counts of premature infants approximately 30–50% lower than term infants.

G. Platelets.

1. Small, non-nucleated, disc-shaped cells aid in hemostasis, coagulation, and thrombus formation.

  a. Derived from megakaryocytes in the bone marrow.

2. After release into the blood stream, will circulate 7–10 days before removal by the spleen.

  a. In the absence of injury, circulate freely without wall adhesion or aggregation with other platelets.

3. Normal range is 100,000–300,000/mm³ in the full-term and premature infant.

H. Blood volume.

1. Volume of blood in cubic millimeters per body weight in kilograms (kg).

2. Factors affecting blood volume.

  a. Gestational age.

    (1) Full-term: approximately 80–100 cc/kg.

Table 17–2
NORMAL LEUKOCYTE VALUES IN PREMATURE AND TERM INFANTS

Age (hrs.)	Total White Cell Count	Neutrophils	Bands/Metas	Lymphocytes	Monocytes	Eosinophils
Term Infants						
0	10.0–26.0	5.0–13.0	0.4–1.8	3.5–8.5	0.7–1.5	0.2–2.0
12	13.5–31.0	9.0–18.0	0.4–2.0	3.0–7.0	1.0–2.0	0.2–2.0
72	5.0–14.5	2.0–7.0	0.2–0.4	2.0–5.0	0.5–1.0	0.2–1.0
144	6.0–14.5	2.0–6.0	0.2–0.5	3.0–6.0	0.7–1.2	0.2–0.8
Premature Infants						
0	5.0–19.0	2.0–9.0	0.2–2.4	2.5–6.0	0.3–1.0	0.1–0.7
12	5.0–21.0	3.0–11.0	0.2–2.4	1.5–5.0	0.3–1.3	0.1–1.1
72	5.0–14.0	3.0–7.0	0.2–0.6	1.5–4.0	0.3–1.2	0.2–1.1
144	5.5–17.5	2.0–7.0	0.2–0.5	2.5–7.5	0.5–1.5	0.3–1.2

Data modified from Xanthou (1970) by Glader (1977).
From Oski, F.A., and Naiman, J.L.: Hematologic Problems in the Newborn, 3rd ed. Philadelphia, W.B. Saunders Co., 1982.

(2) Pre-term: approximately 90–105 cc/kg.
  b. Placental transfusion.
    (1) Timing of cord clamping.
    (2) Position of infant relative to placenta (above or below) prior to cord clamping.
    (3) Timing and strength of uterine contractions.
    (4) Onset of respirations and decrease in pulmonary vascular resistance.
    (5) Cord compression.
  c. Maternal-fetal or fetal-maternal transfusion.
  d. Twin-twin transfusion.
  e. Placenta previa or abruptio.
  f. Nuchal cord.

Coagulation

Hemostasis is accomplished by biochemical and physiological events initiated to stop the flow of blood when vessel injury occurs (Corrigan, 1990a, 1990b; Oski and Naiman, 1982; Ryan, 1986).

A. **Deficiencies in newborn clotting mechanisms**.
1. Transient diminished platelet function.
2. Transient deficiency of clotting Factors II, VII, IX, X, XI, XII.
  a. Immaturity of hepatic enzymes responsible for production.
  b. Transient deficiency of vitamin K needed for synthesis of Factors II, VII, IX, X.
  c. Factor concentrations are proportional to gestational age.

B. **Hemostatic mechanisms**.
1. Vascular: damaged vessel contracts due to vasospasm.
2. Intravascular: platelet plug formation.
  a. Platelet function is stimulated by exposure to damaged endothelial lining.
    (1) Platelet bloats and develops thorn-like projections.
    (2) Becomes sticky and adheres to subendothelial fibers.
    (3) Secretes adenosine diphosphate (ADP) to trigger swelling and adhesiveness in nearby platelets.
    (4) Platelets aggregate and platelet plug forms.
3. Extravascular.
  a. Pressure effect of surrounding tissue.
  b. Injured tissue releases tissue thromboplastin.

C. **Coagulation process**.
1. Cascade of events, each dependent on the other (Figure 17–2).
2. Thromboplastin formed by activation of the intrinsic or extrinsic systems in conjunction with calcium, iron, and phospholipids.
  a. Intrinsic system triggered by vascular endothelial injury.
  b. Extrinsic system triggered by tissue injury and release of tissue thromboplastin.
  c. Both systems trigger separate mechanisms (see Figure 17–2) until Factor X is activated, beginning the process of prothrombin to thrombin conversion.
    (1) Conversion hydrolyzes fibrinogen (soluble protein in plasma) to fibrin (insoluble, thready polymer) and activates Factor XIII, stabilizing fibrin threads into a meshwork to trap platelets and other cells to form the clot.
3. Massive intravascular clotting controlled by concurrent fibrinolysis.
  a. Inactive plasminogen synthesized by the liver is converted to plasmin, an active enzyme, when a fibrin clot is present.
  b. Plasmin begins fibrin clot dissolution, releasing fibrin degradation products (FDP), also called fibrin split products (FSP), into the circulation.

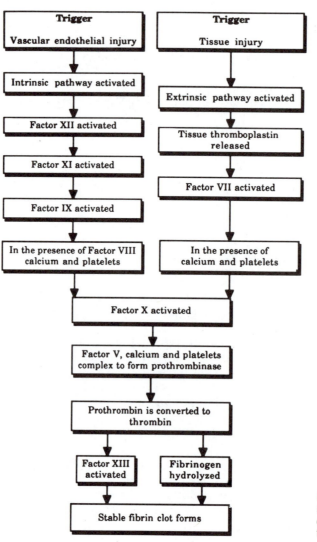

Figure 17–2
Fibrin clot formation through activation of the intrinsic or extrinsic pathways of the coagulation cascade.

    c. FDPs produce an anticoagulant effect by interfering with clot formation and function of platelets, thrombin, and fibrinogen.

D. **Coagulation tests** (Table 17–3).
1. Platelet count assesses platelet number.
2. Bleeding time (BT) assesses platelet function.
3. Prothrombin time (PT) assesses extrinsic and common portions of coagulation cascade.
4. Partial thromboplastin time (PTT) assesses intrinsic and common portions of coagulation cascade.
5. Fibrinogen assesses circulating level of this protein substrate required for clot formation.
6. FDP assesses fibrinolytic activity.
7. Individual clotting factors may be assayed depending on results of above tests.

Anemia

Low hemoglobin concentration and/or decreased number of RBCs diminishes the oxygen-carrying capacity of the blood and the level of oxygen available to the tissues (Blanchette and Zipursky, 1987; Miller, 1990d; Oski and Naiman, 1982).

Table 17-3
NORMAL VALUES FOR TESTS OF HEMOSTASIS

Test of Hemostasis	Normal Adult and Child (>1 yr)	Normal Newborn	Premature Newborn (32-36 wk)
Platelets/μl $\times 10^{-3}$	238 ± 64	310 ± 68	290 ± 70
Bleeding time (Ivy) (min)	<10	<10	<10
Prothrombin time (sec)	13 ± 2	16 (range, 13-20)	17 (range, 12-21)
Partial thromboplastin time (sec)	48 ± 6	55 ± 10	70
Thrombin clotting time (sec)	14 ± 2	12 (range, 10-16)	14 (range, 11-17)
Fibrinogen (Factor I) (mg/deciliter)	283 ± 88	246 ± 55	226 ± 70
Prothrombin (Factor II) (%)	103 ± 21	45 ± 15	35 ± 12
Factor V (%)	94 ± 33	98 ± 40	91 ± 23
Factors VII/X complex (%)	99 ± 15	56 ± 16	39 ± 14
Factor VIII (%)	107 ± 25	105 ± 35	98 ± 40
Factor IX (%)	100 ± 22	28 ± 8	—
Factor XIII (%)	100	100	100
Fibrin(ogen) degradation products, μ/ml	0-7	0-7	0-7
Euglobulin lysis time (min)	140	84	95
Antithrombin III (%)	100	55	48

From McMillan, C.W.: Defects of hemostasis in surgical patients. *In* Holder, T.M., and Ashcraft, K.W. (eds.): Pediatric Surgery. Philadelphia, W.B. Saunders Co., 1980.

A. **Etiological factors.**
1. Hemorrhage.
    a. Fetal-maternal.
        (1) Spontaneous.
        (2) Traumatic amniocentesis.
        (3) External cephalic version.
    b. Twin-to-twin.
        (1) Monozygotic, monochorial (single) placenta.
        (2) >5 gm of hemoglobin/100 ml difference between twins.
    c. Placental/cord.
        (1) Umbilical cord rupture.
        (2) Cord or placental hematoma.
        (3) Anomalous cord insertion.
        (4) Rupture of anomalous vessels of cord or placenta.
        (5) Accidental incision of cord or placenta.
        (6) Placenta previa or abruptio.
    d. Internal.
        (1) Intracranial (subdural, subarachnoid, intraventricular).
        (2) Organ rupture (liver, spleen, adrenal, kidney).
2. Hemolysis.
    a. Blood group incompatibilities.
        (1) Rh incompatibility: erythroblastosis fetalis (Miller, 1990d; Page, 1989).
            (a) Fetal blood cells containing Rh antigen (Rh positive) enter the maternal circulation; maternal red cells have no antigen (Rh negative); maternal immune system produces antibodies against the foreign fetal antigens; maternal antibodies enter fetal circulation and destroy fetal red cells.
            (b) Predisposing factors.
                i. Previous pregnancy, abortion.
                ii. During pregnancy (fetal-maternal hemorrhage).
                iii. Delivery (vaginal, breech, cesarean).
                iv. Amniocentesis, chorionic villus sampling.
                v. External version.

      vi. Manual removal of placenta.
- (c) Infant presentation.
    - i. Anemia secondary to hemolysis increases fetal production of very immature red cells (erythroblasts).
    - ii. Decreased red cell count and decreased oxygen-carrying capacity of immature cells leads to tissue hypoxia, acidosis.
    - iii. Hydrops fetalis (generalized edema): fetal attempts to expand blood volume and cardiac output result in congestive heart failure.
    - iv. Fluid collects in large cavities (ascites, pleural effusion).
    - v. Hepatosplenomegaly secondary to increased extramedullary hematopoiesis.
    - vi. Petechiae (thrombocytopenia accompanies severe anemia).
    - vii. Hypoglycemia secondary to hyperplasia of pancreatric islets and hyperinsulinemia.
    - viii. Positive direct Coombs' test.
- (d) Prophylactic therapy—RhoGAM (anti-D gamma globulin).
    - i. Destroys fetal red cells in maternal circulation, blocking maternal antibody production.
    - ii. 90% effective in prevention of sensitization.
    - iii. Recommended administration within 72 hours after delivery, at 28 weeks' gestation, and following amniocentesis or chorionic villus sampling.
- (2) ABO incompatibility (Miller, 1990d; Ryan, 1986; Wong, 1988).
    - (a) More frequently occurring but less severe hemolytic disease than Rh.
    - (b) Most often seen in mothers with O blood type (absence of antigen) carrying fetus with A or B blood type (Table 17–4 shows all potential incompatibilities).
    - (c) Maternal exposure to naturally occurring A and B antigens in food and bacteria initiates maternal production of anti-A, anti-B antibodies and accounts for severity of disease with first pregnancy.
    - (d) Protective effect against fetal Rh disease if mother is Rh negative due to rapid destruction of fetal A/B cells preventing Rh antigen exposure and maternal antibody production.
    - (e) Infant presentation.
        - i. Mild hemolysis, anemia, reticulocytosis.
        - ii. Hyperbilirubinemia (occasionally requiring exchange).
- b. Enzymatic defect: glucose-6-phosphate dehydrogenase (G6PD) deficiency.
    - (1) Most common inherited disorder of red cells (sex-linked disease affecting mainly male offspring, occasionally female carriers).
    - (2) Interaction of intracellular abnormality (deficiency of red cell enzyme) and extracellular factor (exposure to oxidant stress—drugs, infection) causes hemolysis and shortened erythrocyte life.
    - (3) Occurring most commonly in American black infants (10–15%) and infants of Mediterranean, African, and Far Eastern descent.

Table 17–4
POTENTIAL MATERNAL-FETAL ABO INCOMPATIBILITIES

Maternal Blood Group	Incompatible Fetal Blood Group
O	A or B
B	A or AB
A	B or AB

    c. Infection.
       (1) Intrauterine (viral, protozoan, spirochetal) and post-natal (bacterial) in-
         fection may cause neonatal hemolysis, anemia, thrombocytopenia, and
         DIC.
3. Anemia of prematurity (Stockman, 1986).
    a. Hemoglobin (Hb) concentration at birth varies only slightly in relation to
       gestational age.
    b. During the first 2–3 months, Hb concentration falls to the lowest values that
       occur at any developmental period.
    c. Considered physiological because it is characteristic of healthy infants.
    d. Associated factors.
       (1) Rate of decline and nadir are inversely proportional to gestational age.
       (2) Iron concentration is low secondary to decreased blood volume and
         decreased concentration of circulating Hb iron.
       (3) Improved extrauterine oxygen delivery causes temporarily inactive stage
         of erythropoiesis.
       (4) Erythropoietin production in response to anemia is slightly diminished.
       (5) Slightly shortened red cell life span decreases red cell mass.
       (6) Growth causes dilutional anemia secondary to decreased Hb concentra-
         tion with expanding blood volume.
       (7) In spite of rapid Hb fall, tissue oxygenation is maintained by events
         responsible for right shift of hemoglobin-oxygen dissociation curve.
    e. Some infants do manifest symptoms of hypoxemia (poor feeding and weight
       gain, dyspnea, tachypnea, tachycardia, diminished activity, pallor) in the
       absence of other problems and require transfusion.
    f. No direct correlation has been established between low Hb levels and the
       occurrence of apnea (Blank et al., 1984; Stockman, 1986).
4. Iatrogenic post-natal phlebotomy.
    a. Critically ill infants who require frequent monitoring may have excessive
       amounts of blood removed for diagnostic studies. Removal of >20% of the
       blood volume over 24–48 hours can produce anemia (Blanchette and Zi-
       pursky, 1987).

B. Clinical presentation: varies with the degree of hemorrhage and the time period over which the blood is lost.
1. Acute blood loss.
    a. Pallor.
    b. Shallow, rapid, irregular, respirations.
    c. Tachycardia.
    d. Weak or absent peripheral pulses.
    e. Low or absent blood pressure, low venous pressure.
    f. Hb may be normal initially, with rapid decline over 6–12 hours with
       hemodilution.
2. Chronic blood loss.
    a. Pallor without signs of acute distress.
    b. May demonstrate signs of congestive heart failure with hepatomegaly.
    c. Normal blood pressure, normal or elevated venous pressure.
    d. Hb will be low.

C. Clinical assessment.
1. Family history.
    a. Bleeding, anemia, splenectomy.
    b. Consanguinity.
    c. Ethnic, geographic origins.
    d. Blood group incompatibilities.
2. Maternal history.
    a. Blood type.
    b. Late third-trimester bleeding.

D. Physical exam.
1. Acute or chronic signs of blood loss.
2. Jaundice.
3. Cephalohematoma.
4. Abdominal distention or mass.
   a. Liver, spleen, adrenal, kidney rupture.
5. Petechiae, purpura.
6. Cardiovascular abnormalities.
   a. Tachycardia, murmur, gallop rhythm.
7. Hydropic changes.

E. Diagnostic studies.
1. Hemoglobin.
   a. Venous Hb values <13 g/dl in infants of 34–35 weeks' gestation or older in the first week of life are considered abnormal (Blanchette and Zipursky, 1987; Oski and Naiman, 1982).
      (1) Values vary according to birth weight and post-natal age (Table 17–5).
2. Reticulocyte count.
   a. Reflects erythroid activity and is persistently elevated with increased red cell destruction.
3. Peripheral blood smear.
   a. Evaluates alterations in size, shape, and structure of RBCs.
   b. Identifies fragmentation of RBCs.
4. Blood type.
   a. Identifies most common blood group antigens: A, B, O, Rh.
5. Coombs' test.
   a. Coombs' test is an antiglobulin test that detects antibody attached to the red cell in vivo (direct) or artificially in vitro (indirect).
   b. Positive direct Coombs' indicates presence of maternal IgG antibodies on the red cell surface.
   c. Positive indirect Coombs' detects antibodies in the maternal serum.
   d. Positive reactions are graded from +1 to +4 and approximately quantify the amount of antibody on the cell membrane.
6. Kleihauer-Betke test.
   a. Identifies fetal Hb in maternal blood.
   b. Calculations indicate volume of fetal-maternal hemorrhage.

F. Differential diagnosis.
1. Diseases that diminish oxygen delivery to the tissues (pulmonary, cardiac).
2. Methemoglobinemia.

G. Complications.
1. Inadequate tissue oxygenation, poor growth.
2. Transfusion.

Table 17–5
SERIAL HEMOGLOBIN VALUES (G/DL) IN LOW-BIRTH-WEIGHT INFANTS

Birth Weight (g)	Age (in Weeks)				
	2	*4*	*6*	*8*	*10*
800–1000	16.0 ± 0.6	10.2 ± 3.2	8.7 ± 1.5	8.0 ± 0.9	8.0 ± 1.1
1001–1200	16.4 ± 2.3	12.8 ± 2.5	10.5 ± 1.8	9.1 ± 1.3	8.5 ± 1.5
1201–1400	16.2 ± 1.3	13.4 ± 2.8	10.9 ± 1.2	9.9 ± 1.9	—
1401–1500	15.6 ± 2.2	11.7 ± 1.0	10.5 ± 0.7	9.8 ± 1.4	—

From Oski, F.A.: Hematologic problems. *In* Avery, G.B. (ed.): Neonatology: Pathophysiology and Management of the Newborn. Philadelphia, J.B. Lippincott, 1981.

   a. Transfusion reaction (see Transfusion Therapies).
   b. Overhydration with pulmonary congestion.
H. **Patient care management** (see Transfusion Therapies).
1. Emergency treatment for acute blood loss resulting in hypovolemia.
   a. Whole blood or combination of packed red blood cells (PRBCs) with crystalloid or colloid.
      (1) Group O, Rh negative.
      (2) 10–20 ml/kg.
   b. Fresh frozen plasma (FFP), albumin, or saline if blood unavailable.
2. Non-emergency replacement transfusion.
   a. Clinical decision based on adequacy of tissue oxygenation in the individual infant.
      (1) Adequate oxygen-carrying capacity to maintain cardiopulmonary function can be met by an Hb level of 7 g/dl when intravascular volume is adequate for perfusion (Silberstein et al., 1989).
      (2) Consider gestational and post-natal age; intravascular volume; co-existing cardiac, pulmonary, or vascular conditions.
3. Exchange transfusion.
   a. Treatment of jaundice secondary to blood group incompatibility.
   b. Partial exchange may be required to treat severe anemia of hydrops without increasing intravascular volume.
I. **Outcome**.
1. Improved tissue oxygenation and resolution of symptoms with replacement transfusion.
2. Long-term outcome varies with degree of anemia and underlying cause.

Hemorrhagic Disease of the Newborn

Hemorrhagic disease of the newborn is a hemorrhagic tendency secondary to vitamin K deficiency and decreased activity of Factors II, VII, IX, and X (Corrigan, 1990b; Glader, 1984).

A. **Etiological factors**.
1. Primary vitamin K deficiency.
   a. Required for activation of clotting Factors II, VII, IX, X after liver synthesis.
      (1) Important in the formation of calcium binding sites necessary for activation of factors.
   b. Suppression of bacterial synthesis.
      (1) Intestinal flora required for vitamin K synthesis.
      (2) Newborn intestinal tract virtually bacteria free until feedings begun.
      (3) Antibiotic therapy can alter normal intestinal bacterial colonization.
B. **Clinical presentation**.
1. Bleeding.
   a. Begins at 24–72 hours of age.
   b. May be localized or diffuse.
   c. Rarely life threatening.
C. **Clinical assessment**.
1. Oozing.
   a. Localized.
      (1) Frequently gastrointestinal (hematemesis, melena).
   b. Diffuse.
      (1) Umbilical cord, circumcision, puncture sites.
D. **Physical exam**.
1. Diffuse ecchymosis, petechiae.
2. Oozing puncture sites.

3. Abdominal distention.
4. Jaundice.

E. Diagnostic studies.
1. Response to vitamin K administration establishes the diagnosis.
2. PT/PTT prolonged.
3. Low levels of vitamin K–dependent clotting factors.

F. Differential diagnosis.
1. Decreased absorption of vitamin K.
   a. Biliary atresia.
   b. Cystic fibrosis.
2. Pharmacological antagonism of vitamin K.
   a. Phenytoin (Dilantin), phenobarbital, coumarin compounds.
   b. Bleeding occurs in the first 24 hours secondary to maternal drugs.

G. Complications.
1. Anemia.

H. Patient care management.
1. Prophylactic vitamin K at the time of delivery.
   a. Phytonadione (naturally occurring vitamin K) 0.5–1 mg, IV or IM (premature infants may be given the lower dose).
   b. Adequate serum concentrations of vitamin K have been observed after oral administration of 1–2 mg phylloquinone (vitamin K_1) (Sann et al, 1985; McNinch et al., 1985; O'Connor and Addiego, 1986).
2. Significant bleeding (Hb <12 g/dl).
   a. PRBC infusion may be indicated.
3. Persistent bleeding in premature infant.
   a. FFP infusion may be indicated to replace clotting factors.

I. Outcome.
1. Prophylactic treatment has virtually eliminated the disease.

Disseminated Intravascular Coagulation (DIC)

DIC is an acquired hemorrhagic disorder associated with an underlying disease manifested as an uncontrolled activation of coagulation and fibrinolysis. Consumption of clotting factors is thought to be initiated by release of thromboplastic material from damaged or diseased tissue into the circulation. Fibrinogen converts to fibrin to form microthrombi (Connallon, 1981; Corrigan, 1990b).

A. Common precipitating factors.
1. Maternal.
   a. Pre-eclampsia, eclampsia, abruptio.
   b. Placental abnormalities.
2. Intrapartal.
   a. Fetal distress with hypoxia and acidosis.
   b. Dead twin fetus.
   c. Traumatic delivery.
3. Neonatal.
   a. Infection (bacterial, viral).
   b. Conditions causing hypoxia and acidosis.
   c. Severe Rh incompatibility.
   d. Thrombocytopenia.

B. Clinical presentation (Figure 17–3).
1. Generalized, multiple site bleeding.
   a. Clotting factors and platelets are depleted.
   b. Fibrinolysis is stimulated.
2. Organ and tissue ischemia.

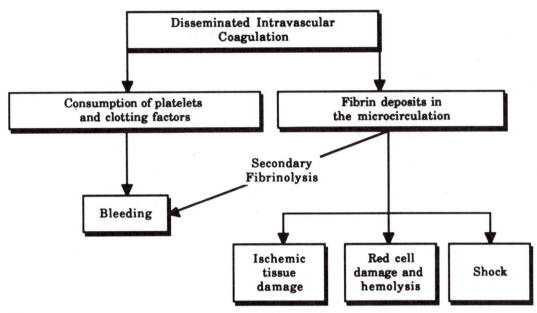

Figure 17-3
Sequence of events in the pathology of disseminated intravascular coagulation (DIC).

     a. Vascular occlusion by fibrin thrombi causes potential ischemia and necrosis of any organ, particularly kidneys.
3. Anemia.
     a. Blood loss.
     b. Red cell fragmentation by fibrin strands.

C. Clinical assessment.
1. Review history for precipitating factors.
2. Concurrent evidence of coagulation and fibrinolysis.

D. Physical exam.
1. Variable signs, depending on the underlying disease process.
2. Prolonged oozing from puncture sites or umbilicus.
3. Petechiae, purpura, ecchymosis.
4. Hemorrhage (pulmonary, gastrointestinal, cerebral).
5. Localized necrosis and gangrene secondary to thrombosis of peripheral vessels.

E. Diagnostic studies (see Table 17-3).
1. Variable diagnostic studies for delineation of the underlying disease process.
2. Platelet count is low.
3. PT/PTT both significantly prolonged.
4. Peripheral blood smear identifies abnormalities of red cell shape, cell fragmentation, and decreased number of platelets.
5. Fibrinogen is low.
6. FDPs significantly increased.

F. Differential diagnosis.
1. Parenchymal liver disease.
2. Vitamin K deficiency.
3. Microangiopathic disease.
4. Primary fibrinogenolysis.
5. Hemophilia.

G. Complications.
1. Organ failure secondary to ischemia and necrosis, especially renal.
2. Intraventricular, parenchymal hemorrhage.

H. Patient care management.
1. Aggressive treatment of the underlying disease.
2. Supportive care.
   a. Replacement transfusion.
      (1) Whole blood for hypovolemia and shock.
      (2) PRBCs for isovolemic anemia.
   b. Maintenance of blood pressure.
3. Measures to control DIC.
   a. Replacement of clotting factors.
      (1) FFP.
      (2) Platelet concentrates.
      (3) Antithrombin III (inhibits coagulation, controls fibrinolysis).
   b. Heparin therapy if treatment of underlying disease and replacement of clotting factors fail to reverse the process or with evidence of significant thrombosis.
      (1) To interrupt fibrin deposition.
      (2) Initial dose of 50–200 units/kg, maintenance dose of 300–600 units/kg per day continuously or divided in 4-hour interval doses.
         (a) Continuous infusion more physiological and safer since intermittent doses may aggravate existing hemorrhage.
      (3) Dose is adjusted to maintain PTT within 60–70 seconds.
   c. Exchange transfusion.
      (1) Replaces clotting factors and removes FDP from circulation.
      (2) Fresh heparinized blood or blood stored <72 hours and preserved with citrate-phosphate-dextrose.
      (3) May be required every 12 hours until clotting studies return to normal.

I. Outcome.
1. Related to the prognosis of the underlying disease and the severity of the DIC.

Thrombocytopenia

Thrombocytopenia is an acquired disease in which there is a significant decrease in the platelet count (<100,000/mm³) of the term or premature infant (Blanchette and Zipursky, 1987; Castle et al., 1986; Corrigan, 1990c).

A. Etiological factors.
1. Platelet destruction.
   a. Maternal autoantibodies.
      (1) Immune thrombocytopenic purpura (ITP), systemic lupus erythematosus (SLE).
         (a) Autoantibodies bind to platelet surface antigens, making them susceptible to premature destruction.
         (b) IgG antibodies cross placenta and destroy fetal platelets.
         (c) Maternal platelet count is low.
   b. Neonatal conditions.
      (1) Isoimmune.
         (a) Analogous to Rh incompatibility.
            i. Fetal platelets contain an antigen lacking in the mother.
            ii. Fetal platelets enter maternal circulation, resulting in maternal production of antibodies against foreign platelets.
            iii. Maternal platelet count remains normal.
      (2) Infection (TORCH,* bacterial).
         (a) Inhibits platelet production in bone marrow.

---

*Toxoplasmosis, hepatitis, rubella, cytomegalovirus, and herpes simplex.

(b) Can cause DIC (platelet consumption).

(c) Activation of reticuloendothelial system (increased platelet sequestration).

(d) Platelets may form antigen-antibody complexes with infectious agent.

(3) Thrombotic disorders.

(a) Large vessel disease (renal vein thrombosis).

(b) Microvascular disease (necrotizing enterocolitis, respiratory distress syndrome).

(4) Birth asphyxia.

(5) Giant hemangiomas.

(a) Mechanical destruction and sequestration.

(6) Exchange transfusion.

(a) Shortened survival of transfused platelets.

2. Impaired platelet production.

a. Congenital malformations.

(1) Bone marrow hypoplasia affects megakaryocyte production.

(2) Trisomy syndromes (13, 18, 21).

(3) Thrombocytopenia with absent radii (TAR) syndrome.

(4) Fanconi anemia (skeletal, renal, and CNS anomalies, café au lait spots).

3. Platelet interference.

a. Maternal drug ingestion.

(1) Interferes with platelet aggregation.

(2) Meperidine (Demerol), promethazine (Phenergan), acetylsalicylic acid, sulfonamides, quinidine, quinine.

b. Infant drug ingestion.

(1) Indomethacin may inhibit platelet function.

B. **Clinical presentation.**

1. Petechiae, purpura.

2. Ecchymosis over presenting part.

3. Cephalohematoma.

4. Bleeding (gastrointestinal, genitourinary, umbilical, puncture sites).

C. **Clinical assessment.**

1. Family history.

a. Bleeding complications in previous children, other family members.

2. Maternal history.

a. History of bruising or bleeding, infections, collagen-vascular disease, splenectomy.

b. Platelet count (low or normal).

c. Peripheral blood smear (may show low platelet count, increased immature forms).

d. Medication history.

D. **Physical exam.**

1. Signs of clinical presentation.

2. Jaundice.

3. Hepatosplenomegaly with infectious etiology (absent with immune etiology).

4. Congenital anomalies consistent with syndromes.

E. **Diagnostic studies.**

1. Platelet count is low.

2. Peripheral blood smear shows low platelet count, increased immature forms.

3. PT/PTT are normal.

4. BT is prolonged.

F. **Differential diagnosis.**

1. DIC.

2. Vitamin K deficiency.

G. Complications.
1. Cranial hemorrhage with neurological sequelae (associated with approximately 12% mortality).
2. Entrapped hemorrhage.
3. Anemia.
4. Hyperbilirubinemia.

H. Patient care management.
1. Cesarean delivery.
   a. Controversial; recommended if maternal platelet count is <100,000/mm³.
2. Platelet transfusion.
   a. Isoimmune: transfusion of maternal platelets (absence of antigen) that have been washed and resuspended in AB-negative plasma.
3. Exchange transfusion.
   a. Autoimmune: exchange transfusion (removal of maternal autoantibodies) followed by platelet transfusions only in infants with life-threatening hemorrhage.
   b. Exchange transfusion may be required for hyperbilirubinemia.
4. Steroids.
   a. May produce a hemostatic effect on the vascular walls and inhibit platelet phagocytosis by the spleen.
   b. May be used in infants with platelet counts <25,000/mm³ and clinical bleeding.
   c. May be administered to mothers with autoimmune disease prenatally and are associated with higher infant platelet counts.
5. Supportive care, treatment of underlying disease.

I. Outcome.
1. Varies with underlying disease, presence of congenital malformations.
2. Autoimmune etiology usually causes only mild, transient problems, with full recovery of platelet count in 8–12 weeks.
3. Isoimmune etiology causes mild to moderate problems, with full recovery of platelet count in 6–8 weeks.

Polycythemia

Polycythemia is a condition in which infants demonstrate an excess in circulating RBC mass. The venous Hb is >22 g/dl or the venous hematocrit is >65% in the first week of life. Blood viscosity increases with hematocrits >60% and leads to a reduction of blood flow to organs (Blanchette and Zipursky, 1987; Miller, 1990b).

A. Etiological factors.
1. Intrauterine hypoxia, placental insufficiency.
   a. Hypoxia stimulates erythropoiesis, increasing fetal red cell mass.
      (1) Maternal pre-eclampsia/eclampsia, placenta previa.
      (2) Post-maturity syndrome, intrauterine growth retardation.
2. Maternal-fetal/twin-to-twin transfusion.
3. Placental hypertransfusion.
4. Maternal diabetes.
   a. Possibly secondary to abnormal fetal erythrocyte deformability.

B. Clinical presentation.
1. Many infants are asymptomatic.
2. Plethora.
3. Cyanosis.
4. CNS abnormalities (lethargy, jitteriness, seizures).
5. Respiratory distress (tachypnea, pulmonary edema, pulmonary hemorrhage).
6. Tachycardia, congestive heart failure.
7. Hypoglycemia.

C. Clinical assessment.
1. History and physical exam usually identify etiology.

D. Physical exam.
1. May be normal except for plethora and, occasionally, cyanosis.
2. Symptoms of clinical presentation not attributable to other disease.
3. Gestational age and intrauterine growth assessment.

E. Diagnostic studies.
1. Venous Hb/hematocrit are elevated.
   a. Hematocrit values should be determined by microcentrifugation rather than automated Coulter counter to avoid falsely low levels (Villalta et al., 1989).

F. Complications.
1. Hyperbilirubinemia.
2. Hyperviscosity syndrome.
   a. Elevated whole blood viscosity associated with reduced blood flow, vascular thrombosis (renal, cerebral, mesenteric), diminished oxygen transport, organ ischemia and failure.
   b. Long-term neurological sequelae.

G. Patient care management.
1. Partial exchange transfusion.
   a. Controversial in asymptomatic infants.
   b. Desired reduction of hematocrit to <60% (blood viscosity relatively normal at this level).
   c. Gastrointestinal symptoms (bleeding, poor feeding tolerance, necrotizing enterocolitis) may follow partial exchange (Black et al., 1985).
2. Supportive treatment of persistent symptoms.

H. Outcome.
1. Gross motor delays, neurological sequelae, fine motor abnormalities, speech delays seen at 2 years (Black et al., 1985).
2. Lower spelling and arithmetic achievement test and gross motor skill scores at 7 years (Delaney-Black et al., 1989).

Blood Products (Depalma and Luban, 1990)

A. Recommendations on use of blood components (Morbidity and Mortality, 1988; FDA Drug Bulletin, 1989; Silberstein et al., 1989).
1. Develop and document criteria indicating need.
2. Use only the blood components required for therapy.
3. Use crystalloid or non-blood colloid whenever possible.
4. Use universal precautions when handling blood products.

B. Whole blood.
1. Indicated in massive hemorrhage and exchange transfusion.
2. Hematocrit approximately 35%.

C. Packed red blood cells (PRBCs).
1. Plasma removed, leaving red cell mass of approximately a whole unit of blood in fluid volume of one-half unit.
2. Hematocrit approximately 60–90%.
3. Indicated to promote delivery of oxygen to tissues during active bleeding or symptomatic anemia.

D. Fresh frozen plasma (FFP).
1. Plasma obtained from a unit of whole blood and frozen within 6 hours of collection.
2. Indicated for replacement of clotting factor deficiency.

E. Granulocytes.
1. Granulocytes are selectively harvested from whole blood.

2. Indicated in life-threatening granulocytopenias.

F. **Platelets**.

1. Platelets are separated from single units of whole blood within 6 hours of collection and suspended in small amounts of plasma.
2. Indicated for treatment of hemorrhage due to thrombocytopenia or platelet dysfunction.

G. **Albumin**.

1. Indicated for volume expansion to treat hypovolemia or decreased colloid oncotic pressure.

Transfusion Therapies (Depalma and Luban, 1990; Silberstein et al., 1989)

A. **Replacement transfusions**.

1. Iatrogenic post-natal phlebotomy in the first week of life and symptomatic anemia.
2. To prevent overhydration, replacement is usually in increments of 10–15 ml/kg per dose.

B. **Partial exchange transfusions**.

1. With normal saline.
   a. Polycythemia (to reduce hematocrit without reducing blood volume).
2. With PRBCs.
   a. Hydrops fetalis (to correct anemia without increasing blood volume).
3. Calculations for total exchange volume:
   a. With normal saline:

$$\frac{\text{Blood Volume} \times (\text{Measured Hematocrit} - \text{Desired Hematocrit})}{\text{Measured Hematocrit}}$$

   b. With PRBCs:

$$\frac{\text{Blood Volume} \times (\text{Desired Hematocrit} - \text{Measured Hematocrit})}{\text{PRBC Hematocrit} - \text{Measured Hematocrit}}$$
$$(70\%)$$

C. **Exchange transfusions**.

1. Single unit of blood (approximately 500 ml) will exchange twice the blood volume and replace 70–85% of the infant's blood.
2. Indications: hyperbilirubinemia, DIC, autoimmune thrombocytopenia.
3. Preservatives provide a significant glucose load; rebound hypoglycemia may occur.
4. Preservatives also contain citrate, which binds calcium and magnesium; hypocalcemia and hypomagnesemia may occur.
5. Potassium level rises as blood ages; blood should be <5 days old.

D. **Erythropoietin transfusions:** Experimental protocol only—not yet approved by the Food and Drug Administration (Christensen et al., 1989.

1. Experimental injections of erythropoietin to correct the diminished erythropoiesis of anemia of prematurity and avoid the need for blood products.
2. Potential hazard: neutrophil production may be diminished due to stem cell competition (erythrocytes, granulocytes, and platelets all derive from a common progenitor).

E. **Transfusion reactions**.

1. Fever, vomiting, hypotension, respiratory distress (cyanosis, tachypnea), hemolysis.

2. Post-transfusion graft-versus-host disease (GVHD) (Sanders and Graeber, 1990; Funkhouser et al., 1991).
   a. Transfused donor lymphocytes (present in erythrocyte and platelet blood products) recognize foreign host antigens and attack organ systems.
   b. Infants at risk for GVHD are those exposed to in utero transfusions or exchange transfusion, extremely premature infants, infants with isoimmune thrombocytopenia, or infants with underlying immunodeficiency.
   c. Clinical symptoms occurring within 100 days of transfusion include rash, diarrhea, hepatic dysfunction, and bone marrow suppression with generalized reduction in all blood cells (pancytopenia).
   d. Recommendations for handling of blood products to prevent GVHD.
      (1) Irradiation of blood products for all infants at risk for GVHD.
      (2) Irradiation of all blood products from directed donors.
         (a) Potential antigen similarities between close family members may impede recognition and destruction of foreign lymphocytes.
      (2) Irradiation with a minimum of 3000–4000 rad will destroy lymphocytes.
         (a) Mature erythrocytes are resistant to radiation damage.
         (b) Irradiation may have some effect on locomotion of WBCs.

Complete Blood Count (CBC) Evaluation

An evaluation of certain components of the CBC may be helpful as an adjunct in the diagnosis of sepsis (Klein and Marcy, 1990; Manroe et al., 1979; Oski and Naiman, 1982).

A. Response to infection.
1. Increased neutrophil release from the bone marrow.
2. Increased number of immature neutrophil forms released into the circulation.
3. Neutropenia rather than neutrophilia commonly results secondary to neutrophil storage pool depletion.
   a. Neutrophil storage pool consists of neutrophils stored outside the circulation in the bone marrow or along vessel walls.
   b. Infant's neutrophil storage pool diminished in size compared with adults.
   c. Disturbed regulation of marrow neutrophil release in neonates.

B. Evaluation of total WBC count: insensitive as a predictor of the infection response.

C. Neutrophil counts: most sensitive indicators of infant sepsis.
1. Factors affecting neutrophil counts.
   a. Birth asphyxia and maternal hypertension (neutropenia in the first 72 hours).
   b. Hemolytic disease (neutrophilia in the first 72 hours).
2. Absolute neutrophil count (ANC).
   a. Normal range.
      (1) Full-term infants: 1750–5400/mm^3.
      (2) Pre-term infants: 1200–5400/mm^3 (Zipursky et al., 1976).
   b. Slightly more sensitive than total WBC count, but as a single indicator of sepsis is only approximately 15% predictive.
3. Absolute band count (ABC).
   a. Normally peaks at 1400/mm^3 by 12 hours of age.
   b. May be elevated early in the response to infection, but is rarely elevated in fatal infection due to rapid exhaustion of marrow reserves and is therefore an insensitive single indicator of sepsis (Christensen et al., 1981).
4. Immature to total neutrophil (I/T) ratio.
   a. Total number of immature neutrophil forms (bands, myelocytes, metamye-

locytes, promyelocytes) is divided by the total number of neutrophils (immature forms plus mature segmented or polymorphonuclear leukocytes; Figure 17–4).

b. More sensitive indicator of sepsis because it considers the number of circulating metamyelocytes, which indicates accelerated release from the neutrophil storage pool.

c. I/T ratio >0.2 may indicate sepsis.

d. I/T ratio >0.8 associated with neutrophil storage pool depletion (Christensen et al., 1981).

e. Complications associated with an increased I/T ratio in the absence of sepsis.
  (1) Maternal fever.
  (2) Maternal oxytocin administration.
  (3) Stressful labor.
  (4) Neonatal asphyxia.
  (5) Pneumothorax.
  (6) Intraventricular hemorrhage.
  (7) Seizures.
  (8) Prolonged crying (≥4 minutes).
  (9) Hypoglycemia (blood glucose ≤30 mg/dl).
  (10) Surgery.

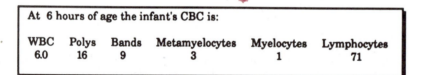

At 6 hours of age the infant's CBC is:

WBC	Polys	Bands	Metamyelocytes	Myelocytes	Lymphocytes
6.0	16	9	3	1	71

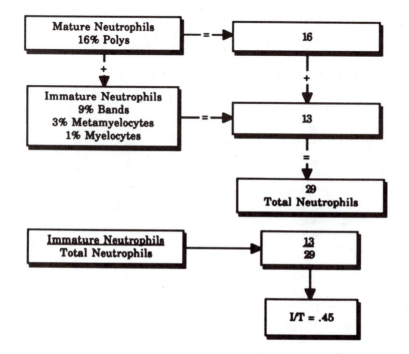

Figure 17–4
Calculation of the immature to total (I/T) neutrophil ratio.

STUDY QUESTIONS

1. Hematopoiesis refers to:
   a. Differentiation of pluripotent cells.
   b. Formation and production of blood cells.
   c. Production of erythrocytes.

2. Hemoglobin values at birth depend on:
   a. Gestational age and volume of placental transfusion.
   b. Maturation of erythroid precursors.
   c. Ratio of fetal hemoglobin (Hb F) to adult hemoglobin (Hb A).

3. Anemia might compromise the infant by causing:
   a. Depletion of clotting factors and platelets.
   b. Inadequate tissue oxygenation and poor growth.
   c. Poor intestinal motility and feeding intolerance.

4. Vitamin K is required for activation of the following clotting factors:
   a. I, III, IV, and VI.
   b. V and VIII.
   c. II, VII, IX, and X.

5. Disseminated intravascular coagulation (DIC) presents as:
   a. Congenital deficiency of Factor VII or Factor IX.
   b. Disturbed regulation of marrow neutrophil release.
   c. Uncontrolled activation of coagulation and fibrinolysis.

6. An important factor in assessment of the thrombocytopenic infant includes:
   a. Determination of the mother's Rh antigen status.
   b. Maternal history of low platelet count.
   c. Timing of administration of vitamin K.

7. Partial exchange transfusion is performed in the polycythemic infant for the purpose of:
   a. Correcting the anemia without increasing the blood volume.
   b. Reducing the bilirubin without reducing the blood volume.
   c. Reducing the hematocrit without reducing the blood volume.

8. According to the current recommendations for the use of blood components, fresh frozen plasma (FFP) is indicated for:
   a. Enhancement of oxygen delivery to the tissues.
   b. Replacement of clotting factors.
   c. Treatment of platelet dysfunction.

9. Post-transfusion graft-versus-host disease (GVHD) can be prevented in infants at risk by:
   a. Bone marrow suppression with steroids.
   b. Irradiation of blood products to destroy donor lymphocytes.
   c. Sequestration of antigens to delay immune responses.

10. The immature to total (I/T) neutrophil ratio may be increased in the absence of sepsis in infants who have:
    a. Bacterial infection.
    b. Neonatal asphyxia.
    c. Isoimmune thrombocytopenia.

11. Prothrombin time (PT) assesses:
    a. Extrinsic and common portions of the coagulation cascade.
    b. Fibrinolytic activity.
    c. Intrinsic and common portions of the coagulation cascade.

Answers to Study Questions

1. b	5. c	9. b
2. a	6. b	10. b
3. b	7. c	11. a
4. c	8. b	

REFERENCES

Baehner, R.L.: Disorders of granulopoiesis. *In* Miller, D.R., and Baehner, R.L. (eds.): Blood Diseases of Infancy and Childhood, 6th ed. St. Louis, C.V. Mosby, 1990, pp. 515–548.

Bhat, A.M., and Scanlon, J.W.: The pattern of eosinophilia in premature infants. J. Pediatr. *98*:612–616, 1981.

Black, V.D., Lubchenco, L.O., Koops, B.L., et al.: Neonatal hyperviscosity: Randomized study of effect of partial plasma exchange transfusion on long-term outcome. Pediatrics, *75*:1048–1053, 1985.

Blanchette, V., and Zipursky, A.: Neonatal hematology. *In* Avery, G.B. (ed.): Neonatology: Pathophysiology and Management of the Newborn, 3rd ed. Philadelphia, J.B. Lippincott, 1987, pp. 638–690.

Blank, J.P., Sheagren, T.G., Vajaria, J., et al.: The role of RBC transfusion in the premature infant. Am. J. Dis. Child. *138*:831–833, 1984.

Castle, V., Andrew, M., Kelton, J., et al.: Frequency and mechanism of neonatal thrombocytopenia. J. Pediatr. *108*:749–755, 1986.

Christensen, R.D.: Recombinant erythropoietic growth factors as an alternative to erythrocyte transfusion for patients with "anemia of prematurity." Pediatrics, *83*:793–796, 1989.

Christensen, R.D., Bradley, P.P., and Rothstein, G.: The leukocyte left shift in clinical and experimental neonatal sepsis. J. Pediatr. *98*:101–105, 1981.

Connallon, M.: Disseminated intravascular coagulation. *In* Perez, R.H. (ed.): Protocols of Perinatal Nursing Practice. St. Louis, C.V. Mosby, 1981, pp 346–370.

Corrigan, J.J.: Hemostasis: General considerations. *In* Miller, D.R., and Baehner, R.L. (eds.): Blood Diseases of Infancy and Childhood, 6th ed. St. Louis, C.V. Mosby, 1990a, pp. 761–776.

Corrigan, J.J.: Coagulation disorders. *In* Miller, D.R., and Baehner, R.L. (eds.): Blood Diseases of Infancy and Childhood, 6th ed. St. Louis, C.V. Mosby, 1990b, pp. 837–899.

Corrigan, J.J. Platelet and vascular disorders. *In* Miller, D.R. and Baehner, R.L. (eds.): Blood Diseases of Infancy and Childhood, 6th ed. St. Louis, C.V. Mosby, 1990c, pp. 777–836.

Delaney-Black, V., Camp, B.W., Lubchenco, L.O., et al.: Neonatal hyperviscosity association with lower achievement and IQ scores at school age. Pediatrics, *83*:662–667, 1989.

Depalma, L., and Luban, N.L.: Blood component therapy in the perinatal period: Guidelines and recommendations. Semin. Perinatol. *14*: pp 403–415, 1990.

FDA Drug Bulletin. Rockville, MD, American Medical Association, July 1989.

Funkhouser, A.W., Vogelsand, G., Zehnbauer, B., et al.: Graft versus host disease after blood transfusions in a premature infant. Pediatrics, *87*:247–249, 1991.

Glader, B.E., and Amylon, M.D.: Hemostatic disorders in the newborn. *In* Taeusch, H.W., Ballard, R.A., and Avery, M.E. (eds.): Schaffer's Diseases of the Newborn, 6th ed. Philadelphia, W.B. Saunders Co., 1991, pp. 777–832.

Klein, J.O., and Marcy, S.M.: Bacterial sepsis and meningitis. *In* Remington, J.S., and Klein, J.O. (eds.): Infectious Diseases of the Fetus and Newborn Infant (3rd ed.). Philadelphia, W.B. Saunders Co., 1989, pp 601–656.

Manroe, B.L., Weinberg, A.G., Rosenfeld, C.R., et al.: The neonatal blood count in health and disease: I. Reference values for neutrophilic cells. J. Pediatr. *95*:89–98, 1979.

McNinch, A.W., Upton, C., Samuels, M., et al.: Plasma concentrations after oral or intramuscular vitamin K_1 in neonates. Arch. Dis. Child., *60*:814–818, 1985.

Miller, D.R.: Origin and development of blood cells and coagulation factors: Maternal-fetal interactions. *In* Miller, D.R., and Baehner, R.L. (eds.): Blood Diseases of Infancy and Childhood, 6th ed. St. Louis, C.V. Mosby, 1990a, pp. 3–25.

Miller, D.R.: Normal blood values from birth through adolescence. *In* Miller, D.R. and Baehner, R.L. (eds.): Blood Diseases of Infancy and Childhood, 6th ed. St. Louis, C.V. Mosby, 1990b, pp. 26–51.

Miller, D.R.: Erythropoiesis, hypoplastic anemias, and disorders of heme synthesis. *In* Miller, D.R. and Baehner, R.L. (eds.): Blood Diseases of Infancy and Childhood, 6th ed. St. Louis, C.V. Mosby, 1990c, pp. 124–169.

Miller, D.R. Hemolytic anemias: Metabolic defects. *In* Miller, D.R. and Baehner, R.L. (eds.): Blood Diseases of Infancy and Childhood, 6th ed. St. Louis, C.V. Mosby, 1990d, pp. 294–357.

Morbidity and Mortality Weekly Report. Rockville, MD, National AIDS Information Clearinghouse, June 24, 1988.

O'Connor, M.E., and Addiego, J.E.: Use of oral vitamin K_1 to prevent hemorrhagic disease of the newborn infant. J. Pediatr. *108*:616–619, 1986.

Oski, F.A., and Naiman, J.L.: Hematologic Problems in the Newborn, 3rd ed. Philadelphia, W.B. Saunders Co., 1982.

Page, S.: Rh hemolytic disease of the newborn. Neonatal Network, *7*(6):31–41, 1989.

Ryan, R.: Hematological conditions. *In* Streeter, N.S. (ed.): High-risk Neonatal Care. Rockville, MD, Aspen, 1986, pp. 409–449.

Sanders, M.R., and Graeber, J.E.: Posttransfusion graft-versus-host disease in infancy. J. Pediatr. *117*:159–163, 1990.

Sann, L., Leclercq, M., Guillaumont, M., et al.: Serum vitamin K_1 concentrations after oral administration of vitamin K_1 in low birth weight infants. J. Pediatr. *107*:608–611, 1985.

Silberstein, L.E., Kruskall, M.S., Stehling, L.C., et al.: Strategies for the review of transfusion practices. J.A.M.A. *262*:1993–1997, 1989.

Stockman, J.A.: Anemia of prematurity. Pediatr. Clin. North Am. *33*(1):111–127, 1986.

Villalta, I.A., Pramanik, A.K., Diaz-Blanco, J., et al.: Diagnostic errors in neonatal polycythemia based on method of hematocrit determination. J. Pediatr. *115*:460–462, 1989.

Whaley, L.F., and Wong, D.L.: Nursing Care of Infants and Children. St. Louis, C.V. Mosby, 1991.

Zipursky, A., Palko, J., Milner, R., et al.: The hematology of bacterial infections in premature infants. Pediatrics, *57*:839–853, 1976.

Josanne M. Paxton

Neonatal Infections

Objectives

1. Differentiate between humoral and cellular immunological responses in the neonate.

2. Calculate the absolute neutrophil count and immature to total cell ratio from a complete blood count and differential.

3. Identify the common gram-positive and gram-negative organisms responsible for bacterial infections in the neonatal period.

4. Name six antimicrobial agents used to treat neonatal sepsis and discuss indications and risks of their use.

5. Differentiate between pseudomembranous, systemic, and cutaneous candidiasis.

6. List several clinical manifestations associated with congenital viral infection.

7. Define human immunodeficiency virus and acquired immunodeficiency syndrome.

Infection is a major cause of demise during the first month of life, contributing to 13–15% of all neonatal deaths. A review of immunology assists the nurse in understanding neonatal host defense limitations. Interpretations of hematological studies and identification of risk factors and clinical manifestations can aid in the early detection of neonatal infection.

Group B streptococci, *Escherichia coli,* and *Listeria monocytogenes* are currently responsible for the majority of early-onset sepsis. Antibiotic therapy for bacterial infections must be based on the susceptibility of the organism and achievement of bactericidal concentrations. Congenital viral infections may be asymptomatic at birth or manifest with a host of multisystem involvements. Finally, the human immunodeficiency virus has become a leading cause of immunodeficiency in the neonate, with maternal-infant transmission accountable for the majority of neonatal acquisitions.

This chapter provides the nurse with a comprehensive review of neonatal infection.

Immunology

A. **Humoral immunity**.

1. Immunoglobulins.
   a. A specific antibody-mediated response that functions most effectively if there has been previous exposure.
   b. Antibodies are derived from B cells, which have been activated by T cells and antigens (Figure 18-1).
      (1) B cells mature and are stored in lymph tissue and bone marrow.
      (2) B cells also produce memory cells that recognize antigens on subsequent exposures and initiate an antibody response.
      (3) Antibody functions include:
         (a) Recognition of bacterial antigens.
         (b) Neutralization or opsonization of foreign substances, rendering them susceptible to phagocytosis.
2. Types of immunoglobulins.
   a. Immunoglobulin G (IgG).
      (1) Major immunoglobulin of serum and interstitial fluid.
      (2) Provides immunity against bacterial and viral pathogens.
      (3) Placental transfer to fetus may be an active or passive process.
      (4) Increases gradually until 40 weeks' gestation.
      (5) Pre-term infants have decreased levels proportional to their gestational age.
      (6) Postmature and small-for-gestational-age infants have decreased levels, suggesting inhibition of transfer with placental damage.
   b. Immunoglobulin M (IgM).
      (1) Does not cross the placenta.
      (2) Synthesis begins early in fetal life, with detectable levels at approximately 30 weeks' gestation.
      (3) May see increased levels (>20 mg/ml) with intrauterine infection.
      (4) Serum levels rapidly increase after birth.
   c. Immunoglobulin A (IgA).
      (1) Most common immunoglobulin in gastrointestinal tract, respiratory tract, human colostrum and breast milk.
      (2) Does not cross the placental barrier.
      (3) Intrauterine synthesis is minimal in an uninfected fetus and does not become detectable in the newborn until 2–3 weeks of life.
      (4) May see an increase in levels with certain congenital viral infections.

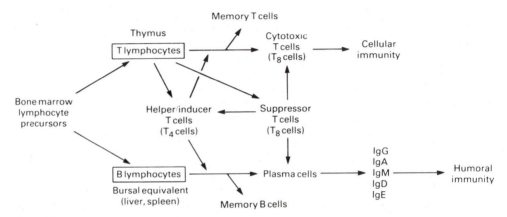

Figure 18-1
The development of cellular and humoral immunity. (From Ganong, W.F.: Review of Medical Physiology, 14th ed. E. Norwalk, CT, Appleton & Lange, 1989.)

   d. Immunoglobulin E (IgE).
      (1) Present in very small amounts in serum and secretions.
      (2) Major role is in allergic reactions.

B. **Cellular immunity**.
1. Specific cellular immunity is mediated by T lymphocytes, which serve to enhance the efficiency of phagocytic responses.
   a. T lymphocytes migrate to the thymus where they begin differentiation (see Figure 18-1).
   b. They are activated by antigens to which they have been sensitized and subsequently become memory or activated T cells.
      (1) Memory cells respond at a later time to the same antigen.
      (2) Activated T cells (three types).
         (a) Cytotoxic: kill foreign or virus-infected cells.
         (b) Helper: enable B or T cells to respond to antigens and activate macrophages.
         (c) Suppressor: repress responses of specific T and B lymphocytes to antigens.
   c. T lymphocytes modify the behavior of phagocytic cells and increase their antimicrobial activity.
   d. Depressed T-cell function may occur as a consequence of neonatal viral infection, hyperbilirubinemia, corticosteroid therapy, or maternal medications taken late in pregnancy.
2. Non-specific cellular immunity is an inflammatory response involving phagocytosis and includes neutrophils, monocytes, and complement.
   a. Neutrophils are the most numerous of the leukocytes.
      (1) Neutrophils mature from the bone marrow committed phagocyte stem cell.
      (2) They are the first line of defense against bacterial infection.
      (3) In a well neonate, a neutrophil reserve is present and exceeds the circulating pool; however, in a septic neonate, the neutrophil reserve pool quickly becomes depleted due to the following:
         (a) Decrease in proliferation or reproduction.
         (b) Decrease in the neutrophil storage pool.
         (c) Decrease in the number of neutrophils that reach the site of infection.
   b. Monocytes are important in the defense against fungal and bacterial infections and are found mainly in the connective tissue.
   c. Complement is the mediator of antigen-antibody reactions.
      (1) Is activated by an antibody-dependent mechanism (classic pathway) or antibody-independent mechanism (alternate pathway).
      (2) Serves to:
         (a) Increase neutrophil mobilization from the bone marrow.
         (b) Draw neutrophils to the site of infection.
         (c) Opsonize bacteria for improved phagocytosis.

C. **Summary of neonatal host defense limitations**.
1. Humoral immunity.
   a. Decreased antibody levels.
      (1) Poor response to antigenic stimuli.
      (2) Do not produce type-specific antibodies.
   b. Decreased opsonic activity.
      (1) Impaired circulating antibody.
      (2) Depressed complement pathways.
2. Neutrophil response.
   a. Decrease in neutrophil storage pool.
   b. Failure to increase stem cell proliferation during infection.
   c. Altered neutrophil function with respect to chemotaxis, phagocytosis, and bacterial killing.

Transmission of Bacterial Organisms

A. **Vertical:** mother to infant.
1. Transplacental infection crosses from the placenta to the fetus, an uncommon event as the environment is usually sterile.
2. Ascending infection occurs near the time of delivery when the cervical mucus plug, chorion, and amnion are less than optimal barriers.
3. Intrapartum infection occurs at delivery during passage of the fetus through a birth canal that is host to a variety of bacteria, chlamydia, fungi, yeast, and viruses.

B. **Horizontal:** passes from nursery personnel and the hospital environment to the infant.

Clinical Assessment

Identification of predisposing risk factors.

A. **Maternal.**
1. Antepartum.
    a. Poor prenatal care.
    b. Poor nutrition.
    c. Low socioeconomic status.
    d. Recurrent abortion.
    e. Substance abuse.
2. Intrapartum.
    a. Prolonged rupture of membranes (>24 hours).
    b. Maternal fever.
    c. Chorioamnionitis.
    d. Prolonged or difficult labor.
    e. Premature labor.
    f. Urinary tract infection.

B. **Neonatal.**
1. Low birth weight.
2. Prematurity.
3. Difficult delivery.
4. Birth asphyxia.
5. Meconium staining.
6. Resuscitation.
7. Foreign bodies.
8. Congenital anomalies, i.e., spinal and abdominal wall defects.

Clinical Manifestations

A. **Unusual general presentation:** may be the infant who just doesn't look right to the nurse or mother with subtle changes in feeding and activity.

B. **Problems with thermoregulation.**
1. Fever.
2. Hypothermia.

C. **Neurological manifestations.**
1. Lethargy.
2. Jitteriness.
3. Irritability.
4. Seizures.
5. Hypotonia or hypertonia.

6. Bulging fontanelles.
7. High-pitched cry.

D. **Respiratory abnormalities**.
1. Grunting.
2. Retractions.
3. Cyanosis.
4. Apnea.
5. Tachypnea.

E. **Cardiovascular manifestations**.
1. Tachycardia.
2. Arrhythmias.
3. Hypotension or hypertension.
4. Cold, clammy skin.
5. Decreased peripheral perfusion.

F. **Gastrointestinal signs**.
1. Poor feeding.
2. Vomiting.
3. Diarrhea.
4. Abdominal distention.
5. Increasing residuals.

G. **Skin**.
1. Rash.
2. Pustules.
3. Jaundice.
4. Pallor.
5. Vasomotor instability.
6. Petechiae.

H. **Internal organ response**.
1. Hepatomegaly.
2. Splenomegaly.

Hematological Evaluation

A. **Complete blood count**.
1. White blood count (WBC): interpretation is difficult due to the wide range of normal in the neonate (9000–30,000/mm³).
   a. Leukocytosis: an elevated WBC; may be a normal finding in the newborn.
   b. Leukopenia: a depressed WBC, generally an abnormal finding in the newborn.
2. Differential (Figure 18–2).
   a. Neutrophil count.
      (1) Absolute neutrophil count (ANC).
         (a) Calculated as:

$$\frac{(\% \text{ segs} + \% \text{ bands} + \% \text{ immature cells}) \times \text{total WBC}}{100}$$

         (b) Manroe et al (1979) developed a reference range for the absolute neutrophil count (Figure 18–3).
      (2) Neutropenia: <1500/mm³.
         (a) Most accurate predictor of infection.
         (b) May be associated with maternal hypertension, confirmed periventricular hemorrhage, severe asphyxia, and reticulocytosis (after 14 days' postnatal age).

Neutrophil: Stages of Maturation

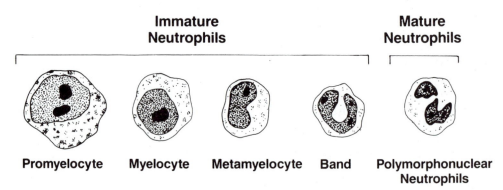

Immature Neutrophils

Mature Neutrophils

Promyelocyte   Myelocyte   Metamyelocyte   Band   Polymorphonuclear Neutrophils

Figure 18–2
Neutrophils represent a percentage of the total white blood count and are reported as the differential on a complete blood count.

      (3) Neutrophilia.
          (a) Although less predictive, may also suggest presence of an infection.
          (b) May be elevated at birth due to the neonate's increased neutrophil production and rates of release and demargination from the circulating neutrophil pool.
          (c) Other clinical conditions associated with neutrophilia include hemolytic disease, asymptomatic hypoglycemia, use of oxytocin during labor, maternal fever, stressful labor, pneumothorax, and meconium aspiration.
    b. Immature to total neutrophil (I/T) ratio.
      (1) Less specific than ANC.

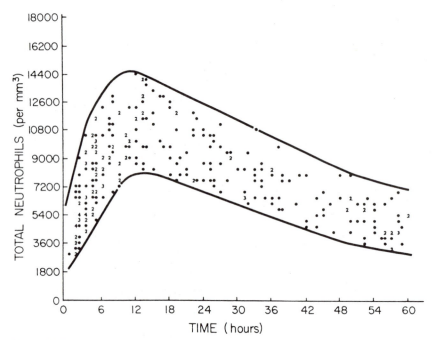

Figure 18–3
The total neutrophil count reference range in the first 60 hours of life. (From Manroe, B.L., Weinberg, A.G., Rosenfeld, C.R. and Browne, R.: The neonatal blood count in health and disease. J. Pediatr., *95*:91, 1979.)

(2) An increase in the I/T ratio is also known as a left shift and reflects an increase in immature neutrophils.

(3) An I/T ratio >.16–.20 may suggest infection (Figure 18–4).

(4) Calculation for I/T ratio:

$$\frac{\% \text{ bands} + \% \text{ immature forms}}{\% \text{ mature} + \% \text{ bands} + \% \text{ immature forms}}$$

c. Platelet count.

(1) Normal = 150,000–400,000.

(2) Thrombocytopenia may be associated with bacterial sepsis or viral infection.

(3) Severe thrombocytopenia may be associated with disseminated intravascular coagulation (DIC).

B. Additional diagnostic aids.

1. Detection of bacterial antigens.

   a. Provides a rapid method of diagnosis, although a negative result does not exclude an infectious process.

   b. Identifies antigens in the blood, urine, and cerebral spinal fluid (CSF) for *Neisseria meningitides, Haemophilus influenzae, Streptococcus* pneumonia, and group B streptococci.

   c. Does not rely on viable organisms; therefore, it is possible to obtain positive results even after initiation of appropriate antimicrobial therapy and until suppression of antigen activity has occurred.

   d. Counter-immunoelectrophoresis (CIE) and latex particle agglutination (LPA) are the most common methods for the identification of antigen response.

2. Hematological evidence of infection.

   a. Erythrocyte sedimentation rate (ESR): although false positives can occur and rates vary widely, may see a rise in levels above the 95th percentile during an infectious process.

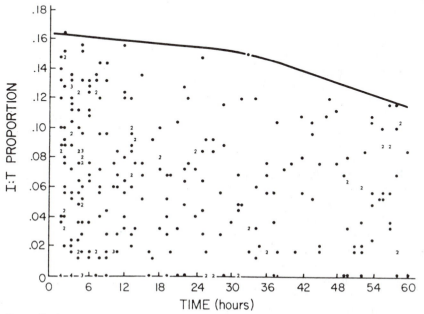

Figure 18–4
The reference range for the proportion of immature to total neutrophils in the first 60 hours of life. (From Manroe, B.L., Weinberg, A.G., Rosenfeld, C.R., and Browne, R.: The neonatal blood count in health and disease. J. Pediatr., *95*:95, 1979.)

    b. C-reactive protein (CRP).
        (1) Acute-phase reactant that appears in the blood during an inflammatory process.
        (2) Poor response when infection occurs during the first day of life or in infections caused by group B streptococci.
        (3) Most useful in determining effectiveness of treatment, resolution of disease, and duration of antibiotic therapy.
    c. IgM levels: may see a rise in the presence of bacterial and/or viral infections.

Diagnostic Evaluation

A. **Cultures:** isolation of a pathogen is essential for the absolute diagnosis of infection.
1. Blood.
    a. Culture may be obtained from peripheral vein or umbilical vessel.
    b. Procedure.
        (1) Carefully clean with an antiseptic such as povidone iodine solution 10%.
        (2) Allow to dry for 30 seconds before inserting needle and obtaining culture for maximal bactericidal effect.
        (3) A minimum of 0.5–1.0 ml of blood should be obtained to improve chances for detection of bacteremia.
2. Cerebrospinal fluid.
    a. Abnormal CSF findings include the following:
        (1) A leukocyte count of $100/mm^3$, especially if greater than 60% are polymorphonucleocytes.
        (2) Protein count >100 mg/dl.
        (3) CSF glucose less than 50% of a serum level (obtain serum level before spinal tap to allow for equilibrium to occur between CSF and blood).
        (4) Presence of micro-organisms on Gram stain.
    b. Culture.
        (1) Repeat the CSF tap every 24–36 hours until culture is sterile.
        (2) There is a direct correlation between adverse neonatal outcome and persistence of bacteria in CSF.
    c. Urine.
        (1) High incidence of contamination with urine obtained by an external collection bag.
        (2) If urine is obtained by urethral catheterization, a count >50,000–100,000 organisms per milliliter suggests infection.
        (3) When culture is positive, a percutaneous bladder tap should be performed because the urine obtained via bladder tap is presumed to be sterile.
    d. Superficial cultures.
        (1) Indicates colonization; however, does not diagnose bacteremia or sepsis.
        (2) 4+ bacteria in a gastric aspirate and an elevated WBC may suggest acquisition of an organism from the fetal amniotic fluid.
        (3) May have sepsis in the absence of a positive surface culture.
        (4) Common sites for obtaining surface cultures include the nares, deep ear, throat, axilla, umbilicus, and rectum.
B. Follow-up.
1. If a positive culture has been obtained in blood, CSF, or urine, a follow-up culture should be obtained to document sterilization.
2. Persistent bacteremia may be caused by:
    a. Resistance to antibiotics.
    b. Incorrect administration of antibiotics.
    c. An occult site of infection that may require surgical intervention (e.g., abscess).

Bacterial Infection

A. **Epidemiological history**.
1. 1930s and 1940s: a high incidence of group A streptococcus.
2. 1940s and 1950s: *E. coli* was responsible for the majority of infections.
3. 1950s and 1960s: the emergence of *Staphylococcus aureus*.
4. 1970s and 1980s: group B streptococci, *E. coli*, and *L. monocytogenes* are responsible for the majority of sepsis during the first week of life.
5. 1980s: *H. influenzae* and *Staphylococcus epidermidis* emerging as a cause of neonatal sepsis.

B. **Common sites of bacterial infection** include the blood, CSF, lungs, and urinary tract.
1. Sepsis.
   a. Incidence of neonatal sepsis is approximately 1 in 1000 live, full-term births and 1 in 250 live, pre-term births.
   b. 50% of neonates with bacterial sepsis will also present with meningitis.
   c. The most common organisms responsible for septicemia are *E. coli*, *S. aureus*, *S. epidermidis*, group B streptococci, and *L. monocytogenes*.
   d. Presentation is often non-specific, with subtle signs of temperature instability, lethargy, poor feeding, and glucose instability.
2. Meningitis.
   a. Occurs more frequently during the neonatal period than at any other time.
   b. Group B streptococci and *E. coli* account for the majority of pathogens identified in neonatal meningitis.
   c. Acquisition includes direct invasion, contamination between CSF space and integumental surfaces, and bacterial dissemination from infected structures.
   d. Clinical manifestations.
      (1) May present with general signs and symptoms of infection.
      (2) Can see specific CNS symptoms, including increased irritability, alteration in consciousness, poor tone, tremors, seizures, and bulging fontanel.
   e. CSF culture.
      (1) May have a positive CSF culture even though blood culture is negative.
      (2) If the CSF is positive, must repeat culture in 24–36 hours after initiation of treatment to ensure adequate therapy.
   f. Prompt initiation of antibiotic therapy is crucial to optimizing outcome, and may be administered prior to obtaining CSF.
   g. Significant sequelae develop in 20–50% of infants who survive, including motor and mental disabilities, convulsions, hydrocephalus, and hearing loss.
3. Pneumonia.
   a. Transmission.
      (1) Vertical.
         (a) Onset usually from birth to 7 days.
         (b) Most common bacterial pathogens responsible for pneumonia include group B streptococci and *L. monocytogenes*.
      (2) Horizontal.
         (a) Onset beyond 1 week of life.
         (b) *Pseudomonas aeruginosa* is the most common bacterial organism transmitted nosocomially and can result in a serious nursery outbreak.
      (3) Clinical manifestations may be general but often involve specific symptoms of respiratory distress.
      (4) Diagnosis.
         (a) Tracheal aspirate culture of the lower respiratory tract.
         (b) Presentation on chest X-ray can be varied and may include asymmetrical densities, pleural effusions, or pulmonary granularity, which is most often associated with group B streptococci.

4. Urinary tract infections.
   a. *E. coli* is the most common organism responsible for urinary tract infections, with *Klebsiella* and *P. aeruginosa* less common and gram-positive bacteria a rare cause.
   b. Clinical manifestations.
      (1) General signs are often nonspecific and may include temperature instability, poor weight gain, poor feeding, cyanosis, abdominal distention, hematuria, and proteinuria.
      (2) Localized signs consist of a weak urinary stream and/or bladder distention.
   c. Antimicrobial agents should be administered parenterally.
      (1) Oral absorption is erratic.
      (2) There is a 30% association between urinary tract infection and septicemia.
   d. Follow-up.
      (1) Repeat urine culture should be sterile within 36–48 hours after initiation of antimicrobial therapy.
      (2) If a urinary tract infection has been documented in an infant, a voiding cystourethrogram should be performed to evaluate the possibility of any congenital abnormalities of the urinary tract system.
5. Neonatal ophthalmia.
   a. May be caused by a variety of organisms, including *S. aureus*, *P. aeruginosa*, *Neisseria gonorrhoeae*, and *Chlamydia trachomatis*.
   b. Manifestations usually include discharge from the eye and conjunctivitis.
   c. Diagnosis is made by a culture and Gram stain, which reveals leukocytes and organisms.
   d. Ophthalmic antibiotics: methicillin is the drug of choice for *S. aureus* and a combination of carbenicillin and gentamicin are used when *P. aeruginosa* has been identified (also refer to *N. gonorrhoeae* and *C. trachomatis*).

Specific Bacterial Pathogens

A. **Gram-positive organisms.**
1. Group B streptococci.
   a. Common bacterial organism in the adult female genital tract.
   b. Colonization to disease ratio is approximately 100–200:1.
   c. Most common organism isolated in the neonate.
   d. Infection may be asymptomatic bacteremia or present as septicemia, pneumonia, or meningitis.
   e. Early onset.
      (1) Fulminant presentation occurring in the first 72 hours of life.
      (2) Acquired by vertical transmission.
      (3) Clinical manifestations include respiratory distress, hypotonia, poor feeding, hypoxemia, and shock.
   f. Late onset.
      (1) Insidious presentation usually occurring after 7–10 days.
      (2) Horizontal transmission.
      (3) Symptoms include fever, lethargy, and bulging fontanel.
2. Staphylococcus.
   a. *S. aureus*.
      (1) A nosocomial pathogen, with the major source of infection being hospital personnel, although also associated with umbilical catheters, endotracheal tubes, and central lines.
      (2) Colonization occurs in 40–90% of neonates by the fifth day of life.
      (3) May have widespread manifestations, including osteomyelitis, mastitis, and septicemia.
      (4) If resistant to penicillin or methicillin, vancomycin is antibiotic of choice.

    b. *S. epidermidis.*
      (1) Often regarded as a contaminant; however, coagulase-negative staphylococci may be important pathogenic organisms, and one should therefore evaluate for other clinical signs of sepsis.
      (2) Associated with use of invasive procedures, i.e., central line, endotracheal intubation.
      (3) Vancomycin is most effective antimicrobial agent.
    c. *L. monocytogenes.*
      (1) Short gram-positive rod.
      (2) May be acquired transplacentally or from the vaginal canal of a colonized mother.
      (3) Should suspect in a pre-term infant who has had passage of meconium or if maternal history includes prior stillbirth or repeated spontaneous abortions.
      (4) Can present as a fulminant disseminated disease with multi-organ involvement.
      (5) Symptoms commonly include hypothermia, lethargy, and poor feeding or may have a characteristic salmon-colored rash.
      (6) Sensitive to ampicillin.

B. **Gram-negative organisms**.
1. *E. coli.*
    a. Most common gram-negative organism in neonatal period.
    b. Found in female genital tract with high incidence of colonization in the neonate.
    c. Association between *E. coli* possessing the K1 capsular polysaccharide antigen and bacteremia.
    d. In addition to septicemia, may cause localized infection, including cellulitis, pneumonia, septic arthritis, urinary tract infection, and otitis media.
2. *P. aeruginosa.*
    a. Known as the "water bug" and is a common inhabitant of respirators and moist oxygen circuits.
    b. An infant on a respirator and receiving antibiotics is particularly susceptible to colonization and the subsequent development of pneumonia.
3. *H. influenzae.*
    a. Gram-negative bacillus.
    b. Low rate of maternal genital colonization, although passage to fetus is via ascending transcervical route.
    c. Chorioamnionitis occurs in all placentas but appears more severe among survivors.
    d. 50% chance of symptomatic infection in the colonized infant.
    e. Early-onset fulminant presentation with pneumonia, respiratory distress, hypotension, and leukopenia.
    f. Mortality may be as high as 50%, especially in the very-low-birth-weight infant.
4. *N. gonorrhoeae.*
    a. Infant presents with unilateral or bilateral conjunctivitis 2–5 days after birth.
    b. Diagnosis is made by Gram stain, which reveals gram-negative intracellular diplococci.
    c. Silver nitrate (1%) aqueous solution or erythromycin (0.5%) ophthalmic ointment in the eyes of all vaginally delivered infants is recommended. (*Note:* eye prophylaxis only minimizes the risk of infection but does not guarantee prevention of disease.)

C. **Bacterial parasites**.
1. *C. trachomatis* is commonly found in the adult female genital tract.
2. Delivery through an infected vaginal canal may result in neonatal infection.
3. Inclusion conjunctivitis of the newborn.

a. Presentation usually occurs 5–12 days after birth.
b. Discharge with crusting and slight edema of the eyelid may be the only signs of the disease.
c. Prophylactic use of erythromycin ophthalmic ointment after delivery may reduce the risk of the infection.
d. If diagnosed, treat with erythromycin ophthalmic ointment 50 mg/kg/day in four divided doses for 14 days.
e. May recur even after adequate treatment.
4. Chlamydial pneumonia of the newborn.
   a. Presentation usually occurs between 3 and 11 weeks of age.
   b. Symptoms include a persistent cough, rales, and wheezing.
   c. Chest radiograph may reveal hyperinflation.
   d. Chronic disease may persist even after acute phase of disease is over.
   e. Treat with erythromycin 40 mg/kg/day orally for 14 days.

Intervention

A. Antibiotic therapy (Table 18–1).
1. Ampicillin is commonly used in combination with an aminoglycoside for initial treatment of suspected or confirmed bacterial infection.
2. If meningitis is suspected, ampicillin and cefotaxime are the antibiotics of choice until a specific organism has been identified.
3. Ultimate choice of antibiotics must be based on:
   a. Sensitivity of organisms—may vary from institution to institution.
   b. Possible adverse side effects.
   c. Achievement of bactericidal concentration.
4. Third-generation cephalosporins, including cefotaxime and ceftazidime, have increased antimicrobial activity against gram-negative bacilli.

B. Transfusions.
1. Intravenous immune globulin (IVIG).
   a. Administration of IVIG appears to be effective in preventing nosocomial infections in pre-term low-birth-weight infants and may decrease mortality.
   b. Acts to neutralize viruses, promote phagocytosis, increase opsonization, and enhance polymorphonucleocyte migration and prevents neutrophil storage pool depletion.
   c. Prophylactic use has been recommended in pre-term infants due to their quantitative and qualitative deficiency of immunoglobulin.
   d. Study by Kyllonen et al. (1989) suggests a dose of 900 mg/kg every 2 weeks if birth weight is 501–1000 kg; 700 mg/kg every 2 weeks if birth weight is 1000–1500 kg.
   e. Although clinical trials are not yet completed, IVIG is generally well tolerated in the neonate; however, side effects may include nausea, vomiting, and fever.
2. Neutrophil transfusion.
   a. May improve survival in septic infants with a decreased neutrophil storage pool (Christensen et al., 1982).
   b. Transfuse with 10–15 ml/kg of irradiated granulocytes.
   c. Process may be time consuming and expensive.
   d. Risks include fluid overload, graft versus host disease, infections, and blood-group sensitization.
3. Exchange transfusion.
   a. Used widely prior to 1980; however, prospective studies have not been done to support its effectiveness (Vain et al., 1980).
   b. Adverse reactions include hypoglycemia, acid-base imbalance, thrombocytopenia, and infection.

Table 18-1
NEONATAL ANTIMICROBIAL THERAPY

Agent	Dose	Indication	Risks
Ampicillin	100–200 mg/kg/day IM, IV q 12 hours	Therapy for sepsis or meningitis gram-positive organisms	Seizures in high doses
Cefotaxime	100 mg/kg/day (third generation) IV q 12 hours	Sepsis, meningitis caused by gram-negative organisms, e.g., *E. coli, H. influenzae*	Nephrotoxicity, neutropenia, eosinophilia
Ceftazidime	100–150 mg/kg/day IM, IV q 8–12 hours over 30 minutes	Sepsis or meningitis caused by gram-negative organisms, e.g., *E. coli, H. influenzae,* and *Klebsiella*	Rash, diarrhea, eosinophilia
Chloramphenicol	25 mg/kg/day IV q 24-hours; monitor serum levels	Gram-positive and negative organisms, Chlamydia, and ampicillin-resistant strains; no primary indication for use	Gray baby syndrome, anorexia, vomiting, abdominal distention, ashen gray color, death
Erythromycin	40 mg/kg/day po q 6 hours	Chlamydia	None
Gentamicin	5 mg/kg/day IV q 12 hours	Aminoglycoside, initial choice of therapy for sepsis or meningitis; monitor serum levels; gram-negative organisms	Ototoxicity, nephrotoxicity
Methicillin	100 mg/kg/day IV q 12 hours	Use if penicillin-resistant *S. aureus* organism	Nephrotoxicity, eosinophilia
Nafcillin	50 mg/kg/day IV q 12 hours	Penicillin-resistant *S. aureus* organisms	Nephrotoxicity, eosinophilia
Penicillin	100,000–150,000 units/kg/day IV q 12 hours	Gram-positive anaerobes	Rare neuromuscular side effects and nephrotoxicity
Tobramycin	4 mg/kg/day IV q 12 hours	Aminoglycoside with broad gram-negative coverage	Possible nephrotoxicity and ototoxicity
Vancomycin	20–40 mg/kg/day IV q 12 hours	Most gram-positive cocci and rods, methicillin-resistant *S. aureus*	Nephrotoxicity, ototoxicity, rash, neutropenia, eosinophilia

Fungal Infections

A. Candidiasis.
1. Significant neonatal pathogen with *Candida albicans* as the most common species.
2. Can cause localized disease in any organ system.
3. Neonates at risk include those that are premature, immunocompromised, receiving total parenteral nutrition, or have been on broad-spectrum antibiotics.
4. Thrush (acute pseudomembranous candidiasis).
   a. Most common form of candidiasis in newborns.
   b. Acquired during passage through the birth canal or from mothers during breast feeding.
   c. Appears as pearly white material on the buccal mucosa, dorsum and lateral areas of tongue, gingivae, and pharynx.

    d. Treat with nystatin oral suspension 100,000–200,000 units every 6 hours for 1 week.

5. Acute disseminated (systemic) candidiasis.
    a. Most frequent sites of infection include the lungs, kidneys, liver, spleen, and brain and may involve several sites simultaneously.
    b. Presentation includes respiratory deterioration, abdominal distention, apnea, acidosis, carbohydrate intolerance, hypotension, skin abscesses, temperature instability, or erythematous rash.
    c. Formation of fungus in urine may lead to urinary tract infection.
    d. Antibiotic therapy.
      (1) Amphotericin B 0.25–1 mg/kg/day as a daily infusion over 4–6 hours for 3–4 weeks is the treatment of choice, with close monitoring of hematological and renal function.
      (2) 5-Fluorocytosine 100–150 mg/kg/day in four divided doses for 3–4 weeks, especially if severe infection or CNS involvement.

6. Cutaneous candidiasis.
    a. Presence of oral candida is strongly associated with the development of cutaneous candidiasis in the perineal region.
    b. May appear initially as erythematous and vesiculopapular lesions, then develop into fine white, scaly collarettes.
    c. Management.
      (1) Use of topical agents such as nystatin four times per day and continued 2–3 days after rash has cleared.
      (2) Simultaneous treatment with oral nystatin to minimize the risk of recurrence.
      (3) Maintain area free from moisture and stool.

Viral Infections

A. Mode of transmission.
1. Congenital: acquired in utero during maternal viral infection with exposure to the fetus. Infant presents with disease at birth or shortly thereafter.
2. Intrapartum: acquired at birth with organisms present in the genital tract and onset of neonatal symptoms within 5–7 days or longer, depending on the incubation period.
3. Postnatal: acquired during the neonatal period and may be transmitted in breast milk (e.g., cytomegalovirus, hepatitis B), blood transfusions (e.g., cytomegalovirus, hepatitis B), or from hospital personnel or family (e.g., enterovirus, respiratory syncytial virus [RSV]).

B. Viral organisms.
1. Rubella.
    a. Teratogenic virus that often results in congenital malformations.
    b. The severity of neonatal disease is increased if infection occurs during the first trimester.
    c. There may be no initial symptoms, although most infected infants will have long-term sequelae.
    d. Early manifestations include intrauterine growth retardation, thrombocytopenia, hepatomegaly, jaundice, congenital heart disease (patent ductus arteriosus, peripheral pulmonary artery stenosis, arterial or ventricular septal defects), interstitial pneumonia, cataracts, bone lesions, microphthalmia, lethargy, irritability, bulging fontanel, and late-onset seizures.
    e. Diagnosis is made with detection of specific rubella IgM antibody.
    f. Prevention via maternal rubella vaccine prior to pregnancy.
    g. No treatment.
2. Cytomegalovirus (CMV).

    a. Most common congenital viral infection and member of the herpesvirus group.

    b. May be congenitally acquired or transmitted through blood transfusion.

    c. 90–95% of neonates are asymptomatic at birth; however, 10% of these may have long-term sequelae, including decreased intelligence, hearing loss, and microcephaly.

    d. Risk of severe congenital disease in the neonate is greatest when a primary maternal infection occurs during pregnancy.

    e. Severity may be decreased in a recurrent infection; however, the virus may be transmitted despite maternal immunity.

    f. Presentation may include hepatosplenomegaly, chorioretinitis, and cerebral calcification.

    g. Diagnosis is made by early isolation of the virus from the infant.

    h. No treatment.

3. Herpes simplex virus (HSV).

    a. Types.

        (1) HSV-1—non-genital type, although can infect the genital area.

        (2) HSV-2—genital type, more often associated with neonatal disease.

    b. Transmission.

        (1) Intrapartum or postnatal transmission can occur even without evidence of maternal lesions.

            (a) If there is primary maternal infection, neonatal infection is 10–20 times more likely.

            (b) Presentation includes vesicular lesions, thermal instability, lethargy, respiratory distress, vomiting, poor feeding, cyanosis, and, if there is CNS involvement, irritability, bulging fontanel, seizures, opisthotonos, and coma.

        (2) Congenital transmission.

            (a) Occurs less commonly than intrapartum or postnatal transmission.

            (b) Presentation includes early vesicular rash, small for gestational age, low birth weight, chorioretinitis, diffuse brain damage, microcephaly, intracranial calcifications.

        (3) Diagnosis is made when a positive culture is obtained from vesicular fluid, blood, or cerebrospinal fluid.

        (4) Treatment.

            (a) Systemic infection.

                i. Acyclovir 10 mg/kg/dose every 8 hours for 2–3 weeks.

                ii. Side effects include nephrotoxicity, lethargy, tremors, and seizures.

            (b) Ocular involvement should be treated with a topical ophthalmic drug such as 3% vidarabine, in addition to parenteral antiviral therapy.

        (5) High mortality rate if untreated.

        (6) If positive maternal history, prevention includes the following:

            (a) Weekly virological and clinical screening, beginning at 32 weeks.

            (b) Cesarean section if lesions or positive culture at the time of delivery.

            (c) Vaginal delivery if no clinical or virological evidence.

4. Hepatitis B.

    a. DNA double-shelled virus.

    b. Prenatal transmission occurs when mothers are hepatitis B surface antigen (HBsAg) positive and/or hepatitis Be antigen (HBeAg) positive.

    c. Prevention of perinatal transmission by routine screening of all pregnant women.

    d. Treatment of the infant born to a HBsAg-positive mother is 85–95% effective in preventing the development of the hepatitis B carrier state and should include the following:

(1) Careful bathing of the neonate to remove blood and secretions that may be contaminated and gastric wash to remove blood from stomach.

(2) Administration of hepatitis B immune globulin (HBIG), 0.5 ml intramuscularly as soon as possible within 12–24 hours of birth.

(3) Administration of hepatitis B (HB) vaccine 0.5 ml IM at birth and at 1 and 6 months after the first dose.

5. Human immunodeficiency virus.

   a. Definitions.

     (1) Human immunodeficiency virus (HIV): agent causing viral infection that is the leading cause of immunodeficiency in the neonate.

     (2) Acquired immunodeficiency syndrome (AIDS): severe, late manifestations resulting from HIV infection.

     (3) AIDS-related complex (ARC): refers to those infants who present with symptoms but whose manifestations do not meet the Centers for Disease Control (CDC) definitions of AIDS.

   b. Etiology.

     (1) HIV is a cytopathic human retrovirus.

     (2) Utilizes reverse transcriptase enzyme to produce viral DNA and integrates this into the DNA of the T-helper cells.

     (3) Suppresses the T-helper lymphocytes resulting in B-cell and suppressor T-cell dysfunction with subsequent defects in cell-mediated immunity and development of opportunistic infections.

     (4) Virus may also infect monocytes and macrophages.

     (5) Can have an HIV infection with absence of symptoms, suggesting that other factors (e.g., genetic predisposition, nutritional status) may contribute to development of infection.

   c. Epidemiology.

     (1) Humans are the only known carriers.

     (2) Neonatal transmission.

       (a) Transfusion of blood or blood products.

       (b) Mother-to-infant transfer is thought to be the most common method of transfer, although time of transmission is uncertain.

         i. Transplacental transmission has been demonstrated.

         ii. Intrapartum transmission during exposure to infected maternal blood or genital tract secretions is presumed.

     (3) Risk of infection to an infant born to an HIV-seropositive mother is 20–65%.

       (a) HIV may be transmitted during more than one pregnancy, although an infant delivered after an infected sibling may be uninfected.

       (b) Evidence of congenitally acquired infection may not be evident until 12–18 months of age.

     (4) HIV may be transmitted through human milk.

     (5) No evidence of transmission through intimate contact among family members.

   d. Diagnosis.

     (1) Difficult to interpret serologic data in the neonate as it will reflect maternal infectious status.

     (2) Must have documentation of previous opportunistic infection.

     (3) Must exclude primary or secondary immunodeficiency disease.

       (a) Primary include DiGeorge syndrome, graft versus host disease, neutropenia, neutrophil function abnormality, etc.

       (b) Secondary associated with immunosuppressive therapy, lymphoreticular malignancy, or starvation.

   e. Clinical presentation.

     (1) Although uncommon, lymphadenopathy and hepatomegaly can be seen at birth, with an opportunistic infection occurring during the first month of life.

(2) Symptoms most often become evident between 4 and 6 months of age.
(3) Common clinical manifestations.
   (a) Failure to thrive.
   (b) Persistent oral candidiasis.
   (c) Generalized lymphadenopathy.
   (d) Hepatosplenomegaly.
   (e) Recurrent diarrhea.
   (f) Recurrent bacterial infections.
   (g) Opportunistic infections.
   (h) Encephalopathy.
   (i) Cardiomyopathy.
   (j) Hepatitis.
   (k) Nephrotic syndrome.
(4) Uncommon for infants to develop Kaposi's sarcoma and opportunistic infections from toxoplasmosis and tuberculosis.
f. Management.
(1) Prompt intervention during bacterial and treatable opportunistic infections.
(2) Adequate nutrition.
(3) Antiretroviral therapy.
   (a) Zidovudine (formerly azidothymidine or AZT).
      i. Nucleotide analog; thought to function by inhibition of reverse transcriptase and/or by chain termination.
      ii. Demonstrated toxic side effects in the neonate include macrocytosis, anemia, and neutropenia.
   (b) Ribovirin and dideoxycytidine are undergoing clinical trials.

Other Infections

A. **Toxoplasmosis** (Parasite).
1. Maternal transmission from consumption of poorly cooked meat or by ingestion of infected cat feces.
2. Congenitally acquired.
   a. Manifestations may include maculopapular rash, hepatomegaly, splenomegaly, jaundice, and thrombocytopenia.
   b. CNS involvement includes microcephaly or hydrocephalus accompanied by convulsions; mav see cerebral calcifications on radiographs.
   c. Sequelae include mental retardation, learning disabilities, impaired vision, or blindness.
   d. May be asymptomatic at birth but manifest as intellectual impairment in late infancy and childhood.
3. Diagnosis is made by serological tests.
4. Treatment includes pyrimethamine, trisulfapyrimidines, and a folic acid supplement to prevent bone marrow suppression.

B. **Syphilis** (*Treponema pallidum*).
1. May be asymptomatic or present with florid disease at birth.
2. Classic presentation of congenital syphilis includes petechiae, skin lesions, hepatosplenomegaly, respiratory distress, CNS involvement, rhinitis, and periostitis of long bones with guarding of extremities.
3. CNS involvement.
   a. CNS status is affected in 30–50% of all infants, although many will have a normal neurological exam at birth.
   b. If suspect congenital syphilis, one should obtain cerebrospinal fluid to determine if neurosyphilis is present.
4. Evaluation.
   a. U.S. Public Health Service recommends that all pregnant women be

screened with Venereal Disease Research Laboratory (VDRL) or Rapid Plasma Reagin (RPR) test early in pregnancy and at the time of delivery.
b. Diagnosis of active disease in the neonate.
  (1) High VDRL titer (four times higher than maternal titer).
  (2) Reactive RPR.
  (3) Serum IgM level greater than 20 mg/dl.
  (4) Confirm with a positive fluorescent treponema antibody absorption (FTA-ABS) test.
c. Uninfected infants possess maternally acquired antibodies at concentrations similar to those infected, and it may be difficult to interpret neonatal lab data; therefore, it is important to determine adequacy of maternal treatment, possibility of re-exposure, and family compliance for follow-up.
5. Treatment.
  a. Benzathine penicillin G 50,000 units/kg IM once if asymptomatic with normal cerebrospinal fluid.
  b. Procaine penicillin G 50,000 units/kg IM once daily for 10–14 days if symptomatic with abnormal cerebrospinal fluid findings.
  c. If uncertain of maternal treatment or if the treatment was within last 4 weeks of pregnancy, neonatal therapy should be instituted.

Infection Control

A. **Universal precautions**—CDC guidelines designed to prevent skin and mucous membrane exposure to pathogens when in contact with blood or body fluids.

B. **Body substance isolation** (BSI)—utilizes barrier precautions; however, encompasses all body sites and is intended to reduce the risk of nosocomial infections in both patients and personnel. Recommendations include the following:
1. Gloves before contact with mucous membranes, moist body surfaces, and non-intact skin.
2. Additional barriers, i.e., gowns, mask, and goggles when splashes are likely.
3. Handwashing before each new patient contact and whenever hands are soiled.
4. Non-recapping of sharps and needles; disposal in puncture-resistant plastic containers.

STUDY QUESTIONS

1. The only immunoglobulin to cross the placenta and provide passive immunity to the neonate is:
   a. IgA
   b. IgG
   c. IgM

2. The most accurate hematological predictor of neonatal infection is:
   a. Leukocytosis
   b. Neutropenia
   c. Neutrophilia

3. Which of the following statements about *Staphylococcus epidermidis* is false?
   a. Can be associated with the use of invasive procedures.
   b. Is usually a contaminant and requires no further evaluation.

   c. Vancomycin is the most effective antimicrobial agent.

4. Persistent bacteremia may be caused by:
   a. Meconium aspiration.
   b. Occult site of infection.
   c. Sensitivity to antibiotics.

5. Infants at risk for acquisition of systemic candidiasis include those who are:
   a. Intrauterine growth retarded.
   b. Premature and immunocompromised.
   c. Postmature and meconium stained.

6. The most common congenitally acquired viral infection is:
   a. Cytomegalovirus.
   b. Herpes simplex virus.
   c. Syphilis.

Answers to Study Questions

1. b	3. b	5. b
2. b	4. b	6. a

REFERENCES

American Academy of Pediatrics: Report of the Committee on Infectious Diseases. Elk Grove Village, IL, Author, 1988.

Avery, G.B.: Neonatology: Pathophysiology and Management of the Newborn. Philadelphia, J.B. Lippincott, 1987.

Baly, J.E., Kliegman, R.M., Boxerbaum, B., et al: Fungal colonization in the very low birth weight infant. Pediatrics, 78:225–232, 1986.

Baly, J.E., Kliegman, R.M., and Fanaroff, A.A.: Disseminated fungal infection in the very low-birth-weight infant: Therapeutic toxicity. Pediatrics, 73:153–157, 1984.

Baumgart, S., Hall, S.E., Campos, J.M., et al: Sepsis with coagulase-negative staphylococi in critically ill newborns. Am. J. Dis. Child., 137:461–463, 1983.

Boyd, R.F.: General Microbiology. St. Louis, Times Mirror/Mosby, 1988.

Butler, K.M., and Baker, C.J.: Candida: An increasingly important pathogen in the nursery. Pediatr. Clin. North Am., 35:543–563, 1988.

Butler, K.M., Rench, M.A., and Baker, C.J.: Amphotericin B as a single agent in the treatment of systemic candidiasis in neonates. Pediatr. Infect. Dis. J., 9:51–56, 1990.

Campognone, P., and Singer, D.B.: Neonatal sepsis due to non-typable Haemophilus influenzae. Am. J. Dis. Child., 140:117–121, 1986.

Cario, M.S.: Neonatal neutrophil host defense: Prospects for immunologic enhancement during neonatal sepsis. Am. J. Dis. Child., 143:40–46, 1989.

Centers for Disease Control: Sexually transmitted disease treatment guidelines. MMWR, 38:1–43, 1989.

Centers for Disease Control: Recommendations for prevention of HIV transmission in health-care settings. MMWR, 36:3S–5S, 1987.

Cerase, P.A.: Neonatal sepsis. J. Perinatal Neonatal Nurs., 3:48–54, 1989.

Christensen, R.D., Rothstein, G., Anstall, H.B., et al: Granulocyte transfusions in neonates with bacterial infection, neutropenia and depletion of mature marrow neutrophils. Pediatrics, 70:1–6, 1982.

Conway, S.P., Gillies, D.R.N., and Doherty, A.: Neonatal infection in premature infants and use of human immunoglobulin. Arch. Dis. Child., 62:1252–1256, 1987.

Dagbjartsson, A., and Ludvigsson, P.: Bacterial meningitis: Diagnosis and initial antibiotic therapy. Pediatr. Clin. North Am., 34:219–230, 1987.

Donowitz, L.S., Haley, C.E., Gregory, W.W., et al.: Neonatal intensive care unit bacteremia: Emergence of gram-positive bacteria as major pathogens. Am. J. Infect. Control, 15:141–147, 1987.

Falloon, J., Eddy, J., Wiener, L., et al.: Human immunodeficiency virus infection in children. J. Pediatr., 114:1–30, 1989.

Fanaroff, A.A., and Martin, R.J.: Neonatal-perinatal Medicine: Diseases of the Fetus and Newborn. St. Louis, C.V. Mosby, 1987.

Feigin, R.D., and Cherry, J.D.: Textbook of Pediatric Infectious Diseases. Philadelphia, W.B. Saunders Co., 1987.

Fisher, G.W.: Therapeutic uses of intravenous gammaglobulin for pediatric infection. Pediatr. Clin. North Am., 35:517–533, 1988.

Ganong, W.F.: Review of Medical Physiology, 14th ed. E. Norwalk, CT, Appleton and Lange, 1989.

Haggerty, L.: TORCH: A literature review and implications for practice. J. Gynecol. Neonat. Nurs. 14:124–126, 1985.

Henneberry, C.: Candida sepsis in the very low birthweight infant. Neonatal Network, 5(6):39–45, 1987.

Inglis, A.D., and Lozano, M.: AIDS in the neonatal ICU. Neonatal Network, 5(3):39–43, 1986.

Johnson, J.P., Nair, P., Hines, S.E., et al: Natural history and serologic diagnosis of infants born to human immunodeficiency virus-infected women. Am. J. Dis. Child., 143:1147–1153, 1989.

Kraune, P.J., Herson, V.C., Eisenfeld, L., et al.: Enhancement of neutrophil function for treatment of neonatal infections. Pediatr. Infect. Dis. J., 8:382–389, 1989.

Kyllonen, K.S., Clapp, D.W., Kliegman, R.M., et al.: Dosage of intravenously administered immune globulin and dosing interval required to maintain target levels of immunoglobulin G in low birth weight infants. J. Pediatr., 115:1013–1016, 1989.

Lynch, P., Cummings, M.J., Roberts, P.L., et al.: Implementing and evaluating a system of generic infection precautions: Body substance isolation. Am. J. Infect. Control, 18:1–12, 1990.

Manroe, B.L., Weinberg, A.G., Rosenfeld, C.R., et al.: The neonatal blood count in health and disease. Pediatrics, 95:89–98, 1979.

McCracken, G.H., and Nelson, J.D.: Antimicrobial therapy for newborns. New York, Grune and Stratton, 1983.

Merenstein, G.B., and Gardner, S.L.: Handbook of Neonatal Intensive Care. St. Louis, C.V. Mosby, 1989.

Pizzo, P.A., Eddy, J., Falloon, J., et al: Effect of continuous intravenous infusion of azidothymidine (AZT) in children with asymptomatic HIV infection. N. Engl. J. Med., 319:889–896, 1988.

Prober, C.G., Sullender, W.H., Yasukawa, L.L., et al.: Low risk of herpes simplex virus infections in neonates exposed to the virus at the time of vaginal delivery to mothers with recurrent genital herpes simplex virus infections. N. Engl. J. Med., *316*:240–244, 1987.

Remington, J.S., and Klein, J.O.: Infectious Diseases of the Fetus and Newborn Infant. Philadelphia, W.B. Saunders Co., 1990.

Streeter, N.: High-risk neonatal care. Rockville, MD, Aspen Publishers, 1986.

Vain, N.E., Nazlumian, J.R., and Swarner, O.W.: Role of exchange transfusion in neonatal septicemia. Pediatrics, *66*:693–697, 1980.

Wallace, R.J., Baker, C.J., Quinones, F.J., et al.: Non-typable Haemophilus influenza and a neonatal, maternal and genital pathogen. Rev. Infect. Dis., *5*:123–136, 1983.

Weese-Meyer, D.E., Fondriest, D.W., Brovillette, R.T., et al.: Risk factors associated with candidemia in the neonatal intensive care unit: A case-control study. Pediatr. Infect. J., *6*:190–196, 1987.

Weintzen, R.L., and McCracken, G.H.: Pathogenesis and management of neonatal sepsis and meningitis. Curr. Prob. Pediatr., *8*:3–61, 1977.

Wender, G.D.: Gestational and congenital syphilis. Clin. Perinatol., *15*:287–303, 1988.

Wilson, C.B.: Immunologic basis for increased susceptibility of the neonate to infection. J. Pediatr., *108*:1–12, 1986.

Janice Bernhardt

Renal/Genitourinary Disorders

Objectives

1. Relate congenital renal/genitourinary disorders to embryological development.

2. Apply knowledge of normal renal anatomy and physiology to renal pathophysiology that presents in the neonatal period.

3. Explain the etiology of selected neonatal renal/genitourinary disorders.

4. Describe clinical manifestations and complications that may be associated with selected neonatal renal/genitourinary disorders.

5. Determine the appropriate management of each disorder discussed.

6. Formulate an appropriate plan of care for each disorder discussed.

The genitourinary system has the highest percentage of anomalies, congenital or genetic, of all the organ systems. These anomalies frequently present in the neonatal period (Portman et al., 1989). Pre-natal diagnosis of some renal/genitourinary disorders is possible with the use of ultrasound. Renal/genitourinary anomalies have been found to account for 14–57% of malformations detected during prenatal screening (Horger and Pai, 1983; Sarda et al., 1983). There have even been attempts at in utero treatment (Appleman and Golbus, 1986; Manning, 1986).

Because a variety of renal/genitourinary disorders can present in the neonatal period, accurate assessment and early intervention are essential. This chapter presents embryology and anatomy and physiology of the kidney as a base from which to discuss selected neonatal renal/genitourinary disorders.

Embryology

A. **Introduction.**

1. Embryological development of the urinary system begins within the first weeks after conception and progresses through three stages.

2. Both the urinary and genital system develop from the same germ layer of the embryo.

B. **Kidney.**
1. Pronephros, "fore kidneys."
    a. Plays a primary role in normal organogenesis.
    b. Appears during 3–4 weeks' gestation.
    c. Degenerates by the fifth week.
2. Mesonephros, "mid-kidneys."
    a. Originates during 4–5 weeks' gestation, just prior to degeneration of the pronephros, and is fully developed by 37 days.
    b. Consists of 30–40 glomerulotubular units.
    c. Capsule and glomerulus form mesonephros (renal) corpuscle.
    d. Develops into genital glands.
    e. Regresses at the end of the second month.
3. Metanephros, "hind kidneys."
    a. Develops early in the fifth week and functions within a few weeks.
    b. Permanent kidney/metanephros develops from the metanephros diverticulum (ureteric bud) and metanephros mesoderm.
    c. Normal differentiation of ureteric bud is essential for initiation of branching that leads to formulation of urinary collecting system and initiation of nephron formation.
    d. Nephrons form from proximal end of renal/metanephric tubules beginning at about 8 weeks and continuing until approximately 34–36 weeks, resulting in the formation of approximately 800,000 nephrons.
    e. Minor calyces and their communicating papillary ducts are well delineated and resemble those of a mature kidney by 13–14 weeks' gestation.
    f. By 4 months, the kidney contains 14–16 lobes, which is the same number as that in the mature kidney.
    g. The kidney begins to secrete urine by approximately 3 months' gestation.

C. **Urinary tract.**
1. Differentiation of the urinary tract occurs synchronously with the early stages of metanephric development.
2. Urinary bladder develops at approximately 6 weeks' gestation.
3. Formation of the urethra is completed by the end of the first trimester.
4. Fetal ureter does not open functionally into the bladder until the ninth week.

D. **Development of vascular supply.** The vascular pattern of the fetal kidney resembles that of the mature kidney by 14–15 weeks' gestation.

Gross Renal Anatomy

A. **Cortex:** outermost portion of the kidney, which contains the glomeruli, proximal and distal convoluted tubules, and collecting ducts of the nephron.

B. **Medulla:** middle section of the kidney, which contains renal pyramids, straight portions of tubules, loops of Henle, vasa recta, and terminal collecting ducts.

C. **Renal sinus and pelvis:** renal sinus and pelvis comprise the innermost portion of the kidney. The renal sinus contains the uppermost part of renal pelvis and calyces, surrounded by some fat in which branches of the renal vessels and nerves are embedded. The renal pelvis is formed as the major calyces unite.

D. **Ureter:** excretory duct of the kidney, which transports urine from kidney to bladder.

Microscopic Renal Anatomy

A. **Nephron.**
1. Structural and functional unit of the kidney.
2. Approximately 1,000,000 per kidney.

3. All nephrons are present at birth; functional maturation occurs later.
4. Functional component of the nephron is the renal corpuscle/malpighian body, which consists of the glomerulus and glomerular (Bowman's) capsule.
   a. Glomerulus is formed by a capillary network.
   b. Glomerular/Bowman's capsule is a membrane surrounding the glomerulus, which serves as a filter mechanism through which non-protein components of blood plasma can enter the renal tubules.
5. Renal tubular system.
   a. Located in the cortex and medulla.
   b. Consists of proximal convoluted tubule, loop of Henle, distal convoluted tubule, and collecting duct.

Renal Hemodynamics

A. **Renal blood flow.**
1. Renal blood flow comprises 4–6% of the cardiac output during the first 12 hours of life and 8–10% of the cardiac output during the first week of life.
2. Increased renal blood flow that occurs with maturation is mainly caused by decreased afferent and efferent vascular resistance.
3. Renal plasma flow.
   a. 150 ml/minute/1.73 m² at term and increases to 200 ml/minute/1.73 m² in the first weeks of life.
   b. The low renal plasma flow in the neonate is mainly due to the high renal vascular resistance, but also to the low perfusion pressure.

B. **Regulation of renal blood flow.**
1. Autoregulation.
   a. Myogenic mechanism is the response of arterial smooth muscle to changes in vascular wall tension to maintain normal blood flow.
   b. Tubuloglomerular feedback mechanism is an alteration in distal tubular flow causing the juxtaglomerular apparatus to release renin, convert it to angiotensin II, and thus mediate changes in vascular resistance.
2. Hormonal regulation of renal blood flow.
   a. Renin-angiotensin-aldosterone system (RAAS).
      (1) Major renal hormonal system.
      (2) Well developed in the newborn; renin is present from 3 months' gestation onward.
      (3) Involved with regulation of systemic blood pressure, sodium and potassium balance, and regional blood flow.
      (4) Stimulation of the RAAS leads to vasoconstriction, sodium retention, and increased extracellular fluid volume.
   b. Prostaglandins.
      (1) Involved in regulation of fetal renal growth and morphogenesis.
      (2) Synthesized in both the cortex and medulla.
      (3) Principal renal prostaglandin is prostaglandin E_2 (PGE_2).
      (4) Major effects of renal prostaglandins.
         (a) Vasodilation.
         (b) Greater intrarenal blood flow to inner versus outer cortical area.
         (c) Maintenance of glomerular filtration rate via regulation of renal blood flow and perfusion pressure.
         (d) Natriuresis.
         (e) Stimulation of renin release and antagonism of angiotensin II.
         (f) Vasodilation and inhibition of the distal tubule's response to antidiuretic hormone (ADH).
         (g) Regulation of electrolyte and fluid balance.
   c. Kallikrein-kinin system.
      (1) Influences renal hemodynamics.
      (2) Involved in regulation of sodium due to increasing tubular reabsorption.

Renal Physiology

A. **Post-natal changes.**
1. Increased GFR.
2. Decreased fractional excretion of sodium due to increasing tubular reabsorption.
3. Increasing ability to concentrate urine.
4. Renal vasoactive hormones are initially increased.
5. Several rapid post-natal changes in renal function reflect major changes in renal hemodynamics and morphology.
6. Decreased renal vascular resistance.
7. Increased renal blood flow.

B. **Glomerular filtration.**
1. As blood passes through the capillaries, plasma is filtered through glomerular capillary walls. Filtrate is collected in Bowman's space and enters tubules where composition is modified, according to the body's need, until it is excreted as urine.
2. The force for ultrafiltration stems from the systemic arterial blood pressure and is modified by the tone of the afferent and efferent arterioles.
3. GFR is autoregulated over a range of arterial blood pressure by changes in vascular resistance.
4. Factors that affect GFR.
   a. Capillary surface area.
   b. Permeability of capillary basement membrane.
   c. Rate of renal plasma flow.
   d. Changes in renal blood flow.
   e. Changes in glomerular capillary hydrostatic pressure.
   f. Changes in blood pressure.
   g. Changes in afferent or efferent arteriolar vasoconstriction.
   h. Changes in hydrostatic pressure in Bowman's capsule.
   i. Ureteral obstruction.
   j. Edema of kidney.
   k. Changes in the concentration of plasma proteins.
      (1) Dehydration.
      (2) Hypoproteinemia.
   l. Increased permeability of the glomerular filter.
   m. Decrease in total area of glomerular capillary bed.
5. Glomerular filtration rate.
   a. Doubles in the first 2 weeks of life to 30–40 ml/minute/1.73 m^2.
   b. Increases to adult values of 100–120 ml/minute/1.73 m^2 between 1–2 years of life.
   c. Factors that may contribute to decreased GFR at birth:
      (1) Small glomerular capillary area available for filtration.
      (2) Structural immaturity of glomerular capillary, which is associated with decreased water permeability.
      (3) Decreased blood pressure.
      (4) Increased hematocrit.
      (5) Renal vasoconstriction, which results in decreased glomerular plasma flow.
   d. Infants less than 34 weeks' gestation have low GFR (0.5 ml/minute) until nephrogenesis is completed.
   e. Factors responsible for increasing GFR:
      (1) Expansion in filtration surface area.
      (2) Decreased renal vascular resistance.

C. **Tubular function.**
1. Modification of glomerular ultrafiltrate leading to production of urine.

2. Major functions.
   a. Reabsorption: movement of substance into the peritubular capillary plasma from the tubular epithelium.
   b. Tubular secretion: movement of substances into the tubular epithelium from the peritubular capillary plasma.

D. **Concentration and dilution mechanism.**
1. Major function of kidney is to maintain osmolality of extracellular fluid within the narrow range compatible with optimal cellular function.
2. Sites of urinary concentration and dilution.
   a. Loop of Henle.
   b. Collecting duct.
3. Factors responsible for the limited ability of the neonatal kidney to concentrate urine.
   a. Decreased glomerular filtration rate.
   b. Relatively short loops of Henle in the mid-cortical and juxtamedullary glomeruli.
   c. Deficient transport of sodium chloride in the incompletely developed loops of Henle.
   d. Decreased response of the distal nephron to ADH.
4. Normal range of neonatal specific gravity is 1.002–1.010.
5. Maximum concentrating ability.
   a. 700 mOsm/kg of water (full-term infants).
   b. 600–700 mOsm/kg of water (pre-term infants).
6. Capacity for urine dilution.
   a. 30–50 mOsm/kg of water.

E. **Acid-base balance.**
1. Kidneys regulate acid-base balance in conjunction with the lungs and blood buffers.
   a. Reabsorption of bicarbonate.
   b. Secretion of hydrogen ions.
   c. Production of buffers.
2. Renal response to acidosis.
   a. Reabsorption of bicarbonate in the proximal tubule.
   b. Secretion of hydrogen ions is increased in the distal convoluted tubule.
   c. Production of ammonia.
3. Renal response to alkalosis.
   a. Excretion of bicarbonate.
   b. Production of ammonia is decreased.
   c. Hydrogen ion secretion in the distal tubule is decreased.
4. Neonatal limitations.
   a. Decreased serum bicarbonate level in the neonate is due to decreased renal threshold for bicarbonate in the proximal tubule.
   b. Urinary pH in the neonate is greater than that of the child or adult.
   c. Rapid post-natal maturation results in a urine pH as low as that of a child or adult by the end of the first 2 weeks.

Acute Renal Failure

A. **Definition:** acute decrease in renal function resulting in solute and water retention, alteration in acid/base balance, and accumulation of nitrogenous waste products.

B. **Etiology.**
1. Pre-renal: renal hypoperfusion caused by a reduction in circulating blood volume or by failure of the heart to provide adequate circulation.
   a. Hypotension.

  b. Hypoperfusion caused by hemorrhage.
  c. Sepsis.
  d. Dehydration.
  e. Hypoxia.
  f. Respiratory distress syndrome.
  g. Congestive heart failure.
  h. Renal artery thrombosis.
2. Renal parenchymal: renal cellular damage involving functional compromise to the glomerular, tubular, and collecting system due to prolonged pre-renal insult or from use of nephrotoxic agents.
  a. This may occur in the form of cortical, tubular, medullary, or papillary necrosis.
  b. Classification.
    (1) Congenital.
       (a) Hypoplasia.
       (b) Dysplasia.
       (c) Polycystic kidney disease.
       (d) Nephrotic syndrome.
    (2) Inflammatory.
       (a) Congenital infection.
       (b) Pyelonephritis.
    (3) Vascular.
       (a) Cortical/medullary necrosis.
       (b) Arterial or venous thrombosis.
       (c) Intravascular coagulation.
    (4) Ischemia necrosis.
       (a) Asphyxia/hypoxia.
       (b) Dehydration.
       (c) Hemorrhage.
       (d) Sepsis.
       (e) Respiratory distress syndrome.
    (5) Nephrotoxic drugs.
       (a) Aminoglycoside antibiotics.
       (b) Radiological contrast media.
3. Post-renal: obstruction to urinary flow involving the urinary flow distal to the kidney.
  a. Posterior urethral valves.
  b. Bilateral ureteropelvic junction obstruction.
  c. Imperforate prepuce.
  d. Urethral structure.
  e. Urethral diverticulum.
  f. Megaureter.
  g. Ureterocele.
  h. Ureteropelvic/ureterovesical obstruction.
  i. Neurogenic bladder.

C. **Incidence.**
1. Reported to comprise up to 8% of intensive care nursery admissions (Portman et al., 1989).
2. Pre-renal acute renal failure is the most commonly encountered type of acute renal failure in neonates.

D. **Disease states.**
1. Intrapartal asphyxia.
2. Infection.
3. Congenital renal abnormality.

E. **Clinical presentation.**
1. Oliguria/anuria: less than 0.5–1.0 ml/kg/hour sustained for at least 24 hours.

2. Azotemia: blood urea nitrogen (BUN) greater than 20 mg/dl or rising more than 10 mg/dl/day.
3. Elevated serum creatinine: greater than 1 mg/dl or rising more than 0.2 mg/dl/day.

F. Clinical assessment.
1. Perinatal history.
   a. Low Apgar score.
   b. Perinatal asphyxia.
   c. Renal abnormalities observed on antenatal ultrasound.
   d. History of oligohydramnios.
2. Urine output: less than 1 ml/kg/hour, after 48 hours, lasting at least 24 hours.
3. Daily weight: increase in daily weight greater than that predicted based on infant's condition and caloric intake.
4. Edema.
5. Blood pressure.
   a. Hypotension may be a factor in the development of acute renal failure.
   b. Hypertension may be observed in established cases of acute renal failure.

G. Diagnostic studies.
1. Urine.
   a. Urinalysis.
      (1) pH often > 6.
      (2) Specific gravity usually decreased.
      (3) Hematuria.
      (4) Casts.
      (5) Tubular cells.
      (6) Proteinuria.
   b. Sodium: increased with intrinsic renal failure.
   c. Osmolality: decreased.
   d. Creatinine: decreased.
   e. Culture: rule out urinary tract infection/sepsis.
   f. Urinary indices lose their diagnostic usefulness after therapy for oliguria has begun, particularly with diuretics.
2. Blood.
   a. BUN > 20 mg/dl or rise > 1.0 mg/dl/day.
   b. Creatinine > 1 mg/dl or rise > 0.2 mg/dl/day.
   c. Osmolality: increased.
   d. Electrolytes.
      (1) Hyperkalemia.
      (2) Hyponatremia.
      (3) Hypocalcemia.
      (4) Hyperphosphatemia.
   e. Glucose: increased.
   f. Total protein: decreased.
   g. Albumin: decreased.
3. Ultrasound: to determine intrinsic or post-renal cause. It will rule out urinary tract obstruction, renal vein thrombosis, congenital renal abnormality, and cystic disease.
4. Intravenous pyelogram (IVP): rule out obstructive disease.
5. Voiding cystourethrography (VCUG): rule out obstructive disease and reflux.

H. Differential diagnosis.
1. Pre-renal acute renal failure.
2. Renal parenchymal acute renal failure.
3. Post-renal acute renal failure.
4. Differentiation between types.
   a. Assess for specific etiological factors.
   b. Pre-renal versus renal parenchymal.

(1) Renal failure index (RFI) =

$$\frac{\text{Urine Na concentration} \times \text{plasma creatinine}}{\text{Urine creatinine}}$$

(2) Fractional excretion of Na (FENa) =

$$\frac{\text{Urine Na}}{\text{Plasma Na}} \times \frac{\text{plasma creatinine}}{\text{urine creatinine}} \times 100$$

(3) RFI or FENa > 3 suggests intrinsic failure. These values will have limited significance in neonates less than 32 weeks' gestation because of these infants' limited ability to conserve sodium.

(4) BUN/creatinine ratio: disproportionate rise in the BUN/creatinine ratio suggests a pre-renal etiology, while a proportionate rise indicates a renal parenchymal etiology.

(5) Fluid challenge: crystalloid or plasma (20 ml/kg) intravenously over 1–2 hours. If oliguria persists, follow with furosemide (1–2 mg/kg), intravenously.

    (a) A rapid and sustained diuresis within 1–2 hours indicates a pre-renal cause.

    (b) Urine output < 2 ml/kg/hour after furosemide suggests a parenchymal or post-renal cause.

(6) Presence of casts, tubular cells, and proteinuria is suggestive of parenchymal renal failure.

  c. Renal parenchymal versus post-renal.

    (a) Ultrasound.

    (b) Voiding cystourethrography.

I. **Complications.**

1. Electrolyte imbalance.
2. Hyperproteinemia.
3. Anemia.
4. Thrombocytopenia.
5. Hemorrhagic diathesis.
6. Metabolic acidosis.
7. Edema.
8. Hypertension.
9. Congestive heart failure.

J. **Patient care management.**

1. Treat primary cause.
2. Strict intake and output: restrict fluids to insensible water loss, urine output, and other losses.
3. Monitor specific gravity.
4. Monitor urine pH.
5. Monitor urine for hematuria, proteinuria, and glucosuria.
6. Monitor urine osmolality and sodium.
7. Monitor body weight once or twice daily.
8. Monitor serum glucose and electrolytes; treat imbalances — sodium and potassium intake may need to be restricted.
9. Treat acidosis.
10. Restrict protein to 0.5 g/kg/day.
11. Provide adequate nutrition.
12. Monitor blood pressure and treat hypertension.
13. Observe for signs and symptoms of congestive heart failure.
14. Assess for bleeding diathesis.
15. Avoid nephrotoxic medication.
16. Peritoneal dialysis.
17. Continuous arteriovenous hemofiltration: a method of extracorporeal filtration that is capable of removing retained fluid more rapidly than peritoneal

dialysis or hemodialysis. It may be initiated if the patient is unresponsive to peritoneal dialysis.

K. **Outcome.**
1. Largely dependent on etiology, extent of other organ damage, and management.
2. Reversal of underlying condition is the most important factor in determining prognosis.
3. Recognition and correction of renal hypoperfusion lead to rapid restoration of kidney function.
4. Best prognosis is for patients with non-oliguric acute renal failure.
5. Chronic renal failure occurs in approximately 40% of cases (Portman et al., 1989).
6. Renal tubular abnormalities have been seen.
7. Hypertension may be evident.
8. Renal growth can be affected.
9. Mortality is reported as 14–75% (Portman et al., 1989).

Hypertension

A. **Etiology.**
1. Renal/vascular: renal vascular disease appears to be the leading cause of neonatal hypertension, with thromboembolic occlusion of the renal artery secondary to umbilical artery catheterization the most frequently implicated factor.
2. Medication.
3. Other.

B. **Incidence:** 1.2–5% of intensive care nursery admissions (Portman et al., 1989).

C. **Disease states.**
1. Renal.
   a. Renal dysplasia/hypoplasia.
   b. Polycystic kidney disease.
   c. Renal failure.
   d. Obstructive uropathy.
   e. Reflux nephropathy.
   f. Pyelonephritis.
   g. Glomerulonephritis.
   h. Tumors.
2. Endocrine.
   a. Adrenogenital syndrome.
   b. Cushing's disease.
   c. Hypoaldosteronism.
   d. Thyrotoxicosis.
3. Vascular.
   a. Renal artery stenosis.
   b. Renal artery thrombosis.
   c. Coarctation of the aorta.
   d. Hypoplastic abdominal aorta.
   e. Arterial calcification.
4. Other.
   a. Closure of abdominal wall defect.
   b. Fluid overload.
   c. Genitourinary surgery.
   d. Hypercalcemia.
   e. Increased intracranial pressure.
   f. Renal infection.
   g. Central nervous system disorders.

h. Seizures in pre-term infants.
 i. Bronchopulmonary dysplasia.
 u. Pneumothorax.
 k. Infants of drug-dependent mothers.
 l. Medications.
   (1) Corticosteroids.
   (2) Ocular phenylephrine.
   (3) Theophylline.
   (4) Deoxycorticosterone.

D. Clinical presentation (Feld and Springate, 1988).
1. Term infants:
   a. Birth: bp > 90/60.
                       mean bp > 70.
   b. 7 days: bp > 92/60.
                       mean bp > 77.
   c. 8 days–1 month: bp > 106/74.
                       mean bp > 85.
2. Premature infants less than 1 kg:
   a. Birth: bp > 60/40.
   b. 7 days: mean bp > 57.
   c. 1 month: mean bp > 63.
3. Premature infants greater than 1 kg:
   a. Birth: bp > 80/50.
                mean bp > 60.
   b. 7 days: mean bp > 65–70.
   c. 1 month: mean bp > 71–76.

E. Clinical assessment.
1. Arterial blood pressure: elevated.
2. Serum creatinine: may be within normal limits or elevated.
3. BUN: elevated with renal involvement.
4. Serum electrolytes: assess for values indicative of renal involvement.
5. Urine output: may be decreased.
6. Urinalysis: may be normal or show hematuria or proteinuria.
7. Urine culture: rule out renal infection.
8. Presence of unilateral/bilateral abdominal mass: rule out tumor or polycystic kidneys.
9. Cardiac status: size, rate, rhythm, murmur, signs and symptoms of congestive heart failure.
10. Assess femoral pulses: rule out coarctation of the aorta.
11. Perinatal history: assess for presence of umbilical artery catheter, renal disease, or congenital heart disease.
12. Failure to thrive.

F. Diagnostic studies.
1. Renal ultrasound, renal scan, IVP: rule out renal disease.
2. Chest x-ray: rule out cardiac involvement.
3. EKG: rule out cardiac involvement.
4. Arteriography: rule out renal vascular hypertension.

G. Complications.
1. Congestive heart failure.
2. Left ventricular hypertrophy.
3. Hypertensive retinopathy.
4. Intracranial hemorrhage.
5. Cerebrovascular accident.
6. Encephalopathy.

H. Patient care management.
1. Direct arterial blood pressure monitoring.

2. Diuretic, prn.
3. Sodium restriction.
4. Medications.
   a. Antihypertensives.
      (1) Hydralazine: IV or IM 0.1–0.5 mg/kg every 3–6 hours to a maximum of 2 mg/kg every 6 hours for BP control.
      (2) Propranolol: starting dose, 0.25–1.0 mg/kg/day divided every 6–12 hours; maximum, 2 mg/kg/day, IV or PO.
   b. Angiotensin I converting enzyme inhibitors: captopril: initial dose, 0.5 mg/kg or 0.45 mg/kg/day divided TID, PO; maintenance dose, 0.1–0.4 mg/kg every 6–24 hours as required for BP control, PO.

I. **Outcome.**
1. Prognosis good if blood pressure is controlled.
2. Poor growth of kidney affected with renal artery disease.
3. Infants with hypertension associated with bronchopulmonary dysplasia do well.
4. Infants with hypertension secondary to renal artery thrombosis from umbilical artery catheters do well, if they survive.
5. Renal scans tend to be persistently abnormal.
6. Death occurs in approximately 30% of infants with uncontrolled hypertension.

Potter's Syndrome

A. **Bilateral renal agenesis with Potter's facies** (Fig. 19–1).

B. **Etiology.**
1. Failure of development or early degeneration of ureteric bud.
2. Failure of formation of the urogenital ridge.
3. Absence of the nephrogenic blastema.
4. Failure of vascularization.

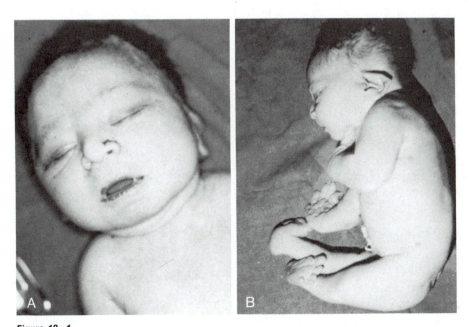

Figure 19–1
A and B, Potter's syndrome. (From Avery, G.B. (ed.): Neonatology: Pathophysiology and Management of the Newborn, 3rd ed. Philadelphia, J.B. Lippincott, 1987, p. 1045.)

C. **Incidence.**
1. 1:4000 births (Potter, 1965).
2. Male predominance.

D. **Clinical presentation.**
1. Anuria.
2. Potter facies.
   a. Blunted nose.
   b. Receded chin.
   c. Prominent depression between lower lip and chin.
   d. Low-set ears.
   e. Widely spaced eyes.
   f. Depressed nasal bridge.
   g. Prominent skin fold arising from epicanthus progressing interiorly and extending laterally beneath the eyes.
3. Small for gestational age.
4. Pulmonary hypoplasia.
5. Excessively dry skin.
6. Relatively large and claw-like hands.
7. Bell-shaped chest.
8. History of oligohydramnios.
9. Legs may be bowed and clubbed.

E. **Clinical assessment.**
1. Urinary output: anuria after the first 24 hours without bladder distention.
2. Potter's facies.
3. Signs and symptoms of respiratory distress.
4. Perinatal history of oligohydramnios.
5. Presence of other associated anomalies.
   a. Abnormal genitalia.
   b. Gastrointestinal malformations.

F. **Physical examination:** palpation of abdomen for presence of kidneys.

G. **Diagnostic studies.**
1. Renal ultrasound: rule out renal agenesis.
2. Renal scan, if ultrasound inconclusive.
3. Umbilical artery angiography: rule out presence of renal arteries.

H. **Differential diagnosis:** acute renal failure.

I. **Complications.**
1. Respiratory distress.
2. Pneumothorax.
3. Complications associated with acute renal failure.

J. **Patient care management** consists of comfort measures.

K. **Outcome.**
1. Mortality 100% (Perlmutter et al., 1986).
2. 40% stillborn (Perlmutter et al., 1986).
3. Most infants do not survive beyond 24–48 hours.

Infantile Polycystic Kidney Disease

A. **Etiology:** autosomal recessive.

B. **Incidence:** males and females equally affected.

C. **Clinical presentation.**
1. History of oligohydramnios.
2. Bilateral flank masses.
3. Oliguria.

4. Abdominal distention.
5. Respiratory distress.
6. Increased serum creatinine after a few days.
7. Hypertension.
8. Hematuria.
9. Renal insufficiency.
10. Decreased glomerular filtration rate.

D. **Clinical assessment.**
1. Urine output: decreased.
2. Urinalysis.
   a. Proteinuria.
   b. Hematuria.
   c. Decreased specific gravity.
3. Serum creatinine: elevated.
4. BUN: elevated.
5. Serum electrolytes.
   a. Hyperkalemia.
   b. Hyperphosphatemia.
   c. Hypocalcemia.
6. Serum pH: decreased.
7. Serum urea: elevated.
8. Blood pressure: elevated.
9. Respiratory distress.
10. Congestive heart failure.

E. **Physical examination:** bilateral flank masses.

F. **Diagnostic studies.**
1. Renal ultrasound: enlarged nodular kidneys.
2. Urography.
   a. Usually diagnostic when typical sun-ray or streak appearance is noted.
   b. Retention of contrast material in dilated medullary collecting ducts produces linear medullary opacification.
3. Abdominal x-ray: enlarged kidneys.
4. Intravenous pyelogram: delayed appearance of contrast material with mottled irregular nephrogram and distorted calyceal system. May be of limited value in the neonate due to decreased ability to concentrate urine and relatively decreased GFR, resulting in inadequate visualization.

G. **Differential diagnosis.**
1. Multicystic dysplasia.
2. Hydronephrosis.
3. Renal vein thrombosis.
4. Renal tumor.
5. Adult polycystic kidney disease.
6. Tuberous sclerosis.

H. **Complications.**
1. Renal failure.
2. Hepatic failure.
3. Hypertension.
4. Portal hypertension with palpable liver and esophageal varices.
5. Congestive heart failure.

I. **Patient care management.**
1. Genetic counseling.
2. Supportive care.
   a. Treat hypertension.
   b. Treat congestive heart failure.
   c. Nutrition to support normal growth and development.

J. Outcome.
1. Those with severe renal involvement may die in the neonatal period of pulmonary or renal insufficiency.
2. Those who survive the neonatal period may live for years with adequate renal functioning before developing renal insufficiency.

Multicystic Dysplastic Kidney Disease

A. **Renal dysplasia appearing as grape-like clusters.** The abnormal parenchyma contains multiple cysts and decreased nephrons. The proximal ureter is stenotic or non-patent.

B. Etiology.
1. Developmental anomaly.
2. Non-genetic.

C. Incidence.
1. 1:4300 (Gordon et al., 1988).
2. More common in males.
3. Most common form of renal cystic disease in infancy.

D. Clinical presentation.
1. Abnormal mass.
2. History of oligohydramnios.

E. Clinical assessment: assess for signs/symptoms of renal failure.

F. Physical examination.
1. Abdominal palpation.
   a. Irregular mass.
   b. Usually unilateral.
      (1) Appears more often on the left side.
      (2) The contralateral kidney is non-cystic, but there is a risk of another abnormality (usually ureteropelvic junction obstruction).

G. Diagnostic studies.
1. Renal ultrasound.
   a. Multiple cysts.
   b. Ureter usually atretic.
2. Renal scan: absence of renal function.
3. Excretory urogram: non-functioning kidney.

H. Differential diagnosis.
1. Polycystic kidney disease.
2. Hydronephrosis.
3. Renal vein thrombosis.
4. Renal tumor.

I. Complications.
1. Hypertension.
2. Pain.
3. Hematuria.
4. Infection.

J. Patient care management.
1. Non-operative approach.
   a. Follow-up ultrasounds.
   b. Monitor blood pressure.
   c. Monitor for infection.
   d. Monitor for hematuria.
   e. Assess for signs/symptoms of renal failure.
2. Operative approach: nephrectomy.

K. Outcome.
1. Bilateral involvement is incompatible with life.
2. Possible development of malignancy later in life.

Hydronephrosis

A. Definition: usually congenital obstruction that results in dilatation of the pelvis and calyces. Structural abnormalities of the genitourinary tract, other than hydronephrosis, may be evident in the contralateral kidney.

B. Etiology: unknown.

C. Incidence.
1. Approximately 1:1000 fetuses have been reported to have congenital uteropelvic junction obstruction (Grignon et al., 1986).
2. Occurs more frequently in males than in females.

D. Disease states.
1. Ureteropelvic junction obstruction: most common cause of dilatation of the collecting system in the fetal kidney.
2. Posterior urethral values.
3. Vesicoureteral reflux.
4. Prune-belly syndrome.

E. Clinical presentation.
1. Abdominal distention.
2. Urinary tract infection.
3. Poor urinary stream.
4. History of oligohydramnios.
5. Potter's facies.
6. Respiratory distress.
7. Failure to thrive.

F. Clinical assessment.
1. Decreased urinary output.
2. Urinary tract infection common.
3. Urinalysis.
   a. May be within normal limits.
   b. Proteinuria.
   c. Hematuria.
   d. Leukocyturia.
4. Serum creatinine: may be elevated.
5. BUN: may be elevated.
6. Antenatal ultrasound: evidence of hydronephrosis.

G. Physical examination.
1. Abdominal palpation reveals enlarged kidney.
2. Observe for associated anomalies that may occur outside the urinary tract.
   a. Imperforate anus.
   b. Congenital vertebral anomalies.
   c. Facial skeletal anomalies.
   d. Malformed ears.
   e. Myelodysplasia.
   f. Absent or decreased abdominal musculature.
   g. Unexplained pneumonia.
   h. Absence or dysplasia of the radius.
   i. Hypoplasia of the pelvis.
   j. Unexplained septicemia.
   k. Severe hypospadias.

H. Diagnostic studies.
1. Ultrasound.
2. Renal scan.
3. Voiding cystourethrography.
   a. Rule out obstruction.
   b. Rule out vesicoureteral reflux.
4. Excretory urography: rule out reflux.
5. IVP.

I. Differential diagnosis.
1. Renal cystic disease.
2. Renal vein thrombosis.
3. Tumor.
4. Megacalycosis.
5. Uteropelvic junction obstruction.
6. Posterior urethral valves.
7. Vesicoureteral reflux.

J. Complications.
1. Urinary tract infection.
2. Hypertension.
3. Damage to renal parenchyma.

K. General patient care management.
1. Strict intake and output.
2. Urinalysis.
   a. Hematuria.
   b. Proteinuria.
   c. Leukocyturia.
3. Monitor specific gravity.
4. Monitor urine for hematuria and proteinuria.
5. Urine culture.
6. Monitor serum electrolytes.
7. Serum creatinine.
8. BUN.

L. Specific patient care management.
1. Uteropelvic junction obstruction: pyeloplasty.
2. Posterior urethral valves.
   a. Catheterize initially.
   b. Correct fluid/electrolyte or other metabolic imbalances.
   c. Treat anemia.
   d. Treat acidosis.
   e. Assess for rickets.
   f. Fulguration of valves after 1 year or direct transurethral ablation.
3. Vesicoureteral reflux.
   a. Catheterize initially.
   b. Long-term antibiotic treatment until surgery.
   c. Surgical repair.
4. Obstruction at ureterovesical junction: excision of stenotic segment and ureteric reimplantation.

M. Outcome.
1. Depends on extent of renal damage and degree of pulmonary hypoplasia.
2. Posterior urethral valves.
   a. Prognosis of the newborn depends on the degree of pulmonary hypoplasia and the potential for renal recovery.
   b. Patients do well after prompt, early, effective drainage and appropriate management.
   c. There is some degree of urinary incontinence in up to 50% of children after treatment; however, this improves with age (Behrman et al., 1987).

d. Of those who survive the neonatal period, approximately one-half will have some degree of renal insufficiency and many will eventually need a transplant (Behrman et al., 1987).

Renal Vein Thrombosis

A. **Precipitating factors.**
1. Maternal diabetes.
2. Toxemia.
3. Maternal thiazide therapy.
4. Polycythemia.
5. Placental insufficiency.
6. Congenital heart disease.
7. Birth asphyxia.
8. Respiratory distress syndrome.
9. Sepsis.
10. Dehydration.
11. Hypovolemia.
12. Hyperosmolality.
13. Umbilical artery/venous catheter.

B. **Incidence.**
1. 1.9–2.7% of neonatal deaths (Arneil, 1973).
2. Occurs more frequently in males.

C. **Disease states.**
1. Congenital heart disease.
2. Congenital renal anomalies.
3. Severe pyelonephritis.
4. Sepsis.
5. Respiratory distress syndrome.

D. **Clinical presentation.**
1. Hematuria.
2. Anemia.
3. Oliguria/anuria.
4. Microangiopathic hemolytic anemia.
5. Thrombocytopenia.
6. Increased fibrin split products.
7. Decreased fibrinogen.
8. Decreased Factors V and VII.
9. Uremia.
10. Azotemia.
11. Metabolic acidosis.
12. Hyperosmolality.
13. Abdominal distention.
14. Proteinuria.
15. Rarely present at birth; usually presents within 24 hours.

E. **Clinical assessment.**
1. Perinatal history.
   a. Infant of a diabetic mother.
   b. Asphyxia.
2. Decreased urine output.
3. Variable blood pressure.
4. Urinalysis.
   a. Hematuria.
   b. Proteinuria.
   c. Leukocyturia.
5. Urine culture: rule out urinary tract infection.

6. CBC: rule out microangiopathic hemolytic anemia.
7. Platelet count: decreased.
8. BUN: increased.
9. Serum electrolytes.
   a. Hyponatremia.
   b. Hyperkalemia.
10. Serum pH: decreased.
11. Blood culture: positive in cases of sepsis.

F. **Physical examination: palpation of smooth, enlarged kidney.**

G. Diagnostic studies.
1. Renal ultrasound: enlarged kidney with a disordered central collection of echoes.
2. IVP: decreased urinary function.
3. Renal scan: non-functioning kidney.

H. **Differential diagnosis.**
1. Hydronephrosis.
2. Cystic disease.
3. Tumors of renal/adrenal origin.

I. **Complications.**
1. Renal tubular dysfunction.
2. Hypertension.
3. Some degree of renal atrophy.
4. Chronic renal infection.

J. **Patient care management.**
1. Treat underlying illness.
2. Correct electrolyte imbalances.
3. Antibiotics prn.
4. Treat symptoms.
   a. Hydration: assess volume and correct deficits.
   b. Oliguria: treat as for acute renal failure.
   c. Treat intravascular coagulation.
   d. Peritoneal dialysis for fluid overload, severe electrolyte imbalance, acidosis, or bilateral thrombosis with anuria.

K. **Outcome.**
1. Kidney may recover or show signs of damage; depends in part on severity of underlying medical condition.
2. Mortality has been reported as 12.5% (Schmidt, 1988).

Urinary Tract Infections

A. **Etiology.**
1. Abnormality of the urinary tract.
2. Sepsis: in the neonatal period, bacteria reach the urinary tract via the blood stream, whereas later in life, they ascend from below.
3. Most common organism is *Escherichia coli*.
4. Incidence: 1.4–5:1000 live births (Belman, 1987).

B. **Disease states.**
1. Sepsis.
2. Urinary tract anomalies.

C. **Clinical presentation.**
1. May be asymptomatic.
2. Non-specific signs and symptoms of sepsis.
   a. Abnormal weight loss during the first days of life.
   b. Poor feeding.

    c. Irritability.
    d. Lethargy.
    e. Cyanosis.
    f. Jaundice.
3. Septicemia.
4. Dehydration.

D. Diagnostic studies.
1. Urine culture.
2. Urinalysis.
    a. Leukocyturia.
    b. Hematuria.
    c. Casts suggests renal involvement.
3. Blood culture.
4. CBC with differential.
5. Abdominal ultrasound: rule out urinary tract anomalies.
6. Renal scan: rule out vesicoureteral reflux, obstructive uropathy.
7. Cystourethrography: rule out urinary tract malformation.

E. Differential diagnosis.
1. Sepsis.
2. Urinary tract obstruction.

F. Complications.
1. Renal scarring.
2. Recurrence of urinary tract infection.

G. Patient care management.
1. Antibiotics (ampicillin and aminoglycoside) for 14 days.
2. Follow-up urine culture 3 days after antibiotics are discontinued.
3. Supportive.

H. Outcome: excellent with prompt and adequate treatment.

Patent Urachus

Patent urachus is a communication between the bladder and the umbilicus.

A. Etiology: failure of normal closure of epithelialized urachal tube resulting in patent urachus.

B. Incidence: has been reported as approximately 3 : 1,000,000 hospital admissions (Nix et al., 1958).

C. Clinical presentation.
1. Discharge of urine from umbilicus at birth or later.
2. Wet umbilicus.
3. Enlarged/edematous umbilicus.
4. Delayed sloughing of cord.

D. Physical examination: observation of umbilicus.

E. Diagnostic studies.
1. Analysis of fluid for urea and creatinine.
2. Radiographic visualization.
3. Catheterization or probing of urachal tract.
4. IVP and cystography.

F. Differential diagnosis.
1. Patency of vitelline/omphalomesenteric duct.
2. Omphalitis.
3. Simple granulation of a healing umbilical stump.
4. Infected umbilical vessel.
5. External urachal sinus.

G. **Complications.**
1. Urinary tract infection.
2. Excoriation.
3. Infection.

H. **Patient care management.**
1. Non-intervention: spontaneous closure may occur if small defect with intermittent drainage.
2. Operative intervention.
   a. If distal obstructive uropathy is present, treat before surgically closing urachal duct.
   b. Surgical excision of the umbilicus with the entire urachus and a small portion of the bladder.

I. Outcome: good with surgical procedure.

Hypospadias

A. **Urethral meatus on the ventral surface of the penis** (Fig. 19–2).
1. Varies in severity from slightly malpositioned meatus still within glans and without chordee to extreme genital ambiguity with hypoplastic phallus, bifid scrotum, and scrotal or perineal meatus.

B. **Etiology.**
1. Deficient anterior urethral development.
2. Delay or arrest in the normal sequence of development causing the urethra to open proximally and the prepuce to be incomplete ventrally.
3. Probably multifactorial mode of inheritance.

C. **Incidence:** has been reported as 8.2 : 1000 live male births (Sweet et al., 1974).

D. **Clinical presentation.**
1. Urinary meatus located on the undersurface of penis.
2. Deviation of urinary stream.

E. **Clinical assessment.**
1. Direction of urinary stream.
2. Voiding pattern.

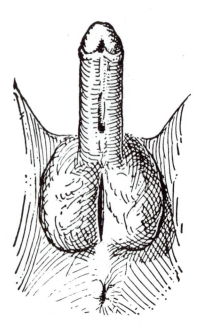

Figure 19–2
Hypospadias showing in one drawing a composite of all three locations. (From Koyle, M.A., and Anand, S.K.: *In* Taeusch, H.W., Balland, R.A., and Avery, M.E. (eds.): Schaffer and Avery's Diseases of the Newborn, 6th ed. Philadelphia, W.B. Saunders Co., 1991, p. 885.)

F. **Physical examination.**
1. Observation of external genitalia.
    a. Meatal location.
    b. Quantity of ventral shaft skin and dorsal foreskin; usually incomplete formation of ventral prepuce.
    c. Chordee: downward curving of the penis.
        (1) Association with chordee variable.
        (2) Severity of chordee generally proportional to degree of hypospadias.
    d. Presence of inguinal hernia.
2. Palpation.
    a. Descent of testes.
    b. Presence of inguinal hernia.

G. **Complications.**
1. Without repair.
    a. Difficulty in voiding while standing.
    b. Presence of chordee may cause painful erection.
    c. Post–surgical repair.
        (1) Urethrocutaneous fistula.
        (2) Balanitis xerotica obliterans.
        (3) Meatal stenosis.
        (4) Urethral stricture.
        (5) Urethral diverticulum.

H. **Patient care management.**
1. Avoid circumcision.
2. Surgical repair.
    a. Move meatus distally.
    b. Improve cosmetic appearance of genitalia.
    c. Straighten curved penis.
    d. Single-stage procedure preferred.
    e. Timing of surgical repair is variable—generally, the penis is of sufficient size by 6–18 months for surgical repair.

I. **Outcome:** good for surgical correction of simple hypospadias.

Exstrophy of the Bladder (Fig. 19–3)

A. **Bladder exposed and protrudes onto the abdominal wall** (Fig. 19–3). The umbilicus is displaced downward and pubic rami are widely separated in the midline. The rectus muscles are separated.
1. Virtually all affected infants have associated epispadias (opening of the urinary meatus onto the dorsal aspect of the penis).
2. The remainder of the urinary tract is usually normal.

B. **Etiology.**
1. Part of the spectrum of conditions resulting from abnormal development of cloacal membrane.
2. Failure of the mesoderm to invade cephalad extension of the cloacal membrane.
3. Position and timing of rupture of the cloacal membrane determine the variant of exstrophy-epispadias complex.

C. **Incidence.**
1. Approximately 1 : 30,000 births (Jeffs, 1987).
2. More common in males.

D. **Disease states.**
1. Exstrophy-epispadias complex.

E. **Clinical presentation.**
1. External presentation of bladder.

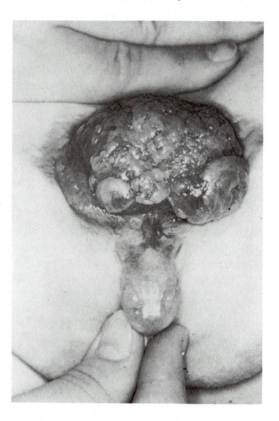

Figure 19-3
Patient with exstrophy of the bladder, associated with complete epispadias. The prominent cystic changes in the bladder mucosa are typical but are of no clinical significance. (From Avery, G.B. (ed.): Neonatology: Pathophysiology and Management of the Newborn, 3rd ed. Philadelphia, J.B. Lippincott; 1987, p. 996.)

2. Epispadias.
3. Anterior displacement of anus.
4. Undescended testes and inguinal hernia common.
5. Separation of symphysis pubis.
6. Lateral rotation of ileum and innominate bone.
7. Umbilical hernia.

F. Clinical assessment.
1. Signs and symptoms of infection.
2. Urine output.

G. Physical assessment.
1. Observation of an external presentation of the bladder.
2. Assessment of associated anomalies.
   a. Epispadias.
   b. Bifid clitoris.
   c. Anteriorly located vagina.
   d. Anteriorly located anus.
3. Palpation.
   a. Testes: to assess descent.
   b. Groin: to assess for presence of inguinal hernias.
   c. Symphysis pubis: to assess widening.

H. Differential diagnosis: complete exstrophy-epispadias complex.

I. Complications.
1. Infections.
2. Postoperative hydronephrosis.
3. Vesicoureteral reflux after bladder closure.
4. Swelling and edema in the bladder wall after surgery that obstructs ureteral drainage. This can lead to anuria, hypertension, or hydroureteronephrosis.

5. Anal incontinence.
6. Malignancy occurring 10 or more years later.

J. **Patient care management.**
1. Cover exposed bladder with Silastic shield or other appropriate dressing to permit drainage but protect bladder (Vaseline gauze is not recommended).
2. Prevent cord clamp from damaging bladder by using cord tie.
3. Surgical closure within 48 hours.
4. Gallows or modified Bryant's traction to immobilize activity for 3–4 weeks of healing.
5. Antispasmodics, analgesics, and sedatives to prevent bladder spasm and excessive crying, which may disrupt closure.
6. Subsequent epispadias repair at about 1-½–2-½ years.
7. Antibiotic therapy.
8. To achieve urinary continence, surgeon performs bladder neck revision with bilateral ureteral reimplantation during 2–3 years of age. Ureteroplasty can also be carried out in the males at this time.

K. **Outcome.**
1. The majority of children with exstrophy can achieve good bladder control with proper management.

Inguinal Hernia

A. **Etiology:** failure of the proximal part of the processus vaginalis to close, producing a hernia sac.

B. **Incidence.**
1. 1–4.4% of the pediatric population (Rajfer, 1986).
2. Occurs in more than 13% of infants <2,000 g at birth (Rajfer, 1986).
3. Occurs more frequently in males.

C. **Disease states.**
1. Cryptorchidism.
2. Presence of multiple congenital anomalies, particularly those involving the lower abdomen, pelvis, or perineum; frequently have inguinal hernias associated with them.

D. **Clinical presentation:** swelling/lump in the inguinal area and/or scrotum.

E. **Physical examination.**
1. Palpation.
   a. Inguinal area and scrotum to determine herniation.
   b. Scrotum to determine testicular descent.
2. Observation.
   a. Transillumination: rule out hydrocele.
3. Gestational age assessment: more common in premature infants because premature birth precedes closure of the processus vaginalis.

F. **Differential diagnosis.**
1. Hydrocele.
2. Testicular torsion.
3. Testicular tumor.

G. **Complications.**
1. Incarceration of hernia.
2. Venous infection of the testicle.

H. **Patient care management.**
1. Herniorrhaphy.
   a. Surgical repair of premature infants should be performed close to the time of discharge, after the infant is stable and has gained weight. The hernia may be monitored and reduced manually until that time.

I. Outcome.
1. Excellent after surgical repair.
2. Rate of complications or recurrence is very small.

Undescended Testicles (Cryptorchidism)

A. Etiology.
1. Endocrine dysfunction of the hypothalamic-pituitary-gonadal axis.
2. Abnormal epididymal development with failure to induce testicular descent.
3. Anatomical abnormality preventing descent.

B. Incidence (Fonkalsrud, 1987).
1. 1.8–4% in full-term neonates.
2. 20–30% in premature neonates.
3. 0.7% after the first year of life.
4. Approximately 70% occur unilaterally on the right side.

C. Disease states.
1. Specific types of cryptorchidism.
   a. Abdominal: testes located inside the internal inguinal ring.
   b. Canalicular: testes located between the internal and external inguinal rings.
   c. Ectopic: testes located away from the normal pathway of descent, between the abdominal cavity and the base of the scrotum.
   d. Retractile: fully descended testicle that moves freely between the base of the scrotum and the groin.
2. Genetic syndromes.
   a. Klinefelter's syndrome.
   b. Noonan's syndrome.
   c. Prader-Willi syndrome.
3. Vasal and/or epididymal abnormalities.

D. Clinical presentation: absence of the testes in the scrotum.

E. Clinical assessment: assess for associated abnormalities. There is an increased incidence with central nervous system abnormalities and hypospadias.

F. Physical examination.
1. Palpation.
   a. Scrotum for presence of testes or associated hernia.
   b. Inguinal area for presence of hernia.

G. Diagnostic studies.
1. Ultrasound: identification of intra-abdominal testes.
2. Computed axial tomography: identification of intra-abdominal testes.

H. Differential diagnosis.
1. Specific type of cryptorchidism.
   a. Abdominal.
   b. Canalicular.
   c. Ectopic.
   d. Retractile.
2. Monorchidism.
3. Anorchidism.

I. Complications.
1. Testicular torsion.
2. Hernia.
3. Infertility.
4. Postoperative complications.
   a. Obstruction of the testicular vascular supply by direct injury.
   b. Compression from twisting of the vascular supply by direct injury.
   c. Tight closure of the abdominal musculature.

d. Narrowing of vessels by placing them under significant tension as the testis is brought into the scrotum.

e. Transient testicular swelling from partial obstruction of lymphatic and venous drainage.

J. **Patient care management.**

1. Orchiopexy.
   a. Surgical procedure that alters the course of the spermatic artery and creates a direct line from the renal pedicle to the scrotum.
   b. Optimum age for surgical repair is 6 months to 2 years of life.
2. Hormonal treatment.
   a. Consists of administration of human chorionic gonadotropin (HCG), or gonadotropin-releasing hormone (GnRH), also referred to as luteinizing hormone–releasing hormone (LHRH).
   b. May be attempted in an effort to avoid orchiopexy.
   c. May make the technical aspects of orchiopexy easier.

K. **Outcome.**

1. Achievement of scrotal placement of virtually all testes is possible.
2. Fertility may be impaired.

Circumcision

A. **Indications:** there is no absolute medical indication for routine circumcision in the newborn period, although the pros and cons of the procedure have been reviewed in the literature (Herzog, 1989; Lohr, 1989; Schoen et al., 1989; Rockney, 1988; Rothberg, 1987; Tedder, 1987; Lincoln, 1986).

B. **Incidence.**

1. 1–1.5 million newborn males per year in the United States (Rockney, 1988).

C. **Physical examination.**

1. Observation.
   a. Assess for the presence of abnormalities of the glans, foreskin, or urethral meatus.
2. Gestational age assessment.
   a. Circumcision should not be performed on premature infants until they meet discharge criteria.

D. **Complications.**

1. Hemorrhage.
2. Infection.
3. Injury to the glans.
4. Meatal stenosis.
5. Urethrocutaneous fistula.
6. Formation of skin bridge.
7. Adhesions.

E. **Patient care management.**

1. Circumcision should not be performed on infants with bleeding disorders or those with abnormalities of the glans, foreskin, or urethral meatus.
2. Vitamin K should be administered within 1 hour after birth.
3. Local anesthesia and dorsal penile nerve block have been shown to alleviate the discomfort associated with the procedure (Masciello, 1990; Stang et al., 1988; Maxwell et al., 1987; Holve et al., 1983; Williamson and Williamson, 1983; Kirya and Werthmann, 1978).
4. Informed consent must be obtained.
5. Postoperative care.
   a. Check the site for bleeding, redness, or pus.
   b. Avoid supine position.

    c. Change diapers frequently.
    d. Apply Vaseline gauze to site for 24 hours.
    e. Apply petroleum jelly to site until healed.
6. Teach parent how to care for circumcision prior to discharge.

F. **Outcome.**

1. Risk of postoperative complications has been reported to range from 0.2 to 0.6% (Harkavy, 1987; Wiswell, 1987; Gee and Ansell, 1976).

STUDY QUESTIONS

1. Post-natal changes in renal physiology include:
   a. Decreased ability to concentrate urine.
   b. Increased glomerular filtration rate.
   c. Increased renal vascular resistance.

2. One mechanism the neonatal kidney employs to respond to changes in acid-base balance is:
   a. Regulation of glomerular filtration rate.
   b. Regulation of hydrogen and bicarbonate.
   c. Regulation of urine output.

3. The neonatal kidney has the following limitation when compared with the older child or adult:
   a. Higher glomerular filtration rate.
   b. Higher specific gravity.
   c. Limited ability to excrete an acid load.

4. An example of each of the three causes of acute renal failure would be:
   a. Hydronephrosis, sepsis, ureteropelvic junction obstruction.
   b. Hypotension, polycystic kidney disease, ureteropelvic junction obstruction.
   c. Posterior urethral valves, multicystic dysplasia, Potter's syndrome.

5. Which of the following blood pressures would be diagnostic of hypertension in the neonatal period?
   a. Premature infant > 1 kg with mean blood pressure of 60 mm Hg at 7 days of age.
   b. Premature infant < 1 kg with mean blood pressure of 80 mm Hg at 1 month of age.

   c. Term infant with blood pressure of 80/50 at birth.

6. Infantile polycystic kidney disease differs from multicystic renal dysplasia in the following manner:
   a. It is an inherited disorder.
   b. It is the most common form of renal cystic disease observed in the neonatal period.
   c. It usually occurs unilaterally.

7. One of the clinical signs of hydronephrosis seen in the neonatal period is:
   a. Abdominal mass.
   b. Increased specific gravity.
   c. Polyuria.

8. Clinical signs of renal vein thrombosis would be:
   a. Bilateral flank masses and anuria.
   b. Hematuria and oliguria.
   c. Thrombocytopenia and hypo-osmolality.

9. Physical assessment of the neonate with hypospadias would include:
   a. Location of urinary meatus, and testicular descent.
   b. Presence of flank mass and presence of chordee.
   c. Urine output and quantity of foreskin present.

10. Post-circumcision nursing care would include:
   a. Application of a pressure dressing.
   b. Assessment of site for bleeding.
   c. Maintaining infant in prone position.

Answers to Study Questions

1. b	5. b	8. b
2. b	6. a	9. a
3. c	7. a	10. b
4. b		

REFERENCES

Appleman, Z., and Golbus, M.S.: The management of fetal urinary tract obstruction. Clin. Obstet. Gynecol., 29(3):483–489, 1986.

Arneil, G.C., MacDonald, A.M., Murphy, A.V., et al.: Renal venous thrombosis. Clin. Nephrol. 1:119, 1973.

Anand, S.K., Aaberg, R.A., and Koyle, M.A.: Renal vascular thrombosis and renal cortical and medullary necrosis. In Taeusch, H.W., Balland, R.A., and Avery, M.E. (eds.): Schaffer and Avery's Diseases of the Newborn, 6th ed. Philadelphia, W.B. Saunders Co., 1991, pp. 898–904.

Belman, A.B.: Abnormalities of the genitourinary system. In Avery, G.B. (ed): Neonatology: Pathophysiology and Management of the Newborn, 3rd ed. Philadelphia, J.B. Lippincott, 1987, pp. 985–1011.

Feld, L.G., and Springate, J.E.: Hypertension in children. Curr. Prob. Pediatr., 18(6):319–379, 1988.

Fonkalsrud, E.W.: Testicular undescent and torsion. Pediatr. Clin. North Am. 34(5):130, 1987.

Gordon, A.C., Thomas, D.F.M., Arthur, R.J., and Irving, H.C.: Multicystic dysplastic kidney: Is nephrectomy still appropriate? J. Urol. (part 2), 140:1231–1234, 1988.

Herzog, L.W.: Urinary tract infections and circumcision. AJDC, 143:348–350, 1989.

Holve, R.L., Bromberger, P.J., Groveman, H.D., et al.: Regional anesthesia during newborn circumcision. Clin. Pediatr., 22(12):813–818, 1983.

Horger, E.O., and Pai, G.S.: Ultrasound in the diagnosis of fetal malformations. Am. J. Obstet. Gynecol., 147:163–170, 1983.

Jeffs, R.D.: Exstrophy, epispadias, and cloacal and urogenital sinus abnormalities. Pediatr. Clin. North Am., 35(5):1233–1257, 1987.

Kirya, C., and Werthmann, M.W.: Neonatal circumcision and penile dorsal nerve block: A painless procedure. J. Pediatr., 92(6):998–1000, 1978.

Lincoln, G.A.: Neonatal circumcision: Is it needed? JOGNN, 15(6):463–466, 1986.

Lohr, J.A.: The foreskin and urinary tract infections. J. Pediatr., 114(3):502–503, 1989.

Manning, F.A.: International fetal surgery registry: 1985 update. Clin. Obstet. Gynecol., 29(3):551–557, 1986.

Masciello, A.L.: Anesthesia for neonatal circumcision: Local anesthesia is better than dorsal penile nerve block. Obstet. Gynecol., 75:834–838, 1990.

Maxwell, L.G., Yaster, M., Wetzel, R.C., and Niebyl, J.R.: Penile nerve block for newborn circumcision. Obstet. Gynecol. (part 1), 79(3):415–419, 1987.

Moore, K.L.: The Developing Human: Clinically Oriented Embryology, 4th ed. Philadelphia, W.B. Saunders Co., 1988.

Nix, J. T., Menville, J.G., Albert, M., and Wendt, D.L.: Congenital patent urachus. J. Urol., 79(2):264–273, 1958.

Pawlak, R.P., and Herfert, L.T. Drug Administration in the NICU: A Handbook for Nurses, 2nd ed. Petaluma, Cal., Neonatal Network, 1990.

Perlmutter, A.D., Retik, A.B., and Bauer, S.B.: Anomalies of the upper urinary tract. In Walsh, P.C., Gittes, R.F., Perlmutter, A.D., and Stamey, T.A. (eds.): Campbell's Urology, 5th ed. Philadelphia, W.B. Saunders Co., 1986, pp. 1665–1759.

Portman, R., Browder, S., and DiStefano, S.M.: Neonatal Nephrology. In Merenstein, G.B., and Gardner, S.L. (eds.): Handbook of Neonatal Intensive Care. St. Louis, C.V. Mosby, 1989, pp. 466–500.

Potter, E.L.: Bilateral absence of ureters and kidneys. Obstet. Gynecol. 25(1):3–12, 1965.

Rafjer, J.: Congenital anomalies of the testis. In Walsh, P.C., Gittes, R.F., Perlmutter, A.D., and Stamey, T.A. (eds.): Campbell's Urology, 5th ed. Philadelphia, W.B. Saunders Co., 1986, pp. 1947–1968.

Rockney, R.: Newborn circumcision. AFP, 38(4):151–155, 1988.

Rothberg, L.: The pros and cons of circumcision. RN, 50(7):30–32, 1987.

Sanders, R.C.: Ultrasonic assessment of genitourinary anomalies in utero. In Sanders, R.C., and James, A.E. Jr. (eds.): The Principles of Ultrasonography in Obstetrics and Gynecology. Norwalk, CT, Appleton-Century-Crofts, 1985, pp. 195–205.

Sarda, P., Bard, H., Teasdale, F., and Grignon, A.: The importance of an antenatal ultrasonographic diagnosis of correctable fetal malformations. Am. J. Obstet. Gynecol., 147:443–445, 1983.

Schmidt, B., and Andrew, M.: Neonatal thrombotic disease: Prevention, diagnosis and treatment. J. Pediatr., 113(2):407–410, 1988.

Schoen, E.J., Anderson, G., et al.: Report of the task force on circumcision. Pediatrics, 84(4):388–391, 1989.

Stang, H.J. Gunnar, M.R., Snellman, L., et al.: Local anesthesia for neonatal circumcision. JAMA, 259(10):1507–1511, 1988.

Sweet, R.A., Schrott, H.G., Kurland, R., and Culp, O.S.: Study of the incidence of hypospadias in Rochester, Minnesota, 1940–1970, and a case control comparison of possible etiologic factors. Mayo Clin. Proc., 49:52–58, 1974.

Tedder, J.L.: Newborn circumcision. JOGNN, 16(1):42–47, 1987.

Williamson, P.S., and Williamson, M.L.: Physiologic stress reduction by a local anesthetic during newborn circumcision. Pediatrics, 71(1):36–40, 1983.

Wiswell, T.E.: Letter. Pediatrics, 79(4):650, 1987.

Zobel, G., Ring, E., and Muller, W.: Continuous arteriovenous hemofiltration in premature infants. Crit. Care Med., 17:534–536, 1989.

BIBLIOGRAPHY

Abman, S.H., Warady, B.A., et al.: Systemic hypertension in infants with bronchopulmonary dysplasia. J. Pediatr., *104*:929–931, 1984.

Anand, S.K.: Acute renal failure in the neonate. Pediatr. Clin. North Am., *29*(4):791–800, 1982.

Aperia, A., and Zetterstron, R.: Renal control of fluid homeostasis in the newborn infant. Clin. Perinatol., *9*(3):523–534, 1982.

Avery, G.B. (ed.): Neonatology: Pathophysiology and Management of the Newborn, 3rd ed. Philadelphia, J.B. Lippincott, 1987.

Avni, E.F., Thou, Y., Lalmond, B., et al.: Multicystic dysplastic kidney: Natural history from in utero diagnosis and postnatal follow-up. J. Urol., *138*:1420–1424, 1987.

Behrman, R.E., Vaughan, V.C., and Nelson, W.E. (eds.): Nelson Textbook of Pediatrics, 14th ed. Philadelphia, W.B. Saunders, Co., 1992.

Bernstein, G.T., Mandell, J., et al.: Ureteropelvic junction obstruction in the neonate. J. Urol. (part 2), *140*:1216–1221, 1988.

Brocklebank, J.T.: Renal failure in the newly born. Arch. Dis. Child., *63*:991–994, 1988.

Burbige, K.A, and Hensle, T.W.: Posterior urethral valves in the newborn: Treatment and functional results. J. Pediatr. Surg., *22*(2):165–167, 1987.

Burns, M.W., Burns, J.L., and Kreiger, J.N.: Pediatric urinary tract infections: Diagnosis, classifications and significance. Pediatr. Clin. North Am., *34*(5):1111–1120, 1987.

Clemente, C.D. (ed.): Gray's Anatomy of the Human Body, 30th ed. Philadelphia, Lea & Febiger, 1984.

Cole, B.R., Conley, S.B., and Stapleton, F.B.: Polycystic kidney disease in the first year of life. J. Pediatr., *111*:693–699, 1987.

DeFossez, S.M., and DeLuca, S.A.: Adult polycystic kidney disease. AFP, *36*(4):157–159, 1987.

Dejter, S.W., Eggli, D.F., and Gibbons, M.D.: Delayed management of neonatal hydronephrosis. J. Urol. (part 2), *140*:1305–1309, 1988.

Elhassani, S.B.: The umbilical cord: Care, anomalies and diseases. South. Med. J., *77*(6):730–736, 1984.

Engle, W.D.: Development of fetal and neonatal renal function. Semin. Perinatol., *10*(2):113–124, 1986.

Filston, H.C., and Izant, R.J.: The Surgical Neonate. Norwalk, CT, Appleton-Century-Crofts, 1985.

Gaudio, K.M., and Seigel, N.J.: Pathogenesis and treatment of acute renal failure. Pediatr. Clin. North Am., *34*(3):771–787, 1987.

Gee, W.F., and Ansell, J.S.: Neonatal circumcision: A ten-year overview: With comparison of the Gomco clamp and the Plastibell device. Pediatrics, *58*(6):824–827, 1976.

Glassberg, K.I., Stephens, F.D., et al.: Renal dysgenesis and cystic disease of the kidney: A report of the Committee on Terminology, Nomenclature and Classification, Section on Urology, American Academy of Pediatrics. J. Urol., *138*:1085–1092 (part 2), 1988.

Gleason, C.A.: Prostaglandins and the developing kidney. Semin. Perinatol., *11*(1):12–21, 1987.

Gonzalez, E.T., Jr.: Urologic considerations in the newborn. Urol. Clin. North Am., *12*(1):43–51, 1985.

Grignon, A. Filion, R., Filiatrault, D., et al.: Urinary tract dilatation in utero: Classification and clinical applications. Radiology, *160*:645–647, 1986.

Guignard, J.P., Gouyon, J.B., and Adelman, R.D.: Arterial hypertension in the newborn infant. Biol. Neonate, 55:77–83, 1989.

Hanna, M.K., and Gluck, P.: Ureteropelvic junction obstruction during the first year of life. Urology, *31*(1):41–45, 1988.

Harkavy, K.L.: Letter. Pediatrics, *79*(4):649–650, 1987.

Hartman, G.E., and Schochat, S.J.: Abdominal mass lesions in the newborn: Diagnosis and treatment. Clin. Perinatol., *16*(1):123–135, 1989.

Horan, M.J., et al.: Report of the second task force on blood pressure control in children. Pediatrics, *79*(1):1–25, 1987.

Kelalis, P.P., King, L.R., and Belman, A.B. (eds.): Clinical Pediatric Urology, 2nd ed. Philadelphia, W.B. Saunders Co., 1985.

McCormick, A., and Sterk, M.B.: Acute renal failure of the neonate. Dimensions Crit. Care Nurs., *5*(3):155–161, 1986.

Merenstein, G.B., and Gardner, S.L.: Handbook of Neonatal Intensive Care. St. Louis, C.V. Mosby, 1989.

Nakayama, D.K. Harrison, M.R., and de Lorimier, A.A.: Prognosis of posterior urethral valves presenting at birth. J. Pediatr. Surg., *21*(1):43–45, 1986.

O'Dea, R.F., Mirken, B.L., Alward, C.T., and Sinaiko, A.R.: Treatment of neonatal hypertension with captopril. J. Pediatr., *113*(2):405–406, 1988.

Paltiel, H.J., and Lebowitz, R.L.: Neonatal hydronephrosis due to primary vesicoureteral reflux: Trends in diagnosis and treatment. Radiology, *170*:787–789, 1987.

Ring, E., and Zobel, G.: Urinary infection and malformations of the urinary tract in infancy. Arch. Dis. Child., *63*:818–820, 1989.

Rudolph, A.M. (ed.): Pediatrics, 18th ed. Norwalk, CT: Appleton & Lange, 1987.

Shaffer, S.E., and Norman, M.E.: Renal function and renal failure in the newborn. Clin. Perinatol., *16*(1):199–218, 1989.

Sheldon, C.A., and Duckett, J.W.: Hypospadias. Pediatr. Clin. North Am., *34*(5):1259–1272, 1987.

Siegal, S.M.: Hormonal and renal interaction in body fluid regulation in the newborn infant. Clin. Perinatol., *9*(3):535–557, 1982.

Thompson, H.C., et al.: Report of the ad hoc committee on circumcision. Pediatrics, *56*(4):610–611, 1975.

Walsh, P.C., Gittes, R.F., Perlmutter, A.D., and Stamey, T.A. (eds.): Campbell's Urology, 5th ed. Philadelphia, W.B. Saunders, Co., 1986.

Wolpert, J.J., Woodard, J.R., and Parrott, T.S.: Pyeloplasty in the young infant. J. Urol., *142*:573–575, 1989.

Mary McCulloch

Neurological Disorders

Objectives

1. Identify the six primary stages of neurodevelopment and the congenital anomalies that result from defective stage development.

2. Define autoregulation.

3. Review a complete neurological examination.

4. Examine birth injuries and patient care management.

5. Differentiate between the different types of intracranial hemorrhages, their origins, clinical presentation, and outcomes.

6. Recognize neonatal seizures, their distinguishing characteristics, and issues in patient care management.

7. Describe hypoxic-ischemic encephalopathy, including periventricular leukomalacia.

8. Distinguish pathophysiological factors, clinical presentation, and patient care management of early- and late-onset meningitis.

The human brain is an intricate, fragile organ requiring precise development from the moment of conception. Several crucial developmental landmarks pinpoint major events in the developing human brain. If interrupted, malformations results.

Neurological problems account for a significant number of admissions into the newborn intensive care unit each year. These problems range from simple, easily treatable problems to major neurological malformations.

This chapter provides a comprehensive review of neurodevelopment, neurophysiology, and neuromalformations. A greater understanding of these concepts may remove some of the mystery and complexity of the brain.

Anatomy of the Neurological System

A. **Embryological development** (Table 20–1).
1. Dorsal induction.

Table 20-1
MAJOR EVENTS IN HUMAN BRAIN DEVELOPMENT AND PEAK TIMES OF OCCURRENCE

Major Developmental Event	Peak Time of Occurrence
Dorsal induction	3-4 weeks' gestation*
Ventral induction	5-6 weeks' gestation
Neuronal proliferation	2-4 months' gestation
Migration	3-5 months' gestation
Organization	6 months' gestation-years post-natal
Myelination	Birth-years post-natal

*Timing of primary neurulation.
From Volpe, J.J.: Neurology of the Newborn, 2nd ed. Philadelphia, W.B. Saunders Co., 1987.

a. Occurs within the first month of life, ending between 24 and 28 days' gestation.
b. Formation of the neural tube, which is created by the invagination and curling of the neural plate distally.
c. Closure of the neural tube gives rise to the central nervous system, including the cranial nerves.
d. This evolution gives rise to the appearance of the skull and vertebrae.
e. Inaccuracies of dorsal induction result in spina bifida, occipital encephalocele, and anencephaly.
2. Ventral induction.
   a. Occurs early in the second month of gestation.
   b. Creates the forebrain; forms the face, thalamus, hypothalamus, cerebral hemispheres, and the basal ganglia.
   c. Disturbance in anterior neural tube closure causes facial and forebrain alternations.
      (1) Holoprosencephaly.
      (2) Midline and midfacial defects.
         (a) Hypertelorism.
         (b) Cyclopia.
         (c) Cleft lip with or without cleft palate.
3. Neuronal proliferation.
   a. Occurs between 2 and 4 months' gestation.
   b. Toxins and inherited diseases can significantly alter the number of neurons.
   c. Chemical and environmental substances can reduce the number of neurons, causing microcephaly vera.
   d. Excess neurons can produce macrocephaly.
   e. Disorders of proliferation of small veins cause Sturge-Weber syndrome.
4. Neuronal migration.
   a. Can occur as early as 2 months; peaks between 3 and 5 months.
   b. By 6 months' gestation, the neurons have migrated to their final, permanent place in the cortex.
   c. Neurons follow glial paths outward.
   d. Cells migrate and differentiate into six cortical layers (Finkel, 1984).
   e. Migration is critical for development of the cerebral cortex and deeper nuclear structure.
      (1) Basal ganglia.
      (2) Hypothalamus.
      (3) Thalamus.
      (4) Brainstem.
      (5) Cerebellum.
      (6) Spinal cord.

f. Dysfunction at this stage results in cortical malformation with neurological function abnormalities.

g. Seizures may be the first clinical manifestation in the early post-natal period.

h. Defects associated with abnormal migration range in severity and may be associated with other neurological development.

5. Neuronal organization.

a. Occurs about 27–28 days' gestation.

b. Provides the basis for brain function and its complex circuitry.

c. Includes cell differentiation, cell death, synaptic development, neurotransmitters and myelination (Finkel, 1984).

d. Achieves stabilization of cell connections.

e. Disorders are not well known, although Down syndrome intellectual problems may be related to inefficient neuronal organization (Volpe, 1987).

6. Myelination.

a. Begins in the second trimester and continues into adult life.

b. Involves myelin deposition around axons.

c. Myelin, a fatty covering, insulates the circuitry; prevents leakage of current; and enables rapid, efficient transmission of nerve impulses.

d. Enhances intercellular communication.

e. Deficiencies occur in some acquired and inherited diseases.

B. Brain anatomy (Fig. 20–1).

1. Cerebellum.

a. Promotes integrative muscle function.

b. Maintains balance.

c. Enables smooth, purposeful movements.

2. Cerebrum.

a. Main components.

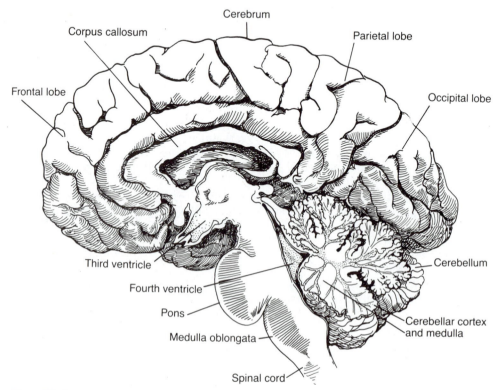

Figure 20–1
Anatomy of the brain.

(1) Cerebral hemispheres.
   (a) Contains four lobes: parietal, frontal, occipital, and temporal lobes.
   (b) Corpus callosum.
      i. Fiber bundles connecting the cerebral hemispheres.
   (c) Cerebral cortex.
      i. Encompasses the mind, the intellect.
      ii. Gray matter.
   (d) Third ventricle.
      i. Fluid-filled space.
   (e) Thalamus.
      i. Integrate sensory input.
   (f) Hypothalamus.
      i. Regulates body temperature.
3. Brainstem.
   a. Relays input and output signals between higher brain centers and the spinal cord.
   b. Three main components.
   (1) Medulla.
      (a) Implicated within cranial nerves VIII, IX, X, XI, and XII.
      (b) Controls areas of the abdomen, thorax, neck, throat, and mouth.
   (2) Pons.
      (a) Carries information between the brainstem and cerebellum.
   (3) Midbrain.
      (a) Involved in eye movements.

Physiology of the Neurological System

A. **Glucose metabolism.**
1. Cerebral metabolism is influenced by the availability of glucose and oxygen.
2. Serum glucose provides the brain with a glucose pool.
3. Glucose supply to the brain is compromised by inadequate cerebral perfusion.
4. The neonatal brain is glucose dependent.
5. The body preferentially pumps glucose against the gradient to the brain.
6. Premature babies have a less efficient glucose uptake mechanism.
7. Glycogen stores are minimal or non-existent in the premature baby.
8. The brain depends on adequate circulation to supply both oxygen and glucose to create enough energy for growth and metabolism.
9. Anaerobic metabolism causes lactic acid build-up.
10. Anaerobic metabolism produces significantly smaller amounts of energy.

B. **Cerebral blood flow.**
1. Cerebral blood flow is affected by pH (controlled by hydrogen ions and carbon dioxide levels), potassium, hypoxemia, osmolarity, and calcium ion concentrations.
   a. The brain increases cerebral blood flow to spare itself inadequacies.
   b. As pH decreases, cerebral blood flow increases.
   c. As potassium levels increase, cerebral blood flow increases.
   d. Hypoxemia causes increase in cerebral blood flow to provide adequate oxygenated blood to the brain.
   e. Increased osmolarity causes increased cerebral blood flow.
   f. An increase in calcium ions causes a decrease in cerebral blood flow.
2. Autoregulation.
   a. Maintains steady-state cerebral blood flow despite systemic blood pressure changes.
   b. Premature infants have limited cerebral autoregulation.
   c. Impaired autoregulation occurs in distressed newborns (Lou, 1980; Lou et al., 1979).

    d. Without cerebral autoregulation, systemic blood pressure regulates cerebral perfusion.

        (1) Hypotension leads to ischemia.

            (a) Ischemia damages blood vessels and surrounding elements supporting the blood vessels.

            (b) Once adequate blood supply resumes, hemorrhage can occur into ischemic areas.

        (2) Hypertension leads to hemorrhage.

Neurological Assessment

A. History.

B. Observation.

1. Determine state (Table 20–2).
2. Note posture.

    a. Gestational age determines posture.

        (1) Premature infants.

            (a) Open, extended position reflecting diminished tone.

        (2) Term infants.

            (a) Flexed position reflecting adequate tone.

    b. Intrauterine position sequelae may be evident.

    c. Abnormal findings.

        (1) Hyperextension.

        (2) Asymmetry.

        (3) Flaccidity.

3. Movements.

    a. Symmetrical body movements.

    b. Note movement quality (jitteriness, seizures, tremors, and clonus).

    c. Quantity (absent or pronounced).

4. Respiratory activity.

    a. Signs of distress.

    b. Hypoventilation (apnea).

C. Complete the physical examination.

1. Check the skull size, shape, symmetry, hair whirls, fontanelles, and sutures.
2. Examine the face for abnormalities in structure.

    a. Placement of ears.

    b. Neck skinfolds.

    c. Spine (intact, openings, masses).

3. Cranial nerve function.

    a. Refer to Table 20–3.

    b. Blink reflex requires intact cranial nerves III and VII.

    c. Corneal reflex requires intact cranial nerves V and VII

        (1) Absent corneal reflex with tonic neck reflex present is associated with severe brain damage (Whaley and Wong, 1979).

Table 20–2
SUMMARY OF NEUROLOGICAL STATES

Neurological State	Physical Findings
Deep sleep	No observable movement
REM sleep	Eye movement, body movement, and irregular respiratory activity
Drowsy	
Quiet-alert	
Active	
Crying	

Table 20–3
CRANIAL NERVES

Cranial Nerve	Bedside Testing Mechanisms
I. *Olfactory* (smell)	Place ammonia under nose; response is startle, grimace
II. *Optic*	Check PERL
III. *Oculomotor* (muscles of the eye)	PERL, EOM full and conjugate
IV. *Trochlear* (superior oblique muscle of the eye)	
V. *Trigeminal* (sensory to face, motor to jaw)	Touch cheek; should turn cheek toward stimulus
VI. *Abducens* (lateral gaze, abducts eyeball)	Rotate infant; eyes look in the direction of travel
VII. *Facial*	Asymmetrical facial movements
VIII. *Auditory*	Infant quiets to voice; blinks to clap of hand
IX. *Glossopharyngeal* (taste)	Strong gag response
X. *Vagus* (pharynx, larynx, esophagus)	Cry is not hoarse
XI. *Accessory* (sternocleidomastoid muscles)	Turn supine infant's head to one side; infant attempts to bring head to midline
XII. *Hypoglossal* (muscles of tongue)	Insert finger in mouth while sucking; note force of tongue; note vesiculations or quivering tongue (uncommon)

PERL, pupils equal and reactive to light; EOM, extraocular movements.
Adapted from Scanlon, J.W., Nelson, T., Grylack, L.J., and Smith, Y.F.: A system of newborn physical examination. Baltimore, University Park Press, 1979; and Whaley, L.F., and Wong, D.L.: Nursing Care of Infants and Children. St. Louis, C.V. Mosby, 1979.

    (2) Cranial nerves IX, X and XII regulate the tongue, suck, swallow, gag, and cry.
4. Muscle tone.
    a. Evaluate head lag, ventral suspension, clonus, and recoil from extension.
    b. Check symmetry; briskness versus flaccidity.
5. Reflexes.
    a. Check grasp (bilaterally), Babinski's, Moro's, and gag.
    b. Evaluate symmetry and strength of response.
    c. Abnormal Moro's reflex: consider clavicular or humeral fractures or brachial plexus injury.
    d. Grasp varies with gestational age; absent grasp, consider nerve damage (refer to Birth Injuries).

Neurological Disorders

A. Anencephaly.
1. Pathophysiology.
    a. Absent neural tube closure exposing neural tissue.
    b. Malfunction of the first stage of neurological development, dorsal induction.
    c. Lack of brain above the brainstem.
    d. Partial absence of skull bones with absent cerebrum with or without missing cerebellum, brainstem, and spinal cord (Avery, 1987).
2. Incidence.
    a. Prevalence varies per country.
    b. United States occurrence rate varies from 0.5 to 2:1000 live births (Volpe, 1987).
    c. British Isles prevalence rates vary from 1 to 6:1000 live births.
    d. Females develop this defect more than males and whites more than blacks (Volpe, 1987).
3. Clinical presentation.
    a. Exposed neural tissue with little definable structure.
    b. The anomalous skull has a frog-like appearance when viewed face-on.
4. Outcome.

        a. 75% stillborn (Volpe, 1987).

        b. Survival is limited to the neonatal period.

   5. Patient care management.

        a. Provide comfort measures for the infant.

        b. Obtain a genetic consult; encourage parents to seek genetic counseling.

        c. Support the grieving process.

        d. Encourage the family to see their baby, since the family's imaginary impression may be worse than reality.

        e. Clinicians must maintain a delicate balance between benefit and harm (Erlen and Holzman, 1988).

B. Microcephaly.

1. Definition.

        a. Small brain.

        b. Occipital frontal circumference (OFC) less than the 10th percentile for gestational age.

2. Pathophysiology.

        a. Neuronal proliferation defect.

        b. Occurs between 2 and 4 months' gestational age (Volpe, 1987).

        c. The most severe microcephaly occurs earlier in utero.

3. Etiology.

        a. Teratogens.

          (1) Irradiation.

          (2) Maternal alcoholism.

         b. Maternal hyperphenylalaninemia.

        c. Genetic (usually autosomal recessive; can be X-linked) (Avery, 1987).

        d. TORCH infections (toxoplasmosis, other, rubella, cytomegalovirus, and herpes) are associated.

        e. Unknown causes.

4. Incidence: not known.

5. Clinical presentation.

        a. Head size is small.

        b. Neurological deficits rarely evident at birth.

6. Diagnostic evaluation.

        a. Perform a complete physical examination including neurological assessment.

        b. Elicit a thorough maternal history.

        c. Utilize tests to confirm or rule out etiologic factors aligned with the maternal history.

7. Patient care management.

        a. Record accurate measurement of OFC, length, and weight weekly.

        b. Note percentiles and alert physician of abnormalities.

        c. Document clearly any deviations from normal.

        d. Obtain tests as ordered; note dates to follow-up results.

        e. Ensure that the family is informed.

        f. Obtain consultations as needed—genetics and infectious disease.

8. Outcome.

        a. Dependent on the severity.

        b. May be associated with developmental delays.

C. Hydrocephalus.

1. Definition.

        a. Excess cerebrospinal fluid (CSF) in the ventricles of the brain.

        b. CSF is in balance between formation and absorption.

        c. CSF is produced at a rate of 1/3 ml/minute from brain parenchyma, cerebral ventricles, areas along the spinal cord, and the choroid plexus (60% is from the choroid plexus).

2. Pathophysiology.

        a. Excessive CSF production (rare).

    b. Inadequate CSF absorption secondary to abnormal circulation.

    c. Excess ventricular CSF secondary to aqueductal outflow obstruction causes obstructive, non-communicating hydrocephalus (refer to Fig. 20–2 for a simplified diagram of the brain).

       (1) Obstructive hydrocephalus may progress rapidly.

    d. Excess ventricular CSF with communication between lateral ventricles and subarachnoid space results in communicating, non-obstructive hydrocephalus.

3. Congenital hydrocephalus.

    a. Precipitating factors.

       (1) Aqueductal stenosis.

       (2) Dandy-Walker cyst (cystic transformation of ventricle IV).

       (3) Arnold-Chiari malformation (herniation of the hindbrain, usually causing obstructive hydrocephalus).

       (4) Congenital masses and tumors.

    b. Associated congenital defects.

       (1) Spina bifida.

       (2) Encephalocele.

    c. Incidence.

       (1) 2:1000 live births (Ment et al., 1984).

    d. Clinical presentation.

       (1) Large head.

       (2) Open sutures.

       (3) Full (bulging) and tense fontanelles.

       (4) Increasing OFC.

       (5) Sunset eyes signify brain tissue damage.

       (6) Visible scalp veins.

    e. Diagnostic studies.

       (1) Positive transillumination.

       (2) Cranial ultrasound.

       (3) Cranial tomography scan (CT scan).

    f. Patient care management.

       (1) Intrauterine diagnosis affords the family more options and allows time for preparation and anticipation.

       (2) Perform a thorough physical examination, assessing for further anomalies.

       (3) Obtain consultation by neurosurgery and genetics.

       (4) Confirm diagnosis and etiology.

       (5) Consider the possible need for reservoir placement versus ventriculo-peritoneal shunt (VP shunt) placement.

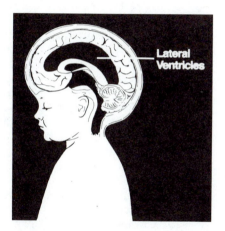

Figure 20–2
Hydrocephalus. (Used and reprinted with permission of the Ross Laboratories, Columbus, OH, 43216, from *New Perspectives on Intraventricular Hemorrhage.* © 1988, Ross Laboratories.)

(6) Support the infant by decreasing noxious stimuli (dim lights, minimize handling).

(7) Position the head carefully.

(8) Waterpillow beds diminish skin breakdown; may provide a source of comfort.

(9) Normalize infant care as much as possible.

(10) Involve parents in infant's care as soon as family is ready.

(11) Position the infant prone for oral feeds.

(12) Allow parents to view an infant with a VP shunt and/or review pictured handouts.

(13) Review VP shunt with parents preoperatively and postoperatively.

(14) Prevent skin breakdown by not allowing the infant to put his or her head on the shunt side postoperatively.

(15) Relieve the infant's probable stiff neck by holding the child's neck on the shunt side during the feeding.

(16) Review signs of infection or blocked shunt with family.

   (a) Irritability.

   (b) Vomiting.

   (c) Increasing head size.

   (d) Lethargy.

   (e) Changes in feeding patterns.

   (f) Bulging fontanelle.

(17) If incision site reddens, position infant on opposite side to relieve pressure from this area.

4. Post-hemorrhagic hydrocephalus (PHH).

  a. Pathophysiology.

    (1) Progressive dilatation of the ventricles following intraventricular hemorrhage (IVH) caused by periventricular white matter injury.

    (2) Two types: acute and chronic.

     (a) Acute.

      i. Rapidly appears within days of the initial bleed.

      ii. Probably occurs secondary to malabsorption of CSF secondary to a blood clot.

     (b) Chronic.

      i. An inhibition of CSF flow.

      ii. Blood from IVH or pus from infection.

  b. Incidence.

    (1) 50% of infants with IVH have no evidence of hydrocephalus (Volpe, 1987).

    (2) 50% of infants with IVH develop hydrocephalus with a mild increase in intracranial pressure (Volpe, 1987).

    (3) Ment and colleagues (1984) reported 25–74% of low birthweight infants with IVH develop hydrocephalus.

  c. Clinical presentation.

    (1) Severe ventricular dilatation.

     (a) Rapid increase in head size.

     (b) Apnea.

     (c) Lethargy.

     (d) Increased intracranial pressure.

     (e) Tense, bulging anterior fontanelle.

     (f) Cranial sutures separating.

    (2) Slow chronic dilatation.

     (a) Relatively asymptomatic.

     (b) As progression occurs, the above signs may become evident.

  d. Diagnostic studies.

    (1) Graph of weekly OFC measurements.

    (2) CT scan.

    (3) Cranial ultrasound.

e. Patient care management.
(1) Obtain daily OFC measurements.
(2) Perform serial cranial ultrasound.
(3) Request a neurosurgical consult.
(4) Perform serial lumbar taps (accelerate removal of protein and blood in CSF) (Kreusser et al., 1985).
(5) Prescribe drugs to diminish CSF production rates: furosemide (Lasix) (1 mg/kg/day) and acetazolamide (Diamox) (up to 100 mg/kg/day) (Kovnar and Volpe, 1982b).
(6) Consider an osmotic agent: glycerol, starting with 1 g/kg PO every 6 hours and slowly increasing over a week to 2 g/kg every 6 hours (Kovnar and Volpe, 1982b). Kovnar and Volpe (1982b) suggested when utilizing any of these drug agents to monitor BUN and electrolytes. They also suggested monitoring serum glucose when prescribing glycerol.
(7) Consider placing a reservoir or VP shunt.
(8) Observe for signs of increasing intracranial hemorrhage and hydrocephalus.
(9) Support the family.
(10) Maintain open communication among all team members and the family.
5. Outcome.
a. Poor outcomes are likely when cerebral decompression does not occur following VP shunt placement (Shankaran et al., 1989).
b. Initial IVH severity is the major determining factor in PHH development.
c. Hydrocephalus partially or completely resolves in 50% of the cases (Volpe, 1987).
d. Hydrocephalus progresses in 50% of the cases (Volpe, 1987).

D. **Myelomeningocele.**
1. Definition.
a. A neural tube defect.
(1) Spina bifida occulta involves vertebral bone.
(2) Invisible (may be found if problems develop in the infant in childhood).
(3) Meningocele is the protrusion of the meninges lying directly under the skin.
(4) Myelocele has the internal surface of the spinal cord and/or nerve roots exposed.
b. Myelomeningocele involves the spinal cord and meninges exposed through the skin into the surface of the back.
c. Myeloschisis involves large areas of spinal cord without dermal or vertebral covering.
2. Pathophysiology.
a. Results from an error of dorsal induction.
b. 80% of cases occur in the lumbar region (the last region of the neural tube to close).
c. Environmental factors, maternal nutrition, genetics, and teratogens, including maternal hyperthermia, are implicated (Fenichel, 1985).
3. Incidence.
a. Varies between 1 and 5:1000 live births, depending on geographical location (Volpe, 1987).
b. Females are affected more often than males (Windham and Edmonds, 1982).
4. Clinical presentation.
a. Myelomeningocele occurs most often (Volpe, 1987).
b. The majority of cases occur in the thoracolumbar, lumbar, and lumbosacral regions (Windham and Edmonds, 1982).
c. A herniated sac, sealed or leaking, protrudes from the back.

    d. Defects include vascular networks surrounding abnormal neural tissue.

    e. Most lesions have incomplete skin coverage.

5. Associated disease states.

    a. Hydrocephalus.

      (1) With OFC > 90th percentile, 95% of infants will have hydrocephalus (Stark, 1971).

      (2) With OFC < 90th percentile, 65% chance of development of hydrocephalus (Stark, 1971).

      (3) With OFC within normal limits, infant may still develop hydrocephalus (Stark, 1971).

    b. Arnold-Chiari malformation.

      (1) Developmental disturbance during neural tube closure (dorsal induction).

      (2) Almost always present with myelomeningocele (Noetzel, 1989).

      (3) 95% of affected infants develop hydrocephalus secondary to obstruction of CSF outflow (Avery, 1987).

      (4) Common features (Noetzel, 1989).

        (a) Reflux and aspiration.

        (b) Laryngeal stridor.

        (c) Central hypoventilation, apnea.

      (5) Patient care management.

        (a) Pre-natal diagnosis helpful.

        (b) Examine lesion and measure size.

        (c) Culture lesion if sac open.

        (d) Wrap the lesion with sterile gauze moistened with warm sterile saline; place a sterile feeding tube within the gauze mesh for intermittent infusion of warm saline.

        (e) Maintain the infant in a prone kneeling position, and protect the knees from skin breakdown.

        (f) Place a drape over the buttocks below the lesion; utilize the drape's adhesive backing to secure the drape to the body (Shaw, 1990).

        (g) Obtain immediate consultation.

          i. Neurosurgery.

          ii. Urology.

      (6) Perform a thorough physical examination to assess the level of the injury, sensory involvement, and anal wink; include an OFC.

      (7) Encourage an open discussion among the family, the consultants, and the primary care team providing the following:

        (a) Underlying physiology.

        (b) Physical examination findings.

        (c) Consultant reports.

        (d) Prognosis.

        (e) Complications.

        (f) Long-term care.

        (g) Options.

      (8) Begin preparing the family for discharge.

        (a) Suggest that the parents contact a support group.

        (b) Involve parents in their infant's care.

      (9) Postoperatively, follow positioning instructions from the neurosurgeon.

      (10) Spend time making eye contact with the infant.

      (11) Watch for signs of hydrocephalus (refer to Hydrocephalus).

      (12) Watch for development of Arnold-Chiari malformation that may present with feeding problems (reflux, aspiration), laryngeal stridor (due to vocal cord paralysis), or central hypoventilation and/or apnea (Cotten, 1984).

      (13) Maintain meticulous hygiene by clearing stool and urine quickly.

      (14) Provide adequate nutrition.

(15) Orthopedic consult appropriate to maximize function of lower extremities.

(16) Physical therapy maximizes range of motion.

6. Outcome.
   a. Incidence of significant mental retardation is less than 20% in children who reach the second decade (Cotten, 1984).
   b. 10% of myelomeningocele infants with Arnold-Chiari malformation will exhibit stridor and a weak suck (Stark, 1971; Cotten, 1984).
   c. Good outlook with meningocele because of normal spinal cord.
   d. Varying degrees of paralysis (commonly the lower extremities).
      (1) Lesions below S-1: infants can learn to walk unaided (Volpe, 1987).
      (2) Lesions between L-4 and L-5: infants may be able to walk with crutches or braces (Volpe, 1987).
      (3) Lesions above L-2: infants usually end up wheelchair dependent (Volpe, 1987).

E. **Encephalocele.**
1. Definition.
   a. Neural herniation.
   b. May or may not contain meninges or brain parenchyma.
2. Pathophysiology.
   a. Precise pathogenesis is unknown (Volpe, 1987).
   b. Occurs in the dorsal induction stage before 28 days' gestation.
   c. 75% occur in the occipital region (Avery, 1987).
3. Precipitating factors.
   a. Environmental and genetic factors.
   b. May be multifactorial.
4. Incidence.
   a. Occurs in females more often than in males (Menkes, 1984a).
   b. 1:10,000 live births (Fenichel, 1985).
5. Clinical presentation.
   a. Protruding midline skin-covered sac from the head or base of neck.
   b. Majority occur in the occipital region.
6. Diagnostic studies.
   a. Cranial ultrasound.
   b. CT scan.
7. Patient care management.
   a. Examine the infant closely.
   b. Obtain a neurosurgical consult.
   c. Educate and support the family.
   d. Treat seizure activity.
8. Outcome.
   a. Early surgery recommended.
   b. Prognosis based on brain involvement.
   c. Possible motor deficits.
   d. Possible impaired intellectual function.
   e. May be complicated by hydrocephalus.

Craniosynostosis

A. **Definition.**
1. Premature closure of cranial sutures.
2. Occurs along one or more suture lines (see Fig. 20–3 for names and placement of cranial sutures).

B. **Pathophysiology.**
1. Etiology unclear.

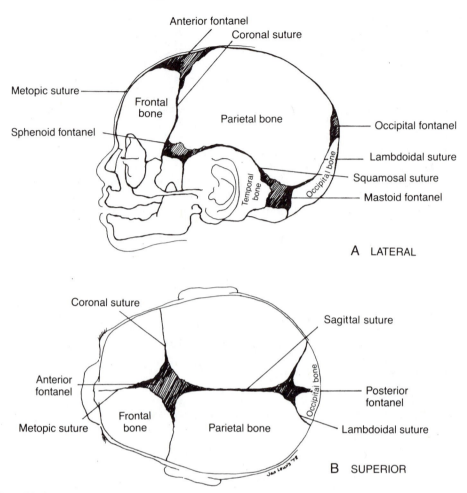

Figure 20-3
A and *B*, Two views of the neonatal skull showing clinically important fontanelles and sutures. (Reprinted with permission from Scanlon, J.W., Nelson, T., Grylack, L.J., and Smith, Y.F.: A System of Newborn Physical Examinations. Baltimore, University Park Press, 1979, p. 47.)

2. Hypothesized that the craniosynostosis results from lack of normal brain growth (Menkes, 1984a).
3. May be secondary to metabolic disorders such as idiopathic hypercalcemia (Menkes, 1984a).

C. **Incidence.**
1. 0.4–1:1000 births.
2. Sagittal craniosynostosis most common (Laurent and Check, 1989).

D. **Clinical presentation.**
1. Cranial suture line reveals bony prominence; even and smooth bilaterally.
2. Inability to move the suture.
3. Abnormal cranial shape.
4. Later signs.
    a. Increased intracranial pressure.
    b. Increased irritability.
    c. Separation of other sutures can occur.

E. **Diagnostic studies.**
1. Skull x-rays.
2. CT scan.
3. Graph OFCs weekly.

F. Patient care management.
1. Thorough physical examination.
2. Obtain neurosurgical consult.
3. Educate and support the family.
4. Watch for signs of increased intracranial pressure.
   a. Irritability.
   b. Lethargy.
   c. Vomiting.
   d. Bulging fontanelle.
5. Early surgical treatment recommended (Laurent and Check, 1989).

G. Outcome.
1. Surgically correctable.
2. Good outcome; possible absence of sequelae.
3. Cosmetically pleasing outcome.

Birth Injuries

A. Definition.
1. Most widely used definition of brain injury:
   a. Any condition that affects the fetus adversely during the entire phase of labor and delivery (Volpe, 1987).

B. Etiology.
1. Abnormal labor time (long or short).
2. Large for gestational age infants.
3. Cephalopelvic disproportion.
4. Prematurity.
5. Birth dystocia.
6. Abnormal presentation (transverse, breech, face, and brow).
7. Instrument-assisted extraction (vacuum or forceps).

C. Incidence.
1. Unknown.

D. Disease states.
1. Cephalohematoma.
   a. Pathophysiology.
      (1) Subperiosteal hemorrhage.
      (2) Does not extend across the cranial suture lines.
      (3) Usually unilateral.
   b. Incidence.
      (1) 1.5–2.5% of deliveries (Menkes, 1984b).
   c. Clinical manifestations.
      (1) Enlarges the first few days after birth.
      (2) Feels firm.
      (3) Does not transilluminate.
      (4) 5–24% of affected infants have x-ray examination revealing linear skull fracture (Korones, 1986).
      (5) No known sequelae (Korones, 1986).
   d. Patient care management.
      (1) Provide supportive care to the family and their baby.
      (2) Watch for hyperbilirubinemia.
      (3) If sudden enlargement occurs, question infection.
      (4) Educate the family.
      (5) Assess neurological status.
   e. Outcome.
      (1) May develop a bony calcified ring that disappears within 6 months.

        (2) Otherwise, usually takes 2 weeks to 3 months for resolution (Hernandez, 1984).

  2. Caput succedaneum.

    a. Pathophysiology.

      (1) Hemorrhagic edema crossing cranial suture lines.

      (2) Commonly seen following vaginal delivery.

    b. Clinical manifestation.

      (1) Evident at birth.

      (2) Hemorrhagic scalp edema causing discoloration at the site.

      (3) Does not grow in size after birth.

    c. Patient care management.

      (1) No treatment.

      (2) Educate and counsel the family.

    d. Outcome.

      (1) Resolution occurs over first few days of life.

  3. Subgaleal hemorrhage.

    a. Pathophysiology.

      (1) Hemorrhage beneath the scalp.

      (2) Can enter the subcutaneous tissue of the neck.

      (3) Marked acute blood loss may occur.

    b. Incidence.

      (1) Much less often than that of caput succedaneum.

    c. Clinical presentation.

      (1) Often a fluctuant mass.

      (2) May increase in size postnatally.

    d. Patient care management.

      (1) Close observation required.

        (a) Observe for indications of bleeding.

        (b) Observe for shock.

        (c) Monitor blood pressure.

      (2) May need blood transfusion emergently.

      (3) Observe for hyperbilirubinemia.

    e. Outcome.

      (1) Once the infant has survived the acute phase, recovery occurs in 2–3 weeks (Volpe, 1987).

  4. Skull fractures.

    a. Pathophysiology.

      (1) Linear fracture can occur.

      (2) Depressed fractures occur secondary to excessive force with forceps and extreme molding (Fenichel, 1985).

    b. Incidence.

      (1) Unknown.

      (2) Linear fracture fairly common finding.

      (3) Depressed fracture much less common than the linear.

    c. Clinical presentation.

      (1) Linear fracture is asymptomatic.

      (2) Depressed fracture.

        (a) Presents with a depressed surface of skull, indented without craniotabes.

        (b) Does not cross the suture lines.

        (c) Adjacent sutures can be markedly separated.

    d. Diagnostic studies.

      (1) X-rays.

      (2) CT scan.

    e. Patient care management.

      (1) Obtain a neurosurgical consult.

      (2) Assess closely for neurological deficits.

(3) If lesion is less than 2 cm and patient is without neurological deficits, follow clinically; spontaneous resolution expected within a few weeks.
  f. Outcome.
    (1) Linear fracture outcome is good.
    (2) Depressed fracture outcome is dependent on cerebral injury and therapy.
5. Brachial nerve plexus injuries.
  a. Pathophysiology.
    (1) Excessive stretching of brachial plexus during delivery.
    (2) Duchenne-Erb paralysis involving cervical nerves 5 and 6 (upper arm paralysis).
    (3) Klumpke's paralysis involving cervical nerve 8 to thoracic nerve 1 (lower arm paralysis).
    (4) Combination of Duchenne-Erb and Klumpke's paralysis involving the entire arm from cervical nerve 5 to thoracic nerve 1 (entire arm paralysis).
  b. Incidence.
    (1) About 4:1000 live births (Molnar, 1984).
  c. Clinical presentation.
    (1) Duchenne-Erb palsy.
      (a) Affected arm is abducted and internally rotated.
      (b) The elbow is extended with arm pronation and wrist flexion (waiter's tip position).
      (c) Asymmetrical Moro's reflex (absent in the affected arm) with a normal grasp.
    (2) Klumpke's paralysis.
      (a) Extremely rare.
      (b) Involves intrinsic muscles of the hand.
      (c) No grasp in the affected hand.
    (3) Entire arm paralysis.
      (a) A combination of the above.
      (b) Occurs more often than isolated Klumpke's paralysis.
      (c) Entire affected arm is flaccid.
      (d) Moro and grasp reflexes absent.
  d. Diagnostic studies.
    (1) X-ray of affected arm and shoulder.
    (2) Serial electromyographic (EMG) studies.
    (3) Rule out fracture of the clavicle or humerus.
    (4) Rule out shoulder dislocation.
    (5) Rule out cerebral injury.
    (6) Rule out bone or soft tissue impairment of the affected shoulder or upper arm (Coulter, 1980).
  e. Patient care management.
    (1) No treatment (Smith, 1989).
    (2) Obtain neurology consult.
      (a) Immobilizing the affected arm may comfort the infant.
    (3) Obtain serial EMG examinations to note improvements.
    (4) Begin passive range of motion, beginning after the swelling and inflammation subsides (Molnar, 1984).
    (5) Exercise the arm with every diaper change.
    (6) Request a physical therapy consult (infant may be able to benefit from splints at some point).
    (7) Educate and support the entire family.
  f. Outcome.
    (1) Generally spontaneous recovery results (Smith, 1989).
      (a) Definite improvement within 1–2 weeks is probably a sign that full recovery is ahead.

> (b) Lack of improvement by 6 months suggests permanent damage.
> (c) Majority resolve the first 3–4 months of life.
>> (2) Mild Erb's palsy.
>>> (a) May only last 1 day.
>>> (b) Majority resolve over the first 3 weeks after birth (Hernandez, 1984).

6. Phrenic nerve paralysis.
   a. Pathophysiology.
      (1) Diaphragmatic paralysis involving cervical nerves 3, 4, and 5.
      (2) Results from torn nerve sheaths with edema and hemorrhage.
   b. Clinical presentation.
      (1) Varies, depending on severity.
      (2) Episodes of cyanosis.
      (3) Breath sounds decreased on the affected side.
      (4) Irregular labored breathing.
      (5) Usually unilateral.
      (6) May be associated with an Erb's palsy on the same side.
   c. Diagnostic studies.
      (1) Chest x-ray.
      (2) Fluoroscopy.
      (3) Ultrasound (especially for serial evaluation).
   d. Patient care management.
      (1) Administer oxygen and ventilatory support as needed.
      (2) Place the infant affected side down (splint the affected side).
      (3) Follow physical examination closely to note improvements.
      (4) Counsel and teach the family.

7. Traumatic nerve palsy.
   a. Pathophysiology.
      (1) Trauma causes hemorrhage and edema into the nerve sheath rather than a true disruption of the nerve fiber (Volpe, 1987).
      (2) Weakness of the facial muscles results.
   b. Incidence.
      (1) 0.3 : 1000 live births (Fenichel, 1985).
   c. Clinical manifestations.
      (1) Varies with the degree of nerve involvement.
      (2) Usually presents the first two days after birth.
      (3) Persistently open eye on the affected side.
      (4) Suck with drooling.
      (5) Mouth is drawn to the normal side when baby is crying.
      (6) The corner of the mouth does not pull down on the affected side.
      (7) The eyeball may roll up behind the open eyelid.
   d. Patient care management.
      (1) Artificial tears for the open eye.
      (2) Support parents.
      (3) Watch for signs of improvement.
   e. Outcome.
      (1) High rate of spontaneous recovery by 7–10 days, especially between 1 and 3 weeks.
      (2) Detectable deficits are rarely evident after several months.

Intracranial Hemorrhages

A. Subdural hemorrhage.
1. Definition.
   a. Tears of cerebral veins (most common).
   b. Tears of venous sinuses.
   c. Occurs with or without laceration of the dura.

2. Etiology.
   a. A large fetal head compared with the size of the birth canal, rigid pelvic structures (Volpe, 1987).
   b. Abnormal labor duration (Volpe, 1987).
   c. Vaginal breech delivery (Volpe, 1987).
   d. Malpresentation (breech, face, brown, foot) (Volpe, 1987).
   e. Difficult instrument-assisted delivery (Volpe, 1987).
3. Incidence.
   a. Uncommon occurrence.
   b. Usually affects term infants.
4. Clinical presentation.
   a. Often normal.
   b. Seizure activity may occur on day 2 or 3 of life with focal third cranial nerve malfunction on the side of the hemorrhage (see Table 20–3 for review of cranial nerves).
   3. More severe cases: lethargy may progress to coma.
   d. Dilated, poorly reactive pupil on the same side as the hemorrhage.
   e. Doll's eye maneuver normal to abnormal.
5. Diagnostic studies.
   a. CT scan.
6. Outcome.
   a. If tear or rupture is large, outlook is poor.
   b. If condition worsens, outlook is poor.
   c. Hydrocephalus rarely develops.
   d. High percentage of infants do well.

B. **Subarachnoid hemorrhage (primary).**
1. Pathophysiology.
   a. Bleeding of venous origin in the subarachnoid space.
   b. May be precipitated by prematurity, trauma, hypoxia (Volpe, 1987).
2. Incidence.
   a. The most common of the neonatal intracranial hemorrhages (Volpe, 1987).
3. Clinical presentation.
   a. Ranges from normal to seizure activity beginning on day 2 of life.
   b. Infant looks healthy between seizures.
   c. Recurrent apnea (more common in pre-term infants) (Kovnar and Volpe, 1982b).
   d. Hydrocephalus may occur.
4. Diagnostic studies.
   a. CT scan.
5. Outcome.
   a. Good.
   b. Sequelae very uncommon (Kovnar and Volpe, 1982b).

C. **Intracerebellar hemorrhage.**
1. Pathophysiology.
   a. Subpial and subependymal locations.
   b. Results from primary bleed or extension of hemorrhage into the cerebellum.
   c. An association exists with respiratory distress, perinatal asphyxia, and prematurity.
   d. Three factors of greatest significance (Volpe, 1987):
      (1) Large volume of blood present with IVH.
      (2) Increased intracranial pressure.
      (3) Incomplete myelination of the cerebellum.
2. Incidence.
   a. 5–10% of autopsied neonatal deaths (Volpe, 1987).
   b. Higher in pre-term infants than in term.
3. Clinical presentation.
   a. Apnea.

    b. Bradycardia.

    c. Decreasing hematocrit and bloody CSF.

 4. Diagnostic studies.

    a. Cranial ultrasound (lack of symmetrical echogenicity may be important) (Volpe, 1987).

    b. CT scan.

    c. Autopsy.

D. **Periventricular-intraventricular hemorrhages.**

1. Pathophysiology.

    a. Prematurity <34 weeks' gestation.

    b. Associated with increasing arterial blood pressure and perinatal asphyxia (Goddard-Finegold, 1986).

    c. Associated clinical factors (Carey, 1983).

        (1) Prematurity.

        (2) Maternal general anesthesia (probably due to the indication for the anesthesia rather than the anesthesia itself) (Bada et al., 1990.

        (3) Low 5 minute Apgar score.

        (4) Asphyxia.

        (5) Low birthweight (Bada et al., 1990).

        (6) Acidosis.

        (7) Hypotension and hypertension.

        (8) Low hematocrit (Bada et al., 1990).

        (9) Respiratory distress requiring mechanical ventilation.

      (10) Rapid sodium bicarbonate administration.

      (11) Rapid volume expansion.

      (12) Infusion of hyperosmolar solution.

      (13) Coagulopathy.

      (14) Pneumothorax.

      (15) Patent ductus arteriosus ligation.

    d. See Figure 20–4 for description and grading system.

2. Incidence.

    a. 32–44% of infants with birthweight less than 1500 grams (Shinnar et al., 1982).

    b. 20–30% occur during the first hours of life (Bada et al., 1990).

    c. 50% occur on the first day of life (Volpe, 1987).

    d. The majority occur during the first 72 hours of life.

    e. Significant predictive variables for developing severe periventricular-intraventricular hemorrhage.

        (1) Low birthweight.

        (2) Low 5 minute Apgar score.

3. Clinical presentation.

    a. Presentation ranges from unnoticeable to dramatic.

        (1) Sudden deterioration.

        (2) Oxygen desaturation.

        (3) Bradycardia.

        (4) Metabolic acidosis.

        (5) Hematocrit significantly decreases.

        (6) Hypotonia.

        (7) Shock.

        (8) Hyperglycemia.

        (9) Tense anterior fontanelle.

    b. Symptomatology of worsening bleed.

        (1) Full, tense fontanelles.

        (2) Increased ventilatory support.

        (3) Seizures.

        (4) Apnea.

        (5) Decrease in level of consciousness and/or activity.

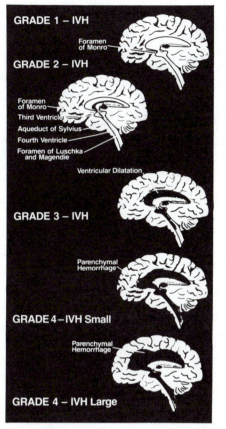

GRADE 1 – IVH

Foramen of Monro

GRADE 2 – IVH

Foramen of Monro
Third Ventricle
Aqueduct of Sylvius
Fourth Ventricle
Foramen of Luschka and Magendie

Ventricular Dilatation

GRADE 3 – IVH

Parenchymal Hemorrhage

GRADE 4 – IVH Small

Parenchymal Hemorrhage

GRADE 4 – IVH Large

Grade I IVH: Subependymal hemorrhage in the Periventricular Germinal Matrix. Often localized at the Foramen of Monro.

Grade 2 IVH: Partial filling of lateral ventricles without ventricular dilatation.

Grade 3 IVH: Intraventricular hemorrhage with ventricular dilatation.

Grade 4 IVH (small and large): Parenchymal involvement or extension of blood into the cerebral tissue itself. Can be present to a lesser degree.

Correlation between the severity or extent of involvement and subsequent impairment is not absolute. Because outcomes are so varied, assessment of early symptoms and the practice of purposeful interventions are extremely important.

Figure 20–4
Quantifying the extent of intraventricular hemorrhage (IVH). Four grades of hemorrhagic involvement categorized IVH as differentiated by Papile and Burstein. (Used and reprinted with permission of Ross Laboratories, Columbus, OH 43216, from *New Perspectives on Intraventricular Hemorrhage*. © 1988, Ross Laboratories.)

4. Diagnostic studies.
   a. Cranial ultrasound
   b. CT scan.
   c. Lumbar puncture (CSF studies show elevated red blood cells, increased protein concentration, xanthochromia, and decreased glucose concentration) (Kovnar and Volpe, 1982b).
   d. Rule out septic shock or meningitis.
5. Outcome.
   a. Morbidity and mortality have decreased secondary to decreased incidence as well as severity (Shinnar et al., 1982; Enzmann, 1989).
   b. An important cause of low birthweight morbidity and mortality (Kosmetatos et al., 1980).
   c. Hemorrhage alone does not account for all the neurological deficits.
   d. Conditions involving infarction, porencephaly (the ventricles of the brain and the subarachnoid space are connected by a small opening), and parenchymal damage most closely account for neurological deficits (Enzmann, 1989).
   e. Approximately 20–40% exhibit progression of hemorrhage (Volpe, 1987).
   f. Predictive prognosis can be based on the grade of the hemorrhage, the placement of the hemorrhage, and the underlying etiology.
6. Patient care management.
   a. Prevent pre-term births, perinatal asphyxia, and birth trauma.
   b. Promote in utero transports.

   c. Promote a non-stressful intrapartum course.
   d. Provide efficient, expedient intubation.
   e. Minimize handling; cluster scheduled patient cares.
   f. Avoid noxious procedures when possible.
   g. Avoid events associated with abrupt hypertension.
      (1) Seizures.
      (2) Excess motor activity.
   h. Avoid administration of hyperosmolar solutions.
   i. Prevent blood pressure swings: give volume replacement slowly.
   j. Avoid overventilation leading to pneumothorax.
   k. Use two people for endotracheal suctioning.
   l. Monitor Po_2 and Pco_2 with transcutaneous monitoring (maintain within normal limits).
   m. Correct abnormal clotting.
   n. Be alert to signs of a bleed.
   o. Educate and support the parents.

Seizures

A. Definition.
1. A seizure is a symptom of a neurological dysfunction (not a disease).
B. Pathophysiology.
1. Seizures result from excessive simultaneous electrical discharge or depolarization of neurons.
2. Metabolic encephalopathies.
   a. Decreased adenosine triphosphate (ATP) production.
      (1) Ischemia.
      (2) Hypoxemia.
      (3) Hypoglycemia.
   b. Hypo- or hypernatremia.
   c. Hypocalcemia, hypomagnesemia.
   d. Inborn errors of metabolism.
   e. Pyridoxine dependency.
   f. Hyperammonemia.
3. Structural.
   a. Intraventricular hemorrhage (IVH).
   b. Intrapartum trauma.
   c. Cerebral cortical dysgenesis.
      (1) Secondary to abnormal neuronal migration.
   d. Hypoxic-ischemic encephalopathy.
4. Intracerebral meningitis.
   a. Bacterial infection.
      (1) Group B beta-streptococci and *Escherichia coli* account for 65% of the cases (Avery, 1987).
      (2) *Listeria monocytogenes.*
   b. Non-bacterial infection.
      (1) TORCH.
5. Withdrawal from maternal drugs.
   a. Uncommon cause of seizures.
   b. Onset occurs during first 3 days of life.
   c. Drugs.
      (1) Narcotic-analgesics.
      (2) Sedative-hypnotics.
      (3) Alcohol.
6. Familial (genetic).
   a. Onset second and third days of life.

  b. Infant appears well between seizures.
  c. Self-limiting (within 1–6 months, seizures stop).
  d. Autosomal dominant inheritance.

C. Clinical presentations.
1. Subtle.
  a. Most frequent of neonatal seizures.
  b. Often unrecognized.
  c. Presentation varies.
    (1) Tonic.
    (2) Horizontal deviation of the eyes.
    (3) Pedalling movements.
    (4) Swimming movements.
    (5) Eye blinking or fluttering.
    (6) Non-nutritive sucking.
    (7) Smacking lips.
    (8) Drooling.
    (9) Apnea (convulsive apnea usually does not occur by itself).
2. Tonic.
  a. Characteristic in premature infants weighing < 2500 g.
  b. Often seen with severe IVH.
  c. Generalized tonic extension of all extremities or flexion of upper limbs with extension of lower extremities.
  d. Often mimics decorticate posturing.
3. Multifocal clonic.
  a. Characteristic in full-term infants with hypoxic-ischemic encephalopathy (Avery, 1987).
  b. Clonic movements migrating from one limb to another without a specific pattern.
4. Focal clonic.
  a. Uncommon.
  b. Presents as localized clonic jerking.
5. Myoclonic.
  a. Very rare in the neonatal period.
  b. Multiple jerks of upper or lower limb flexion.

D. Diagnostic studies.
1. Perform physical examination.
  a. Rule out jitteriness.
    (1) Characterized by trembling of hands and feet.
    (2) Does not involve eye movements.
    (3) Stopped by gentle passive flexion of the affected extremity.
  b. Note infant's history, which may provide a predisposed underlying etiology.
2. Lab work.
  a. Check serum glucose level.
  b. Electrolyte levels (sodium, potassium, chloride, calcium, magnesium).
  c. Arterial blood gas analysis.
3. Perform septic work-up.
  a. Lumbar puncture.
  b. Culture blood, urine, and CSF; bacterial and viral.
  c. Complete blood count and platelet count.
4. Electroencephalogram, CT scan, cranial ultrasound.
5. Obtain skull films if etiology is trauma (Torrence, 1985).
6. Request 12 lead EKG (Torrence, 1985).
7. Possibly test hepatic function.
  a. ALT and AST.
  b. Serum ammonia.
8. Obtain neurological consultation.

E. **Patient care management.**

1. Determine underlying etiology.
2. Resuscitate as necessary.
3. Obtain diagnostic studies as ordered.
4. Provide pharmacological therapy (Young and Mangum, 1990).
   a. Phenobarbital.
      (1) Load 20 mg/kg slow IV over 15–20 minutes.
      (2) Maintenance.
         (a) 3–5 mg/kg/day every 12 hours after the loading dose.
      (3) Therapeutic range 15–30 μg/ml.
      (4) Excretion.
         (a) 70% metabolized by liver.
         (b) 30% unchanged in urine.
   b. Phenytoin.
      (1) Load 15–20 mg/kg IV (over 30 minutes or longer).
      (2) Maintenance.
         (a) 4–8 mg/kg/day.
         (b) Recommended administration routes.
            (i) IV slow push.
            (ii) By mouth.
      (3) Therapeutic range.
         (a) 6–15 μg/ml.
         (b) 10–20 μg/ml.
      (4) Excretion.
         (a) Protein bound (90%).
         (b) Displaced by bilirubin.
   c. Lorazepam.
      (1) 0.05–0.1 mg/kg slow push IV.
      (2) Repeated based on clinical response.
      (3) Excretion.
         (a) By kidneys.
         (b) Lipid soluble.
5. Monitor oxygenation and vital signs.
6. Document precisely.
7. Educate and inform the family.
8. Provide support as needed.

F. **Outcome.**

1. Related to underlying etiology.
2. Refer to Table 20–4.

Table 20–4
PROGNOSIS OF NEONATAL SEIZURES—RELATION TO NEUROLOGICAL DISEASE

Neurological Disease*	Normal Development (%)
Hypoxic-ischemic encephalopathy	50
Intraventricular hemorrhage	<10
Primary subarachnoid hemorrhage	90
Hypocalcemia	
Early onset	50
Later onset	100
Hypoglycemia	50
Bacterial meningitis	50
Developmental defect	0

*Prognosis is for those cases with the stated neurological disease when seizures are a manifestation (thus, value usually will differ from *overall* prognosis for the disease).

From Volpe, J.J.: Neurology of the Newborn, 2nd ed. Philadelphia, W.B. Saunders Co., 1987.

Hypoxic-Ischemic Encephalopathy (HIE)

A. **Definition.**
1. Term infant with a history of perinatal asphyxia who exhibits clinical signs of acute brain injury (Papile, 1987).
2. Multisystem disease (Papile, 1990).

B. **Pathophysiology.**
1. Asphyxia.
   a. Hypoxemia and ischemia follow.
   b. Cardiac output is redistributed, cerebral blood flow is increased, and autoregulation is impaired or lost (Kovnar and Volpe, 1982a).
   c. Asphyxial state is prolonged, cardiac output is decreased, and autoregulation is lost, causing cerebral blood flow to fall, resulting in neurological impairment (Pearlman, 1989).
   d. Total acute asphyxia.
      (1) Abruptio placentae.
      (2) Complete cord compression.
   e. Partial asphyxia (Brann, 1986).

C. **Incidence.**
1. Unknown.
2. 0.5–4% of term infants (Papile, 1987).
3. Timing of occurrence (Hill and Volpe, 1989a).
   a. 20% antepartum.
   b. 30% intrapartum.
   c. 35% antepartum and intrapartum.
   d. 10% post-partum.

D. **Clinical presentation (Fenichel, 1985).**
1. Mild encephalopathy.
   a. Maximum presentation of symptoms occurs in the first 24 hours post-partum.
   b. Improvement to normal by 1 week of age.
   c. Characteristic features.
      (1) Brief lethargy.
      (2) Jitteriness.
      (3) Hyperalert state.
      (4) Irritability.
      (5) Hyper-responsiveness to stimulation.
      (6) Tachycardia.
      (7) Dilatation of pupils.
      (8) Decreased secretions.
      (9) Transient hypoglycemia.
      (10) No convulsions (unless due to hypoglycemia or pre-existing conditions that predisposed the infant to the perinatal distress).
      (11) EEG is within normal limits.
2. Moderate encephalopathy.
   a. The first 12 hours post-partum.
      (1) Lethargy.
      (2) Hypotonia.
      (3) Decreased spontaneous movement.
      (4) Jitteriness.
      (5) Discrepant muscle strength between the shoulder and pelvic regions.
   b. Critical period.
      (1) 48–72 hours post-partum.
      (2) The infant either improves or deteriorates.
   c. Deterioration indicated by:
      (1) No signs of improvement.

(2) Development of:
    (a) Seizures.
    (b) Cerebral edema.
    (c) Lethargy.
    (d) Abnormal EEG.
  d. Recovery.
    (1) No further seizure activity.
    (2) EEG returns to normal.
    (3) Transient jitteriness.
    (4) Improving level of consciousness.
3. Severe encephalopathy.
  a. Post-partum course.
    (1) Level of consciousness deteriorates from obtunded to stupor to comatose.
    (2) Mechanical ventilation required to sustain life.
  b. Symptoms.
    (1) Apnea.
    (2) Seizures appearing within the first 12 post-natal hours.
    (3) Tonic and multifocal clonic seizures within the first day of life.
    (4) Severe hypotonia.
    (5) Absent reflexes.
    (6) Doll's eye movements present.
    (7) Reactive pupils.
  c. Deterioration.
    (1) 24–72 hours.
    (2) Pupils become unreactive.
    (3) Seizures increase in severity and frequency.
    (4) Cerebral edema.
    (5) EEG shows burst-suppression pattern.
    (6) Death may ensue.
  d. Survivors.
    (1) Remain stuporous.
    (2) Severe neurological handicaps.

E. **Diagnostic studies.**
1. Precise detailed history.
2. Complete neurological examination.
3. Lumbar puncture.
4. Electroencephalogram (EEG).
5. Brainstem auditory evoked response (BAER).
6. Creatinine kinase.
7. CT scan.
8. Cranial ultrasound.
9. Radionuclide brain scan.

F. **Patient care management.**
1. Prevent perinatal asphyxia.
2. Perform prompt, efficient resuscitation by trained staff.
3. Maintain sufficient oxygenation, normal Pco_2 and pH.
4. Maintain normal metabolic state.
  a. Glucose.
  b. Calcium.
  c. Sodium.
5. Monitor blood pressure; avoid blood pressure swings.
6. Maintain adequate perfusion.
7. Replace volume slowly.
8. Restrict fluid.
9. Treat seizures.
10. Perform a thorough neurological examination.

11. Monitor and manage disturbances of other body organs.
    a. Pulmonary.
    b. Cardiac.
    c. Hepatic.
    d. Renal.
12. Raise the head of the bed up 30 degrees (Fenichel, 1985).
13. Educate and support the family.
14. Obtain neurological consultation.
15. Document appropriately.

G. **Outcome.**
1. Important cause of death (Hans, 1980).
2. Single most important predisposing factor in the newborn with neurological deficits (Percy, 1986).
3. Selective neuronal necrosis (Volpe, 1987).
4. 20% (term infants) develop severe neurological disorders (Papile, 1987).
5. Factors associated with poor outcome.
   a. Seizures for > 48 hours post-partum.
   b. CT scan revealing diffuse hypodensity.
   c. Abnormal radionuclide brain scan at 3 weeks post-natal life.
6. Seizures early and/or difficult to control are associated with poorer prognosis (Hill and Volpe, 1989a).
7. High mortality rates with severe encephalopathy (Svenningsen et al., 1982).
8. Hyperactivity and attention difficulties seen in infants with less severe encephalopathy (Kovnar and Volpe, 1982a).
9. Rapid initial improvement indicative of better outcomes (Volpe, 1987).
10. Long-term sequelae based on:
    a. Site.
    b. Extent of the cerebral injury (Kovnar and Volpe, 1982a).

Periventricular Leukomalacia (PVL)

A. **Definition.**
1. Ischemic-necrotic periventricular white matter.
2. Mild cases.
   a. Small areas with ventricular dilatation (Volpe, 1987).
3. Severe cases.
   a. Multicystic encephalomalacia (Volpe, 1987).

B. **Pathophysiology.**
1. Predisposition.
   a. Loss of cerebral autoregulation.
   b. Periventricular regions where vasodilatation capacity is lacking in the pre-term infant's brain.
2. Occurs secondary to inadequate cerebral perfusion.
3. Manifestation of hypoxic-ischemic encephalopathy in preemies.

C. **Incidence.**
1. 80–90% of PVL occurs in premature infants (Hill and Volpe, 1989b).
2. Increased incidence is associated with increased length of patient stay.

D. **Clinical presentation.**
1. Weakness of lower extremities (Volpe, 1987).

E. **Diagnostic studies.**
1. Autopsy.
2. Cranial ultrasound (Enzmann, 1989).

F. **Outcome.**
1. Spastic quadriplegia.
2. Visual impairment.

3. Lower limb weakness.
4. Based on:
   a. Location.
   b. Severity (Hill and Volpe, 1989b).

Meningitis

A. Definition.
1. Infection of the central nervous system.
2. Early-onset infection from pathogens in vaginal flora (e.g., group B beta-streptococci and *Escherichia coli*).
3. Late-onset infection from environmental microbes found in the nursery environment (e.g., *Pseudomonas aeruginosa* and *Staphylococcus aureus*).

B. Pathophysiology.
1. Organisms reach the fetus.
   a. Transplacental organisms lead to congenital infection.
   b. Ascending organisms from the vagina or cervix lead to early-onset infection.
   c. Infants infected by passing through the birth canal develop late-onset infection.
   d. Organism introduction after birth from the surrounding environment leads to iatrogenic infection.
2. Precipitating factors.
   a. Maternal infection.
   b. Prolonged ruptured membranes.
   c. Prematurity.
3. Organisms.
   a. Bacteria.
      (1) Aerobic.
         (a) Group B beta-streptococci (most common).
         (b) *Escherichia coli* (second most common).
         (c) *Listeria monocytogenes* (third most common).
      (2) Anaerobic.
   b. Viruses.
      (1) TORCH infection.
      (2) Enterovirus.
   c. Fungi.

C. Incidence.
1. Bacterial meningitis.
   a. Occurs 0.3 : 1000 live births (Volpe, 1987).
   b. Accounts for 4% of all neonatal deaths (Fenichel, 1985).

D. Congenital presentation.
1. Congenital viral infection.
   a. Pre-term delivery.
   b. Infant may have low birth-weight.
   c. Blueberry muffin rash.
   d. Inflammation of other affected organs.
   e. Microcephaly.
2. Early-onset bacterial meningitis.
   a. Presents in the first 24 hours with shock.
   b. May progress rapidly to shock.
   c. Respiratory distress.
   d. Hypotension.
   e. Apnea.
   f. Seizures.
   g. Temperature instability.
   h. Diarrhea.

    i. Hepatomegaly.
    j. Jaundice.
3. Late-onset meningitis.
    a. Non-specific symptoms.
    b. Lethargy.
    c. Feeding intolerance.
    d. Irritability.
    e. Posturing.
    f. Temperature instability.
    g. Apnea.
    h. Bradycardia.
    i. Bulging fontanelles.
    j. Nuchal rigidity.

E. **Diagnostic studies.**
1. CSF.
    a. Organism found on Gram's stain.
    b. Low glucose level.
    c. Elevated protein and white blood cell count.
    d. Culture for specific identification.
    e. Counterimmune electrophoresis (CIE).
2. Complete septic work-up.

F. **Patient care management.**
1. Promote prevention.
2. Detect early and treat.
3. Perform through physical examination.
4. Observe for seizure activity.
5. Obtain infectious disease consult.
6. Provide pharmacological agents (Nelson, 1989; Nelson, 1991).
    a. Initial therapy.
        (1) Ampicillin or penicillin G (IV) *and*:
        (2) Aminoglycoside (IV or IM).
        (3) Ampicillin and cefotaxime recommended for aminoglycoside-resistant organism.
    b. Group B beta-streptococcus.
        (1) Ampicillin or penicillin G (IV or IM) *and*:
        (2) Gentamicin (IV or IM) (discontinue if sensitivities warrant).
        (3) Treat for 14 days.
    c. Coliform bacteria (like *Escherichia coli*).
        (1) Aminoglycoside (IM or IV) *and*:
        (2) Ampicillin (IV).
        (3) Treat for 21 days.
    d. *Listeria monocytogenes* and enterococci.
        (1) Ampicillin (IV or IM) *and*:
        (2) Aminoglycoside (IV or IM).
        (3) Treat for 14 days.
    e. *Staphylococcus epidermidis.*
        (1) Vancomycin (IV or IM).
        (2) Treat for 10–14 days (or longer).
    f. *Staphylococcus aureus.*
        (1) Methicillin (IV or IM).
        (2) Treat for 10–14 days.
        (3) If methicillin-resistant strain, use vancomycin.
    g. *Pseudomonas aeruginosa.*
        (1) Mezlocillin or ticarcillin (IV or IM) *and*:
        (2) Aminoglycoside (IV or IM).
        (3) Treat for 10–14 days (or longer).
    h. *Bacteroides fragilis* (anaerobic).

(1) Metronidazole, clindamycin, mezlocillin, or ticarcillin (IV or IM).

(2) Treat for 14–21 days.

(3) For CNS infection, metronidazole recommended.

7. Sample CSF at specific intervals until sterile.

8. Treat at least 2 weeks after sterilization of CSF.

9. Obtain and test CSF sample 48 hours after antibiotic therapy discontinued.

10. Educate and support the family.

G. Outcome.

1. Dependent on rapidity of detection and initiation of adequate drug therapy.

2. 50% of survivors of bacterial meningitis develop significant neurological sequelae (Fenichel, 1985).

a. Hydrocephalus.

b. Seizures.

c. Sensorineural hearing loss.

d. Visual losses.

e. Mental and motor disabilities.

STUDY QUESTIONS

1. A defect arising from abnormal dorsal induction is:
   a. Cyclopia.
   b. Macrocephaly.
   c. Myelomeningocele.

2. Autoregulation is a means of regulating:
   a. Cerebral blood flow.
   b. Ischemia.
   c. Systemic blood pressure.

3. An asymmetrical Moro's reflex can result from all *but*:
   a. Clavicular fracture.
   b. Duchenne-Erb palsy.
   c. Skull fracture.

4. A subperiosteal bleed that does not cross suture lines is:
   a. Caput succedaneum.
   b. Cephalhematoma.
   c. Subgaleal hemorrhage.

5. The brachial nerve plexus injury presenting with an absent grasp is:
   a. Duchenne-Erb palsy.
   b. Klumpke's palsy.
   c. Traumatic nerve palsy.

6. A subependymal germinal matrix hemorrhage with intraventricular blood but no ventricular dilatation is:
   a. Grade I.
   b. Grade II.
   c. Grade III.

7. The incidence of periventricular-intraventricular hemorrhage in infants less than 1500 g:
   a. 30–40%.
   b. 50–60%.
   c. 70–80%.

8. A frequently observed neonatal seizure is:
   a. Multifocal clonic.
   b. Subtle.
   c. Tonic.

9. Periventricular leukomalacia is characterized by:
   a. Germinal matrix hemorrhage.
   b. Intraventricular hemorrhage.
   c. Ischemic-necrotic periventricular white matter.

Answers to Study Questions

1. c	4. b	7. a
2. a	5. b	8. b
3. c	6. b	9. c

REFERENCES

Avery, G.A.: Neonatology: Pathophysiology and Management of the Newborn, 3rd ed. Philadelphia, J.B. Lippincott, 1987.

Bada, H.S., Korones, S.B., Perry, E.H., et al.: Frequent handling in the neonatal intensive care unit and intraventricular hemorrhage. J. Pediatr., 117(1):part 1:126–131, 1990.

Brann, A.W.: Hypoxic-ischemic encephalopathy (asphyxia). Pediatr. Clin. North A., 33(3):451–464, 1986.

Carey, B.E.: Intraventricular hemorrhage in the preterm infant. J. Obstet. Gynecol. Neonat. Nurs., (Supplement) 12(3):60s–67s, 1983.

Cotten, J.M.: A comprehensive nursing approach to the neonate with myelomeningocele. Neonatal Network, 2(4):7–16, 1984.

Coulter, D.M.: Birth trauma. In Cloherty, J.P., and Stark, A.R. (eds.): Manual of Neonatal Care. Boston, Little, Brown, 1980, pp. 251–255.

Enzmann, D.R: Imaging of hypoxic-ischemic cerebral damage. In Stevenson, D.K., and Sunshine, P. (eds.): Fetal and Neonatal Brain injury: Mechanisms, Management and the Risks of Practice. Philadelphia, B.C. Decker, 1989, pp. 196–220.

Erlen, J.A., and Holzman, I.R.: Anencephalic infants: Should they be organ donors? Pediatr. Nurs., 14(1):60–63, 1988.

Fenichel, G.M.: Neonatal Neurology, 2nd ed. New York, Churchill Livingstone, 1985.

Finkel, R.S.: Neurodevelopmental anatomy and physiology. Paper presented at the meeting of neonatal nurse practitioner students, The Children's Hospital, Denver, December 1984.

Goddard-Finegold, J.: Intracranial hemorrhage in the neonate. In Fishman, M.A. (ed.): Pediatric Neurology. Orlando, Grune & Stratton, 1986, pp. 45–56.

Hans, C.L: Perinatal hypoxic-ischemic brain damage and intraventricular hemorrhage. Arch. Neurol., 37:585–587, 1980.

Hernandez, J.A., Birth injuries. Paper presented at the meeting of neonatal nurse practitioner students, The Children's Hospital, Denver, October 1984.

Hill, A., and Volpe, J.J.: Hypoxic-ischemic encephalopathy of the newborn. In Swaiman, K.F. (ed.): Pediatric Neurology: Principles and Practice (Vol. 1). St. Louis, C.V. Mosby, 1989a, pp. 373–392.

Hill, A., and Volpe, J.J.: Perinatal asphyxia: Clinical aspects. Clin. Perinatol., 16(2):435–457, 1989b.

Korones, S. B.: High-risk Newborn Infants: The Basis for Intensive Nursing Care, 4th ed. St. Louis, C.V. Mosby, 1986.

Kosmetatos, N., Dinter, C., Williams, M.L., et al.: Intracranial hemorrhage in the premature. Its predictive features and outcome. Am. J. Dis. Child., 134:855–859, 1980.

Kovnar, E., and Volpe, J.J.: Current concepts in neonatal neurology. Part 1. Hypoxic-ischemic brain injury. Perinatology-Neonatology, 6(4):51–63, 1982a.

Kovnar E., and Volpe, J.J.: Current concepts in neonatal neurology. Part 2. Periventricular-intraventricular hemorrhage. Perinatology-Neonatology, 6(5):81–92, 1982b.

Kreusser, K.L., Tarby, T.J., Kovnar, E., et al.: Serial lumbar punctures for at least temporary amelioration of neonatal posthemorrhagic hydrocephalus. Pediatrics, 75(4):719–723, 1985.

Laurent, J.P., and Check, W.R.: Craniosynostosis. In McLaurin, R.L., Schut, L., Venes, J.L., and Epstein, F. (eds.): Pediatric Neurosurgery: Surgery of the Developing Nervous System, 2nd ed. Philadelphia, W.B. Saunders, 1989, pp. 107–133.

Lou, H.C.: Perinatal hypoxic-ischemic brain damage and intraventricular hemorrhage. Arch. Neurol. 37:585–587, 1980.

Lou, H.C., Lassen, N.A., and Friis-Hansen, B.: Impaired autoregulation of cerebral blood flow in the distressed newborn infant. J. Pediatr., 94:118–121, 1979.

Menkes, J.H.: Malformations of the central nervous system. In Avery, M.E., and Taeusch, H.W., Jr. (eds.): Schaffer's Diseases of the Newborn, 5th ed. Philadelphia, W.B. Saunders Co., 1984a, pp. 680–702.

Menkes, J.H.: Perinatal trauma and asphyxia. In Avery, M.E., and Taeusch, H.W., Jr. (eds.): Schaffer's Diseases of the Newborn, 5th ed. Philadelphia, W.B. Saunders Co., 1984b, pp. 661–679.

Ment, L.R., Duncan, C.C., Scott, D.T., and Ehrenkranz, R.A.: Posthemorrhagic hydrocephalus. J. Neurosurg., 60:343–347, 1984.

Molnar, G.E.: Brachial plexus injury in the newborn infant. Pediatr. Rev., 6(4):110–115, 1984.

Nelson, J.D.: Pocketbook of Pediatric Antimicrobial Therapy, 8th ed. Baltimore, Williams & Wilkins, 1989.

Nelson, J.D.: Pocketbook of Pediatric Antimicrobial Therapy, 9th ed. Baltimore, Williams & Wilkins, 1991.

Noetzel, M.J.: Myelomeningocele: Current concepts of management. Clin. Perinatol., 16(2):311–329, 1989.

Papile, L.: Neonatal brain injury and its assessment. Paper presented at the meeting of The Fetus and Newborn: State of the Art Care, San Diego, September 1987.

Papile, L.: Hypoxic/ischemic encephalopathy: Diagnosis and management. Paper presented at the meeting of the National Association of Neonatal Nurses, Phoenix, September, 1990.

Pearlman, J.M.: Systemic abnormalities in term infants following perinatal asphyxia: Relevance to long-term neurologic outcome. Neonat. Neurol. 16(2):475–484, 1989.

Percy, A.K.: Neonatal asphyxia and static encephalopathies. In Fishman, M.A. (ed.): Pediatric Neurology. Orlando, Grune & Stratton, 1986, pp. 57–70.

Shankaran, S., Koepke, T., Woldt, E., et al.: Outcome after posthemorrhagic ventriculomegaly in comparison with mild hemorrhage without ventriculomegaly. Fetal Neonat. Med., *114*(1):109–114, 1989.

Shaw, N.: Common surgical problems in the newborn. J. Perinat. Neonat. Nurs., *3*(3):50–65, 1990.

Shinnar, S., Molteni, R.A., Gammon, K., et al.: Intraventricular hemorrhage in the premature infant. New Engl. J. Med. , *306*(24):1464–1468, 1982.

Smith, S.A.: Peripheral neuropathies in children. *In* Swaiman, K.F. (ed.): Pediatric Neurology: Principles and Practice, Vol. 2 St. Louis, C.V. Mosby, 1989, pp. 1105–1123.

Stark, G.D.: Neonatal assessment of the child with a myelomeningocele. Arch. Dis. Child., *46*:539–548, 1971.

Svenningsen, N.W., Blennow, G., Lindroth, M., et al.: Brain-oriented intensive care treatment in severe neonatal asphyxia. Arch. Dis. Child., *57*:176–183, 1982.

Torrence, C.: Neonatal seizures: Part II. Recognition, treatment, and prognosis. Neonatal Network, *4*(2):21–28, 1985.

Volpe, J.J.: Neurology of the Newborn, 2nd ed. Philadelphia, W.B. Saunders Co., 1987.

Whaley, L.F., and Wong, D.L.: Nursing Care of Infants and Children. St. Louis, C.V. Mosby, 1979.

Windham, G.C., and Edmonds, L.D.: Current trends in the incidence of neural tube defects. Pediatrics, *70*(3):333–337, 1982.

Young, T.E., and Mangum, O.B.: Neofax: A manual of Drugs Used in Neonatal Care, 3rd ed. Columbus, OH, Ross Laboratories, 1990.

BIBLIOGRAPHY

Allan, W.C., and Volpe, J.J.: Periventricular-intraventricular hemorrhage. Pediatr. Clin. North Am., *36*(1):47–63, 1986.

Ashwal, S.: Brain death in the newborn. Clin. Perinatol., *16*(2):501–518, 1989.

Ashwal, S., and Schneider, S.: Brain death in the newborn. Pediatrics, *84*(3):429–437, 1989.

Bartoshesky, L.E., Haller, J., Scott, M., and Wojick, C.: Seizures in children with meningomyelocele. Am. J. Dis. Child., *139*:400–402, 1985.

Carter, B.S., Portman, R.J., Gaylord, M.S., and Merenstein, G.B.: Prospectively predicting asphyxial severity. Clin. Res., *35*(1):75A, 1987.

Carter, B.S., Portman, R.J., Gaylord, M.S., et al.: Prediction of perinatal asphyxial severity. Pediatr. Res., *20*:376A, 1986.

Charney, E.B., Weller, S.C., Sutton, L.N., et al.: Management of the newborn with myelomeningocele: Time for a decision-making process. Pediatrics, *75*(1):58–64, 1985.

Cole, C.H. (ed.): The Harriet Lane Handbook, 10th ed. Chicago, Year Book Medical Publishers, 1984.

DeVries, S.L., Dubowitz, L.M.S., Dubowitz, V., et al.: Predictive value of cranial ultrasound in the newborn baby: A reappraisal. Lancet, *137*(2):137–140, 1985.

Diebler, C., and Dulac, O.: Pediatric Neurology and Neuroradiology: Cerebral and Cranial Diseases. Berlin, Springer-Verlag, 1987.

Drugs and therapeutics, a medical letter on drugs for viral infections. The Medical Letter, 1000 Main Street, New Rochelle, NY 10801, Vol. 32 (ISSN 824), 1990.

Dubowitz, L.M.S., Dubowitz, V., Palmer, P.G., et al.: Correlation of neurologic assessment in the preterm newborn infant with outcome at 1 year. J. Pediatr., *105*(3):452–456, 1984.

Ellison, P.H., Largent, J.A., and Bahr, J.P.: A scoring system to predict outcome following neonatal seizures. J. Pediatr., *99*(3):455–459, 1981.

Emery, J.R., and Peabody, J.L.: Head position affects intracranial pressure in newborn infants. J. Pediatr., *103*(6):950–953, 1983.

Freeman, J.M.: Neonatal seizures: Diagnosis and management. Fetal Neonat. Med., *77*(4):701–708, 1970.

Freitag-Koontz, M.J.: Parents' grief reaction to the diagnosis of their infants' having severe neurologic impairment and static encephalopathy. J. of Perinat. Neonat. Nurs., *2*(2):45–57, 1988.

Guyton, A.C.: Textbook of Medical Physiology, 8th ed. Philadelphia, W.B. Saunders Co., 1991.

Hambleton, G., and Wigglesworth, J.S.: Origin of intraventricular hemorrhage in the preterm infant. Arch. Dis. Child., *51*:651–659, 1976.

Hayden, P.W.: Adolescents with meningomyelocele. Pediatr. Rev. *6*(8):245–252, 1985.

Ho, E.: Neural tube defects. Nurs. Mirror, *156*(9):iv–vi, 1983.

Hoffman, H.J., and Raffel, L.: Craniofacial surgery. *In* McLaurin, R.L., Schut, L., Venes, J.L., and Epstein, F. (eds.): Pediatric Neurosurgery: Surgery of the Developing Nervous System, 2nd ed. Philadelphia, W.B. Saunders Co., 1989, pp. 120–144.

Kalbus, B.H., and Neal, K.G.: A Laboratory Manual and Study Guide for Human Anatomy. Long Beach, California, ELOJ Publishing, 1978.

Kinney, M.R., Dear, C.B., Packa, D.R., and Voorman, D.M.N. (eds.): AACN's Clinical References for Critical Care Nursing. New York, McGraw-Hill, 1981.

Kurtzke, J.F., Goldberg, I.D., and Kurland, L.T.: The distribution of death from congenital malformations of the nervous system. Neurology, *23*(5):483–496, 1973.

Labson, L.H.: Newborn exam: Neurologic evaluation. Patient-Care, March 1983, pp. 121–123, 127, 130–132.

Lemire, R.J.: Neural tube defects. JAMA, *259*(4):558–561, 1988.

Levine, M.G., Holroyde, J., Woods, J.R., et al.: Birth trauma: Incidence and predisposing factors. Obstet. Gynecol., *63*(6):792–795, 1984.

Lou, H.C., Lassen, N.A., and Friis-Hansen, B.: Impaired autoregulation of cerebral blood flow in the distressed newborn infant. J. Pediatr., *94*(1):118–121, 1979.

Luciano, D.S., Vander, A.J., and Sherman, J.H.: Human Function and Structure. New York, McGraw-Hill, 1978.

Lupton, B.A., Hill, A., Roland, E.H., et al.: Brain swelling in the asphyxiated term newborn: Pathogenesis and outcome. Pediatrics, *82*(2):139–146, 1988.

McLaughlin, J.F., Shurtleff, D.B., Lamers, J.Y., et al.: Influence of prognosis on decisions regarding the care of newborns with myelodysplasia. N. Engl. J. Med., *312*(25):1589–1594, 1985.

Ment, L.R., Duncan, C.C., Ehrenkranz, R.A., et al.: Intraventricular hemorrhage in the preterm neonate: Timing and cerebral blood flow changes. J. Pediatr., *104*(3):419–425, 1984.

Ment, L.R., Scott, D.T., Ehrenkranz, R.A., and Duncan, C.C.: Neurodevelopmental assessment of very low birth weight neonates: Effect of germinal and intraventricular hemorrhage. Pediatr. Neurol., *1*(3):164–168, 1985.

Mizrahi, E.M.: Consensus and controversy in the clinical management of neonatal seizures. Clin. Perinatol., *16*(2):485–500, 1989.

Painter, M.J., Bergman, I., and Crumrine, P.: Neonatal seizures. Pediatr. Clin. North. Am., *33*(1):91–109, 1986.

Painter, M.J., Pippenger, C., Wasterlain, C., et al.: Phenobarbital and phenytoin in neonatal seizures: Metabolism and tissue distribution. Neurology, *31*:1107–1112, 1981.

Papile, L., Burstein, J., Burstein, R., and Koffler, H.: Incidence and evolution of subependymal and intraventricular hemorrhage: A study of infants with birth weights less than 1,500 grams. J. Pediatr., *92*(4):529–534, 1978.

Passo, S. Positioning infants with myelomeningocele. Am. J. Nurs., *74*(9):1658–1660, 1974.

Passo, S.: Malformations of the neural tube. Nurs. Clin. North Am., *15*(1):5–21, 1980.

Perlman, J.M., Goodman, S., Kreusser, K.L., and Volpe, J.J.: Reduction in intraventricular hemorrhage by elimination of fluctuating cerebral blood-flow velocity in preterm infants with respiratory distress syndrome. N. Engl. J. Med., *312*(21):1353–1357, 1985.

Raimondi, A.J.: Cystic transformation of the IV ventricle (the Dandy-Walker cyst). *In* Hoffman, H.J., and Epstein, F. (eds.): Disorders of the Developing Nervous System: Diagnosis and Treatment. Boston, Blackwell Scientific Publications, 1986, pp. 235–246.

Reproductive toxicology, a medical letter on environmental hazards to reproduction. Reproductive Toxicology Center, 2524 L Street, Washington, D.C. 20037, ISSN 0736-5098, 1987.

Rhoads, G.G., and Mills, J.L.: Can vitamin supplements prevent neural tube defects? Current evidence and ongoing investigations. Clin. Obstet. Gynecol., *39*(3):569–578, 1986.

Rubin, A.: Birth injuries: Incidence, mechanisms and end results. Obstet. Gynecol., *23*(2):218–221, 1964.

Sarnat, H.B., and Sarnat, M.S.: Neonatal encephalopathy following fetal distress. Arch. Neurol., *33*(10):696–705, 1976.

Scher, M.S., and Painter, M.J.: Controversies surrounding neonatal seizures. Pediatr. Clin. North Am., *36*(2):281–310, 1989.

Steer, C.R.: Barbiturate therapy in the management of cerebral ischemia. Develop. Med. Child Neurol., *24*(2):219–231, 1982.

Sykes, G.S., Molloy, P.M., Johnson, P., et al.: Do Apgar scores indicate asphyxia? Lancet, *1*:494–496, 1982.

Thorns, S.: Controversy, treatment and care. Nurs. Mirror, *154*(24):32–33, 1982.

Torrence, C.: Neonatal seizures: Part I. A developmental and clinical understanding. Neonatal Network, *4*(1):9–16, 1985.

Vandar, A.J., Sherman, J.H., and Luciano, D.S.: Human Physiology: The Mechanisms of Body Function, 2nd ed. New York, McGraw-Hill, 1970.

Volpe, J.J.: Perinatal hypoxic-ischemic brain injury. Pediatr. Clin. North Am., *23*(3):383–397, 1976.

Volpe, J.J.: Intraventricular hemorrhage and brain injury in the premature infant: Diagnosis, prognosis and prevention. Clin. Perinatol., *16*(2):387–411, 1989.

Volpe, J.J.: Intraventricular hemorrhage and brain injury in the premature: Neuropathology and pathogenesis. Clin. Perinatol., *16*(2):361–386, 1989.

Pamela Creger

Developmental Support in the NICU

Objectives

1. Identify intervention strategies to maximize an infant's capacity for behavioral organization.

2. Describe predictable, sequential patterns of neuromotor maturation.

3. Demonstrate supportive positioning-handling strategies to encourage the development of normal motor patterns in an infant.

4. List six common feeding problems encountered in high-risk infants.

5. Explain the limitations and advantages of each of the four major tools used to screen neonatal hearing.

6. Identify intervention strategies to promote parent-infant interaction.

7. Design a developmental care plan to communicate an infant's unique needs with regard to environmental modifications, positioning techniques, and promotion of self-quieting behaviors.

Developmental support in the neonatal intensive care unit (NICU) integrates the developmental needs of infants with intensive medical care. Development occurs along a continuum, with the usual course of development being interrupted by the birth of a pre-term or ill newborn. Care providers now recognize that an infant responds to and interacts with the environment using different "cues" and is able to communicate on many different levels. Understanding an infant's developmental needs and learning how to provide the interventions necessary to support development are essential in providing optimal care for these infants. This chapter provides information on the developmental needs of the newborn and discusses strategies for providing this care.

Concepts of Developmental Care

A. **Key concepts** facing neonatal health professionals and parent educators.
1. How to provide needed care in the least disruptive way.
2. How to optimize an infant's developmental potential and outcome, given the medical constraints of the NICU.

3. How to have a more positive impact on the quality of life high-risk infants will go on to share with their families.

B. **Provision of developmentally supportive care** involves the following:
1. Assessing infant behavior according to the synactive theory of development (Als et al., 1982).
   a. Physiological or autonomic system: behaviorally observable in respiratory pattern, color changes, and visceral responses (emesis, gagging, hiccups, bowel movements).
   b. Motor system: behaviorally observable in posture, tone, and overall movements.
   c. State organizational system: behaviorally observable in range of states, pattern of state transitions, and clarity of states.
   d. Attention and interactional system: observable in ability to be attentive and take in cognitive and social information from the environment.
   e. Self-regulatory system: behaviorally observable in strategies infant uses to maintain or return to state of balance and relaxation.
2. Assessing an infant's *unique* behavioral style.
3. Adapting intervention goals to the medical constraints of the NICU.
4. Facilitating an infant's neurosocial behavioral organization by:
   a. *Recognizing* and *responding* to the infant's behavioral cues.
   b. Effecting change within the physical and social environment of the NICU.
   c. Providing individualized intervention programs.
5. Implementing appropriate intervention strategies to foster parent-infant interaction and enhance parents' understanding of their infant as an individual.

Behavioral Organization

A. **Behavioral organization:** ability to maintain a balance among autonomic, motor, state, attention-interactional, and self-regulatory subsystems of behavioral maturation as infant deals with a variety of sensory and postural demands imposed on him or her (Als et al., 1982).

B. **Infant's capacity for behavioral organization** is reinforced and enhanced by caregivers who recognize and respond to infant's behavioral cues by:
1. Providing "time-out" when infant demonstrates *avoidance* behaviors (Als et al., 1982; Figure 21–1).

SELF REGULATION PARAMETERS									
	CATALOG OF REGULATION MANEUVERS					CATALOG OF REGULATION MANEUVERS			
	Spit-ups	Gags	Hiccoughs	Bowel Mvt		Tongue Extension	Hand on Face	Sounds	
	Grimace	Arching	Finger Splay	Airplane		Hand Clasp	Foot Clasp	Fingerfold	Tuck
WITHDRAWAL OR AVOIDANCE BEHAVIOR	Salute	Sitting on Air			APPROACH OR GROPING BEHAVIOR	Body Movement	Hand to Mouth	Grasping	Leg/Foot Bracing
	Sneezing	Yawning	Sighing	Coughing		Mouthing	Suck Search	Sucking	Hand Hold
	Averting	Frowning				Ooh Face	Locking	Cooing	

Figure 21–1
Approach and avoidance behaviors. (From Als, H., Brazelton, T.B., Lester, B.M., and Tronick, E.Z.: Manual for the assessment of preterm infants' behavior (APIB). *In* Fitzgerald, H.E., Lester, B.M., and Yogman, M.W. (eds.): Theory and Research in Behavioral Pediatrics. New York, Plenum Press, 1982, p. 70.)

2. Supporting and enhancing infant's *approach* behaviors (Als et al., 1982; Figure 21–1).

C. **Points to consider when assessing** an infant's levels of behavioral stability or organization.
1. What experiences upset the infant during the daily caregiving routine?
2. When and with what help does the infant function smoothly?
3. Does a particular position agitate the infant more than another?
4. How much handling can the infant tolerate before losing control?
5. How is the infant most readily consoled?
6. What support is necessary to help the infant maintain self-control?
7. Can the timing and organization of medical and nursing procedures be altered to help decrease the infant's level of stress and increase his or her organization?

D. **Intervention strategies** to help infant manage stress and organize behavior.
1. Autonomic system.
   a. Signs of stress: changes in vital signs or color, hiccups, spitting, sneezing.
   b. Intervention strategies.
      (1) Modify environment (light, noise, traffic).
      (2) Decrease handling.
      (3) Use therapeutic positioning techniques.
2. Motor system.
   a. Signs of stress: generalized hypotonia, frantic flailing, finger splaying, hyperextension of extremities.
   b. Intervention strategies.
      (1) Handle slowly, gently.
      (2) Use therapeutic positioning techniques.
3. State system.
   a. Provides context for any interaction between infant and environment; used by infant to control how much and what kind of input received from the environment.
   b. Six sleep-awake states.*
      (1) Sleep states.
         (a) *State 1A:* Infant in deep sleep with momentary regular breathing, eyes closed, no eye movements under closed lids; relaxed facial expression; no spontaneous activity, oscillating fairly rapidly with isolated startles, jerky movements or tremors and other behavior characteristic of State 2 (light sleep).
         (b) *State 1B:* Infant in deep sleep with predominantly regular breathing, eyes closed, no eye movements under closed lids, relaxed facial expression; no spontaneous activity except isolated startles.
         (c) *State 2A:* Light sleep with eyes closed; rapid eye movements can be observed under closed lids; low activity level with diffuse or disorganized movements; respirations are irregular and there are many sucking and mouthing movements, whimpers, facial twitchings, much grimacing; the impression of a "noisy" state is given.
         (d) *State 2B:* Light sleep with eyes closed; rapid eye movements can be observed under closed lids; low activity level with movements and dampened startles; movements are likely to be of lower amplitude and more monitored than in State 1; infant responds to various internal stimuli with dampened startle. Respirations are more irregular, mild sucking and mouthing movements can occur off and on; one or two whimpers may be observed, as well as an isolated sigh or smile.

*Section b. is reprinted from Als, H., Brazelton, T.B., Lester, B.M., et al.: Manual for the assessment of preterm infants' behavior (APIB). *In* Fitzgerald, H.E., Lester, B.M., and Yogman, M.W. (eds.): Theory and Research in Behavioral Pediatrics. New York, Plenum Press, 1982, pp. 65–132; with permission.

(2) Transitional states.

    (a) *State 3A:* Drowsy or semi-dozing; eyes may be open or closed, eyelids fluttering or exaggerated blinking; if eyes open, glassy veiled look; activity level variable, with or without interspersed, mild startles from time to time; diffuse movement; fussing and or much discharge of vocalization, whimpers, facial grimacing, etc.

    (b) *State 3B:* Drowsy, same as above but with less discharge of vocalization, whimpers, facial grimacing, etc.

(3) Awake states.

    (a) *State 4:* Alert.

        i. *4AL:* Awake and quiet, minimal motor activity, eyes half open or open but with glazed or dull look, giving impression of little involvement and distance; or focused, yet seems to look through, rather than at, object or examiner; or the infant is clearly awake and reactive but has his eyes open intermittently.

        ii. *4AH:* Awake and quiet, minimal motor activity, eyes wide open, "hyperalert" or giving the impression of panic or fear; may appear to be hooked by the stimulus, seems to be unable to modulate or break the intensity of the fixation.

        iii. *4B:* Alert with bright shiny look; seems to focus attention on source of stimulation and appears to process information actively and with modulation; motor activity is at a minimum.

    (b) *State 5:* Active.

        i. *5A:* Eyes may or may not be open, but infant is clearly awake and aroused, as indicated by his motor arousal, his tonus, and his mildly distressed facial expression, grimacing, or other signs of discomfort; fussing is diffuse.

        ii. *5B:* Eyes may or may not be open, but infant is clearly awake and aroused, with considerable, well defined motor activity. Infant is also clearly fussing but not crying.

    (c) *State 6:* Crying.

        i. *6A:* Intense crying, as indicated by intense grimace and cry face, yet cry sound may be very strained or very weak or even absent.

        ii. *6B:* Rhythmic, intense crying which is robust, vigorous, and strong in sound.

c. Signs of stress: diffuse sleep states (twitching, grimacing, glassy eyed, gaze aversion, panicked look, irritability).

d. Intervention strategies.

    (1) Cluster care.

    (2) Primary nursing: allows for more reliable reading of subtle behavioral cues.

    (3) Time care appropriately.

    (4) Use therapeutic positioning techniques.

    (5) Evaluate immediate environment from *infant's* viewpoint.

4. Attention-interactional system.

  a. Signs of stress: same as autonomic, motor, and state systems.

  b. Intervention strategies.

    (1) Time interactions appropriately.

    (2) Offer one mode of stimuli at a time.

    (3) Respect infant's avoidance behaviors (time-out cues).

5. Self-regulatory system.

  a. Behaviorally exemplified by postural change, grasping, hand-to-mouth, sucking, visual locking.

  b. Intervention strategies.

    (1) Use therapeutic positioning techniques.

    (2) Modify environment.

    (3) Time care appropriately.

(4) Provide momentary time-out from incoming stimuli, allowing infant to draw fully on self-regulatory abilities.

Neuromotor Development

A. **Neuromotor maturation** follows *predictable sequence* as premature infant progresses to 40 weeks of age.
1. Generalized hypotonia progresses to flexion.
2. Random movements become purposeful and controlled.
3. Primary reflexes become consistent and complete.
4. Gradual perfection of primary reflexes proceeds cephalocaudally.
5. Muscle tone proceeds caudocephally.

B. **Sequential patterns of maturation** identified by examining the following:
1. Resting postures (Amiel-Tison, 1968).
   a. Generalized hypotonia.
   b. Thigh flexion.
   c. Hip flexion.
   d. Frog-like position.
   e. Total body flexion.
   f. Hypertonia.
2. Resistance to passive movement (Amiel-Tison, 1968).
   a. Full, passive range of motion.
   b. Extreme head lag with attempt to right head when pulled to sit.
   c. Places some weight on feet when held in a supported stand.
   d. Stepping and placing responses are complete.
3. Active movements (Amiel-Tison, 1968).
   a. Spasmodic, random movements.
   b. Reflexive movements.
   c. Reciprocal movements.
   d. Wide variety of smooth and purposeful movements.

C. **Sequence of development** is predictable; however, *timing* is *individual* and may be affected by:
1. Level of medical support required.
2. Medications.
3. Timing of exam.
4. Infant's own biological clock.

Positioning Techniques: Therapeutic Handling

A. **Positioning** should be selected to accomplish the following (Anderson and Auster-Liebhaber, 1984):
1. Support infant's developing perceptual and sensorimotor abilities.
2. Counteract emerging stereotypical or abnormal postures.
3. Provide positive input during time spent without direct physical contact.
4. No interference with necessary medical interventions.

B. **General goals** of developmentally supportive positioning (Biber, Creger, Kolar, et al., 1989).
1. Promote newborn flexion.
   a. Physiological flexion develops in last trimester of pregnancy in response to decreased space in utero and as an active process in neurological development (Moore, 1966); infants born prematurely do not have opportunity to develop physiological flexion.
2. Facilitate midline orientation (hand-to-mouth activity) and symmetrical positioning.

3. Enhance self-quieting skills and behavioral organization.
4. Encourage relaxation and improve digestion.
5. Prevent bony deformities and skin breakdown.
6. Increase awareness of body in space.
7. Facilitate visual and auditory skill development.
8. Facilitate development of head control.

C. **General principles** (Biber, Creger, Kolar, et al., 1989).
1. Infant is capable of demonstrating most competent motor behavior when in an organized, quiet, alert state. Techniques to help infant organize movement and orient to stimulation include the following:
    a. Swaddle.
    b. Provide non-nutritive sucking activity.
    c. Prevent visual or auditory stimulus.
    d. Elicit rooting, sucking, or grasping reflexes.
    e. Shade infant's eyes or position away from bright lights.
2. Handling is any touch, movement, or caregiving activity requiring contact, e.g., medical procedures, diapering, dressing, etc., through which the infant receives sensory-motor information.
3. With certain high-risk infants, handling must be kept to a minimum to avoid further medical compromise and help the infant conserve energy.
4. Provision of developmentally supportive positioning interventions may promote a calm state and physiological stability for the high-risk infant.
5. If the infant is motorically stressed, help him or her reorganize by holding extremities in flexion close to body until calm, thereby decreasing unnecessary energy expenditure and encouraging self-regulation. Swaddling, non-nutritive sucking, or rhythmic vestibular input also may help soothe and reorganize the infant.
6. Providing momentary time-out from incoming stimuli when a baby is stressed and disorganized allows him or her time to draw fully on self-regulatory abilities.
7. Observe for avoidance behaviors in response to movement transitions or particular positions, i.e., gaze aversion, regurgitation, crying, increased extension patterns, etc.
8. When repositioning an infant, contain the limbs to help the infant maintain stability and stay in control; use slow, gentle movements.
9. Encourage positions that allow the infant to place his or her hands near the mouth.
10. Knowledge of an infant's individual sensitivities and responses will facilitate the caregiver's selection of the most effective consoling technique. Communication of this information can be enhanced through primary nursing and the use of a developmental care plan.

D. **Positioning strategies** (Biber, Creger, Kolar, et al., 1989).
1. A variety of positioning options are available; certain positions are required for medical reasons. It is often possible to modify these positions to be developmentally supportive.
2. Benefits of positioning options must be measured in terms of impact on total infant, not just one subsystem. It is essential to monitor infant's physiological and behavioral responses to various positioning strategies, i.e., gains in motor and state control systems may be offset by unstabilizing effects to heart rate, respiratory rate, blood pressure, etc.
3. Use as little external support as possible to properly position infant, but recognize that some infants require maximal support to be comfortable. Infant should look comfortable and in control.
4. Premature infants often engage in intentional movements aimed at making and maintaining contact with a stable surface in their immediate environment (Newman, 1981). This is a coping strategy used to maintain organizational

balance through containment. Provide these infants with "boundaries" at their head, side, and feet, i.e., "nesting."
5. Prone position.
   a. Benefits.
      (1) Facilitates flexion (Connally and Montgomery, 1987).
      (2) Facilitates development of early head control (Bobath and Bobath, 1972).
      (3) May improve oxygenation due to mechanical advantages on chest wall expansion (Martin et al., 1979).
   b. Principles.
      (1) Hips and knees should be flexed, knees under hips, hips higher than shoulders.
      (2) Arms flexed with hands near head, hand on face side near mouth.
6. Side-lying position.
   a. Benefits.
      (1) May facilitate flexion.
      (2) Encourage hand-to-mouth activity, a self-quieting behavior.
      (3) May be used to discourage arching or opisthotonus by providing boundaries to support flexion.
   b. Principles.
      (1) Hips and knees should be flexed.
      (2) Arms "cuddled" forward at shoulders and softly flexed.
      (3) Head in line with body or slightly flexed.
7. Supine position.
   a. Frequently necessary due to medical interventions, i.e., ventilator, arterial lines, chest tubes, etc. Infants maintained in this position may have difficulty developing flexor patterns because:
      (1) Supine position facilitates extension.
      (2) Difficult for infant to flex against gravity.
   b. Principles.
      (1) Hips and knees slightly flexed up toward abdomen.
      (2) Shoulders flexed forward with hands on chest or abdomen.
      (3) Arms and legs symmetrical.
      (4) Head in midline or comfortably turned to one side.

E. **Potential indications for referral** to occupational therapist, physical therapist, or neurodevelopmental therapist (Biber, Creger, Kolar, et al., 1989; Figure 21–2).
1. Questionable or abnormal tone or posturing, i.e., poor head and trunk control, asymmetries, hypertonicity or hypotonicity.
2. Marked prematurity.
3. Prolonged hospitalization.
4. Feeding or suck-swallow difficulties.
5. Congenital malformations.
6. Sensory impairments.
7. Disorganized behavior, i.e., irritability, inability to self-quiet, jitteriness, excessive startle or hyperexcitability.

F. **Areas in which therapists can offer treatment** to infant (Biber, Creger, Kolar, et al., 1989).
1. Normalizing muscle tone.
2. Increasing infant's tolerance for touch and/or handling.
3. Improving oral-motor control for sucking.
4. Preventing limitations in movement.
5. Developing normal movement patterns.
6. Developing more mature movement patterns.
7. Integrating normal infant movement patterns into caregiver's daily activities.
8. Developing more normal righting and equilibrium reactions.
9. Promoting relaxation.

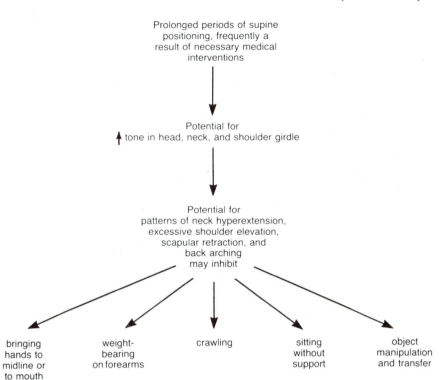

Prolonged periods of supine
positioning, frequently a
result of necessary medical
interventions

↓

Potential for
↑ tone in head, neck, and shoulder girdle

↓

Potential for
patterns of neck hyperextension,
excessive shoulder elevation,
scapular retraction, and
back arching
may inhibit

bringing	weight-	crawling	sitting	object
hands to	bearing		without	manipulation
midline or	on forearms		support	and transfer
to mouth				

Figure 21–2
"Red alert" indicators for consultation and follow-up. (From Biber, P. et al.: Developmentally supportive positioning and therapeutic handling strategies. *In* Creger, P. (ed.): Infant Interaction Program, Module 5: Developmentally Supportive Positioning and Therapeutic Handling of the Hospitalized Infant. Denver, CO, The Children's Hospital Association, 1989, p. 36.)

Assessment of Feeding Abilities

A. Sucking response.
1. Simple and rhythmical motor reflex (Wolff, 1968).
2. Comprised of a pattern of bursts and pauses that allow infant to rest, regroup, socialize, and process cognitive information (Brazelton, 1987).
3. Neurodevelopmental progression of sucking response.
    a. 9.5 weeks post-conceptional age (PCA): Perioral stimulation produces opening of mouth; lips do not protrude as in the sucking reflex (Humphrey, 1964).
    b. 14 weeks PCA: Basic taste bud morphology and its nerve supply are established (Bradley, 1972).
    c. 17 weeks PCA: Sucking response (Dubignon et al., 1969) and swallowing (Heird and Anderson, 1977) have been observed.
    d. 24 weeks PCA: Ganglion cells have innervated entire GI system, allowing for motility (Heird and Anderson, 1977).
    e. 28 weeks PCA: Rooting, sucking, and swallowing reflexes are well established, but response may be slow and imperfect (Amiel-Tison, 1968).
    f. 32 weeks PCA: Gag reflex is present and serves as a protective mechanism for feeding (Fanaroff and Klaus, 1986).
    g. 34 weeks PCA: Coordination of suck-swallow-breathe (Bragdon, 1983) possible due to myelinization of the medulla (Logan and Bosma, 1967).

B. Successful oral feeding experiences (Biber, Creger, and Kolar, 1989).
1. Goals.
    a. Safe: caregiver should feel infant's risk of aspiration is minimal.

   b. Functional: infant should consume enough formula in reasonable amount of time to assure adequate caloric intake and growth.

   c. Pleasurable: feeding interaction should provide positive reinforcement to infant and caregiver.

2. Variables affecting success:

   a. Infant's gestational age and weight.

   b. Infant's physiological stability and overall medical status.

   c. Infant's muscle tone.

   d. Infant's energy level and endurance.

   e. Previous oral experiences of the infant.

   f. Physical demands of the infant's daily routine.

   g. Caregiver's attitude and experience.

   h. Overall environmental atmosphere.

C. **Nutritive sucking**.

1. Requires greater coordination between suck-swallow-breathe than non-nutritive sucking.

2. Goal is to encourage as normal a suck-swallow pattern as possible while infant maintains physiological, motor, and state stability.

3. Four nutritive sucking patterns.

   a. Mature: long sucking bursts of 10 or more with breathing interspersed with suck-swallow.

   b. Immature: short sucking bursts of less than 5 with swallowing occurring before or after the sucks.

   c. Disorganized: reflects lack of rhythm in total sucking response rather than incoordination of specific response (Braun and Palmer, 1985/1986).

   d. Dysfunctional: reflects problem nippling due to abnormal movements of tongue and jaw (Braun and Palmer, 1985/1986).

4. Criteria to assess prior to initiating nutritive sucking (VandenBerg, 1987).

   a. Ability to organize physiological, motor, and state systems.

   b. Receptivity to non-nutritive sucking opportunities.

   c. Ease with which rooting reflex is elicited.

   d. Coordination of suck and swallow during non-nutritive sucking.

   e. Presence or absence of "hungry" behaviors (crying, rooting, hand-to-mouth activity); satiation may inhibit sucking behavior (Satinoff and Stanley, 1963).

   f. Physical demands of infant's daily routine: energy reserves are limited.

   g. Ability to maintain body temperature outside of Isolette.

   h. Growth curve: gaining weight consistently over time while on gavage feeds.

   i. General muscle tone: infant with trunkal hypotonia may also have decreased oral-motor tone.

   j. Oxygen requirement: supplemental oxygen may make a difference between success and failure.

5. Setting the scene for nutritive sucking (VandenBerg, 1987).

   a. Negotiate with health care team members to plan stressful treatments and procedures at times not associated with feedings.

   b. Allow sufficient time to give infant "undivided attention."

   c. Position self comfortably.

   d. Plan to assess infant's color, heart rate, respiratory rate and effort, muscle tone, and state; apnea or bradycardia during feeding may indicate infant is not ready for nutritive sucking.

   e. Be aware of environmental factors (sounds, lights, movements) that may disorganize infant.

   f. Assess infant's response to environment. Is capacity for behavioral organization enhanced by:

     (1) Avoiding conversation with the infant or around the immediate area?

     (2) Avoiding eye contact?

     (3) Facing wall to inhibit visual stimulation?

        (4) Use of privacy screen?

        (5) Dimming lights?

    g. Use infant cues to determine timing of feedings.

    h. Consider swaddling infant to minimize extraneous movements and to provide external stability; swaddling encourages flexion, which facilitates sucking (Connally and Montgomery, 1987).

    i. Primary nursing facilitates consistency of caregiver and feeding techniques.

6. Mechanical considerations (nonbreast-feeding infants) (VandenBerg and Goderez, 1987).

    a. Nipple characteristics to assess.

        (1) Size of nipple.

            (a) Affects infant's ability to close mouth around nipple.

            (b) Affects how far back into throat formula is ejected.

        (2) Shape of nipple.

            (a) Affects seal of infant's lips around nipple.

            (b) Affects how far back into throat formula is ejected.

            (c) Determines "fit" inside infant's mouth.

        (3) Firmness of nipple.

            (a) Affects strength of suck required to extract formula.

            (b) Affects amount of formula ejected per suck.

        (4) Size of hole in nipple.

            (a) Affects amount of formula ejected per suck.

            (b) Affects rate of flow of formula.

            (c) Affects strength of suck required to extract formula.

    b. Temperature of formula.

        (1) Affects rate of flow of formula.

        (2) Warmer the liquid, faster the flow.

    c. Thickness of formula.

        (1) Affects strength of suck required to extract formula.

        (2) Affects amount of formula ejected per suck.

        (3) Affects degree of tactile feedback in mouth.

        (4) May give infant more control of formula, but may also require more energy to extract formula.

    d. Infant characteristics to assess.

        (1) Muscle tone.

        (2) Strength of suck.

        (3) Sucking organization and coordination.

        (4) Energy level.

        (5) Gag reflex.

    e. There is no "recipe" approach to determine what nipple works for what infant.

7. Common feeding problems (Biber, Creger, and Kolar, 1989).

    a. Poor coordination of suck-swallow-breathe.

        (1) Infant may first require assistance with general systems organization.

        (2) Coordination not expected less than 34 weeks' PCA.

        (3) Position with head midline, slightly flexed, arms "cuddled" forward; too much neck flexion compromises breathing; extension opens airway and can result in aspiration.

        (4) Swaddling may provide external support needed to maintain "soft" flexion position and promote infant's capacity for behavioral organization and control.

        (5) Environmental stimuli may need to be reduced or eliminated.

        (6) Select nipple designed to optimize individual infant's sucking ability: evaluate shape, size, firmness, and size of hole in nipple.

        (7) Note gagging and spitting: may be indicative of incoordination between suck-swallow-breathe.

    b. Fatigue.

        (1) Feeding process can be very tiring for pre-term or disorganized infant.

Sucking is comprised of a pattern of bursts and pauses. Help parents distinguish between fatigue and pauses (rest periods), which are normal part of sucking activity.

(2) Monitor physiological parameters and/or clinical indicators during feeding to prevent fatigue.

(3) Swaddle to provide external support and minimize unnecessary movements.

(4) Consider use of supplemental oxygen during feeding.

(5) Limit number of bottle feedings per day until organization and endurance improve.

(6) Provide light jaw support (gentle pressure under infant's chin) to lessen fatigue from wasted jaw movements.

(7) Evaluate firmness of nipple used: affects strength of suck required.

(8) Assess infant's feeding regime. Would he or she tire less if fed:

(a) More frequently, smaller volume?

(b) Less frequently, larger volume?

(c) Less frequently, smaller volume and increase caloric density?

c. State disorganization.

(1) Feeding behavior is affected by infant state, or level of arousal (Meier and Pugh, 1985). Infants pursue feedings more eagerly and demonstrate more organized nutritive sucking pattern if awake and active first.

(2) Cue-based feeding may be more profitable than rigid schedule.

(3) Clinical conditions that affect infant state, e.g., anemia, may influence feeding behavior (Meier and Pugh, 1985) as evidenced by:

(a) Slower sucking rate.

(b) Longer but less interactive pauses between sucking bursts.

(c) Feeding with eyes closed.

(d) Fewer non-nutritive feeding behaviors.

d. Poor lip closure around nipple.

(1) Provide light jaw support: lessens fatigue from wasted jaw movements and encourages better lip closure.

(2) Provide light cheek support.

e. Sustained closure of jaws/pursing of lips tightly closed.

(1) Gentle massage of infant's cheeks to encourage relaxation of mouth.

(2) Shifting infant's position to allow for slight neck extension may increase receptivity.

f. Weak, arrhythmical suck.

(1) This infant frequently has an eager non-nutritive sucking pattern.

(2) Once a suck is performed, gently tugging at the bottle as if to pull it out of the infant's mouth may help smooth out the sucking pattern and strengthen the suck. Must not pull bottle too much or it will cause infant to lose seal around nipple.

8. "Stop" signs.

a. Infants with significant feeding difficulties are at risk for speech and language abnormalities (Illingworth, 1969). The same muscles necessary for successful nutritive sucking activity are used in speech production.

b. "Stop" sign behaviors.

(1) Increased biting.

(2) Lack of jaw closure.

(3) Tongue thrusting.

(4) Gagging and hiccupping repeatedly.

(5) Inability to suck.

(6) Irritability without the ability to self-quiet.

(7) Sucks eagerly on pacifier but demonstrates weak or arrhythmical nutritive suck.

(8) Aversive behavior (squirming, hyperextension, turning head away, pursing of lips, crying) occurring consistently after the infant takes a few nutritive sucks.

   c. Short rest period may deter above behaviors; if not, referral to occupational and physical therapy may be indicated.

9. Breast-feeding the pre-term infant (Biber, Creger, and Kolar, 1989).

   a. Indicators of readiness (Meier and Pugh, 1985).

     (1) Post-conceptional age of 34–35 weeks (to allow for mature suck-swallow reflex).

     (2) Demonstrated ability to bottle feed safely.

     (3) Ability to maintain infant's body temperature while being held.

     (4) Mother's readiness to breast-feed.

   b. Improving chances for success.

     (1) Assess infant state.

       (a) Level of arousal is associated with infant's ability and eagerness to breast-feed (Meier and Pugh, 1985).

       (b) Pre-term infants pursue the breast more eagerly and demonstrate more organized nutritive sucking pattern if awake and active first.

       (c) Feed the infant based on cue rather than according to a rigid schedule.

     (2) Provide assistance.

       (a) Provide privacy.

       (b) Assist mother with finding a comfortable position.

       (c) Guide infant's head onto breast; simultaneously encourage wider opening of infant's mouth to encompass areola.

     (3) Assess daily fluid balance and weight gain.

       (a) Must allow the infant to consume more volume in one feeding than another when using cue-based schedule (Meier and Pugh, 1985).

       (b) Monitor daily fluid balance and weight gain over time rather than specific volume intake every 3–4 hours.

     (4) Allow total feeding time flexibility.

       (a) Breast-feeding sessions frequently last longer than bottle-feeding sessions: infant independently paces breast-feeding session, sucking, and pausing as individually necessary.

       (b) Breast-feeding infants integrate nutritive sucking, rest periods, and social behaviors, thereby lengthening overall feeding time (Meier and Anderson, 1987).

       (c) Help the pre-term infant control breast-feeding experiences by monitoring physiological and/or clinical indicators to prevent fatigue.

     (5) Provide anticipatory guidance.

       (a) Mothers are easily disappointed and discouraged when infant will not awaken to breast-feed (Meier and Pugh, 1985).

       (b) Offer consultation with lactation specialist to address any foreseeable problems.

       (c) Some infants may be able to consistently organize nutritive sucking and interactional periods; others demonstrate more variable feeding patterns, ranging from organized sucking to little nutritive feeding activity.

     (6) Breast-feeding recommendations must be applied to pre-term infant and family on an individual basis.

Auditory Assessment and Follow-Up of Infant at Risk for Impairment

A. Background.

1. Hearing loss: 2.1–9.7% of infants in NICU (Schulman-Galambos and Galambos 1979; Bergman et al., 1985).

2. Hearing impaired: 1 : 1000 to 1 : 3000 normal newborns (Feinmesser and Tell, 1976; Coplan, 1987).

a. Demonstrate limited speech production skills (Osberger et al., 1986).
b. Significantly delayed receptive and expressive language skills (Moeller et al., 1986).
c. Reduced academic achievement, especially language related areas (Allen, 1986).

B. Types of hearing loss (Biber, Creger, Mediavilla, et al., 1989).
1. Conductive loss.
   a. Caused by interference in sound transmission from external auditory canal to inner ear.
   b. Inner ear capable of normal function.
   c. Associated with frequent ear infections.
   d. Sounds muffled or faint.
   e. Loss for air-conducted sounds; sounds transmitted in inner ear by bone conduction of the skull and temporal bone are heard normally.
   f. May resolve spontaneously: most can be corrected medically or surgically.
2. Sensorineural loss.
   a. Caused by damage to sensory end organ (cochlear hair cells) or by dysfunction of auditory nerve.
   b. Sounds distorted or muffled.
   c. Air and bone conduction thresholds usually equal.
   d. High tones inaudible.
   e. Loss usually irreversible.
   f. Loss treated with hearing aid and speech therapy.
3. Mixed loss.
   a. Combination of conductive and sensorineural loss.
   b. Bone-conduction thresholds below normal, air conduction even more so.
   c. Gap between air- and bone-conduction threshold levels should disappear after conductive loss is treated.
   d. Hearing levels not likely to return to normal.
4. Central auditory dysfunction.
   a. Sounds are transmitted normally but interpreted incorrectly by brain.
   b. Manifested by decreased auditory comprehension.

C. Four major tools used to screen neonatal hearing.
1. High-Risk Register: A.B.C.D.'s of Deafness (Downs and Silver, 1972); infant with any of following seven factors in prenatal, perinatal, or neonatal history has an increased chance of hearing impairment.
   a. *A:* Asphyxia (may include infants with Apgar scores of 0–3 who fail to exhibit spontaneous respirations by 10 minutes, and those with hypotonia existing to 2 hours of age.
   b. *B:* Bacterial meningitis (especially *Haemophilus influenzae*).
   c. *C:* Congenital perinatal infections (cytomegalovirus, rubella, herpes, toxoplasmosis, syphilis).
   d. *D:* Defects of the head or neck.
   e. *E:* Elevated bilirubin exceeding indications for exchange.
   f. *F:* Family history of childhood hearing impairment.
   g. *G:* Gram birth weight <1500 g.
2. Behavioral observation audiometry.
   a. Observation of infant response to high-intensity auditory stimuli.
   b. Variance of infant responses (i.e., generalized startle, eye widening, changes in facial expression) and examiner subjectivity make results difficult to interpret.
   c. Not reliable for follow-up screening of newborns failing High-Risk Register screening.
3. Crib-O-Gram.
   a. Monitors relatively diffuse respiratory and/or motor movements.
   b. Low-cost procedure.

c. Questionable reliability and validity in NICU population.
4. Auditory brain stem response (ABR).
   a. Non-invasive measurement of electrophysiological response of brainstem auditory pathways to an acoustic response.
   b. ABRs can be recorded in infants of very low stimulus levels: reduces possibility of passing infant with mild to moderate hearing loss.
   c. Can identify unilateral or asymmetrical hearing impairment.
   d. Requires audiologist for testing and interpretation of results.

D. **Ototoxic hearing loss**.
1. Damage to cochlea and/or vestibular part of inner ear, resulting in permanent sensorineural hearing loss; loss is usually bilateral and symmetrical.
2. Drugs implicated in ototoxicity.
   a. Aminoglycoside antibiotics.
      (1) Streptomycin.
      (2) Neomycin.
      (3) Gentamicin.
      (4) Kanamycin.
      (5) Tobramycin.
      (6) Amikacin.
      (7) Vancomycin.
   b. Diuretics.
      (1) Edecrin.
      (2) Lasix.
3. Factors that may enhance risk of ototoxicity.
   a. Increased serum drug level.
   b. Decreased renal function.
   c. Use of more than one ototoxic drug simultaneously or in consecutive courses.
   d. Use of ototoxic drug in increased daily doses for extended period.

E. **Implications for caregivers** (Biber, Creger, Mediavilla, et al., 1989).
1. "Listen" to environment from infant's viewpoint; assess appropriateness of existing or additional auditory stimulation.
2. Points to consider when designing care plan. *Note:* not every item will be appropriate for every infant, and no single item will be appropriate for a particular infant all of the time.
   a. High-frequency sounds usually arouse attention.
   b. Low-frequency sounds may produce sleep.
   c. Sudden loud noises may induce agitation and/or crying, producing physiological signs of stress.
   d. Simulate diurnal noise levels.
   e. Provide auditory stimulation from different locations: Does infant quiet? Anticipate sounds when repeated? Document observations.
   f. Behavioral assessment of infant and evaluation of interventions must be on-going.

F. **Follow-up and management** (Biber, Creger, Mediavilla, et al., 1989).
1. Parents of all newborns.
   a. Should receive information about normal auditory, speech, and language development.
   b. Benefit from information about expected milestones in communication development, enhancing their ability to detect abnormal auditory, speech, and language development.
   c. Should be informed of importance of early audiological evaluation of suspected hearing problems.
2. Hearing of at-risk infants should be evaluated by an audiologist: prior to discharge or no later than 3 months of age (Figure 21–3).
3. Habilitation of hearing impaired infant should begin by 6 months of age.

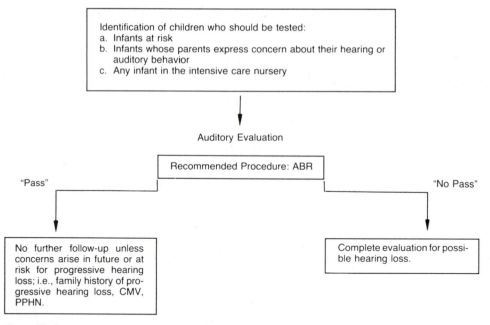

Figure 21-3
Identification and assessment of infants at risk for hearing impairment. (From Hayes, D.: Identification and assessment of infants at risk for hearing impairment. *In* Creger, P. (ed.): Infant Interaction Program, Module 4: Assessment of the Auditory System and Follow-Up of the Infant at Risk for Hearing Loss. Denver, CO, The Children's Hospital, 1989, p. 29.)

Fostering Parent-Infant Interaction (Biber, Bradley, et al., 1989)

A. **Key to supporting mutually satisfying parent-infant interaction** is to give parents the ability to understand their infant's level of communication through the infant's behavior. Once parents understand their infant's behavior, they will be in a better position to respond to and interact with their infant in a developmentally supportive manner.

B. **Intervention strategies**.
1. Teach parents to recognize and use infant states.
2. Encourage parental sensitivity to infant cues.
3. Help parents identify consoling measures unique to their infant.
4. Help parents recognize and respond to their infant's stress behaviors and time-out signals.
5. Help parents identify the most effective techniques for interacting with their infant.
6. Place parent in situations where they will succeed in interacting positively with their infant.
7. Help parents recognize their infant's capabilities by highlighting the strengths of their infant's behavioral repertoire.
8. Recommend specific activities when appropriate, i.e., verbal interaction, eye contact, use of toys, recorded tapes of parent's voice.
9. Suggest appropriate parental actions to assist their infant in coping with the environment.
10. Identify infant feedback to parent actions.
11. Encourage parents to assume caregiving responsibilities when appropriate.
12. Discuss parents' expectation and goals for themselves and their infant.
13. Discuss discrepancies between expectations and reality.
14. Be aware of and involve the family's support system.
15. Provide anticipatory guidance.

The Developmental Care Plan

A. **Is a written communication** to help health care providers support an individual infant's capacity for behavioral organization.

B. **Should coordinate input** from multidisciplinary team: medicine, nursing, occupational therapy, physical therapy, respiratory therapy, social services, and parents.

C. **Allows infant's primary nurse to make specific recommendations** regarding environmental modifications, positioning techniques, calming measures, and the promotion of self-quieting abilities.

STUDY QUESTIONS

1. An infant's capacity for behavioral organization is supported by:
   a. Clustering all necessary care.
   b. Providing minimal stimulation when acutely ill.
   c. Recognizing and responding to the infant's behavioral cues.

2. To quiet an upset pre-term infant, parents should be encouraged to:
   a. Leave the infant alone because he is already overstimulated.
   b. Pat the infant gently on the back while talking softly.

   c. Place their hand at the infant's feet and gently hold them close to the infant's body.

3. The infant who fatigues rapidly with the nutritive feeding process:
   a. Requires careful monitoring of physiological parameters and/or clinical indicators while nipple feeding.
   b. Should be limited to gavage feedings until stronger.
   c. Should not be given a pacifier with gavage feedings as this will increase caloric expenditure.

Answers to Study Questions

1. c
2. c
3. a

REFERENCES

Allen, T.: Patterns of academic achievement among hearing impaired students: 1974 and 1983. *In* Schildroth, A., and Karchmer, M. (eds.): Deaf Children in America. San Diego, College-Hill Press, 1986, pp. 161–206.

Als, H., Brazelton, T.B., Lester, B.M., et al.: Manual for the assessment of preterm infants' behavior (APIB). *In* Fitzgerald, H.E., Lester, B.M., and Yogman, M.W. (eds.): Theory and Research in Behavioral Pediatrics. New York, Plenum Press, 1982, pp. 65–132.

Amiel-Tison, C.: Neurological evaluation of the maturity of newborn infants. Arch. Dis. Child., 43:89–93, 1968.

Anderson, J., and Auster-Liebhaber, J.: Developmental therapy in the neonatal intensive care unit. Phys. Occupat. Ther. Pediatr., 4:89–106, 1984.

Bergman, I., Fria, T., Hirsch, R., et al.: Cause of hearing loss in the high-risk premature infant. Pediatrics, *106*:95–101, 1985.

Biber, P., Bradley, D.A., Collins, S.A., et al.: Intervention strategies to foster parent-infant interaction. *In* Creger, P. (ed.): Infant Interaction Program, Module 1: Developmental Interventions and the Special Care Infant. Denver, Children's Hospital Association, 1989.

Biber, P., Creger, P., and Kolar, D.: The promotion of positive feeding experiences. *In* Creger, P. (ed.): Infant Interaction Program, Module 6: Neurodevelopmental Assessment of Feeding Abilities and Follow-up of the Disorganized Feeder. Denver, Children's Hospital Association, 1989, pp. 7–8.

Biber, P., Creger, P., Kolar, D., et al: Developmentally supportive positioning and therapeutic handling strategies. *In* Creger, P. (ed.): Infant Interaction Program, Module 5: Developmentally Supportive Positioning and Therapeutic Handling of the Hospitalized Infant. Denver, Children's Hospital Association, 1989, pp. 11–28.

Biber, P., Creger, P., Mediavilla, K., et al.: Four basic types of hearing impairments: General implications for caregivers. *In* Creger, P. (ed.): Infant Interaction Program, Module 4: Assessment of the Auditory System and Follow-up of the Infant at Risk for Hearing Loss. Denver, Children's Hospital Association, 1989.

Bobath, B., and Bobath, K.: The neurodevelopmental approach to treatment. *In* Pearson, P., and Williams, C. (eds.): Physical Therapy Services in the Developmental Disabilities. Springfield, IL, Charles C. Thomas, 1972.

Bradley, R.N.: Development of the tastebud on gustatory papillae in human fetuses. *In* Bosma, J.F. (ed.): Third Symposium on Oral Sensation and Perception: The Mouth of the Infant. Springfield, IL, Charles C Thomas, 1972, pp. 137–162.

Bragdon, D.B.: A basis for the nursing management of feeding the premature infant. J. Obstet. Gynecol. Neonat. Nurs., 12:515–575, 1983.

Braun, M.A., and Palmer, M.M.: A pilot study of oral-motor dysfunction in "at risk" infants. Phys. Occupat. Ther. Pediatr., 5:13–25, Winter 1985/1986.

Brazelton, T.B.: Behavioral competence of the newborn infant. *In* Avery, G.B. (ed.): Neonatology: Pathophysiology and Management of the Newborn, 3rd ed. Philadelphia, J.B. Lippincott, 1987, pp. 379–399.

Connally, B.H., and Montgomery, P.C. (eds.): Therapeutic Exercise in Developmental Disabilities, 1st ed. Chattanooga, Chattanooga Corporation, 1987.

Coplan, J.: Deafness: Ever hear of it? Delayed recognition of permanent hearing loss. Pediatrics, 79:206–213, 1987.

Downs, M.P., and Silver, H.K.: The "A.B.C.D.'s" to H.E.A.R.: Early detection in nursery, office and clinic of the infant who is deaf. Clin. Pediatr., 11:563–566, 1972.

Dubignon, J.M., Campbell, D., and Patington, M.W.: The development of nonnutritive sucking in premature infants. Biol. Neonate, 14:270–278, 1969.

Fanaroff, A., and Klaus, M.: Feeding and selected disorders of the gastrointestinal tract. *In* Klaus, M., and Fanaroff, A. (eds.): Care of the High-Risk Neonate. Philadelphia, W.B. Saunders Co., 1986, pp. 113–146.

Feinmesser, M., and Tell, L.: Neonatal screening for detection of deafness. Arch. Otolaryngol., 102:297–299, 1976.

Hayes, D.: Identification and assessment of infants at risk for hearing impairment. *In* Creger, P. (ed.): Infant Interaction Program, Module 4: Assessment of the Auditory System and Follow-Up of the Infant at Risk for Hearing Loss. Denver, Children's Hospital Association, 1989, p. 29.

Heird, W., and Anderson, T.: Nutritional requirements of the low birth weight infant. *In* Behrman, R.E. (ed.): Neonatal Perinatal Medicine: Diseases of the Fetus and Infant. St. Louis, C.V. Mosby, 1977.

Humphrey, T.: Embryology of the central nervous system with some correlations with functional development. Ala. J. Med. Sci., 1:60–64, 1964.

Illingworth, R.: Sucking and swallowing difficulties in infancy: Diagnostic problem of dysphagia. Arch. Dis. Child., 44:655–665, 1969.

Logan, W.J., and Bosma, J.F.: Oral and pharyngeal dysphasia in infancy. Pediatr. Clin. North Am., 14:47–61, 1967.

Martin, R.J., Herrell, N., Rubin, D., et al.: Effect of supine and prone positions on arterial oxygen tension in the preterm infant. Pediatrics, 63:528–531, 1979.

Meier, P., and Anderson, G.C.: Responses of small preterm infants to bottle and breastfeeding. Matern. Child Nurs. J., 12:97–105, 1987.

Meier, P., and Pugh, E.J.: Breastfeeding behavior of small preterm infants. Matern. Child Nurs. J., 10:396–401, 1985.

Moeller, M., Osberger, M., and Eccarius, M.: Receptive language skills. *In* Osberger, M. (ed.): Language and Learning Skills in Hearing Impaired Students. ASHA Monogr., 23:41–53, 1986.

Moore, K.L., and Nilsson, L.: A Child is Born. New York, Dell Publishing, 1966.

Newman, L.F.: Social and sensory environment of low birth weight infants in a special care nursery. J. Nerv. Mental Dis., 169:448–455, 1981.

Osberger, M., Moeller, M., Eccarius, M., et al: Expressive language skills. *In* Osberger, M. (ed.): Language and Learning Skills of Hearing Impaired Students. ASHA Monogr., 23:54–56, 1986.

Satinoff, E., and Stanley, W.C.: Effect of stomach loading on sucking behavior in neonatal puppies. J. Comp. Physiol. Psychol., 56:66–68, 1963.

Schulman-Galambos, C., and Galambos, R.: Brainstem evoked response audiometry in newborn hearing screen. Arch. Otolaryngol., 105:86–90, 1979.

VandenBerg, K.A.: Neurodevelopmental assessment of feeding problems and interventions for the disorganized feeder in NICU and follow-up. Developmental Intervention in Neonatal Care Conference Syllabus, Developmental Interventions in Neonatal Care Conference. San Francisco, Contemporary Forums, July 1987.

VandenBerg, K.A. and Goderez, L.: Neurodevelopmental assessment of feeding problems and interventions for the disorganized feeder in NICU and follow-up, handout "Feeding Variables." Developmental Interventions in Neonatal Care Conference Syllabus, Developmental Interventions in Neonatal Care Conference. San Francisco, Contemporary Forums, July 1987.

Wolff, P.H.: The serial organization of sucking in the young infant. Pediatrics, 42:943–956, 1968.

Sharon Kuhrt
Lynn Hornick

Fetal Anomalies: Diagnosis and Management

Objectives

1. Define birth defects and possible causes.

2. Identify the number of chromosomes in a normal human cell.

3. Describe the characteristics and causes of structural and numerical chromosomal abnormalities, modes of inheritance of single gene disorders, and multifactorial inheritance.

4. Describe what prenatal diagnostic tests are available and which anomalies they detect.

5. Describe the components and benefits of genetic counseling.

6. Identify three patient care management issues in genetic counseling.

7. Verbalize the systematic process used to evaluate the malformed infant.

8. List common congenital malformations and possible mechanisms of cause.

Congenital malformations commonly have multiple causes. This chapter includes information on basic genetics, characteristics and causes of some common fetal anomalies, as well as a systematic process for evaluation of the malformed infant. Commonalities of patient care management issues are addressed, with the understanding that every family requires individualized care.

Basic Genetics

DEFINITIONS

A. **March of Dimes' definition of birth defects:** "an abnormality of structure, function or metabolism whether genetically determined or a result of environmental interference during embryonic or fetal life. A congenital defect may cause disease from the time of conception through birth or later in life."

B. **Chromosome:** structural elements in cell nucleus that carry the genes and convey genetic information.

1. Each cell (except red blood cells) in the body contains all the chromosomes received from both parents within its nucleus.
2. There are 23 pairs of chromosomes for a total of 46 chromosomes, with one maternal and one paternal chromosome creating each pair.

C. **Gene:** the smallest unit of inheritance of a single characteristic, responsible for physical, biochemical, and physiological traits and located in linear sequence along the chromosome.

D. **Genotype:** the hereditary composition of an individual.

E. **Autosome:** one of 22 chromosomes that do not determine the sex of the individual.

F. **Sex chromosomes:** the X and Y chromosomes that are responsible for sex determination—XX for female and XY for male.

G. **Diploid:** containing a set of maternal and a set of paternal chromosomes, for a total of 46 chromosomes.

H. **Gamete:** one of two cells, containing 23 chromosomes (haploid number), with the union of a male and female gamete required during sexual production to create a new individual (with diploid number of chromosomes).

I. **Haploid:** state of having half the number of chromosomes found in the person's cells; characteristic of the gametes.

J. **Locus:** the position that the gene occupies on a chromosome.

DOMINANCE AND RECESSIVENESS

A. **Phenotype:** observable characteristics of an individual.

B. **Heterogeneous chromosomes:** differing pair of chromosomes, one from each parent, arraying differing genes for specific traits. When there are unlike genes on a locus, one gene dominates.

C. **Homologous chromosomes:** a matched pair of chromosomes, one from each parent carrying the genes for the same traits.

D. **Dominant gene:** a gene that is expressed in the heterozygous state. In a dominant disorder, the mutant gene overshadows the normal gene.

E. **Recessive:** both genes of a set of homologous chromosomes at the given locus must be abnormal to show the disease. In a heterozygote (carrier), the normal gene overshadows the mutant gene.

F. **Possible combinations of chromosomes** include the following:
1. Both genes can be dominant—AA (homozygous).
2. Both genes can be recessive—aa (homozygous).
3. One gene can be dominant and one can be recessive—Aa (heterozygous).

G. **Autosomal dominant characteristics:** there are more than 1218 identified disorders.
1. Males and females are both affected equally; either parent can pass the gene on to sons or daughters.
2. An affected offspring has an affected parent if it is not a new mutation.
3. Half the sons and half the daughters of an affected parent can be anticipated to have the disorder.
4. Unaffected offspring of an affected parent will have all normal offspring if the mate is with an unaffected person (assuming complete penetrance).
5. If two affected persons mate, three-fourths of their offspring will be affected. If any of their offspring get a double dose of the mutant gene, it will result in a lethal anomaly (except in the case of Huntington's disease).
6. A positive family history with a vertical route of transmission through successive generations from one side of the family is present (if not a new mutation).
7. Examples of autosomal dominant disorders include myotonic dystrophy, neurofibromatosis, and coronary artery disease.

H. **Autosomal recessive characteristics:** there are approximately 947 identified disorders.

1. Both males and females are affected equally.
2. Parents of affected offspring are rarely affected and are usually heterozygous carriers.
3. After the birth of an affected offspring, there is a 25% chance of having another affected offspring and a 50% chance that the offspring will be a carrier.
4. There may be a distant relative with the disorder.
5. Affected persons who mate with unaffected persons will have offspring who will be heterozygous carriers.
6. If two affected persons mate, all offspring will be affected.
7. A negative family history is present—a horizontal route of transmission in the same generation.
8. Examples of autosomal recessive disorders include sickle cell anemia, Tay-Sachs disease, thalassemia major.

I. **X-linked dominant disorder characteristics:** there are 171 known disorders.

1. Both sexes can be affected, and because females have a double chance of receiving the mutant X chromosome, they have twice the risk to be affected.
2. Affected males will have all affected daughters and no affected sons.
3. Affected females transmit the disorders the same as with autosomal dominant patterns.
4. Two-thirds of the time, affected females have an affected mother and one-third of the time have an affected father.
5. A positive family history with no father-to-son transmissions.
6. Vitamin D–resistant rickets is one example.

J. **X-linked recessive disorder characteristics**.

1. Only male offspring are affected, with rare exceptions. A female offspring will be affected if she has both a carrier mother and affected father.
2. Carrier females transmit the disorder.
3. Affected males will have all normal sons.
4. Affected males will have all daughters that are carriers.
5. Heterozygous females transmit the gene to one-half their sons, who will be affected, and to one-half their daughters, who will be carriers.
6. There is a horizontal transmission among males in the same generation. There is also a skipping of generations to another group of second-generation males.
7. Examples include Duchenne's muscular dystrophy, hemophilia, color blindness, and glucose-6-phosphate dehydrogenase deficiency.

Chromosomal Defects

ABNORMAL NUMBER

A. **Polyploidy:** more than two sets of homologous chromosomes showing multiples of the haploid number.

B. **Non-multiples** are designated by the suffix "somy"—monosomy is one less than the diploid number (45), and trisomy is one more than the diploid (47).

C. **Causes**.

1. Non-disjunction: failure of separation of paired chromosomes during cell division.
2. Chromosome lag: failure of a chromosome to travel to the appropriate daughter cell.
3. Anaphase lag: chromosome lag during third state of division of a cell nucleus in meiosis/mitosis.

D. **Mosaicism:** non-disjunction of an anaphase lag that occurs during mitosis after fertilization resulting in two different cell lines in the same person.

ABNORMAL STRUCTURE

A. Deletion: loss of a chromosomal segment.

B. Translocation: the occurrence of a chromosome segment at an abnormal site, either on another chromosome or the wrong position on the same chromosome (i.e., an inversion).

C. Polygenic defects: the type of inheritance in which a trait is dependent on many different gene pairs with cumulative effects.

D. Environmental influences: inadequate nutritional intake, certain drugs, irradiation, viruses are examples that could alter the genetic makeup of an offspring while in vitro. Multifactorial—genes plus environment.

E. Basic generalizations.
1. Loss of an entire autosome is usually incompatible with life.
2. One X chromosome is necessary for life and development.
3. If the male-determining Y chromosome is missing, life and development may continue but will follow female pathways.
4. Extra entire chromosomes, the translocation of extra chromatin material, or the insertion of extra chromatin material are often compatible with life and development.
5. Multiple congenital structural defects are present when gross aberrations are present.
6. Incidence.
   a. Autosomal aberrations: 5:1000 births.
   b. Sex chromosome aberrations: 2:1000 births.
   c. 60% of spontaneous abortions are associated with chromosomal aberration.

Prenatal Diagnosis

ADVANTAGES

A. Knowledge that the fetus is unaffected.

B. Time to explore options and prepare for an affected newborn.

C. Opportunity electively to abort an affected fetus.

MATERNAL SERUM ALPHA-FETOPROTEIN (MSAFP)

A. Screening test done at 16–18 weeks' gestation for amount of protein produced by fetus that normally is found in amniotic fluid. Smaller amounts that normally cross the placenta and enter the mother's blood. This test is uninterpretable after 22 weeks' gestation.

B. Preparation: explain to client that this is a screening test, *not* a diagnostic test. Explain that an abnormal result does not indicate an abnormality, but will indicate the possible need for a diagnostic test to rule out abnormalities.

C. Reasons for high MSAFP (≥ 2 multiples of the median).
1. Greater gestational age than expected (incorrect due date).
2. Multiple gestation.
3. Risk of fetal complications, including spontaneous abortion, premature labor, or baby who will not attain full birthweight.
4. Fetal structural defect: neural tube, abdominal wall, esophageal or intestinal obstructions, or renal anomalies.
5. Undetermined reason with subsequent normal outcome of newborn.

D. Reasons for low MSAFP (≤ 0.5 multiples of the median).
1. Less gestational age than expected (incorrect due date).
2. Chromosomal birth defect, Down syndrome being the most common.

3. Undetermined reason with subsequent normal outcome of newborn.

E. **If the MSAFP is abnormal**, perform an ultrasound to confirm estimated gestational age and assess for anomalies.

F. **If gestational age was overestimated or underestimated**, recalculate MSAFP based on corrected age; provide client with preliminary revised due date and the recalculated MSAFP. Reschedule follow-up ultrasound in 2–3 weeks to confirm new due date.

G. **If gestational age confirmed by ultrasound, subsequent to a high MSAFP**, repeat the MSAFP, schedule genetic counseling, and offer amniocentesis for fetal chromosomes, amniotic fluid alpha$_1$-fetoprotein, (AFP) and acetylcholinesterase (ACHE).

H. **If gestational age is confirmed by ultrasound, subsequent to a low MSAFP**, schedule genetic counseling and offer client amniocentesis for chromosomes and AFP. This ultrasound should include Down screening for frontal lobe findings, mild ventriculomegaly, nuchal edema, cardiac defects, mild renal pelvis dilatation, and abnormalities of the fetal hand.

ULTRASOUND

A. **Ultrasound preparation:** explain to the client that a transducer coated with ultrasonic gel will be placed on her abdomen, using high-frequency sound waves to display sectional planes of the uterine contents on a monitor. Explain that an ultrasound cannot detect all anomalies and cannot guarantee the outcome of the fetus.

B. **Initial assessment:** is recommended to occur by 16–20 weeks for gestational age verification and evaluation.

C. **Ultrasonographer** (trained expert) can detect abnormalities of fetus, placenta, amniotic fluid, and uterus and can monitor changes in anatomy and growth with serial ultrasounds.

D. **Diagnostic capability** only as good as the person's training, not just contingent on the equipment.

E. **No known harmful effects**.

F. **Critical to safety of amniocentesis:** chorionic villus sampling and percutaneous blood sampling.

G. **Anatomical landmarks** commonly observed: fetal spine, kidneys, bladder, stomach, three-vessel cord, cord insertion, four-chambered heart, face, upper lip, biparietal diameter, head circumference, abdominal circumference, femur length, transcerebellar diameter, placenta, amount of amniotic fluid, uterus, and adnexa.

H. **Detectable anomalies are many**, including those indicative of various syndromes.
1. Examples: Anencephaly, atrial septal defect, cardiac anomalies, choroid plexus cyst, cleft lip, craniosynostosis, cystic hygroma, cystic kidneys, encephalocele, gastroschisis, hydrocephalus, microcephaly, myelomeningocele, omphalocele, skeletal dysplasia.

I. **If an anomaly is identified** during the ultrasound, point it out on the monitor to the client, explaining its implications. Initiate grief counseling and discuss options.

AMNIOCENTESIS (AMNIO)

A. **Removal of 10–30 cc of amniotic fluid** through a needle placed into the woman's abdomen, for the purpose of chromosomal analysis and other biochemical tests as indicated.

B. Preparation: Review risks and benefits of the procedure, discuss options based on current information, and arrange to obtain amnio results. Explain that normal results from an amnio do not guarantee a good fetal outcome. Obtain written consent for this procedure. Obtain client's blood type prior to procedure. If she is Rh negative, obtain father's blood type.

C. 16–18 gestational weeks is usual timing of procedure, but amnio can be performed at later gestation and as early as 14 weeks.

D. Indications include the following:
1. Woman of advanced maternal age (≥35 at time of expected delivery).
2. Previous fetus with Down syndrome.
3. Previous fetus with a neural tube defect.
4. Both parents are known heterozygous carriers for autosomal recessive chromosome.
5. Both parents are known carriers of a sex-linked recessive disorder.
6. Client or partner has a balanced chromosomal translocation of his or her chromosomes.
7. High or low MSAFP with accurate gestational age.

E. Fluid analysis requires 2–3 weeks for cells to grow adequately for accurate analysis.

F. Risks: overall risk to mother or fetus is 1%.
1. Spontaneous abortion occurs in approximately 0.5% of cases.
2. Hemorrhage.
3. Infection.
4. Premature labor.
5. Rh sensitization from fetal bleeding into maternal circulation.
6. Trauma to fetus or placenta.

G. Analysis
1. Fetal sex is determined through special staining techniques, karyotype, or amniotic fluid testosterone levels, providing risk information for X-linked disorder.
2. Alpha-fetoprotein: abnormally high or low levels are concerning (see earlier section on MSAFP).
3. Biochemical: metabolism disorders can be discovered by 20 weeks' gestation, including Tay-Sachs disease (a lipid disorder) and amino acid, carbohydrate, and mucopolysaccharide metabolism disorders.
4. Chromosomes: abnormalities, including Down syndrome, other trisomies, and other chromosomal abnormalities, can be detected at 16 weeks' gestation by a karyotype.

H. Post-amniocentesis care.
1. Assess fetal heart activity.
2. Cleanse insertion site and apply bandage.
3. Instruct client to rest for 24 hours, to include lifting of no more than 10 pounds and no straining.
4. Administer RHOgam if client is Rh negative and father of the fetus is either Rh positive or of unknown blood type. Do not give RHOgam if Rh sensitized.
5. When results are available, explain their implications.

CHORIONIC VILLUS SAMPLING (CVS)

A. Transvaginal or transabdominal sampling of the chorionic villi to obtain fetal cells for the purpose of chromosomal analysis and other biochemical tests. It cannot identify neural tube defects.

B. Preparation: Review risks and benefits of the procedure, discuss options, and arrange to obtain CVS results. Obtain written consent for this procedure.

C. 8–10 weeks' gestation is usual timing of procedure.

D. Indications.
1. Client prefers to make decisions regarding pregnancy in first trimester.
2. Severe oligohydramnios.

E. Contraindications.
1. Multiple gestation.
2. Uterine bleeding during this pregnancy.
3. Active genital herpes infection or other cervical infection.
4. Uterine fibroids.

F. Fetal cell analysis requires 24–48 hours for initial results.

G. Risks overall 2–3%.
1. Infection.
2. Bleeding.
3. Cervical lacerations.
4. Miscarriage 1–5%.

H. Vaginal CVS: catheter is inserted through the vagina and cervix into the chorion outer tissue of the embryonic sac, and a tiny amount of the chorionic villi is aspirated by suction or cut with forceps.

I. Abdominal CVS: needle is inserted through the abdomen into the chorion to obtain the chorionic villus sample.

J. Post-CVS care.
1. Same recommendations as the amniocentesis care.
2. Nothing in the vagina (tampon, douche, intercourse) for 24 hours.
3. If transvaginal sample, apply sanitary napkins as needed for 24–48 hours.

PERCUTANEOUS UMBILICAL BLOOD SAMPLING (PUBS)

A. Removal of fetal blood through a needle placed into the woman's abdomen and into the umbilical vein.

B. Preparation: Same as that recommended for CVS.

C. 18 weeks to term.

D. Indications.
1. Client wants fast results to support her decision making regarding pregnancy.
2. Abnormality identified by ultrasound late in pregnancy.
3. Exposed to infectious disease that could affect development of the fetus.
4. Blood incompatibility (Rh disease).
5. A drug or chemical level in the fetal blood needs to be assessed.

E. Risks.
1. Same as amnio: infection, bleeding, isoimmunization, miscarriage, trauma to the fetus for overall 1–5% risk factor.
2. Perforation of uterine arteries, clotting in fetal cord.
3. Premature delivery.

F. Fetal blood analysis takes 3 days.

G. Post-PUBS care.
1. Same as amnio care.

GENETIC COUNSELING

A. Definition by the Ad Hoc Committee on Genetic Counseling: a communication process that deals with the human problems associated with the occurrence or the risk of occurrence of genetic disorders in a family. This process involves collaboration of multiple disciplines (physician, ultrasonographer, nurse, genetic counselor, social worker, neonatologist, and pediatric specialty services as indicated) for family support.

B. **Principles of genetic counseling**.
1. Based on correct diagnosis and pattern of inheritance.
2. Non-directive.
3. Reinforcement of information.
4. Communication with the primary care physician.

C. **Indications**.
1. Previously affected child, parent, grandparent.
   a. Congenital malformation.
   b. Sensory defect.
   c. Metabolic disorder.
   d. Mental retardation.
   e. Known or suspected chromosome abnormality.
   f. Neuromuscular disorder.
   g. Degenerative CNS disease.
2. Previous affected cousins.
   a. Muscular dystrophy.
   b. Hemophilia.
   c. Hydrocephalus.
3. Cousin marriages.
4. Hazards of ionizing radiation.
5. Recurrent miscarriages.
6. Concern for teratogenic effect.
7. Advanced maternal age.
8. High or low MSAFP.

D. **Methods**.
1. Questionnaire.
2. Pedigree.
3. Medical records.
4. Physical exam.
5. Laboratory tests.
6. Carrier detection.

E. **Provide medical facts** with differential diagnosis and risks to fetus and mother; probable course of the disorder; recommended management for prenatal course; type and timing of delivery; neonatal, pediatric and long-term care requirements.

F. **Explain hereditary factors** that contribute to the disorder.

G. **Discuss with parents** all alternatives.
1. Home care of newborn.
2. Institutionalization.
3. Adoption.
4. Appropriate method of termination for the gestational age.
5. Provide only objective information regarding fetus/newborn status. Provide statistical risk factors as they relate to this individual fetus.
6. Identify which normal characteristics can exist in the affected fetus, and point these out in pictures to promote awareness of total condition of fetus.
7. Assist parents to understand causes, risks of recurrence, and limits of current treatments.
8. Discuss options available for dealing with risk of recurrence.
9. Provide parents with written information and support groups.
10. Explain recommended obstetrical care, mode and timing of delivery and newborn care.

Newborn Care Management

DIAGNOSIS

A. **A complete diagnosis** is important in planning care. Consideration for the infant's overall problems, in addition to the defect, is essential.

PREVENT PHYSICAL PROBLEMS

A. **Respiratory problems**.
1. Teach percussion and postural drainage.
2. Emphasize importance of infant's position.
3. Promote use of cool-mist vaporizer.
4. Instruct suctioning of nose.
5. Promote good mouth care.

B. **Feeding difficulties in the newborn**.
1. Provide small, frequent feeding schedule.
2. Stress that tongue thrust does not indicate refusal of food.
3. Calculate caloric needs on height and weight, not chronological age.

Evaluation of the Malformed Infant

EVALUATE HISTORY

A. **Family history**.
1. Record three generations of history.
2. Be aware of defects in the family history related to the problem in the child.
3. Medical records and/or photos of similarly affected relatives.
4. History of consanguinity.
5. Reproductive history, such as frequent spontaneous abortions.
6. Look for patterns of inheritance of the problems.

B. **Prenatal history**.
1. Length of gestation.
2. Fetal activity level.
3. Maternal exposures: to infections, illness, high fevers, medications, x-ray examinations, known teratogens, alcohol, smoking, street drugs.
4. Obstetrical factors: uterine malformations, complications of labor, presenting fetal part.
5. Neonatal factors: birthweight, length, head circumference, Apgar scores.

C. **Systematically conduct a physical exam** of the infant.
1. Face: observe for configuration, centered features with normal spacing, round, triangular, flat, bird-like, elfin, coarse, or expressionless characteristics.
2. Head: assess size of anterior fontanel, third ventricle, prominence of frontal bone, flattened or prominent occiput, abnormalities in shape (proportionally large or small).
3. Eyes: structure and color of iris, centering and spacing of epicanthal folds (hypotelorism or hypertelorism), slanting, eyelash length.
4. Ears: protruding or prominent shape, location, low set, unilateral or bilateral defect.
5. Nose: beaked, bulbous, pinched, upturned, misshapen, two nares, flattened bridge, patency, centered on face.
6. Oral: natal teeth; shape and size of tongue, mouth, jaw.
7. Neck: short and/or webbed, redundant folds.
8. Hands and feet: broad, square, or spade-like shape, polydactyly, clinodactyly,

syndactyly, abnormal creases in the palm of the hand (simian or sydney creases), contractures, abnormally large or small, over-riding fingers, proximally placed thumb.

D. Consider causation of defect.
1. Identify the primary abnormality.
2. Recognize etiological heterogeneity (a defect having more than one cause).
3. Determine category of congenital malformation, according to its etiology.
   a. Malformation: poor formation of tissue may be caused by chromosomal disorders and single gene disorders.
   b. Deformation: unusual force on normal tissue may be caused by intrauterine constraint.
   c. Disruption: breakdown of normal tissue may be caused by amniotic bands, vascular accidents, infections.

E. Family care management for all genetic syndromes or disorders.
1. Grief counseling: acknowledge short- and long-term grief, promote awareness that each of the parents may be in a different stage of grief process, creating additional stress. Recommend that parents communicate their needs to each other and ask for support when needed.
2. Genetic counseling.
3. Facilitate family use of support systems: social services, Aid to Families with Dependent Children, Women-Infant-Children (WIC) program, March of Dimes, clergy, mental health services, support groups.
4. Provide unconditional emotional support. Allow parents and siblings to verbalize feelings.
5. Identify normal aspects of newborn that can co-exist with the syndrome or disorder.
6. Promote parent involvement in care. Offer choices in care and interventions.
7. Discuss treatment options, their risks, benefits.
8. Provide literature.
9. Obtain legal and ethical counsel when parents prefer not to pursue medical interventions.

Beckwith-Wiedemann Syndrome

ETIOLOGY AND PRECIPITATING FACTORS

A. Unknown.
B. 60% are females.

INCIDENCE

A. 100 cases have been reported.

CLINICAL PRESENTATION

A. Large muscle mass with subcutaneous tissue and birthweight greater than 3200 g.
B. Head: microcephaly.
1. Prominent occiput.
2. Large fontanel.
3. Malocclusion with mandibular prognathism (projection forward of the jaw).
4. Unusual linear fissures in lobe of external ear.
   e. Prominent eyes.
   f. Strabismus.
C. Omphalocele or other umbilical anomaly.

D. Cryptorchidism.

E. Large tongue.

F. Other major manifestations.

1. Accelerated osseous maturation.
2. Mild to moderate mental deficiency; can be of normal intelligence.
3. Large kidneys with renal medullary dysplasia.
4. Pancreatic hyperplasia.
5. Fetal adrenocortical cytomegaly.
6. Interstitial cell hyperplasia.
7. Pituitary hyperplasia.
8. Neonatal polycythemia.
9. Hypoglycemia usually after the first day of life.

G. Care management.

1. Facilitate feeding with use of a large, soft nipple.
2. Place infant on side to facilitate breathing; may need oral airway.
3. Treat hypoglycemia.
4. Consider partial exchange for polycythemia greater than 65%.

H. Complications and outcome.

1. Hypoglycemia may be severe enough to cause death or slow development.
2. Feeding difficulties due to large tongue.
3. Polycythemia.
4. Pneumonia.
5. Individuals who survive infancy are healthy.

Cleft Lip and Palate

ETIOLOGY AND PRECIPITATING FACTORS

A. Defective development of embryonic primary palate may cause clefts of the lip and anterior maxilla.

B. Defective development of the embryonic secondary palate may cause clefts of the hard and soft palate and often appear in persons with cleft lip.

C. There are at least 50 recognized syndromes that involve cleft lip and/or palate as a characteristic.

D. Cleft lip and/or palate may be caused by mutant genes, chromosomal aberrations, teratogen, or multifactorial inheritance.

INCIDENCE

A. Cleft lip and/or palate.

1. 1:1000 births in Caucasian population.
2. 2:1000 births in Japan.
3. 0.5:1000 births for American blacks.
4. About twice as frequent in males than females.
5. Associated with phenytoin (Dilantin) use during pregnancy.

CLEFT PALATE

A. 1:2500 births.

B. More often in females than males.

C. Clinical presentation.

1. Cleft lip with or without cleft palate is usually apparent at birth.
2. There may be variations in the degree of the malformations.
3. Cleft lip may be unilateral or bilateral.

4. If cleft lip is unilateral, two-thirds are on the left side.
5. If cleft lip is bilateral, it is often accompanied by a cleft palate.
6. Varying degrees of nasal distortion with deformed or absent teeth may be present.
7. Cleft palate may occur as a single defect and is less apparent at birth.
8. Assessment can be made by placing the examiner's fingers on the palate.
9. Infant may have difficulty in feeding due to the inability to create suction.

COMPLICATIONS AND OUTCOME

A. **Upper respiratory infections** and recurrent otitis media due to inefficient function of the eustachian tube may result in impaired hearing.

B. **Impaired social adjustment** can be minimized if surgery is successful.

C. **Impaired speech and hearing.**

D. **Aspiration.**

E. **Orthodontic problems.**

F. **Good outcome** with surgical correction.

CARE MANAGEMENT

A. **Feeding:** special nipples such as lamb's nipple, medicine droppers, or spoon feeding may be indicated.

B. **Post-operative care.**
1. Prevent trauma to suture line.
   a. Position in car seat or on back.
   b. Restrain arms with elbow restraints.
   c. Discourage from sucking.
2. Prevent infection.
   a. Rinse mouth after feedings.
   b. Gently cleanse suture line.
   c. Apply antibiotic ointment or light mineral oil.
3. Facilitate airway.
   a. Suction gently.
   b. Elevate head of bed.
4. Provide adequate nutritional intake.
5. Provide comfort measures to avoid stress on suture line for general infant comfort.
6. Teach parents postoperative and continued care to minimize long-term complications.
7. Speech therapy.

Cornelia de Lange Syndrome

ETIOLOGY AND PRECIPITATING FACTORS

A. Unknown.

INCIDENCE

A. 1:150,000 births.

CLINICAL PRESENTATION AND PHYSICAL EXAM

A. **Very small in stature**, not due to skeletal dysplasia.

B. **Irregular hairline.**

C. Narrow forehead.

D. Thick eyebrows meeting midline.

E. Long eyelashes.

F. Flat nasal bridge.

G. Short, upturned nose with anteverted nares.

H. Prominent philtrum.

I. Small mandible.

J. Short, tapering extremities.

K. Short, tapering digits with incurved fifth finger.

L. Hirsutism.

M. Congenital heart disease.

N. Microcephaly.

O. Growling cry.

COMPLICATIONS AND OUTCOME

A. Aspiration in infancy.

B. Increased susceptibility to infections.

C. Failure to thrive.

D. Many die during infancy due to poor feeding and growth.

E. Survivors usually have severe mental defects.

Craniosynostosis (premature closure of sutures)

ETIOLOGY AND PRECIPITATING FACTORS

A. Unknown.

INCIDENCE

A. 0.4–1:1000 births.

CLINICAL PRESENTATION

A. Premature stenosis of the sagittal suture is the most common form (50% of all cases).

B. Some or all of the sutures are closed.

COMPLICATIONS AND OUTCOME

A. Increased cerebral pressure.

B. Retardation and significant facial and cranial distortion and asymmetry may occur.

C. Good outcome if corrected early in infancy.

CARE MANAGEMENT

A. Surgical intervention may be indicated, with preoperative and postoperative teaching.

Crouzon Syndrome

ETIOLOGY AND PRECIPITATING FACTORS

A. Autosomal dominant.

INCIDENCE

A. Unknown.

CLINICAL PRESENTATION

A. Ocular proptosis due to shallow orbits.

B. May have divergent strabismus, hypertelorism.

C. Hypoplasia of maxilla.

D. May have curved, parrot-like nose.

E. Craniosynostosis of coronal, lambdoid, and sagittal sutures leading to a short anterior, posterior, and wide lateral dimensions of the cranium.

COMPLICATIONS AND OUTCOME

A. May lead a normal life.

PATIENT CARE MANAGEMENT

A. Provide emotional support for patients.

B. May have surgery if craniosynostosis is present with increased intracranial pressure.

Trisomies

TRISOMY 21

A. Incidence and etiology.
1. Maternal age

(yr)	Incidence
15–29	1 : 1500
30–34	1 : 800
35–39	1 : 270
40–44	1 : 100
>45	1 : 50

2. Accounts for 15–20% of severe mental retardation cases.
3. Risk increases with maternal age.
4. 25% of Down syndrome infants receive an extra chromosome from their father.
5. 47 chromosomes.
6. Extra chromosome fits into group G 21, 22.
7. Extra chromosome results from nondisjunction during meiosis.
8. Non-disjunction occurs as a more frequent accident in aging laboratory subjects than in young.
9. May occur unrelated to mother's age and appear as:
   a. 46 chromosomes.
   b. Translocation of chromosome 21.
   c. Familial transmission is autosomal dominant.

     d. No abnormalities if they are balanced. There is one 21 and one 14 chromosome.

     e. Balanced carriers may produce unbalanced gametes and should consider prenatal diagnosis.

10. There have been reported infants who are mosaics for trisomy 21 or translocation 14/21 or 21/22.

     a. Some have all of the defects.

     b. Some have only a few of the defects.

     c. Some of this group may have normal intellectual ability.

11. Clinical presentation defects that may be present.

     a. Size: small; 20% are premature.

     b. Skull: short and round with a flat occiput.

     c. Eyes: slant upward and outward.

     d. Prominent epicanthal fold.

     e. Flat face.

     f. Brushfield's spots present (iris may be speckled with ring of round, grayish spots in light-colored eyes).

     g. Cheeks: red.

     h. Palate: narrow and short.

     i. Nose: short with flat bridge.

     j. Tongue: protrudes; can become dry and wrinkled.

     k. Skin: loose around lateral and dorsal aspects of neck.

     l. Hands.

        (1) Fingers are short.

        (2) Hands appear square.

        (3) Thumb is low set, separated more than usual from the second finger.

        (4) Fifth finger is short and curves inward.

        (5) Single or bilateral simian crease (present in 40% of Down syndrome).

     m. Umbilicus: herniated.

     n. Feet.

        (1) Wide space between great and second toe.

        (2) Deep crease that starts between the great toe and the second toe and curves to the medial edge of the sole.

     o. Muscular hypotonia.

     p. Narrow acetabular angle.

     q. Narrow iliac index.

     r. Broadened iliac bones.

     s. Retarded psychomotor development.

     t. Heart: 50% have a ventricular septal defect or other congenital heart defects.

     u. Duodenal atresia.

B. **Complications and outcome.**

1. Congestive heart failure due to congenital heart disease.

2. Upper respiratory tract infections.

3. Developmentally delayed.

4. Mildly to severely mentally retarded, IQ ranges from 25 to 70.

TRISOMY 18

A. **Etiology and precipitating factors.**

1. Non-disjunction most frequent, but may have partial trisomy, translocation, or mosaicism.

2. Advanced parental age.

B. **Incidence.**

1. 1:3500 births.

C. **Clinical presentation:** numbers 1–7 below appear in most cases. Numbers 8–14 below may also appear.

1. Weight: low birth weight in term infant.
2. Ears: low set and/or abnormal shape.
3. Micrognathia and microstomia.
4. Mental retardation.
5. Hands.
   a. Clenched hand with flexed fingers.
   b. Flexion contraction of the two middle digits.
   c. Underfolded thumb.
6. Heart: usually ventricular septal defect with patent ductus arteriosus.
7. Feet: rocker bottom.
8. Eyes: ptosis of one or both eyelids.
9. Syndactyly.
10. Head: abnormally prominent occiput.
11. Genitourinary defects.
12. Hernias.
13. Simian crease appears in 25%.
14. Arches on seven or more fingers in 80% of cases.

D. Complications and outcome.
1. 30% die within 2 months of birth, usually from heart failure.
2. 10% survive the first year with severe mental retardation.

E. Care management.
1. No treatment beyond supportive care.
2. Gavage feeding as needed for poor feeding.
3. Oxygen as needed for respiratory distress.

TRISOMY 13

A. Incidence and etiology.
1. Unknown: may be related to older maternal age.
2. 1:5000 births.

B. Clinical presentation.
1. Psychomotor retardation.
2. Ears: malformed.
3. Hands: flexion deformities of hand, fingers, and wrist; postaxial polydactyly.
4. Heart: usually ventricular septal defect, patent ductus arteriosus, or rotational anomalies such as dextroposition.
5. Feet: rocker bottom.
6. Simian creases.
7. Eye: microphthalmos, colobomata of iris, cataracts.
8. Nose: broad and flattened, cleft lip and palate.
9. Umbilicus: hernia, omphalocele.
10. Genitalia.
    a. Female: bicornate or septate uterus.
    b. Male: cryptorchidism, small scrotum with anterior placement.
11. Kidneys: polycystic.
12. Cutaneous hemangiomas.
13. Brain: gross defects, grand mal seizures, myoclonic jerks.
14. Hematological abnormalities such as increased frequency of nuclear projections in neutrophils and/or persistence of embryonic and/or fetal-type hemoglobin.

C. Complications and outcome.
1. 44% die within the first month.
2. 18% survive the first year.
3. Severe mental retardation.

D. Care management.
1. No treatment beyond supportive care.

Turner's Syndrome

ETIOLOGY AND PRECIPITATING FACTORS

A. **Chromosomal aberration:** absence of the X chromosomes caused by non-disjunction resulting in 45 chromosomes.

B. **Incidence.**
1. 1:5000.

C. **Clinical presentation** and physical exam.
1. Short stature, mean birth weight 2900 g.
2. Webbed neck.
3. Low posterior hairline.
4. Micrognathia.
5. Low-set and sometimes malformed ears.
6. Widely spaced hypoplastic nipples on a shield-shaped chest.
7. Increased carrying angle at the elbow.
8. Cardiac anomalies: coarctation of the aorta or aortic valvular stenosis.
9. Learning difficulties: intelligence is normal.
10. Abnormal growth patterns.
11. Congenital lymphedema of hands and feet.
12. Broad nasal bridge.
13. Ptosis of the eyelids.
14. Epicanthal folds.
15. Lack of secondary sexual characteristics.
16. Gonadal dysplasia.
17. Horseshoe kidney.
18. Unilateral renal agenesis.

D. **Complications and outcome.**
1. Most raised as females with good outcome despite failure of sexual development.

E. **Care management.**
1. Estrogen treatment.
2. Counseling and psychiatric support.

Vater Association

ETIOLOGY AND PRECIPITATING FACTORS

A. Unknown.

INCIDENCE

A. Unknown.

CLINICAL PRESENTATION

A. **Three or more of the following defects** are present.
1. Vertebral anomalies.
2. Ventricular septal defects or other cardiac defects.
3. Anal atresia with or without fistula.
4. Tracheoesophageal fistula with esophageal atresia.
5. Radial dysplasia including thumb or radial hypoplasia, polydactyly, syndactyly.
6. Renal anomaly.
7. Single umbilical artery.

COMPLICATIONS AND OUTCOME
A. Failure to thrive.

B. May lead normal life after slow mental development during infancy.

CARE MANAGEMENT
A. Postoperative care.

STUDY QUESTIONS

1. The March of Dimes' definition of birth defects states:
   a. All abnormalities of structure, function or metabolism only due to genetic disorders
   b. An abnormality of structure, function or metabolism whether genetically determined or a result of environmental interference during embryonic or fetal life
   c. An environmental interference or a genetic disorder that only affects structure

2. The correct number of chromosomes in a normal human cell is:
   a. 23
   b. 43
   c. 46

3. If there is an autosomal-dominant disorder present, the following will apply to the affected parent:
   a. Half the sons and half the daughters can be anticipated to have the disorder
   b. Offspring will always be male
   c. There is usually a positive family history with a horizontal route of transmission

4. If two persons with the same autosomal-recessive disorder mate, their offspring will be:
   a. Affected 50% of the time
   b. Always affected
   c. Never affected

5. Chromosomal defects can be a result of an abnormal number of chromosomes. Multiples is (are):
   a. A term for pairs of chromosomes
   b. Called polyploidy and are multiples of the haploid number

   c. Called polyploidy and are multiples of the diploid number

6. Trisomy means the number of chromosomes are:
   a. One more than the diploid number
   b. Multiple of the haploid number
   c. Multiple of the diploid number

7. Amniocentesis is the removal of amniotic fluid for study. Types of disorders that can be detected are:
   a. Biochemical disorders
   b. Cardiac anomalies
   c. Hydrocephalus

8. The purpose of genetic counseling is:
   a. For research studies on genetic defects
   b. To help people to make responsible decisions concerning reproduction
   c. To provide support to married couples who would like to divorce after having an infant with a defect

9. When considering patient care management issues:
   a. Consideration for the infant's overall problems and not just defect is essential
   b. Parents do not usually need any support
   c. Try to isolate each defect

10. What steps should be taken when evaluating a malformed infant:
    a. Evaluate family and prenatal history and systematically conduct a physical exam of the infant
    b. Systematically conduct a physical exam of the infant
    c. Evaluate family history and conduct a physical exam of the infant

Answers to Study Questions

1. b	5. b	8. b
2. c	6. a	9. a
3. a	7. a	10. a
4. b		

BIBLIOGRAPHY

Avery, G.: Neonatology, Pathophysiology and Management of the Newborn, 3rd ed. Philadelphia, J.B. Lippincott, 1987.

Avery, M.: Schaffer's Diseases of the Newborn, 6th ed. Philadelphia, W.B. Saunders Co., 1991.

Blatt, R.: Prenatal Tests. New York, Vintage Books, 1988.

Cunningham, F., MacDonald, P., Grant, N.: Williams Obstetrics, 18th ed. Norwalk, CT/San Mateo, CA, Appleton & Lange, 1989.

Goodman, R., and Gorlin, R.: The Malformed Infant and Child. New York, Oxford University Press, 1983.

Jones, K.: Smith's Recognizable Patterns of Human Malformation, 4th ed. Philadelphia, W.B. Saunders Co., 1988.

McAteer, J.: Inherited disorders and counseling families with inherited disorders. *In* Streeter, N. (ed.): High Risk Neonatal Care. Rockville, MD, Aspen Publications, 1986, pp. 451–474.

National Genetics Foundation: Clinical Genetics Handbook. Oradell, NJ: Medical Economics Books, 1987.

Nyhan, W., and Sakati, N.: Diagnostic Recognition of Genetic Disease. Philadelphia, Lea & Febiger, 1987.

Romero, R., Pilu, G., Jeanty, P. et al.: Prenatal Diagnosis of Congenital Anomalies. Norwalk, CT/San Mateo, CA, Appleton & Lange, 1988.

Scipien, G., Barnard, M., Chard, M., et al.: Comprehensive Pediatric Nursing. New York, McGraw-Hill, 1975.

Spranger, J., Benirschke, K., Hall, J., et al.: Errors of morphogenesis: Concepts and terms. J. Pediatr. *100*(1):160–165, 1982.

Whaley, L., and Wong, D.: Nursing Care of Infants and Children. St. Louis, C.V. Mosby, 1987.

Williams, J.: Evaluating the dysmorphic child. Pediatr. Nurs., *9*(4):241–248, 1983.

Leann Sterk

Neonatal Orthopedic Conditions

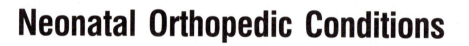

Objectives

1. Discuss perinatal factors that may place the child at risk for development of orthopedic abnormalities.

2. Demonstrate awareness of need for accurate, comprehensive orthopedic assessment.

3. Identify common neonatal orthopedic conditions and assessment and interventions of those conditions.

Development and maturation of the musculoskeletal system is an ongoing and complex process. Abnormalities within the system range from minor to devastating. Accurate assessment, treatment, and referral are essential if maximal outcome for the child and family is to occur.

Skeletal System

A. **Axial skeleton:** head and trunk.
1. Formation begins with 4th gestational week.
2. Consists of vertebral column, sternum, ribs, and skull.
B. **Appendicular skeleton:** limb bones, pelvic and pectoral girdles.
1. Limb formation proceeds within 4th gestational week.
2. Limbs develop from outpouching of the embryonic wall and proceed proximal to distal.
3. Developmental progression: buds to paddles to plates to digital rays to digits.
4. Position and attitude of extremities change with developmental stages: close anatomical approximation if present by week 8.
C. **Joints.**
1. Three types of joints identified: synovial, hyaline, fibrous.
2. Joints develop from mesenchymal cells found between developing bone.

Muscular System

A. **Joints develop from intra-embryonic mesoderm**. Progressive differentiation of mesoderm yields myoblast; end result is specialized muscle groups.
1. Skeletal muscle: striated voluntary muscle develops from myofibrils, myofilaments, and other cytoplasmic organelles.
2. Smooth muscle: nonstriated involuntary muscle develops from myofibrils; form sheets and bundles of smooth muscle.
3. Cardiac muscle: striated involuntary muscle develops from myofibrils.

Clinical Assessment

A normal uterine environment is vital to the development of the fetus. Any event that negatively changes the environment can affect normal orthopedic development and function. The fetus may be exposed to conditions that alter growth, positioning, and movement in utero and may risk harm in passage to extrauterine life. The fetus may also be exposed via the placenta to nearly all drugs taken by the mother that exert a systemic effect. These events can have lasting orthopedic consequences. Obtaining a comprehensive history is vital to the understanding of possible cause-and-effect relationships.

A. **Perinatal factors**.
1. Abnormal ultrasound findings: altered growth patterns.
2. Bleeding during pregnancy.
3. Exposure to teratogenic agents: irradiation, drugs.
4. Fetal position: breech.
5. Infection: type, course, treatment received.
6. Oligohydramnios.
7. Pattern of fetal movement.
8. Traumatic delivery, birth asphyxia.

B. **Family history**.
1. Familial musculoskeletal disorders.
2. Maternal uterine abnormalities.

C. **Medication history.**
1. Current use of sedatives, anticonvulsants, neuromuscular agents.
2. Maternal exposure to recreational drugs, alcohol, tranquilizers, anticonvulsants.

D. **Physical exam.**
1. Assessment achieved through inspection, palpation, and auscultation.
   a. General assessment of position, body symmetry, range of motion, level of alertness, and responsiveness.
   b. Accurate measurements of length and occipital and frontal circumferences.
2. Systems assessment.
   a. Head and neck.
      (1) Skull: configuration, proportion, fontanelles, suture lines.
      (2) Neck: shape, proportion, range of motion, body abnormalities, webbing, excessive skin.
   b. Trunk and spine.
      (1) Anterior chest.
         (a) Chest: symmetrical appearance and movement; number of and placement of nipples; masses.
         (b) Abnormal musculature: prune belly.
         (c) Abnormal umbilical cord: appearance, insertion, number of vessels, anomalies such as gastroschisis or herniation.
      (2) Posterior chest.

(a) Spinal curvature: scoliosis, kyphosis, lordosis.
(b) Trunk: symmetrical passive flexion, extension, and lateral bending.
(c) Rib cage: shape, obvious bony deformities.
(3) Upper extremities.
(a) Limbs: present, complete, equal length, amputations.
(b) Clavicles: inspected for size, contour, masses, fractures.
(c) Spontaneous movement: fingers, wrists, elbows, and shoulders; contractures.
(d) Bones: number, contour, size.
(e) Hands: shape, size, posture, number of digits.
(f) Nails: shape, presence, surface defects.
(g) Skin: palmar creases, finger loops, whorls, ridges.
(4) Lower extremities.
(a) Limbs: present, complete, equal length, symmetrical, amputations.
(b) Bones: number, contour, size; fractures, dysplasia, absence syndromes.
(c) Spontaneous movement: feet, ankles, hips; birth injuries, fractures.
(d) Passive movement: feet, ankles, hips; contractures, reflexes normal.
(e) Knees: contour, presence, range of motion, location of patella.
(f) Ankles and feet: range of motion, spontaneous movement.
(g) Digits: number, size, spacing, sole creases, amputations.
(h) Fore and hind foot: range of motion — equinovarus deformity.

Pathological Conditions

A. **Limb abnormalities** originate within critical embryonic period days 22–24. Expression of abnormality dependent on timing within this period. Amelia occurs during week 4. Meromelia occurs during weeks 5 and 6.

B. **Etiology and precipitating factors.**
1. Minor limb abnormalities common, defects usually correctable. May serve as an indicator of more serious abnormalities.
2. Causes linked to genetic, environmental, or chromosomal factors or a combination.

C. **Polydactyly**: presence of more than ordinary number of digits.
1. Present in otherwise normal infants. Extra digits often incompletely formed, lack usual muscular development, and often useless. Border digits frequently involved.
2. Inherited as a dominant trait: stimulus causes limb bud duplications.
3. Physical exam reveals variety of defects: soft-tissue only, partial duplication of digit, or complete duplication.
4. Radiological studies valuable to delineate bone structure, especially if webbing or fusion of digits exists.
5. Intervention: surgical removal of extra digit. Removal dependent on digit attachment and vascular involvement.
6. Complications: limited to cosmetic or nerve damage.
7. Parental education is centered on understanding and acceptance of abnormality.

D. **Syndactyly**: partial or complete fusion of fingers or toes.
1. The most common limb abnormality: involves feet more often than hands.
2. Inherited as simple dominant or recessive trait. Failure of webbing between digits to degenerate.
3. Physical exam essential to rule out osseous syndactyly.
4. Radiological exam: demonstrates presence and extent of bony fusion.
5. Intervention: depends on physical findings. If function is not limited, no treatment is needed. Complex fusion states are treated surgically at 2–3 years of age.

6. Complications: rare and are related to surgical relief.
7. Parental involvement: foster informational and emotional support.

E. Absent radius: complex deformity resulting in partial or complete absence of radius.
1. Associated anomalies occur without any set pattern. Riordan (1986) lists cleft palate, clubfoot, hydrocephalus, hernia, kyphosis, scoliosis, and rib deformities as associated anomalies.
2. Etiology believed to be genetic.
3. Absence of the radius distal half is the most common; 50% of the defects are bilateral.
4. Physical exam reveals three deformities: radial deviation of the hand 90 degrees or more, shortening of the forearm, general underdevelopment of entire extremity.
   a. Muscles usually involved: abnormal origin and insertion of pectoralis minor and major biceps, brachialis, and extensors.
   b. Thumb may be absent, present, or hypoplastic.
5. Radiological exam: reveals reduction in scapular size, shortened ulna, abnormalities of the clavicle, scapula, and humerus.
6. Intervention: centered on casting and splinting soon after delivery. Surgical repair at 2 to 18 months of age. Purpose of the surgery is to centralize the wrist on the ulna. Long-term splinting is needed to prevent recurrence.
7. Complications: related to surgical relief.
8. Parental involvement: vital through casting and splinting period.

F. Amniotic bands: constrictive bands of fibrous tissue encircling body parts result in malformation of the extremities.
1. Amniotic bands believed to be caused by localized rupture of the amniotic sac with subsequent entanglement of body parts by amniotic threads.
2. Banding can occur on any body surface: distal extremities commonly affected, especially middle, index, and ring fingers.
3. Incidence approximately 1:15,000 births.
4. Physical exam: Bayne and Costas (1990) place deformities into four groups.
   a. Simple ring constrictions.
   b. Constrictions with bony fusion.
   c. Constrictions with fusion of soft-tissue parts.
   d. Intrauterine amputations: depth of constriction varies from minor involvement to strangulation of the affected part.
5. Radiological exam: vital to identify type and involvement of defect.
6. Intervention: severe bands released surgically as infant's condition allows or if circulation is compromised. Less severe bands corrected at 1–2 years of age.
7. Complications: related to loss of vascular and nerve supply. Severe defects with lymphedema may result in joint stiffness.
8. Parental educational information and support essential in fostering acceptance.

Neck Abnormalities

Abnormalities can be either muscular or bony. The embryonic critical period is 22–28 days. Causes are diverse, congenital or acquired.

A. Torticollis: tilting of head and neck secondary to muscular or bony defect (Fig. 23–1).
1. Muscular defect secondary to fibrosis and shortening of sternocleidomastoid muscle on one side. Etiology related to tearing and bleeding into the muscle. Mass is then palpable at approximately 2 weeks of age.
   a. Breech, forceps, primipara deliveries at risk.
   b. Lesion most commonly right sided.
2. Congenital bony or skeletal torticollis (wryneck) caused by variety of agents,

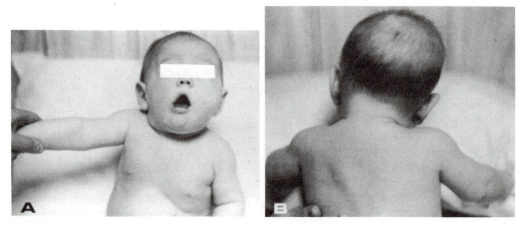

Figure 23-1
A, Congenital torticollis affecting the right sternocleidomastoid muscle in a 3 month old baby. *B*, Note the flattening of the left occiput and right head tilt. (From Avery, G.B. (ed): Neonatology: Pathophysiology and Management of the Newborn, 3rd ed. Philadelphia, J.B. Lippincott, 1987, p. 1163.)

associated with other abnormalities. The muscle is not shortened. Symptoms do not usually occur until adulthood and are progressive.

3. Physical exam: muscular defect identified by non-tender mobile mass within body of sternocleidomastoid muscle. Palpable muscle contracture and torticollis are present. Bony defect–torticollis is without palpable mass.

4. Radiological exam: difficult to obtain secondary to head position. Laminograms and flexion-extension stress films may be helpful. Need to rule out abnormalities of cervical spine.

5. Intervention: muscular defects treated conservatively with stretching of the muscle or by surgical resection of a portion of the muscle followed by stretching. Bony defects are treated non-operatively because defect is a fixed bony deformity.

6. Parental involvement: education and active participation are essential.

B. **Klippel-Feil syndrome:** defective segmentation of cervical vertebrae.

1. Results as a failure of segmentation; may extend beyond cervical spine.

2. Etiology uncertain: associated with genitourinary, cardiopulmonary, and auditory defects.

3. Physical exam: reveals low posterior hairline, limitation of neck movement, and shortened neck.

4. Radiological exam: flexion-extension views most valuable—confirm a decrease in number or fusion of two or more vertebrae.

5. Treatment: depends on level and extent of defect. Ranges from no treatment to surgical stabilization of cervical vertebrae. Mechanical problems of joint irritation treated with traction, cervical collar, bracing.

6. Complications can be extensive, depending on other associated defects. Quadriplegia can result from minor injury if cervical vertebrae are unstable.

7. Parental involvement: awareness of long-term effects and of need for orthopedic and neurological follow-up is essential because associated defects tend to worsen with time. Outcome depends on individual lesions.

Lower Extremities

A. **Critical period for lower limb development** exists between 26–44 days. Abnormalities of limbs originate depending on the timing within this period. Causes of defects are multifactorial, result from genetic, chromosomal, mutant genes, or environmental factors.

1. Talipes equinovarus: developmental deformity of hind part of foot — clubfoot.
   a. Defect occurs in 1:1000 births — males affected twice as often as females.
   b. Occurs bilaterally in 50% of infants; accounts for 95% of clubfoot anomalies.
2. Causative factors: genetic and environmental. Although most cases occur sporadically, Beaty (1991) describes clubfoot as being an autosomal dominant trait with incomplete penetrance. Development of defect may be secondary to primary soft-tissue abnormalities within neuromuscular units, and resulting bony changes or primary germ plasma defect in the talus. Results in prolonged plantar flexion and inversion of bone and soft-tissue changes (Beaty, 1991). Defects are generally believed to be related to uterine pressure exerted during critical period on a fetus who is genetically predisposed.
3. Physical exam: common findings are forefoot adduction, varus of hind foot, and equinus of the ankle. Foot held at right angle to ankle and tibia. Affected foot is smaller, associated with calf muscle atrophy. Vital to obtain measurement of angles as they correlate well with clinical appearance of foot and result following non-surgical or surgical relief. Rules out other bone abnormalities.
4. Radiological exam: identifies abnormal talocalcaneal, tibiocalcaneal, talometatarsal angles on anteroposterior and lateral x-rays.
5. Intervention: centered initially on serial casting every 2 weeks until child is approximately 3–6 months of age. Surgical relief is required in 50% of infants to lengthen contracted tendons and divide ligaments.
6. Outcome: depends on early intervention. Some defects require repeat surgeries, braces, or casting to maintain treatment or prevent recurrence.
7. Parental support vital to success through casting, bracing, surgery.

B. **Metatarsus adductus:** incurving of foot (Fig. 23–2).
1. Incidence: 1:1000 births, exists as positional or structural abnormalities, usually bilateral.
2. Causative factors multifactorial: combination of genetic and environmental.
3. Physical exam: findings are specific as to type of defect.
   a. Structural defects reveal heel in varus position; forefoot flexible, abducts beyond midline.

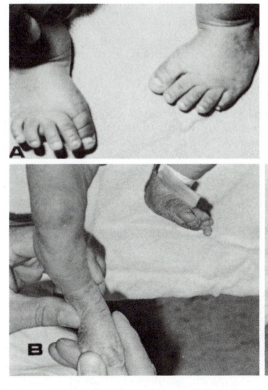

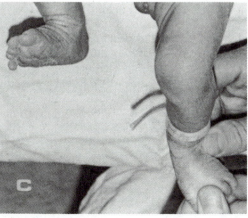

Figure 23–2
A, Structural metatarsus adductus. *B*, Structural metatarsus adductus. The forefoot does not abduct beyond neutral. *C*, Positional metatarsus; the forefoot abducts beyond the midline. (From Avery, G.B.: Neonatology: Pathophysiology and Management of the Newborn, 3rd ed. Philadelphia, J.B. Lippincott, 1987, p. 1061.)

4. Radiological exam: pinpoints type of defect and rules out other abnormalities.
5. Intervention: guided by type of deformity; supple positional defects require no treatment or only gentle passive range of motion exercises. Rigid structural defects require serial castings. Extreme cases may require surgical realignment.
6. Complications: related to recurrence of defect or the surgical procedure.
7. Active participation by parents is essential for successful treatment.

C. **Congenital hip dislocation:** dislocation of the femoral head outside the acetabulum.
1. Occurs in 1.3:1000 births only; more common in North American Indians, Japanese, Central and Southern European groups. Females affected 4–6 times more often than males.
2. Affected hip: left 50%; right 30%; bilateral 20%.
3. Factors of origin are genetic, hormonal, and mechanical.
4. Two types identified.
   a. Typical or common: occurs at or around birth. Child has no bony abnormalities or underlying pathology.
   b. Teratogenic: occurs early in fetal life; results in severe joint abnormality. Abduction of hips limited; thighs appear short in relation to lower legs — perineum appears wider.
5. Physical exam: examination is positive when femoral head lies outside the acetabulum with no contact between articular surfaces. Subluxation demonstrates as inability to abduct the affected thigh.
   a. With infant positioned supine, thighs flexed to right angle, attempt to bring them outward and downward one at a time. When a sharp click is felt and heard consistently on one side, this click is termed *Ortolani's sign.*
6. Radiological exam: changes evident only after long-standing dislocation. Anteroposterior views with legs extended and in neutral abduction.
7. Interventions: aimed at restoration of anatomical alignment of hip. Early detection vital. Treatment consists of abduction-flexion braces for 2–4 months — goal is to hold hips reduced while not interfering with care.
8. Complications: rare; avascular necrosis of part or all of the femoral epiphysis.
9. Outcome: with common lesions, good; with teratogenic lesions, poor.
10. Parents must be aware of need for continuing support and follow-up.

D. **Arthrogryposis multiplex congenita:** non-progressive, multiple, congenitally rigid joints.
1. Characterized by loss of function of major motor groups with no associated sensory defect.
2. Etiology unknown, related to failure of anterior spinal cord formation. Joint contractures result secondary to lack of fetal movement.
3. Physical exam: wide range of expression, depending on involvement. Drennan (1990) relates symptoms as limitation of active and passive motion, joint fixed in flexion or extension, decreased muscle mass, tense skin, webbing, and decreased deep tendon reflexes.
4. Radiological exam: limited value — rules out bony abnormalities.
5. Intervention: aimed toward maximizing potential. Splinting and gentle range of motion provided early. Surgical relief for repair of clubfeet and realignment of joints increases ambulatory and self-care potential.
6. Complications: recurrence common; improvements deteriorate over time; scoliosis may develop in later childhood.
7. Outcome: variable.
   a. Clients may have adequate function despite loss of function.
   b. Life span not usually affected.

E. **Osteogenesis imperfecta:** complex disorder resulting in multiple fractures and widespread organ involvement.
1. Heritable disease with great phenotypic expression range. Etiology believed to be both autosomal dominant and recessive.
2. Physical exam: features vary with disease severity.
   a. Bone: soft, fragile; stature usually decreased, scoliosis common; the skull is

soft; facies are triangular; vertebrae fracture easily; fracture and skeletal deformities at birth common.
   b. Skin: thin, translucent, easily distensible.
   c. Teeth: delayed, defective, soft, translucent.
   d. Joints: dislocate easily.
   e. Neurological: hydrocephalus and intracranial hemorrhage common.
3. Radiological exam: identifies fracture, scoliosis, diaphyseal abnormalities. Generalized osteopenia common.
4. Intervention: no effective systemic therapy exists. Treatment aimed toward treatment of acute fractures, maintenance of ambulation.
5. Complications: as disease affects nearly all organ systems, complications are multiple. Respiratory involvement frequent.
6. Outcome: dependent on degree of expression—minor to life-threatening.
7. Parental involvement and support are essential for understanding and acceptance.

F. **Fractured clavicle:** fracture occurring along clavicular line.
1. Two types identified: undisplaced (or greenstick) and displaced (or symptomatic).
2. Etiology related to consequences of difficult delivery.
3. Physical exam: findings vary with fracture type.
   a. Asymptomatic: detected as a lump over clavicle 7–10 days following delivery.
   b. Exam of displaced fracture reveals decreased or absent movement of arm, discoloration over fracture site, crepitus, tenderness, irregularity along clavicle.
4. Radiological exam: done to confirm the fracture (see Chapter 33).
5. Intervention: consists of shoulder immobilization and arm abduction.
6. Complications rare.
7. Parental involvement centered on educational and infant care issues.

STUDY QUESTIONS

1. A perinatal factor that may lead to orthopedic abnormalities is:
   a. Fetal position.
   b. Maternal activity.
   c. Maternal diet.

2. Formation of the appendicular skeleton begins at:
   a. Fourth gestational week.
   b. Second gestational week.
   c. Sixth gestational week.

3. The most common limb abnormality is:
   a. Absent radius.
   b. Polydactyly.
   c. Syndactyly.

4. Klippel-Feil abnormality is defined as:
   a. Defective segmentation of cervical vertebrae.
   b. Tilting of the head and neck.
   c. Webbing of the neck.

5. Treatment of metatarsus adductus is primarily:

   a. Casting and surgery.
   b. Exercise and casting.
   c. Exercise and stretching.

6. A common etiology of congenital hip dislocation is:
   a. Genetic factors.
   b. Gender related.
   c. Race related.

7. Osteogenesis imperfecta is characterized by:
   a. Fractures and skeletal deformities at birth.
   b. Stiffness of joints and hypoplasia of muscles.
   c. Thick and parchment-like skin.

8. Examination of a displaced fracture of the clavicle reveals:
   a. Decreased or absent movement of the arm.
   b. No identifiable symptoms.
   c. No irregularity along clavicular line.

Answers to Study Questions

1. a	4. a	7. a
2. a	5. c	8. a
3. c	6. b	

REFERENCES

Bayne, L., and Costas, B.: Malformations of the upper limb. *In* Morrissy, R.T. (ed.): Lovell and Winters Pediatric Orthopedics, 3rd ed. Philadelphia, J.B. Lippincott, 1990, pp. 563–605.

Beaty, J.H.: Congenital anomalies of the lower and upper extremities. *In* Canale, S.T. and Beaty, J.H. (eds.): Operative Pediatric Orthopedics. St. Louis, Mosby Year Book, 1991, pp. 73–98.

Drennan, J.C.: Neuromuscular disorders. *In* Morrissy, R.T. (ed.): Lovell and Winters Pediatric Orthopedics, 3rd ed. Philadelphia, J.B. Lippincott, 1990, pp. 381–453.

Riordan, D.C., and Bayne, L.G.: The upper limb. *In* Lovell, W.W. and Winter, R.B. (eds.): Pediatric Orthopedics, 2nd ed. Philadelphia, J.B. Lippincott, 1986, pp. 549–556.

BIBLIOGRAPHY

Chung, S.M.: Hip Disorders in Infants and Children. Philadelphia, Lea & Febiger, 1981.

Langmen, J.: Skeletal system and ossification. *In* Medical Embryology: Human Development—Normal and Abnormal, 3rd ed. Baltimore, Williams & Wilkins, 1975, pp. 137–152.

Moore, K.: The skeletal system, the muscular system, the limbs. *In* The Developing Human: Clinically Oriented Embryology, 4th ed. Philadelphia, W.B. Saunders Co., 1988, pp. 334–363.

Scoles, P.V.: Pediatric Orthopedics in Clinical Practice. Chicago, Year Book Medical Publishers, 1988.

Catherine L. Witt

Neonatal Dermatology

Objectives

1. Name five functions of the skin.

2. Describe two ways in which the skin of a newborn or pre-term infant differs from that of an adult.

3. Identify three factors that affect the appearance of the newborn's skin.

4. Identify two factors important in the care of the pre-term infant's skin.

5. Recognize three common skin lesions that are normal variations in the newborn. Describe their appearance and treatment, if any.

6. Describe three common vascular lesions in the newborn, their appearance, and appropriate treatment.

7. Identify two syndromes associated with vascular lesions.

8. Evaluate two pigmented lesions occurring in the newborn and list implications associated with each.

9. List four types of infectious skin lesions and select the appropriate treatment.

Careful assessment of the skin is an essential element of the newborn physical examination. The appearance of the skin can give the nurse important clues regarding gestational age, nutritional status, function of organs such as the heart and liver, and the presence of cutaneous or systemic disease. It is important for the clinician to be familiar with normal variances in the skin of the newborn, as well as those that signify disease.

Proper care of the neonate's skin can directly affect mortality and morbidity in the pre-term infant. The skin is the first line of defense against infection. Proper skin care can protect the integrity of the skin and prevent breakdown.

Anatomy and Physiology

A. **Anatomy of the skin** (Fig. 24–1).
1. Three main layers of skin.

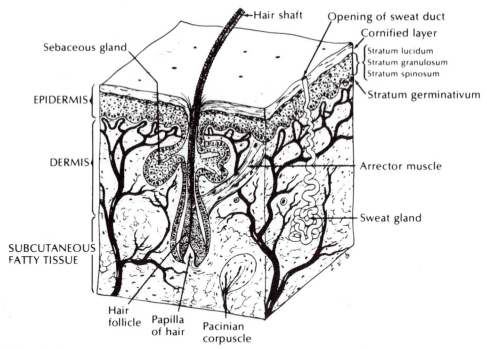

Figure 24 – 1
The several layers and structures of human skin. (Reproduced by permission from Francis, C.C., and Martin, A.H.: Introduction to Human Anatomy, 7th ed. St. Louis, The C.V. Mosby Co., 1975.)

    a. Epidermis: outermost layer, subdivided into five layers.
        (1) Stratum corneum: outermost layer consisting of closely packed dead cells that are consistently brushed off and replaced by lower levels of the epidermis.
        (2) Lower layers of epidermis: contain keratin-forming cells that create the outer layer of skin; as well as melanocytes, which produce melanin, or pigment.
    b. Dermis: directly under epidermis, 2 – 4 mm thick at birth (Francis and Martin, 1975).
        (1) Composed of fibrous and elastic tissue.
        (2) Contains a rich supply of blood vessels and many nerves that carry sensations of heat, touch, pain, and pressure from the skin to the brain.
        (3) Also contains sweat glands, sebaceous glands, and hair shafts.
    c. Subcutaneous layer: fatty tissue functioning as insulation, protection of internal organs, and calorie storage.

B. Functions of the skin.
1. Physical protection.
    a. Provides mechanical, chemical, and bacterial protection for the body.
2. Heat regulation.
    a. Production and evaporation of sweat.
    b. Dilatation and constriction of blood vessels.
    c. Insulation of body by subcutaneous fat.
3. Sense perception.
    a. Heat, touch, pain, pressure.
4. Immunological properties.
    a. Acidic surface of skin has bactericidal properties (Kuller et al., 1983).
5. Self-cleaning.
    a. Constant shedding and replacement of cells.

C. Differences in newborn skin.
1. Newborn/pre-term infant.
   a. Basic structure is same as that of the adult; the less mature the infant, the less mature is the functioning of the skin.
   b. The earlier the gestational age, the more thin and gelatinous is the skin.
   c. Subcutaneous fat is accumulated preponderantly during the third trimester.
      (1) Pre-term babies have little fat, resulting in inability to maintain body temperature.
   d. Immature skin is more permeable.
      (2) An infant, especially the pre-term child, may quickly absorb topically applied drugs and chemicals.
   e. Fewer fibrils connect the dermis and epidermis, and they are more fragile in term or pre-term skin than in the adult. The stratum corneum is thinner in the term or pre-term infant.
      (1) Increased risk of injury from tape, monitors, and handling, especially in the pre-term infant.
   f. Sweat glands are present at birth, but full adult functioning is not present until the second or third year of life.
      (1) The newborn has limited ability to tolerate excessive heat.

Care of the Newborn's Skin

A. The term newborn.
1. Initial bath with water and a mild soap.
   a. Avoid strong alkaline soaps.
   b. Soaps containing hexachlorophene should not be used. The hexachlorophene may be absorbed through the skin.
2. Parents may prefer to give the first bath themselves. Some parents prefer that the vernix not be washed off. They feel it is a natural substance that should be allowed to absorb. Some parents believe vernix has immunological properties, although this has not been proved.
3. More thorough washing may be recommended in cases of suspected or proven maternal infections such as hepatitis or herpes.
4. Avoid puncturing the skin when possible in babies with suspected maternal infections.
5. Dry skin can be treated with a non-perfumed cream or lotion. Perfume may irritate newborn's skin.

B. The pre-term infant.
1. Keep skin clean with water. Mild, non-alkaline soap may be used.
2. Keep handling gentle and to a minimum to avoid trauma.
3. Minimize use of tape as much as possible. Use care when removing tape to avoid tearing of skin.
   a. Safety of adhesive solvents has not been proved. Cotton balls soaked with warm water may be just as effective at loosening tape.
   b. Some nurseries have found it helpful to use pectin-based barriers under all tape.
4. Increased permeability of skin may allow absorption of medications and products such as alcohol, povidone-iodine (Betadine), and benzoin. Cleaning skin with water after using these products is recommended.
5. A tent with warm mist may protect skin and decrease insensible water loss in the very low birthweight infant.
6. Avoid perfumed creams and lotions. Perfumes may irritate the skin, and the chemicals may be absorbed.
7. Use of semipermeable dressings such as Opsite may be useful to heal wounds and protect IV sites.

C. Umbilical cord care.
1. Sterile cutting of cord at delivery and rapid drying of umbilical cord appear to be most effective at preventing umbilical infections (Schuman and Oksol, 1985).
2. Isopropyl alcohol and triple dye are the agents most commonly used for cord care. The above mentioned study showed no difference in infection rate between the two methods.
3. Tub bath should be delayed until cord has fallen off, generally 10–14 days.

Assessment of the Newborn's Skin

A. Factors affecting the appearance of the skin.
1. Gestational age.
   a. The more pre-term the infant, the thinner the skin.
2. Post-natal age.
   a. Skin will be dryer and may peel a few days after birth.
3. Nutritional status and hydration.
4. Racial origin.
5. Type and amount of available light.
6. Hemoglobin and bilirubin levels.
7. Environmental temperatures.
8. Oxygenation status.

B. Definitions used to describe skin lesions (Weston, 1985).
1. Macule: a pigmented, flat spot less than 1 cm in diameter. It is visible but not palpable.
2. Patch: a flat, pigmented spot larger than 1 cm in diameter.
3. Papule: a solid, elevated, palpable lesion, less than 1 cm in diameter.
4. Nodule: a papule larger than 1 cm in diameter.
5. Vesicle: an elevated lesion or blister filled with serous fluid and less than 1 cm in diameter.
6. Bulla: a fluid-filled lesion larger than 1 cm.
7. Pustule: a vesicle filled with cloudy or purulent fluid.
8. Petechiae: subepidermal hemorrhages, pinpoint in size. They do not blanch with pressure.
9. Ecchymosis: a large area of subepidermal hemorrhage.

Common Skin Lesions

A. Normal variations in newborn skin.
1. Cutis marmorata (Fig. 24–2).
   a. Bluish mottling or marbling effect of the skin.
   b. Physiological response to chilling, caused by dilatation of capillaries and venules.
   c. Disappears when infant is rewarmed.
   d. May be sign of stress or overstimulation in newborn.
2. Erythema toxicum (Fig. 24–3).
   a. Small white or yellow papules or vesicles surrounded by erythematous dermatitis.
   b. Benign, found in up to 70% of newborns (Margileth, 1987).
   c. Occurs up to 3 months of age.
   d. Lesions come and go on various sites of face, trunk, and limbs.
   e. Cause unknown but may be exacerbated by handling or chafing of linen.
   f. Differential diagnosis: may resemble a staphylococcal infection. Diagnosis can be confirmed by smear of aspirated pustule showing numerous eosinophils.

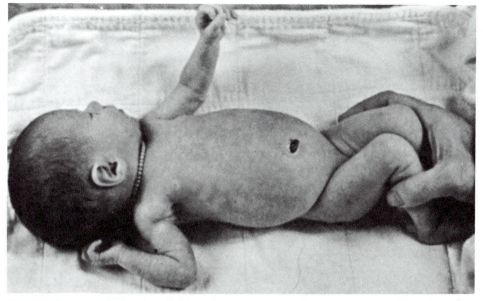

Figure 24-2
Cutis marmorata. (Photo courtesy of Jacinto Hernandez, M.D., The Children's Hospital, Denver, Colorado.)

   g. No treatment necessary. Lotions or creams may exacerbate condition.
3. Milia (Fig. 24-4).
   a. Multiple yellow or pearly white papules about 1 mm in size. They occur on the brow, cheeks, and nose.
   b. Milia are observed in about 40% of full-term infants (Margileth, 1987).
   c. Milia are epidermal inclusion cysts composed of laminated, keratinous material.
   d. No treatment is necessary. They resolve spontaneously during the first few weeks after birth.
4. Epstein's pearls (Fig. 24-5).
   a. Oral counterpart of facial milia. They can be seen on the midline of the palate or on the alveolar ridges.
   b. Epstein's pearls occur in approximately 85% of newborns.

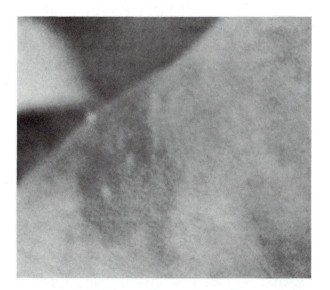

Figure 24-3
Erythema toxicum. (Photo courtesy of Jacinto Hernandez, M.D., The Children's Hospital, Denver, Colorado.)

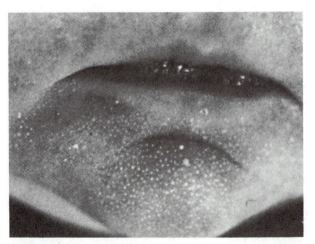

Figure 24–4
Milia. (Photo courtesy of Jacinto Hernandez, M.D., The Children's Hospital, Denver, Colorado.)

5. Sebaceous gland hyperplasia.
   a. Tiny (less than 0.5 mm) white or yellow papules found on the nose, cheeks, and upper lips of newborns.
   b. They involve the sebaceous follicles and are a manifestation of maternal androgen stimulation.
   c. They resolve without treatment within a few weeks.
6. Miliaria.
   a. Miliaria is caused by occlusion of sweat ducts, secondary to excessive heating of the skin. There are two types of miliaria.
      (1) Miliaria crystallina: clear, thin vesicles, 1–2 mm in diameter, that develop in the epidermal portion of the sweat glands. They are seen over the head, neck, and upper trunk in newborns.
      (2) Miliaria rubra: prolonged occlusion of pores leads to release of sweat into the lower epidermis. It appears as papules and vesicles 2–4 mm in diameter, with an erythemic base. The lesions are generally found in the flexure areas such as the neck, groin, and axillae, as well as the face and upper chest.
   b. Treatment consists of avoidance of further sweating and keeping the skin cool and dry.

B. Pigmented skin lesions.
1. Mongolian spots (Fig. 24–6).
   a. Large macule or patch, gray or blue green in color, seen most commonly over the buttocks, flanks, or shoulders.
   b. Most common pigmented lesion seen at birth, occurring in 90% of black, Asian, and Hispanic infants, and in 1–5% of white infants (Margileth, 1987).
   c. Mongolian spots are caused by the presence of melanocytes dispersed in the dermis.

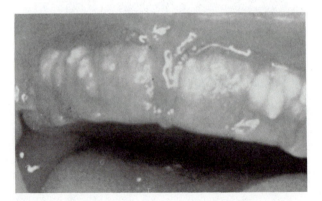

Figure 24–5
Epstein pearls. (Photo courtesy of Jacinto Hernandez, M.D., The Children's Hospital, Denver, Colorado.)

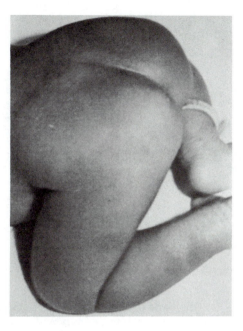

Figure 24–6
Mongolian spots. (Photo courtesy of Jacinto Hernandez, M.D., The Children's Hospital, Denver, Colorado.)

   d. The spots usually fade within the first 2 years after birth.
   e. It is important to document size and location to avoid question of nonaccidental trauma.
2. Pigmented nevus.
   a. Dark brown or black macule that may or may not be hairy. Nevi may occur anywhere on the body, with the "bathing trunk" area being the most common site.
   b. Pigmented nevi are generally benign, but malignant changes occur in approximately 10% of these lesions (Hodgeman et al., 1971).
   c. Close observation for changes in size or shape is indicated, with possible surgical excision.
3. Transient neonatal pustular melanosis.
   a. Superficial vesiculopustular lesions that rupture during the first 12–48 hours after birth, leaving small, brown, hyperpigmented macules. The macules may be surrounded by very fine white scales.
   b. Benign, found in up to 5% of black infants and in about 0.2% of white babies (Ramamurthy et al., 1976).
   c. No treatment is necessary. The macules generally fade during the first few weeks or months after birth.
   d. Aspirating the contents of the vesicles will reveal a variable number of neutrophils and few or no eosinophils.
4. Café au lait spots (Fig. 24–7).
   a. Tan or light brown patches with well-defined borders.
   b. When less than 3 cm in length and less than six in number, they are of no pathological significance.
   c. Six or more spots may be an indication of neurofibromatosis.
     (1) Neurofibromatosis is a condition in which tumors form on cutaneous nerves and along the thorax, brachial, and lumbar nerve trunks. Cranial nerves may also be affected.
     (2) Autosomal dominant disorder; a positive family history is present in 50% of cases (Fienman and Yakovac, 1970).
     (3) Café au lait spots may be the only finding in the newborn period.

C. Vascular lesions.
1. Nevus simplex.
   a. Nevus simplex refers to macular pink areas of distended capillaries found on

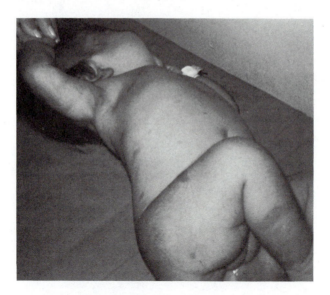

Figure 24-7
Café au lait spots. (Photo courtesy of Jacinto Hernandez, M.D., The Children's Hospital, Denver, Colorado.)

  the nape of the neck, the upper eyelids, the nose, or the upper lip. They have diffuse borders, blanch with pressure, and become pinker with crying.

  b. These are the most common of vascular birthmarks, seen in 30–50% of newborns (Weston, 1985).

  c. The lesions tend to fade by the first or second year, with the exception of those on the nape of the neck, which may persist.

 2. Port-wine stain.

  a. A flat vascular nevus present at birth. It is usually pink in infancy, but it may be red or purple. The nevus may be small or cover almost one-half of the body. It is flat and sharply delineated and blanches minimally. Facial lesions are the most common.

  b. Port-wine stains consist of mature capillaries that are dilated and congested directly below the epidermis.

  c. The nevus does not grow in area or size. It will not resolve and should be considered permanent.

  d. Laser surgery has been somewhat successful at treating smaller port-wine stains. Other methods of surgical excision have been largely unsatisfactory (Apfelberg et al., 1978).

  e. Sturge-Weber syndrome (Fig. 24–8).

   (1) Port-wine stains confined to a pattern similar to that of the branches of the trigeminal nerve may be associated with Sturge-Weber syndrome.

   (2) The central feature of this syndrome is disordered proliferation of endothelial cells, particularly in small veins. It is associated with atrophic changes in the cerebral cortex and calcium deposits in the walls of small vessels and areas of affected cortex (Margileth, 1987).

   (3) Sturge-Weber syndrome is manifested by glaucoma, focal seizures, hemiparesis, and mental retardation.

 3. Strawberry hemangioma (Fig. 24–9).

  a. A strawberry hemangioma is a raised, lobulated, soft, bright red tumor, occurring on the head, neck, trunk, or extremities. These lesions may also occur in the throat, where they can cause airway obstruction.

  b. The lesions are caused by dilated capillaries occupying the dermal and subdermal layers, associated with endothelial proliferation.

  c. 20–30% are present at birth, and 90% are evident by 2 months of age (Margileth, 1987).

  d. The strawberry hemangioma will generally increase in size the first 6 months, then become stable in size before undergoing gradual spontaneous regression. This may take several years.

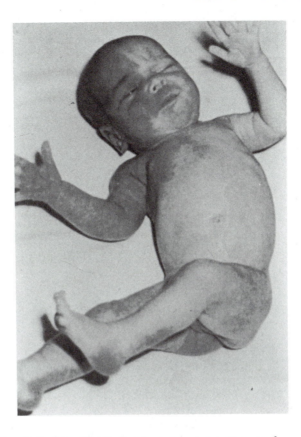

Figure 24–8
Sturge-Weber syndrome. (Photo courtesy of Jacinto Hernandez, M.D., The Children's Hospital, Denver, Colorado.)

    e. Treatment generally consists of allowing the lesion to regress spontaneously. If the lesion is interfering with vision or other vital functions, systemic corticosteroids may be helpful.

    f. The cosmetic concerns of parents require a caring, supportive approach. Pictures illustrating spontaneous regression may be helpful.

  4. Cavernous hemangioma.

    a. This lesion is composed of large venous channels and vascular elements lined by endothelial cells.

    b. It involves the dermis and subcutaneous tissue and appears as a bluish-red discoloration under the overlying skin.

    c. The cavernous hemangioma has poorly defined borders and may feel cystic, like a "bag of worms," when palpated (Ruiz-Maldonado et al., 1989).

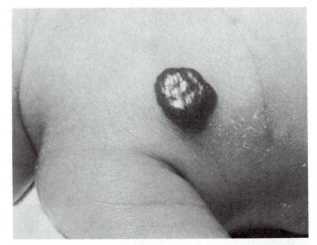

Figure 24–9
Strawberry hemangioma. (Photo courtesy of Jacinto Hernandez, M.D., The Children's Hospital, Denver, Colorado.)

d. Like the strawberry hemangioma, the cavernous hemangioma will increase in size the first 6–12 months and then involute spontaneously.

e. Treatment is not indicated unless the lesion is interfering with vital functioning, in which case systemic corticosteroid treatment may be helpful.

f. Kasabach-Merritt syndrome.
   (1) Giant cavernous hemangiomas may be associated with sequestration of platelets and thrombocytopenia.
   (2) Treatment consists of systemic corticosteroid therapy. Transfusions of platelets and blood are frequently necessary (Solomon and Esterly, 1973).

g. Klippel-Trenaunay-Weber syndrome.
   (1) This syndrome consists of hypertrophy of a limb with associated vascular nevi and hypertrophy of underlying bone and soft structures.
   (2) It is a rare congenital abnormality, seen mostly in males (Margileth, 1987).
   (3) There is no specific treatment for the disease. Severe limb hypertrophy may require orthopedic consultation.

D. Infectious lesions.

1. Thrush
   a. Thrush is a fungal infection of the mouth or throat caused by *Candida albicans*.
   b. Very common in infants.
   c. Presents as patches of adherent white material scattered over the tongue and mucous membranes.
   d. Thrush is treated with oral nystatin (Mycostatin).

2. *Candida* diaper dermatitis.
   a. Fungal infection of skin in the diaper area, which may include the buttocks, groin, thighs, and abdomen.
   b. Caused by the organism *Candida albicans*.
   c. Presents as a moist, erythematous eruption often with satellite pustules, white or yellow in color.
   d. Treatment consists of a nystatin cream applied to the rash several times per day.
      (1) Oral Mycostatin may be recommended in cases of persistent *Candida* dermatitis.

3. Herpes
   a. Neonatal herpes simplex infection is one of the most serious viral infections in the newborn.
   b. Rash appears as vesicular or pustular rash (Fig. 24–10).
   c. 70% of infants with herpes will develop rash, but not necessarily before

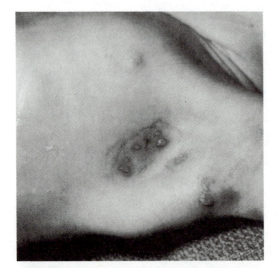

Figure 24–10
Herpes simplex vesicles. (From Margilet, A.: Dermatologic conditions. *In* Avery, G. (ed.): Neonatology: Pathophysiology and Management of the Newborn, 2nd ed. Philadelphia, J.B. Lippincott, 1981, p. 1090.)

other signs and symptoms of illness develop. Therefore, absence of vesicles does not eliminate the possibility of disease (Weston, 1985).

    d. Treatment includes isolation and treatment with an antiviral agent such as acyclovir.

    e. Mortality depends on extent of the illness when treatment is begun, but may be as high as 50–70% (Weston, 1985).

4. Bullous impetigo ("scalded skin").
    a. An inflammatory skin disorder generally caused by staphylococci or streptococci; may follow an upper respiratory infection or otitis media.
    b. Presents as a widespread, tender erythema followed by blisters ranging from small vesicles to large bullae. These rupture, leaving large, raw, scald-like areas. The blisters frequently begin in the diaper area and spread to the rest of the body.
    c. Treatment includes isolation and aseptic handling to prevent further infection in the infected infant and spread of bacteria to others. The infant is treated systemically with penicillin G, unless the organism is resistant; then methicillin may be used. A bacitracin ointment may be applied locally.

5. Congenital rubella.
    a. Petechiae and purpuric macules seen on the head, trunk, and extremities of affected infants. The lesions are often described as "blueberry muffin" spots and are caused by dermal erythropoiesis (Fig. 24–11).
    b. The lesions generally disappear in 2–3 weeks. Treatment is based on the underlying disorder.
    c. Although the lesions are associated with rubella, they may also appear in association with other congenital infections such as cytomegalovirus infections, toxoplasmosis, syphilis, herpes, and gram-negative bacillary infections.
    d. Affected infants may also present with jaundice, hepatosplenomegaly, and thrombocytopenia.

E. **Hereditary and miscellaneous lesions.**

1. Epidermolysis bullosa.
    a. Epidermolysis bullosa is a disease characterized by the formation of vesicles and bullae over various parts of the body. The underlying genetic defect may be autosomal dominant or recessive.
    b. The vesicles may appear spontaneously or in response to minor trauma such as routine handling.
    c. The lesions may appear at birth or a few weeks later.
    d. There are three types that may appear at birth.

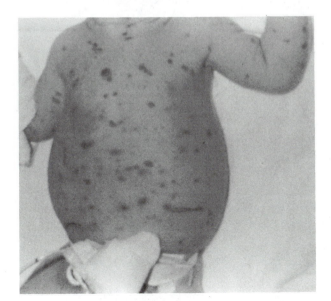

Figure 24–11
Blueberry muffin rash. (Photo courtesy of Jacinto Hernandez, M.D., The Children's Hospital, Denver, Colorado.)

(1) Simple, non-scarring: in this type, the bullae form in small numbers throughout childhood and heal without scarring. It often disappears at puberty. Prevention of trauma and infection is important.

(2) Dystrophic, scarring: this is a more severe form of the disease, with lesions forming scars with loss of nails and contractures. Death may occur from secondary infections.

(3) Epidermolysis bullosa letalis: This is the most severe form, with large, numerous lesions, usually present at birth. Large areas of epidermis are lost, leaving red, weeping erosions. Esophageal lesions may also occur. The lifespan of these patients is generally short. Treatment is supportive care, minimizing trauma and infection (Weston, 1985).

2. Collodion baby.
   a. This describes an appearance rather than a disease. These babies are born covered with a tight, shiny, transparent membrane that cracks and peels off after a few days. A few infants will have no underlying disorder, but many will have some form of ichthyosis (Solomon and Esterly, 1973) (Fig. 24–12).
   b. Treatment consists of liberal application of sterile olive or mineral oil several times a day.

3. Ichthyosis.
   a. Ichthyosis is a disease involving excessive scaling of the skin. There are four types of ichthyosis.
      (1) Ichthyosis vulgaris: an autosomal dominant disease, usually appearing between 1 and 2 years of age. This is the most common and most benign of the ichthyosis disorders and consists of fine white scales and excessively dry skin (Rand and Baden, 1983).
      (2) X-linked ichthyosis: this disorder appears at birth or during the first year of life. It occasionally presents in a collodion baby. The disorder consists of large, thick, dark brown scales over the entire body, with the exception of the palms and soles. It occurs in males only.

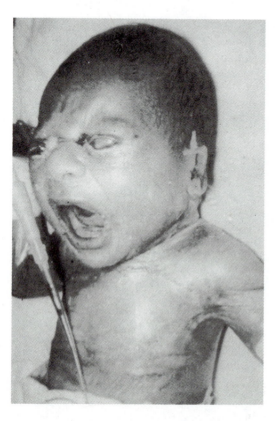

Figure 24–12
Collodion baby. (From Solomon, L.M., and Esterly, N.B.: Neonatal Dermatology. Philadelphia, W.B. Saunders Co., p. 115.)

(3) Lamellar ichthyosis: this is an autosomal recessive trait that presents at birth as bright red erythema and universal desquamation. Some cases present in collodion babies. Scales are large, flat, and coarse and may be less prominent in infancy than they are later in childhood. Eversion of the lips and eyelids may occur, and the palms and soles may be thickened. The large production of scales may be due to an excessive proliferation of epidermal cells (Solomon and Esterly, 1973).

(4) Bullous ichthyosis: this autosomal dominant disorder is characterized by recurrent formation of bullous lesions, erythroderma, and excessive dryness and peeling. As the child grows, the involvement generally becomes limited to small, thick, hard scales, most often found in the flexure regions. Hyperkeratosis may be seen on the palms and soles (Rand and Baden, 1983). Infection in the neonatal period is of primary concern, because of the widespread bullae.

   b. Treatment of ichthyosis is limited to use of topical preparations to hydrate and lubricate the skin. Daily baths with a water-dispersible bath oil are followed by application of ointments, creams, or lotions. Drying soaps and detergents should be avoided.

4. Harlequin fetus.
   a. The harlequin fetus has generally been considered to have a severe form of ichthyosis. Some authors now believe the underlying disorder to be a separate, rare, autosomal recessive disease (Weston, 1985). The harlequin fetus presents with hard, thick, gray or yellow scales that cause severe deformities of skeletal and soft tissues.
   b. The condition is untreatable, and most infants die within a few hours or days of life.

5. Cutis aplasia.
   a. Cutis aplasia refers to the congenital absence of skin, either as a midline defect, posterior scalp defect, or as several small or large defects involving the upper and lower extremities (Fig. 24–13).
   b. The lesions heal slowly over several months, leaving a hypertrophic or atrophic scar.
   c. Cutis aplasia may be associated with other defects such as cleft lip and palate and trisomy 13.

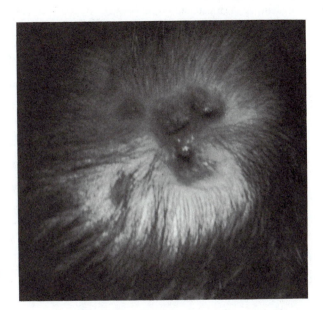

Figure 24–13
Cutis aplasia. (Photo courtesy of Jacinto Hernandez, M.D., The Children's Hospital, Denver, Colorado.)

STUDY QUESTIONS

1. A characteristic of the newborn skin is that:
   a. It contains fully developed sweat glands.
   b. It is more permeable to topically applied chemicals.
   c. It is thicker than adult skin.

2. A vesicle is defined as a:
   a. Flat, pigmented spot smaller than 1 cm in diameter.
   b. Fluid-filled lesion less than 1 cm in diameter.
   c. Solid, elevated lesion greater than 1 cm in diameter.

3. Erythema toxicum can be diagnosed by:
   a. Appearance of papules or vesicles.
   b. Aspiration of pustules showing numerous eosinophils.
   c. Aspiration of pustules showing staphylococci.

4. Port-wine stains may be associated with:
   a. Klippel-Trenaunay-Weber syndrome.
   b. Neurofibromatosis.
   c. Sturge-Weber syndrome.

5. The usual treatment for a strawberry hemangioma is:
   a. Allow it to regress spontaneously.
   b. Surgical removal.
   c. Topically applied steroids.

6. Ichthyosis is caused by:
   a. A genetic defect inherited by various modes.
   b. Infection.
   c. Trauma to the skin.

Answers to Study Questions

1. b	3. b	5. a
2. b	4. c	6. a

REFERENCES

Apfelberg, D.B., Maser, M.R., and Lash, H.: Argon laser treatment of cutaneous vascular abnormalities. Ann. Plast. Surg., 1:14–18, 1978.
Fienman, N.L., and Yakovac, W.C.: Neurofibromatosis in childhood. J. Pediatr., 76:339, 1970.
Francis, C., and Martin, A.H.: Introduction to Human Anatomy, 7th ed. St. Louis, C.V. Mosby, 1975, pp. 413–437.
Hodgeman, J.E., Freedman, R.I., and Levan, N.E.: Neonatal dermatology. Pediatr. Clin. North Am., 18(3):713–754, 1971.
Kuller, J.M., Lund, C., and Tobin, C.: Improved skin care for preterm infants. Maternal Child Nurs., 8:200–203, 1983.
Margileth, A.: Dermatologic conditions. In Avery, C.B. (ed.): Neonatology: Pathophysiology and Management of the Newborn, 2nd ed. Philadelphia, J.B. Lippincott, 1987, pp. 1061–1103.
Ramamurthy, R.S., et al.: Transient neonatal pustular melanosis. J. Pediatr., 88:831–835, 1976.
Rand, R.E., and Baden, H.P.: The ichthyoses: A review. J. Am. Acad. Dermatol., 88:285, 1983.
Ruiz-Maldonado, R., Parish, L.C., and Beare, J.M.: Textbook of Pediatric Dermatology. Philadelphia, Grune & Stratton, 1989.
Schuman, A.J., and Oksol, B.A.: The effect of isopropyl alcohol and triple dye on umbilical cord separation time. Milit. Med., 150(1):49–51, 1985.
Solomon, L.M., and Esterly, N.B.: Neonatal Dermatology. Philadelphia, W. B. Saunders Co., 1973.
Weston, W.L.: Practical Pediatric Dermatology, 2nd ed. Boston, Little, Brown, 1985.

Carla Shapiro

Ophthalmologic Disorders

Objectives

1. Describe the normal anatomy of the eye.

2. Identify the major function(s) of each structure.

3. Describe the components of a nursing assessment of the eyes in the neonate.

4. Describe the nurse's role in assisting the physician with neonatal eye examinations.

5. For each of the following eye disorders of the neonatal period: traumatic injuries to the eye, conjunctivitis, nasolacrimal duct obstruction, cataracts, infections, or "TORCH" diseases:

   a. Provide an overview of the pathogenesis of common disorders of the eye in the neonatal period.
   b. Describe commonly used treatment modalities used and outline the specific nursing care measures designed to meet the needs of neonates with the above disorders.

An examination of the newborn's eyes is an important, though often neglected, portion of a physical assessment. There is a great deal of clinically significant information that the astute nurse can glean from a thorough evaluation of the neonate's eyes. Evidence of intrauterine infection, birth trauma, congenital malformations, disease, and a variety of genetic abnormalities can be detected during the course of the nurse's assessment of the newborn's eyes.

This chapter provides the neonatal nurse with a review of normal eye anatomy together with the major function(s) of each structure; the essential components of an assessment of the newborn's eyes; an overview of the most common eye disorders in the neonate; and common treatment modalities and nursing measures used when caring for various ocular disorders in the newborn.

Anatomy of the Eye (Fig. 25–1)

PROTECTIVE STRUCTURES

A. **The eyelids:** shade the eyes during sleep; protect from excessive light or foreign objects; spread lubricating secretions over the eyeball.

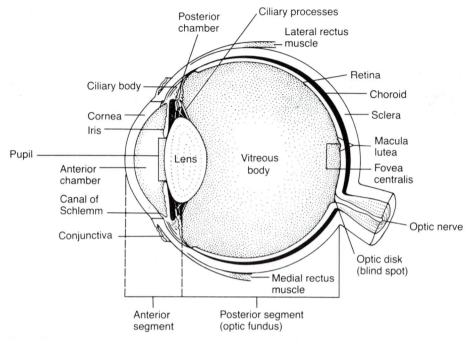

Figure 25-1
Cross-section of the eyeball. (From J. Ophthal. Nurs. Technol., *6*(5):178, 1987. With permission of Burroughs Wellcome Co.)

B. **Conjunctiva:** mucous membrane lining the inner aspect of the eyelids (palpebral), and onto the eyeball to the periphery of the cornea (bulbar).

C. **Lacrimal system:** manufactures and drains away tears; cleans, lubricates, and moistens the eyeball.

D. **Bony orbit or socket:** surrounds and protects the eyeball. Most important opening within the orbit is the optic foramen, through which the optic nerve, ophthalmic artery, and ophthalmic vein from each eye pass through enroute to the brain.

THE EYEBALL

A. **Outer layer (fibrous tunic).**
1. Cornea: transparent; reflects light rays.
2. Sclera: the "white" of the eye; normal bluish appearance in newborns; gives shape to the eyeball and protects the inner parts.

B. **Middle layer (vascular tunic): the uveal tract.**
1. Iris and pupil: a circular pigmented diaphragm with a central hole; controls the amount of light entering the eye.
2. Ciliary body: the anterior portion of the choroid.
3. Choroid: a vascular, pigmented membrane that lines most of the internal surface of the sclera; absorbs light rays, and nourishes the retina.

C. **Inner layer: the retina.**
1. Extends from the ora serrata to the optic nerve.
2. Functions in image formation.
   a. Photoreceptors: rods and cones.
   b. Bipolar cells.
   c. Ganglion cells.

3. Optic disc: retinal blood vessels enter the eye, optic nerve exits the eye. No photoreceptors here, thus a blind spot in the field of vision.
4. Optic nerve: the second cranial nerve.
5. Macula: the exact center of the retina and location of sharpest vision.

D. **Anterior cavity (filled with aqueous humor).**
1. Anterior chamber: behind the cornea, in front of the iris.
2. Posterior chamber: behind the iris, in front of the suspensory ligament and lens.

E. **The lens:** a biconvex, transparent capsule that refracts light. The most important focusing mechanism of the eye.

F. **Posterior cavity (filled with vitreous humor):** lies between the lens and the retina. Contributes to intraocular pressure, gives shape to the eyeball, and holds the retina in place.

EXTRAOCULAR MUSCLES

A. **Musculature and innervation:** six muscles move each globe; innervated by the oculomotor (third cranial) nerve, the abducens (sixth cranial) nerve, and the trochlear (fourth cranial) nerve. Muscles of each eye work in conjunction with each other.

Patient Assessment

HISTORY

A. **Pregnancy:** first trimester infections (e.g., rubella), unknown rashes, fever, venereal disease, vaginal discharge, medications.

B. **Birth history:** gestational age, duration of labor, use of forceps.

C. **Family history:** incidence of ocular disorders, especially retinoblastoma; systemic diseases.

EXAMINATION

The examination is performed with the baby in a quiet, alert state.

A. **External assessment.**
1. General facial configuration: should be symmetrical. Note distance between the eyes. An abnormal width between the eyes is referred to as hypertelorism.
2. Spontaneous eye movements: note range of motion and conjugation (the ability of the eyes to move together). Infants can track and follow objects with both eyes. Erratic or purposeless movements may be observed during the first few weeks of life. Median focal distance for the newborn is about 8 inches (20 cm).

B. **Reaction to light or visual stimuli:** strong blink reflex to bright light or stimulation of the lids, lashes, or cornea. A somewhat unsteady gaze can be observed shortly after birth, with ability to fixate on a stimulus for 4–10 seconds and refixate every 1.0–1.5 seconds. Ability to maintain fixation and follow does not occur until 5–6 weeks of age.

C. **Pupils:** size and reaction to light—should be round and equal; constriction to both direct and contralateral stimulation. The red reflex should be elicited bilaterally. Normally appears as a homogeneous bright red-orange color. Opacities or interruptions may indicate cataracts or retinoblastoma.

D. **Eyelids:** note symmetry, epicanthal folds, bruising or edema, lacerations, ptosis, presence of lacrimal puncta.

E. **Conjunctiva:** should be pink and moist; redness or exudate is abnormal.

F. **Cornea:** may be somewhat less than transparent or slightly hazy in the first few days of life in both premature and full-term infants. Sclera may be bluish in premature or small babies as a result of thinness.

G. **Irises:** should be similar in appearance; note pigmentation. A coloboma or keyhole pupil may be associated with congenital anomalies. Brushfield's spots: silverish-gray spots scattered around the circumference of the iris. Strongly associated with Down syndrome.

H. **Lens:** should be clear and black with direct illumination. Examination of the anterior vascular capsule of the lens is a useful adjunct to determination of gestational age in pre-term infants between 27 and 34 weeks.

I. **Doll's head reflex:** as head is turned on the shoulders, eyes move in the opposite direction.

Pathological Conditions and Management

BIRTH TRAUMA

Pathophysiology

A. Direct result of duration and difficulty of delivery.
B. Improperly applied forceps.
C. Compression of cranial nerves.

Clinical Presentation

A. petechiae; ecchymoses; edema; and/or lacerations of lids, conjunctiva, or globe.
B. bright red patches on conjunctiva (subconjunctival hemorrhage).
C. droopy eyelids.

Complications

A. These injuries are generally mild, transient, and often resolve spontaneously.

CONJUNCTIVITIS

Conjunctivitis is an inflammatory reaction secondary to invasion of conjunctiva by pathological organisms.

Etiology

A wide variety of infectious agents are capable of producing conjunctivitis in the newborn. The most common causes in North America include the following:

A. *Neisseria gonorrhoeae:* peripartum transmission.
B. *Chlamydia trachomatis:* peripartum transmission.
C. *Staphylococcus aureus:* acquired during the neonatal period.
D. *Enteric pathogens.*

Neisseria gonorrhoeae

 Incidence.
1. Reported at less than 0.03%.

2. May be higher in areas with poor perinatal care or irregular antibiotic eye prophylaxis following birth.

B. **Onset of infection:** onset of symptoms usually between days 3 and 5 of life.

C. **Clinical presentation.**
1. Edema of the eyelids.
2. Purulent discharge.
3. Redness/hyperemia of the conjunctiva.

D. **Diagnostic Findings.**
1. History.
   a. Maternal history of sexually transmitted disease.
   b. Age of onset of infection.
2. Physical examination.
   a. Clinical signs of inflammation.
   b. Purulent discharge.
3. Laboratory.
   a. Gram's stain shows gram-negative diplococci.
   b. Positive culture for gonococcus from conjunctival surface or exudate.

E. **Patient management.**
1. Isolate infant in accordance with infection control guidelines.
2. Irrigate eyes with sterile normal saline hourly until discharge is eliminated.
3. Prompt administration of appropriate systemic therapy. Topical antimicrobial therapy is *not* required.
   a. Penicillin-sensitive *N. gonorrhoeae:* aqueous crystalline penicillin G, IV or IM, 50,000–100,000 U/kg/day in two to three divided doses for 7 days.
   b. Penicillin-resistant *N. gonorrhoeae:* ceftriaxone, 125 mg IM in a single dose, or cefixime, 8 mg/kg PO in a single dose.
4. Parents of infected infant should be referred for evaluation and treatment.

F. **Complications.**
1. Infants with gonococcal conjunctivitis are at risk for corneal ulceration, perforation, and subsequent visual impairment.
2. Systemic complications involving the blood, joints, or CNS may occur in a small number of infants.

Chlamydia trachomatis

A. **Incidence.**
1. The most common cause of conjunctivitis in the neonatal period, especially in areas with poor perinatal care or irregular administration of erythromycin eye prophylaxis following delivery.
2. About 50% of babies born to mothers who are colonized with *C. trachomatis* will develop the disease.
3. Prevention of infection in the newborn is dependent upon pre-natal detection and treatment of the mother, or the use of an effective form of eye prophylaxis at birth (e.g., erythromycin ointment).

B. **Onset.**
1. Symptoms usually observed between 5 and 14 days of age.

C. **Clinical presentation.**
1. Symptoms vary from mild conjunctivitis to intense edema of the lids with purulent discharge.

D. **Diagnostic findings.**
1. Identification of chlamydial antigen.
2. Giemsa stains of conjunctival scrapings.
3. Culture of conjunctival scrapings.

E. **Patient management.**
1. Therapy of choice is oral erythromycin.

    a. Infants younger than 7 days: 20 mg/kg/day divided every 12 hours for 2 weeks.

    b. Infants older than 7 days: 30–40 mg/kg/day divided tid or qid for 2 weeks.

2. Topical therapy alone is inadequate to eradicate the organism from the upper respiratory tract.

3. Parents of infected infants should be referred for evaluation and therapy.

F. **Complications.**

1. Spread via the nasolacrimal system to the nasopharynx leading to chlamydial pneumonia.

NASOLACRIMAL DUCT OBSTRUCTION

Pathophysiology

A. **Lacrimal apparatus** consists of structures that produce tears (lacrimal glands) and structures responsible for drainage of tears (upper and lower puncta, canaliculi, lacrimal sac, and nasolacrimal duct). System functions to clean, lubricate, and moisten the eyeball.

B. **Full-term and pre-term newborns have the capacity to secrete tears** (reflex tearing to irritants) but usually do not secrete emotional tears until 2–3 months of age.

C. **Congenital obstruction** is usually caused by an imperforate membrane at the distal end of the nasolacrimal duct.

D. **Congenital nasolacrimal obstruction is the most common abnormality of the newborn's lacrimal apparatus**. Incidence of this condition ranges between 2 and 6% of all newborns.

Clinical Presentation

A. **Usually within the first few weeks of life.**

B. **Persistent tearing (epiphora).** Need to rule out congenital glaucoma.

C. **Crusting or matting of the eyelashes**—"sticky eye."

D. **Tears spill over the lower lid and cheek;** a "wet look" in the involved eye(s).

E. **Absence of conjunctival infection.**

F. **Gentle pressure over the involved nasolacrimal sac may result in mucopurulent material** refluxing from either punctum.

Complications

A. **Acute dacryocystitis:** inflamed, swollen lacrimal sac.

B. **Fistula formation.**

C. **Orbital or facial cellulitis.**

Specific Patient Care

A. **Conservative management**, with daily massage of the nasolacrimal sac in an attempt to rupture the membrane and the lower end of the duct.

B. **Technique**. Technique consists of placing the index finger over the common canaliculus to block the exit of material through the puncta, and stroking down firmly.

C. **Digital pressure increases hydrostatic pressure in the nasolacrimal sac**, which may cause a rupture of the membranous obstruction.

D. **If a mucopurulent discharge is present**, antibiotic eye drops (sodium sulfacetamide) or ointment (erythromycin) may be required.

E. **Cleaning of eyes**. Eyes should be cleaned with moist compresses, and secretions mechanically removed.

F. **Length of conservative management**. Conservative management is advocated for the first year of life.

G. **Resolution**. The majority of nasolacrimal obstructions resolve spontaneously or with medical management (massage) by 1 year of age.

H. **Surgical treatment**. Unresolved obstructions can be successfully surgically treated with tear duct probing under general anesthesia after the first year of life.

CATARACTS

Congenital cataracts are the main treatable cause of visual impairment in infancy. The visual prognosis for the child is improved the sooner in life that the cataracts are removed surgically and proper optics are restored.

Pathophysiology

A. **Lens**. The lens is a biconvex, transparent capsule that refracts light. It is the most important focusing mechanism of the eye.

B. **Cataract**. A cataract is an opacity of any size or degree in the lens of the eye.

C. **Path of light**. Normally, the light from an object passes directly through the lens to a focal point on the retina, producing a sharp image. Cataracts result in production of a degraded image or no image at all.

D. **Cataracts lead to varying degrees of visual impairment**, from blurred vision to blindness, depending upon the location and extent of the opacity.

Etiology or Precipitating Factors

1. Idiopathic: developmental variation, not associated with other abnormalities.
2. Genetically determined.
   a. Most common mode of inheritance is autosomal dominant.
3. Congenital rubella.
   a. Cataracts present in 50% of newborns with congenital rubella syndrome.
4. Other congenital infections.
   a. Toxoplasmosis.
   b. Cytomegalovirus.
   c. Herpes simplex.
   d. Varicella and zoster.
5. Metabolic disorders: e.g., galactosemia.
6. Chromosomal abnormalities: e.g., Down syndrome.
7. Clinical syndromes: e.g., Crouzon's disease, Pierre Robin syndrome.
8. Prematurity.
9. Often transient, disappearing spontaneously within a few weeks.

Clinical Presentation

A. **A white pupil** (leukokoria).

B. **Searching nystagmus** (at 1–2 months of age).

Diagnostic Findings

A. **History**.
1. Family history of ocular disease or systemic disorders.
2. Pregnancy, especially first trimester infections with TORCH diseases. (See Congenital Infections.)

B. **Physical examination**.

1. Normally, the pupils look black to the bare eye of the examiner when light is directed at them.
2. Examine for a white pupil by shining a light into each eye, with the light source held to one side.
3. If the opacity is small, it may only be identified with the pupils dilated, and using an ophthalmoscope.
4. Consider other diseases of the eye that may produce a white pupil, e.g., retinoblastoma.

Complications

A. **Varying degrees of visual impairment**, leading to developmental delay.

B. **Presence and/or severity of associated ocular defects**, such as microphthalmia and glaucoma.

Specific Patient Care

A. **Assist the physician in carrying out a thorough eye examination of the newborn**. This includes the administration of drops necessary to dilate the pupils prior to the examination, and supporting the infant's head to facilitate examination.

B. **Parental education**. In collaboration with the physician, assist parents in understanding the nature, possible etiology and treatment of cataracts in the newborn, and the prognosis for future vision. Surgery is indicated whenever the cataract is likely to interfere with vision.

C. **Explore any feelings of guilt parents may have** related to the cause of the cataracts, and provide appropriate support.

D. **Encourage parent-infant attachment**. Baby may not be able to see the parents but can learn to know their voice, smell, and touch.

E. **Care for the patient postoperatively**.

1. Prevent increased intraocular pressure. Keep baby comfortable, well fed, and free from pain, to decrease crying.
2. Administer eyedrops or ointments as ordered postoperatively.
3. Apply clean eyepatches or protective shields to protect the eye from rubbing or bumping and to prevent irritation from light.
4. Monitor for complications of cataract surgery. These are relatively infrequent, but include infection within the eye, glaucoma, and retinal detachment. Note any increased redness or haziness of the eye, increased tearing, photophobia, or a cloudiness of the cornea. Increased crying, irritability, disruption in sleeping patterns, or rubbing the eye may be indicative of pain.
5. Assist parents in understanding the essential role of optical correction devices such as glasses or contact lenses on their infant's vision and development.
6. Promote appropriate visual stimulation and foster normal infant development by teaching parents about newborn visual preferences (e.g., black and white contrast, or medium-intensity colors; the human face; geometrical shapes; checkerboards).

Outcome

A. **Prognosis**. Visual prognosis depends not only upon the extent of cataracts, age at removal, surgical outcome, and rapid optical correction, but also on the nature of other associated anomalies of the eye or syndromes.

RETINOPATHY OF PREMATURITY (ROP)

Formally referred to as retrolental fibroplasia, ROP is a vasoproliferative retinopathy that occurs primarily in premature infants.

Pathophysiology

A. **The human retina is avascular until 16 weeks' gestation**. After this time, a capillary network begins to grow, starting at the optic nerve and branching outward toward the ora serrata (edge of the retina).

B. **The nasal periphery is vascularized by about 32 weeks' gestation**, but the process is not complete in the more distant temporal periphery until 40–44 weeks.

C. **Following premature birth**, this process of normal vasculogenesis may be arrested as a result of injury from some noxious agent(s) or stressor(s).

D. **Vasoproliferation**. This arrest of normal vasculogenesis is later followed by a phase of rapid, excessive irregular vascular growth and shunt formation (vasoproliferation), stimulated by a "vasoactive factor."

E. **The area of new growth generally forms an abrupt ridge between the vascular and avascular retina**, particularly in the temporal periphery.

F. **Active ROP may resolve if the vasculature in the area recovers and resumes advancing normally**, allowing the retina to become completely vascularized.

G. **If the new vasculature proceeds to develop abnormally**, these capillaries may extend into the vitreous body and/or over the surface of the retina (where they do not belong). Leakage of fluid or hemorrhage from these weak, aberrant blood vessels may occur.

H. **Blood and fluid leakage** into various parts of the eye can result in scar formation and traction on the retina.

I. **Traction may pull the macula out of its normal position, thus affecting visual acuity**. If the macula is slightly out of position, vision will be mildly affected.

J. **Tractional exudative retinal detachment results in blindness**.

Etiology

A. **A complex multifactorial disorder**. Possible risk factors include the following:
1. Prematurity/low birthweight*
2. Hyperoxia.
3. Hypoxia.
4. Blood transfusions.
5. Intraventricular hemorrhage.
6. Apnea/bradycardia spells.
7. Sepsis.
8. Hypercapnia/hypocapnia.
9. Patent ductus arteriosus.
10. Vitamin E deficiency.
11. Lactic acidosis.
12. Pre-natal complications.
13. Duration of mechanical ventilation and oxygen therapy.
14. Exposure to bright light.

Incidence

A. **The incidence appears to increase significantly as birthweight and gestational age decrease**.

B. **Risk**. The risk of ROP rises dramatically from 9 to 32% for infants of 1.0–1.5 kg birthweight to 22–90% for those weighing less than 1 kg at birth.

---

*Denotes the most important clinical factor associated with ROP.

Physical Examination

A. **Examination of the high-risk neonate**. All high-risk newborns (especially those of birthweight less than 1500 g) should have their eyes examined by a trained pediatric ophthalmologist when in stable clinical condition, 4–6 weeks after birth (approximately 32–34 weeks' post-conceptional age).

B. **The infant's pupils should be dilated with a mydriatic agent** prior to examination, to facilitate optimal evaluation.

C. **The location and extent of any retinopathy should be precisely documented and classified** according to the guidelines developed by the International Committee on ROP (1984).

D. **Follow-up examinations**.

1. Infants who are found to have areas of retinal immaturity on initial examination should have repeat examinations every other week, and then later, every 3–4 weeks, until vascularization has reached the ora serrata.
2. If ROP is present during the initial examination, the infant should be examined weekly or every other week, depending on the severity of clinical findings.

Complications

A. Mydriatic eye drops and eye examinations can produce hypertension, reflex bradycardia, and apnea as a result of drug effects and vagal stimulation.

B. **Varying degrees of visual impairment** (e.g., myopia), which may require corrective lenses to improve visual acuity.

C. Strabismus.

D. Glaucoma.

E. Cataracts.

F. Amblyopia.

G. Retinal detachment and blindness.

The majority of babies with ROP have an uneventful recovery and experience no serious complications. Those with progressive R.O.P. may require cryotherapy.

Specific Patient Care

A. **Precautions while using oxygen**. Although the role of oxygen in the pathogenesis of ROP is unclear, cautious and judicious administration and monitoring of oxygen remain one possible preventative measure.

1. Continuous assessment and monitoring of the infant receiving oxygen to control arterial oxygenation. Cautious administration of oxygen while carrying out nursing procedures such as suctioning.
2. Ongoing assessment of the oxygen delivery system, including calibration of O_2 analyzers, monitoring of FIO_2, checking/recording ventilator settings/circuit, and oxygen saturation monitors.
3. Use of oxygen blenders to deliver precise oxygen concentrations.

B. **Results**. At present, no data are available demonstrating a definitive reduction in the incidence of ROP as a result of improved oxygen monitoring.

C. **Provide a variety of forms of sensory stimulation to the infant**, appropriate to level of development and behavioral cues.

D. **Assess newborn's ability to fix and focus**.

E. **Assist the physician in carrying out a safe, minimally stressful eye examination** of the newborn.

F. **Protect the infant's eyes from bright light by shielding the Isolette with a**

blanket and reducing the light levels in the nursery. Do not apply eyepads (except during phototherapy), as the visual system requires sensory stimulation in order to develop normally.

G. **Provide accurate parent education about the possibility of ROP** (when parents are ready to receive information about potential non–life-threatening complications). Ensure that parents understand ROP is essentially a problem of immaturity whose cause is yet unknown.

H. **Provide care for the infant undergoing cryotherapy**.
1. Monitor the infant closely for possible risks of the procedure, including the following:
    a. Risks of undergoing a general anesthetic.
    b. Arrhythmias induced from the use of lidocaine (Xylocaine).
    c. Bradycardia secondary to vagal stimulation created by pressure on the eyeball.
    d. Edema of the eyelids.
    e. Infection.
    f. Intraocular bleeding.
2. Ensure patient safety and comfort during the treatment.
    a. Proper supine positioning of the baby.
    b. Maintain adequate heat source throughout the procedure.
    c. Monitor vital signs and oxygenation status throughout the procedure.
    d. Provide comfort measures and analgesia as needed.
3. Provide postoperative care following the treatment.
    a. Administer eyedrops/ointments as ordered.
    b. Shield the infant from unnecessary direct light.
    c. Observe for signs of feeding intolerance, gastric distention, and/or aspirates when feedings are resumed if mydriatics were used.

I. **Provide emotional support and appropriate community referrals for parents** whose infant will be significantly visually impaired.

Outcome

A. **90% (or more) of cases of acute ROP resolve spontaneously, with little or no visual loss.**

B. **Cryotherapy has been shown to decrease the risk of blinding complications of ROP by 50%.**

Congenital Infections

An infant who is born with an infection acquired in utero may simply present as a baby with intrauterine growth retardation (IUGR), or one who is seriously ill with multisystem involvement. The developing eyes are highly vulnerable to the damaging effects of pre-natal infection, and ocular abnormalities may in fact be the predominant manifestation of the disease. A number of the congenitally acquired infections are associated with abnormal ocular conditions, including cataracts, chorioretinitis, corneal opacities, and glaucoma.

The most common of these infections are referred to by the acronym "TORCH" diseases—toxoplasmosis, rubella, cytomegalovirus, herpes, and other infectious agents (e.g., syphilis).

CONGENITAL RUBELLA SYNDROME

Pathophysiology

A. **Timing of infection**. Consequences of the transplacental infection are determined primarily by the timing of the viral insult.

B. Infection in the first trimester of pregnancy presents the greatest hazard to organogenesis.

Etiology

A. Despite the fact that an effective vaccine to prevent rubella exists, cases of congenital rubella continue to occur.

B. Approximately 10–20% of women in the reproductive age group lack protective antibodies and are at risk for rubella infection.

C. Vulnerable women exposed to the virus in the first or second trimesters of pregnancy are at greatest risk of producing an infant with the disease.

Incidence

A. Ocular abnormalities are the cardinal manifestations of congenital rubella, occurring in 40–62% of patients.

Clinical Presentation

A. Gestational age. Findings in the infant exposed to rubella in utero depend upon the gestational age at which the infection occurred.
1. Ocular manifestations.
   a. Cataracts: present in approximately 50% of patients.*
   b. Pigmentary retinopathy.
   c. Microphthalmia.
   d. Glaucoma: occurs in 10–25% of patients.
2. Other common manifestations:
   a. Intrauterine growth retardation.
   b. Deafness.*
   c. Cardiac defects (patent ductus arteriosus, septal defects, pulmonary artery stenosis).*
   d. Hepatosplenomegaly.
   e. Thrombocytopenia and petechiae.
   f. Microcephaly.
   g. Bone lesions.

Complications

A. This disease is progressive. Although up to 68% of infants show no apparent problems at birth, they may experience consequences of the infection later in life.

B. Hearing loss is the most common defect for neonates.

Specific Patient Care

A. Virus shedding may continue for months following birth. Infants suspected of having congenital rubella should be isolated from other newborns and pregnant women (both in hospital and at home following discharge).

B. Parents need to understand the immediate and long-term effects of this disease.

C. See section on care of patient with cataracts.

---

*Denotes the most common manifestations of congenital rubella syndrome, which often occur together.

Outcome

A. **Prognosis.** Prognosis for infants with rubella syndrome depends upon the severity of symptoms and the number of organ systems involved.

B. **Mortality.** Mortality in the first year of life may approach 80%, when multisystem involvement occurs.

C. **Multiple handicaps are common in surviving infants**.

D. **The consequences of congenital rubella may not be evident at birth**, but may become apparent in subsequent months.

E. **There is a need for ongoing follow-up and evaluation of these infants after discharge from hospital.** Major problems presenting after the newborn period include communication disorders, hearing defects, and mental or motor retardation.

CYTOMEGALOVIRUS (CMV)

Pathophysiology

A. A perinatal viral infection.

B. **Congenital illness is most severe if infection occurs early in pregnancy**, the period of greatest susceptibility to the developing fetus.

Etiology

A. **Cytomegaloviruses are ubiquitous agents that can cause infection in all age groups**.

B. **Route of transmission.** May be acquired transplacentally, during birth (via the cervix), or through breast milk.

C. **An important possible cause of morbidity in premature infants is transfusion-acquired CMV.** All premature infants should receive seronegative blood products.

Incidence

A. **The most common of congenital viral infections, occurring in 1% of all newborns.**

B. **In the presence of primary acute maternal infection, 25–50% of fetuses are affected.**

Clinical Presentation

A. **A diagnosis of congenital CMV infection can rarely be made on the basis of clinical findings alone.** Only 5–10% of neonates infected with CMV will be symptomatic at birth.

B. **Laboratory diagnostic methods must be employed if this condition is suspected** (e.g., isolation of the virus from the urine).

C. **Chorioretinitis:** present in 10–20% of symptomatic infants; is the single most common finding in congenitally infected infants.

D. **Intrauterine growth retardation.**

E. **Hepatosplenomegaly.**

F. **Bleeding disorders.**

G. **Neurological signs.**

H. **Hyperbilirubinemia.**

I. **Other eye abnormalities**, including conjunctivitis, corneal clouding, cataracts, and optic atrophy.

Complications

A. Cytomegalic inclusion disease.

B. Sensorineural hearing loss, the most important late sequela.

Specific Patient Care

A. No effective treatment exists. Supportive nursing care measures, aimed at specific symptoms, are employed.

B. Use of gowns and good handwashing are essential to prevent the spread of infection.

C. Sero-negative pregnant women should not care for infants with known or suspected infection.

D. These infants require long-term follow-up.

Outcomes

A. Mortality. Overall mortality from symptomatic congenital infection is up to 30%.

B. Few survivors are normal. 10–20% of infants asymptomatic at birth may develop neurological sequelae such as mental retardation or sensorineural deafness in the first years of life.

TOXOPLASMOSIS

Pathophysiology

A. Fetal damage occurs as a direct result of inflammation caused by the presence of cysts in the tissue.

Etiology

A. Maternal infection by the protozoan *Toxoplasma gondii* in the first and second trimesters of pregnancy is often associated with transplacental infection of the fetus.

B. Acquisition of infection. Infection is acquired through contact with the excrement of infected cats and ingestion of improperly cooked meat.

Incidence

A. The incidence of maternal infection ranges from 0.15 to 0.64%.

B. Fetal infection occurs in about 0.07–0.13% of all pregnancies.

Clinical Presentation

A. Chorioretinitis: most common.

B. Hepatosplenomegaly.

C. Jaundice.

D. Bleeding disorders.

E. Hydrocephalus.

F. CNS calcifications.

Specific Nursing Care

A. **Pharmaceutical treatment of *Toxoplasma* infection by administering sulfadiazine and pyrimethamine**. These agents will eradicate the cysts, but will not reverse damage already done.

B. **Supportive care of family**, with sensitivity to feelings of guilt they might have.

C. **Teach parents to recognize the signs of visual impairment in infancy** (e.g., failure to fix and focus on objects or faces).

Outcome

A. **Prognosis**. The prognosis for infants with congenital infection is not good.

B. **Mortality**. Mortality is roughly 10–15% of infected infants.

C. **Psychomotor retardation**. 85% of survivors will have severe psychomotor retardation.

D. **Visual disturbances**. 50% of surviving infants will develop visual problems.

STUDY QUESTIONS

1. Shining a bright light in a newborn's eyes should result in:
   a. A prolonged steady gaze.
   b. A strong blink reflex.
   c. Nystagmus.

2. Opacities or interruptions of the red reflex may be:
   a. A variation of normal.
   b. Brushfield's spots.
   c. Congenital cataracts.

3. The most common cause of neonatal conjunctivitis in North America is:
   a. *Chlamydia trachomatis*.
   b. *Neisseria gonorrhoeae*.
   c. *Staphylococcus aureus*.

4. One of the earliest presenting signs of congenital nasolacrimal duct obstruction is:
   a. Conjunctivitis.

   b. Crusting or matting of the eyelashes.
   c. Dry eyes/lack of tears.

5. An important clinical factor associated with retinopathy of prematurity (ROP) is:
   a. Hyperoxia.
   b. Hypoxia.
   c. Prematurity.

6. A number of complications can result from ROP. The majority of babies with ROP will experience:
   a. Blindness.
   b. Little or no visual loss.
   c. Macular degeneration.

7. A common ocular manifestation of congenital rubella infection is:
   a. Cataracts.
   b. Chorioretinitis.
   c. Glaucoma.

Answers to Study Questions

1. b	4. b	6. b
2. c	5. c	7. a
3. a		

BIBLIOGRAPHY

Avery, M.E., and Taeusch, H.W. (eds.): Diseases of the Newborn, 6th ed. Philadelphia, W.B. Saunders Co., 1991.

Bell, T., Sandström, K.I., Gravett, M., et al.: Comparison of ophthalmic silver nitrate solution and erythromycin ointment for prevention of natally acquired *Chlamydia trachomatis*. Sex. Transm. Dis., October–December, *14*(4):195–200, 1987.

Boyd-Monk, H.: The structure and function of the eye and its adnexa. J. Ophthal. Nurs. Technol., 6(5):176–183, 1987.

Bryant, B.G.: Unit dose erythromycin ophthalmic ointment for neonatal ocular prophylaxis. JOGN, 13(2):83–87, 1984.

Calhoun, J.H.: Cataracts in children. Pediatr. Clin. North Am., 30(9):1061–1069, 1983.

Calhoun, J.H.: Problems of the lacrimal system in children. Pediatr. Clin. North Am., 34(6):1457–1465, 1987.

Caputo, A., Schnitzer, R., Lindquist, T., and Sun, S.: Dilatation in neonates: A protocol. Pediatrics, 69(1):77–79, 1982.

Chew, E., and Morin, J.D.: Glaucoma in children. Pediatr. Clin. North Am., 30(6):1043–1060, 1983.

Cohen, K., and Byrne, S.: The role of the nurse in assisting with eye examinations on premature infants. Neonatal Network, 8(2):31–35, 1989.

Crawford, J.S., and Morin, J.D. (eds.): The Eye in Childhood. New York, Grune & Stratton, 1983.

Crom, D., Wilimas, J., Green, A., et al.: Malignancy in the neonate. Med. Pediatr. Oncol., 17:101–104, 1986.

Cryotherapy for retinopathy of prematurity cooperative group: Multicenter trial of cryotherapy for retinopathy of prematurity: Preliminary results. Pediatrics, 81(5):697–706, 1988.

Dennehy, P.J., Warman, R., Flynn, J., et al.: Ocular manifestations in pediatric patients with acquired immunodeficiency syndrome. Arch. Ophthalmol., 107:978–982, 1989.

Eller, A.W., and Brown, G.: Retinal disorders of childhood. Pediatr. Clin. North Am., 30(6):1087–1101, 1983.

Fanaroff, A.A., and Martin, R.J. (eds.): Neonatal-Perinatal Medicine, 4th ed. St. Louis, C.V. Mosby, 1987.

Fisher, M.: Conjunctivitis in children. Pediatr. Clin. North Am., 34(6):1447–1455, 1987.

Flynn, J.: Retinopathy of prematurity. Pediatr. Clin. North Am., 34(6):1487–1516, 1987.

Friendly, D.: Ophthalmia neonatorum. Pediatr. Clin. North Am., 30(6):1033–1042, 1983.

George, D., Stephen, S., Fellows, R., and Bremer, D.: The latest on retinopathy of prematurity. Matern. Child Nurs., 13(4):254–258, 1988.

Gordin, P.C.: Retinopathy of prematurity. NAACOG Update Series, 6:26, 1989. Princeton, New Jersey: Continuing Professional Education Center.

Harley, R.D.: Pediatric Ophthamology, 2nd ed. Philadelphia, W.B. Saunders Co., 1983.

Hittner, H., Hirsch, N., and Rudolph, A.: Assessment of gestational age by examination of the anterior vascular capsule of the lens. J. Pediatr., 91(3):455–458, 1977.

Isenberg S., and Everett, S.: Cardiovascular effects of mydriatics in low-birth-weight infants. J. Pediatr., 105(1):111–112, 1984.

Johnson, L., Quinn, G., Abbasi, S., et al.: Effects of sustained pharmacologic vitamin E levels on incidence and severity of retinopathy of prematurity: A controlled clinical trial. J. Pediatr., 114(5):827–838, 1986.

Kleiman, A.H.: ABC's of pediatric ophthalmology. J. Ophthal. Nurs. Technol., 5(3):86–90, 1986.

Long, C.A.: Cryotherapy: A new treatment for retinopathy of prematurity. Pediatr. Nurs., 15(3):269–272, 1989.

Ludington-Hoe, S.: What can newborns really see? Am. J. Nurs., 83(9):1286–1289, 1983.

Matoba, A.: Ocular viral infections. Pediatr. Infect. Dis., 3(4):358–368, 1984.

McNamara, J.A., Tasman, W., Brown, G.C., and Federman, J.L.: Laser photocoagulation for stage 3+ retinopathy of prematurity. Ophthalmology, 98(5):576–580, 1987.

Nelson, L.B.: Congenital nasolacrimal duct obstruction. J. Ophthal. Nurs. Technol., 6(2):57–60, 1987.

Nucci, P., Capoferri, C., Alfarano, R., and Brancato, R.: Conservative management of congenital nasolacrimal duct obstruction. J Pediatr. Ophthalmol. Strabismus, 26(1):39–43, 1989.

Nurses' Drug Alert: Erythromycin prevents most neonatal eye infections. Am. J. Nurs., 7(2):9, 1983.

Palmer, E.A., Flynn, J.T., Hardy, R.J., et al.: Incidence and early course of retinopathy of prematurity. Ophthalmology, 98(11):1628–1640, 1991.

Pike, M.G., Jan, J., and Wong, P.K.: Neurological and developmental findings in children with cataracts. Am. J. Dis. Child., 143:706–710, 1989.

Reibaldi, A., Santocono, M., Scuderi, A., and Pizzi, G.: Retinopathy of prematurity: Optimal timing of clinical evaluation and standard procedures. Doc Ophthalmol., 74(3):229–234, 1990.

Rettig, P.: Perinatal infections with Chlamydia trachomatis. Clin Perinatol., 15(2):321–350, 1988.

Samson, L.F.: Perinatal viral infections and neonates. J. Perinat. Neonat. Nurs., 1(4):56–65, 1988.

Sandström, I.: Treatment of neonatal conjunctivitis. Arch. Ophthalmol., 105(7):925–928, 1987.

Shapiro, C.: Retrolental fibroplasia: What we know and what we don't know. Neonatal Network, 4(6):33–45, 1986.

Silverman, W.A., and Flynn, J.T. (eds.): Retinopathy of Prematurity. Boston, Blackwell Scientific Publications, 1985.

Smith, J.F., and Nachazel, D.P.: Ophthalmologic Nursing. Boston, Little, Brown, 1980.

Wybar, K., and Taylor, D. (eds.): Pediatric Ophthalmology: Current Aspects. New York, Marcel Dekker, 1983.

Roger G. Martin

Pharmacology in Neonatal Care

Objectives

1. Summarize general nursing responsibilities and interventions when administering drugs to the neonatal intensive care patient.

2. Define the following concepts:

   a. Pharmacotherapy.
   b. Drug.
   c. Pharmacokinetics.

3. Outline the principles that define differences in expression of drug response.

4. Differentiate specific differences between adult and neonatal pharmacology:

   a. Absorption.
   b. Distribution.
   c. Metabolism.
   d. Excretion.

5. Identify specific areas of concern when administering drugs of the following types to neonatal intensive care patients:

   a. Antimicrobials.
   b. Cardiovascular agents.
   c. Diuretics.
   d. Central nervous system drugs.

The study and clinical application of specific knowledge related to neonatal pharmacology can facilitate safe drug administration in the neonatal population. The application of pharmacological principles involves the evaluation of existing knowledge concerning the pharmacodynamic and pharmacokinetic response of the neonatal population to specific drugs. This knowledge must be taken in the context of each patient's gestational age, chronological age, weight, fluid tolerance, and the health-illness state of individual organ systems and evaluated in the context of the desired response to a drug as well as the potential for undesirable drug reactions. The nurse administering drugs to the neonatal intensive care patient is in the ideal position to evaluate these issues and make observations and interventions in the arena where they count most—at the patient's bedside.

The primary focus of this discussion of neonatal pharmacology is intended to bridge the gap between traditional nursing education and other excellent reference materials on drug indications and dose recommendations. Specific, current information on drug dosages and implications for drug administration is given in individual clinical chapters and should also be readily available in any neonatal intensive care unit from a number of other excellent sources. (See Bibliography.)

Principles of Pharmacology

TERMINOLOGY

A. **Pharmacology:** the science studying the actions of chemicals on living systems and molecules; or the origins, nature, and effects of drugs on humans or animals.

B. **Pharmacotherapy**.
1. A branch of pharmacology that focuses on the study of drugs or chemicals used to prevent, diagnose, or treat disease.
2. The administration of a drug or drugs to a patient with the intent of achieving a specific response. This response is limited to augmentation, abolition, or modulation of a normal physiological process.

C. **Drug**.
1. Any substance or mixture of substances intended to be used for the cure, mitigation, or prevention of disease in humans or animals.
2. A non-food substance that affects living protoplasm.

D. **Pharmacodynamics**.
1. The study of how chemicals produce their biological effects on living tissue.

E. **Pharmacokinetics**.
1. The specialized study of the mathematical relationship between a drug dosage regimen and resulting serum concentration.
2. The study of the time course of absorption, distribution, metabolism, and excretion of a drug in humans or animals.

PHARMACODYNAMICS

A. **Receptor concept:** the principle that assumes drugs act by forming a complex with a specific macromolecule in a way that alters that molecule's function. This alteration in function may include inhibition or potentiation of the macromolecule's activity in a way that creates the desired drug effect.
1. Receptor effects.
   a. The drug's affinity for binding to the receptor plays a large part in the determination of the concentration of the drug required to achieve the desired response.
   b. The individual characteristics of the receptor are responsible for the selective nature of drug response.
   c. Receptor theory of drug action allows an explanation of drug antagonists. The antagonist drug may alter the characteristics of the receptor molecule in a way that then limits or inhibits the response to the original drug.
2. There are some drugs that do not appear to act through receptors. Their action is related to a direct response in the recipient.

B. **General mechanisms of drug action**.
1. Based on the nature of the receptor/drug complex.
2. Types of receptor/drug complexes.
   a. There are receptor/drug complexes that regulate gene expression.

(1) One common class of drugs acts by mediating a response that ultimately involves gene expression and new protein synthesis.

(2) These drugs generally do not have a rapid effect following initial administration.

b. There are receptor/drug complexes that change cell membrane permeability.

(1) Many clinically useful drugs act by changing the cell membrane permeability and therefore altering all membrane characteristics.

(2) These drugs may have a very short time lag between administration and response.

c. There are receptor/drug complexes that increase the intracellular concentration of a second messenger molecule.

(1) These drugs increase production and activity of enzyme systems within the cell.

(2) These drugs may stimulate a rapid response in changing cell characteristics.

C. **Relationship between drug dose and clinical response**.

1. Individuals in a population receiving a medication may have a wide range of response to a drug dose.

a. Idiosyncratic drug responses: an abnormal response to a drug that is not usually observed. These unpredictable responses include the following:

(1) Low sensitivity: a patient who, upon receiving the usual drug dose, exhibits a clinical or biological response that is less intense than is usually observed.

(2) Extreme sensitivity: a patient who has a response to the drug that is more intense than is usually observed.

(3) Unpredictable adverse reaction: a patient who exhibits a drug reaction that is substantially different from what would have been predicted. This may include drug reactions that include physiological responses not usually seen.

(4) Tolerance: a diminished response to a given drug dosage that is related to long-term administration of a drug.

(5) Tachyphylaxis: describes rapidly diminished drug response without a drug dosage change. This may be caused by a number of reasons, including limited number of receptor sites or limited numbers of transmitter chemicals.

2. Factors that may affect individual drug response.

a. Alterations in drug concentration: a change from the expected norm in the amount of drug that reaches the receptor molecule.

b. Variation in amounts of antagonistic substances: an unusually large or limited amount of antagonistic substances that alter receptor molecule response.

c. Alterations in numbers or function of receptor molecules: an increased or diminished number of receptor molecules changes the number of potential drug/receptor complexes.

d. Changes in concentration of molecules other than receptor molecules: if drug response is ultimately dependent on an effect on molecules other than the drug/receptor complex, drug response may be limited by the amount of the third molecule type.

D. **Desired versus undesired effects of medications**.

1. No drug causes only one effect: all drugs have several effects that can be divided into three groups.

a. Desired or therapeutic effects: those effects that are the desired outcome of the drug administration.

b. Side effects: those drug effects that result from the drug administration that are in addition to the desired effects. All drugs have some side effects. They vary from very minor and clinically insignificant to major side effects that are sufficiently adverse to require drug discontinuation.

    c. Toxic effects: drug response that results from a drug overdose or unexpected high serum drug concentrations.

2. It is the responsibility of the health care provider to weigh the benefits of the therapeutic effect against the undesirable side effects and the risk of toxic effects and make adjustments accordingly.

PHARMACOKINETICS (Fig. 26–1)

A. Principles of drug absorption.

1. General principles of drug absorption.
    a. The movement of a drug from the site of administration to the blood stream or site of action.
    b. The absorption of a drug is, in large part, dependent on the site of administration. The common sites of administration are as follows:
        (1) Gastrointestinal: commonly used because of convenience.
            (a) Large surface and absorption area of the gastrointestinal tract favor absorption.
            (b) The presence of marked changes in pH from the stomach through the distal gastrointestinal tract, pancreatic, and other digestive enzymes, and intestinal bacterial flora may affect absorption.
            (c) Oral administration of a drug may result in the absorbed drug moving directly from the intestinal absorption site to the liver, where the

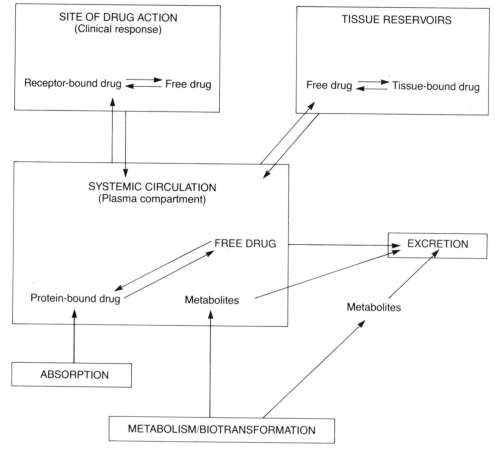

Figure 26–1
Schematic representation of the components of drug movement or pharmacokinetics. Includes absorption, metabolism, excretion, and diagrammatical indication of drug distribution.

drug may be metabolized and excreted in significant amounts. This "first-pass" effect limits the bioavailability of the drug.

(d) Time of response varies, depending upon drug absorption characteristics.

(2) Inhalation: useful for gaseous or easily vaporized drugs.

(a) Large surface area of the alveolar membranes and the generous blood flow favor absorption.

(b) Particular advantage for medications when site of desired action is the tracheobronchial tree.

(c) May have a very rapid drug response.

(d) Useful in some emergency situations when intravenous access is not readily available (e.g., epinephrine, atropine, lidocaine).

(3) Topical: utility limited to drugs whose absorptive characteristics allow permeation through the skin or mucous membranes.

(a) Response may be limited to local area of application.

(b) Some topically applied medications can have a systemic effect (e.g., nitroglycerin).

(c) Rate of absorption is inversely related to membrane thickness and directly related to membrane water content.

(d) Response time variable.

(4) Intramuscular: administration into muscle body.

(a) Bypasses most absorptive barriers.

(b) Limited to drugs that do not cause tissue damage at administration site and are soluble at physiological pH.

(c) Slower response due to time lag between administration and achieving blood concentration.

(d) Dependent on blood flow to muscle.

(5) Subcutaneous: administration into the subcutaneous tissue.

(a) Bypasses most absorptive barriers.

(b) Slower response to achieve significant blood levels.

(c) Limited types and volumes of drug may be used.

(d) Dependent on local blood flow.

(6) Intravenous: direct administration into the blood stream. Bypasses all absorptive barriers.

(a) Hazardous: large amounts of drug may be delivered directly to the target organs as well as to other tissues.

(b) Very rapid response.

2. Drug absorption in the neonate.

a. Oral absorption.

(1) Gastrointestinal surface area: structurally, the neonatal GI tract has a greater surface area ratio in proportion to body mass. This provides a more absorptive surface area.

(2) Immature gastrointestinal system may absorb some substances at a higher rate.

(a) Few studies exist that quantify rates of GI absorption in neonates.

(3) Gastric emptying and intestinal transit times may be prolonged and normally reach adult values at 6–8 months of age.

(a) Gastric and intestinal mobility is dependent on gestational age, illness state, oral intake, and composition of feeding.

(b) Net effect of prolonged GI transit times appears to be, in some cases, increased newborn absorption over adult values.

(c) May also decrease bioavailability because of increased first-pass loss or increased gastrointestinal destruction of drug.

(4) Gastrointestinal tract acidity: a major determinant of drug absorption.

(a) pH of GI tract near neutral at birth.

(b) May not begin to reach normal adult values until two weeks of age and may not be completely to adult pH values of 1 to 3 until 6 to 8 months of age.

(c) Gastric pH is dependent on extrauterine factors. Normal feeding patterns tend to speed normalization of gastric acidity.

(d) The net effect of gastrointestinal acidity is dependent on pH characteristics of the drug and preparation. Drugs that normally may not be absorbed well in the stomach may be absorbed at a higher rate in the neonate because of decreased stomach acidity (e.g., oral insulin has been shown to be absorbed well in the first minutes of life, whereas phenytoin exhibits decreased gastrointestinal absorption in neonates because of increased pH of the GI tract).

(5) Pancreatic enzyme function.

(a) Neonates are deficient in pancreatic enzymes at birth.

(b) This may inhibit absorption of some medications that require pancreatic enzymes for efficient absorption.

(6) Beta-glucuronidase: an enzyme in the neonatal GI tract that may be present up to seven times the adult amounts.

(a) This enzyme deconjugates medications metabolized by the liver. Deconjugated drug may then become available for reabsorption.

(b) May cause a prolonged drug effect.

(7) Bacterial flora: composition and rate of colonization of the GI tract by the normal bacterial flora may affect GI tract motility as well as metabolism of some drugs.

(a) The significance of this effect is highly variable. It is dependent on oral intake and other factors such as antibiotic administration.

(b) Normal colonization in vaginally born, well, term neonates occurs by 4–6 days of age.

(8) Gastrointestinal tract perfusion: in very ill neonates, hypoperfusion of the gut may decrease drug absorption.

b. Rectal absorption.

(1) May be a very efficient means of drug administration to a neonate.

(a) Serum levels of some drugs may be as high or higher than levels obtained through other routes of administration.

(b) Relative volume and fragility of the neonatal rectum must be considered.

c. Inhalation.

(1) Good route for administration of medications whose desired site of action is the tracheobronchial tree (e.g., albuterol, terbutaline).

(2) May be less effective in a newborn with pulmonary hypertension and poor or abnormal pulmonary blood flow.

(3) Excellent route for administration of some drugs used for resuscitation when vascular access is not readily available (e.g., epinephrine).

(4) Used with increasing frequency in neonatal intensive care as various surfactant preparations become available and are more widely used.

d. Topical absorption.

(1) Percutaneous absorption has particular advantages and risks in the newborn.

(a) With increasing gestational age, skin thickness increases and water content decreases.

(b) With increasing gestational age, the ratio of skin surface area to weight decreases, providing relatively less absorptive surface as compared with body mass.

(c) This allows much more efficient percutaneous absorption of drugs in neonates of lower birthweight and gestational age.

(d) Poses a particular hazard in care, as substances that may be safely applied to the skin of a more mature patient may be absorbed in dangerous amounts in the immature neonate.

e. Intramuscular/subcutaneous absorption.

(1) Absorption dependent on local blood flow and muscle activity, which may be affected by many factors in the neonate.

(a) Poor peripheral blood flow and low blood pressure are a common physiological state in newborns. It becomes less common with increasing gestational age but can occur in the presence of many neonatal disease states.

(b) Poor cardiac output frequently occurs with many illness states experienced in the neonatal period.

(c) Subsequent increases in peripheral perfusion following resolution of primary illness states may put the newborn at risk for an increase in the rate and amount of drug absorption.

(d) Limited muscle activity in the ill newborn may limit absorption of drugs administered by this route.

(2) Limited subcutaneous tissue and muscle mass limit these two routes of administration, particularly in the low birthweight newborn.

f. Intravenous absorption.

(1) Bypasses all absorptive barriers.

(2) Most effective and reliable method of drug administration. Drug is delivered directly to the circulating plasma volume.

(3) The ability to reach significant serum drug concentrations rapidly allows for immediate potential drug response. This includes desired as well as undesired or toxic reactions.

(4) May not guarantee adequate and equal distribution to all organs or compartments. Characteristics of some biological membranes may limit drug distribution to body compartments (e.g., cerebral-spinal fluid with meningitis).

(5) Rapid achievement of potentially dangerous serum drug concentrations may require administration of the intravenous medication over a prolonged period.

B. Principles of drug distribution.

1. Distribution: movement of the absorbed drug to and through various body compartments.

a. The extent of this movement, the "size" of the compartment, the number and character of the binding sites, and the amount of the drug administered determine the amount of drug at the desired site of action. When this drug movement reaches a steady state, the volume of distribution is defined as the hypothetical volume of body fluid that would be required to dissolve the total amount of drug as found in the serum.

2. Body compartments.

a. Total body water: approximately .70–.75 liter/kg (70–75% of body weight) in the well, term neonate.

b. Extracellular water: approximately 0.35 liter/kg (35% of body weight) in a well, term neonate.

(1) Large, water-soluble molecules are distributed through this space.

c. Intravascular water: approximately 0.10 liter/kg (10% of body weight) in the well, term neonate.

(1) Very large or tightly protein-bound molecules are distributed through this space.

d. Fat: neonatal values vary widely based on gestational age and intrauterine/post-natal growth patterns.

(1) Highly lipid-soluble molecules are distributed in this space. Low lipid-soluble molecules will not be distributed.

e. Bone: neonatal values not available.

(1) Certain ions are distributed in this space. Most are not distributed in significant amounts.

3. Protein-binding sites.

a. Drugs may also form a complex with other large circulating molecules (usually proteins). This binding to molecules may result in no response or an undesirable drug response because only unbound drug can be distributed to active receptor sites.

b. The amount of drug that binds to these sites has a direct effect on the amount of drug available for the desired pharmacological effect. The more of the drug that is protein bound, the less that is available for the desired drug effect.

c. Primary binding protein in the serum is albumin.

d. This binding may also have the effect of displacing another drug or substance, freeing it for action with another receptor.

4. Drug movement: dependent on two factors:

   a. Blood flow: amount and distribution of blood flow affect the delivery of a drug absorbed into the blood stream to the target organ or cell.

     (1) Continued adequate blood flow is required to maintain an adequate concentration of the drug at the target organ.

   b. Drug solubility: in biological tissues, this refers to the relative ability of the drug to dissolve in biological fluids. Defined by how readily the drug dissolves into the specific tissue and/or body fluids.

     (1) Low lipid-soluble drugs are not distributed well through lipid membranes, although they may be distributed well through the body water spaces, and highly lipid-soluble drugs are distributed readily through most lipid membranes but are not distributed well through body water spaces.

     (2) The relative drug solubility may make some drug use inappropriate. A low lipid-soluble drug will not reach high concentrations in an organ that is primarily fat.

5. Drug distribution in the neonate.

   a. Body compartments: there are significant differences in distribution of body mass in the neonate.

     (1) Total body water: as gestational age increases, total body water, as a percentage of total body mass, decreases.

       (a) Water-soluble drugs have a larger volume of distribution as body water, as a percentage of body mass, increases.

       (b) Because of increased total body water, a less mature neonate may then require a larger, per kilogram, dose to achieve the same drug concentration and effect as an older patient.

       (c) Decreased amounts of body percentage of other body tissues (e.g., body fat) may make the volume of distribution smaller for drugs that are distributed primarily through fatty tissue because of high lipid solubility.

     (2) Extracellular water: the percentage of this physiological volume increases in amounts greater than would be explained by the decrease in total body water percentage as gestational age increases.

       (a) This has an additive effect on the volume of distribution for some drugs.

     (3) In the first several days following birth, neonates may experience rapid changes in volume of distribution for water-soluble drugs related to normal physiology and illness states.

       (a) Normal term and pre-term neonates experience marked decreases in total body water volume in absolute terms as well as a percentage of total body weight.

       (b) Neonates with disease states that alter water excretion may have expansion of body water as a result of this dysfunction (e.g., primary renal disease, secretion of inappropriate antidiuretic hormone [SIADH]).

       (c) The above alterations make drug dosing with medications that are primarily distributed in body water difficult (e.g., aminoglycoside antibiotics such as gentamicin).

       (d) May require frequent drug level monitoring as the neonate experiences the mentioned changes in body compartment volumes.

b. Protein binding.
   (1) There are several factors influencing neonatal protein binding.
      (a) There is decreased total plasma protein/albumin levels in neonates, and more so in premature and ill newborns.
         i. This diminishes potential for circulating plasma protein/drug complexes.
         ii. Serum albumin levels, as the primary serum binding protein, may be markedly decreased in the ill, extremely low birthweight neonate.
         iii. Net effect is to allow more free drug at the same serum concentration. May allow more drug action by formation of receptor/drug complex.
         iv. May allow desired drug response at lower serum concentrations (serum concentration = protein-bound drug + unbound drug).
      (b) Increased plasma, unconjugated bilirubin levels in many neonates.
         i. Have been shown to displace some drugs from albumin-binding sites, which allows more free drug for action.
         ii. In contrast, many drugs displace unconjugated bilirubin from albumin-binding sites. This may promote kernicterus because of increased free, unconjugated bilirubin concentrations.
      (c) Increased serum, free fatty acid concentrations have been shown to displace some drugs from plasma albumin-binding sites.
      (d) Blood pH.
         i. Acidosis is a common finding associated with many neonatal disorders.
         ii. Changes in blood pH have been shown to change albumin-binding characteristics. This may cause drug displacement from albumin.
         iii. May also cause drugs to displace unconjugated bilirubin (see above).
c. Drug movement: an important part of drug distribution involves drug movement from site of administration through the body.
   (1) Dependent on local blood flow.
   (2) Several neonatal conditions affect blood flow. These include the following:
      (a) Hypotension: may affect peripheral drug absorption and/or distribution.
      (b) Distributive shock: seen with septicemia and caused by dilation of the vascular bed. Causes local underperfusion and may limit drug distribution to specific organs.
      (c) Pulmonary hypertension: may impede drug delivery to pulmonary vascular bed.

C. Principles of drug metabolism.

1. General principles of drug metabolism.
   a. Metabolism (bio-transformation): metabolism of a drug into another form. This transformed drug may be pharmacologically active or inactive. Sites of metabolism are as follows:
      (1) Liver: the primary organ of drug metabolism.
         (a) Metabolic activity divided into two main types:
            i. Phase I (non-synthetic-metabolism of drugs: primarily oxidation, reduction, hydrolysis, or hydroxylation reactions that generally occur in the smooth endoplasmic reticulum of the hepatocyte.
            ii. Phase II (synthetic) metabolism of drugs: primarily involves conjugation of the drug with another substance.
         (b) Hepatic uptake of the drug is dependent on the concentration of the drug in the liver (dependent on hepatic blood flow) and the hepato-

cyte concentration of ligandin (Y-protein). This protein is responsible for substrate uptake by hepatic cells.

  (c) First-pass effect: hepatic bio-transformation may markedly alter drug availability by directly metabolizing drugs absorbed from the gastrointestinal tract, before those drugs reach other organs.

  (2) Kidney, intestine, lung, adrenal, and skin are also tissues capable of bio-transformation of certain compounds. These sites of metabolism are much more limited.

2. Metabolism/bio-transformation in the neonate.

  a. Phase I enzyme systems: concentration of enzymes appears to be near adult values.

    (1) Function may be markedly reduced.

    (2) May not reach adult levels of function until several years of age.

  b. Phase II enzyme systems: also immature, based on clinical drug transformation and excretion data.

    (1) Data are limited.

    (2) May not reach adult levels in concentration and function until well after the neonatal period.

    (3) Both enzyme systems may be vulnerable to hypoxic-ischemic insult.

  c. Ligandin (Y-protein): the protein responsible for substrate intake by the hepatocytes.

    (1) Concentrations low at birth.

    (2) May reach near adult values during the neonatal period.

  d. First-pass effect: poor gastrointestinal mobility may increase the potential for first-pass effect. Prolonged gastrointestinal transit times may increase potential for hepatic metabolism and eventual excretion of orally administered drugs.

D. Principles of drug excretion.

1. General principles of drug excretion.

  a. Excretion: final drug elimination from the body. Process of excretion begins with administration of the drug and ends when the drug is completely eliminated from the body. There are several important organs of excretion:

    (1) Minor organs: small amounts of drugs may be excreted through salivary, sweat, and mammary glands.

    (2) Lungs: an important route of excretion of gaseous anesthetics but relatively less important for other drugs.

    (3) Gastrointestinal tract: the large, lipid-soluble surface of the GI tract allows diffusion of drugs from out of the blood stream.

    (4) Liver: the most important site of drug bio-transformation; also serves as an important site of drug excretion. The excretion of bile is an important route of drug elimination.

      (a) Limited bile flow may limit the efficacy of this elimination.

      (b) Metabolite or drug elimination in bile is dependent on solubility characteristics of that substance in bile.

    (5) Kidneys: the primary method of drug elimination. This occurs by two processes:

      (a) Glomerular filtration: the removal of, by passive filtration, small, unbound drug molecules at the glomerulus. Glomerular filtration is dependent on renal blood flow and the characteristics of the glomerular membranes.

      (b) Tubular secretion: the active secretion of large or protein-bound molecules into the tubular urine. Tubular secretion is dependent on the efficiency of tubular function.

      (c) For some drugs, there is significant renal tubular reabsorption of the drug back into the circulating plasma. Renal clearance = (filtration clearance + secretion clearance) $\times$ (1 − fraction reabsorbed).

2. Excretion in the neonate.

a. Minor organs.
   (1) Very limited sweat production makes excretion by this mode insignificant.
b. Lungs.
   (1) Excretion by the lungs is not well studied in the neonatal population.
   (2) Lung disease common in newborns. Adult data indicate that this may affect or limit ability to excrete medications by this method.
c. Gastrointestinal tract.
   (1) Limited mobility: affects excretion as well as increases potential for absorption of drugs or metabolites back into the circulation.
d. Liver.
   (1) Limited oral intake and long-term hyperalimentation may reduce bile flow.
   (2) Reduces the efficacy of this route.
e. Kidney.
   (1) Renal blood flow.
      (a) Limited renal blood flow restricts drug or metabolite delivery to the kidney for excretion.
      (b) Increases with increasing gestational and post-natal age.
   (2) Glomerular filtration: very limited in relationship to adult values. (30% of adult values, per unit of body surface area. Reaches adult values by 2 years of age.)
      (a) Markedly increases with increasing gestational and post-natal age.
      (b) Limited glomerular filtration reduces removal of drugs or metabolites at the glomerulus.
      (c) Has been shown to mature with post-natal age independent of gestational age at birth.
   (3) Tubular secretion.
      (a) Neonates have a relatively small mass of functional tubular cells as well as immaturity of tubular function.
      (b) This limited tubular mass and function causes poor excretion of drugs or metabolites removed by this method.
      (c) Matures much more slowly than glomerular filtration.
      (d) Vulnerable to hypoxic-ischemic insult.
   (4) Urinary flow.
      (a) Because of changes in renal blood flow, glomerular filtration, and tubular secretion in the neonate, urinary output is not a reliable sign of renal excretion of drugs.
      (b) Requires blood level monitoring to ensure safe serum levels of renally excreted medications.

Drug Categories

ANTIMICROBIAL AGENTS

A. **Variety of antimicrobial drugs**. The use of a larger variety of antimicrobial agents in the newborn population has occurred in the last several years because of advancing clinical sophistication in the use of antimicrobial drugs as well as an expanding body of knowledge on the use of such agents in the newborn population.

B. **Definitions**.
1. Antimicrobial drugs: medications that inhibit the growth of or kill microorganisms; includes antibacterial agents, antifungal agents, and antiviral agents.
   a. Bacteriostatic drugs: agents that inhibit the growth of microorganisms, preventing their spread and/or allowing normal body defense mechanisms to control spread of the organism.

   b. Bactericidal drugs: agents whose primary purpose is to kill microorganisms. At lower concentrations, they may be bacteriostatic.
2. Antibiotics are a class of antibacterial agents that are produced from other species of microorganisms (e.g., penicillin). Other antimicrobials are chemicals not produced by other microorganisms.
3. MIC (minimum inhibitory concentration): the lowest concentration of a drug that stops visible spread of organism growth in a laboratory setting. In vivo, this cannot be directly measured and is dependent on achieved tissue concentration and numbers of bacteria present.
4. MBC (minimum bactericidal concentration): lowest concentration of a drug that results in 99.9% or greater decline in microbial number. Measured in laboratory setting. Useful when compared with known potential toxic concentration levels in choosing antimicrobial regimen that does greatest good with minimal adverse or toxic effects.
5. Resistance: the ability of microorganisms to resist the bacteriostatic or bactericidal effects of an antimicrobial agent.
   a. Resistance may occur when the chromosomal make-up of the organism has changed or mutated.
   b. This interferes with drug action either through changes in the microorganism's cellular structure or through production of enzymes that reduce antimicrobial activity.

C. **Basic principles of antimicrobial use.**
1. Must reach target tissue in a concentration adequate to inhibit the growth of or kill the desired microorganism.
   a. This concentration ideally would be such that it would have very limited side or toxic effects on target tissues or the patient as a whole.
   b. This concentration must be readily achievable and sustainable over the desired length of antimicrobial therapy.
2. Choice of antimicrobial regimen must take into account:
   a. Microorganism sensitivity to available antimicrobial agents.
   b. Relative permeability of the target tissue to agent of choice.
   c. Bioactivity of chosen antimicrobial agent in target tissue.
   d. Known MIC/MBC in relation to existing body of knowledge concerning side effects and toxicity in the specific population.
   e. Specific characteristics of the individual patient in relation to the chosen antimicrobial's pharmacokinetics (e.g., in a patient with impaired renal function, a nephrotoxic antimicrobial should be avoided if possible).

D. **Specific considerations in newborn population.**
1. Pharmacodynamics.
   a. Tissue concentration of drug may be altered by clinical/physiological conditions that may increase or decrease bioavailability of the drug in the target tissue. (Example: cerebral spinal fluid penetration by antibiotics may be excellent early during meningitis. As meningeal inflammatory response subsides, penetration of CSF diminishes.)
   b. Differences in response or potential for toxic effects may result from immaturity and/or illness state.
2. Pharmacokinetics.
   a. In seriously ill neonates, greater consideration for clinical status than for gestational or chronological age must be made.
   b. Absorption:
      (1) Changes in GI tract pH affect absorption of oral medication. May be increased or decreased. (Example: oral penicillin G is absorbed better in neonates than in older infants and children because of increased gastric pH.)
      (2) Skin permeability changes with the extremely immature neonate may allow topically applied antimicrobial agents to be absorbed systemically.
   c. Distribution.

(1) Decreasing body water and increasing body fat concentration in more mature neonates affect volume through which antimicrobial agent is distributed. This may make dosage adjustments necessary in the first days of life.

(2) Blood flow changes may affect absorption and distribution of antimicrobials administered intramuscularly or subcutaneously. (Example: repeated IM administration of aminoglycosides to premature babies may result in local tissue damage and unacceptably variable rates of absorption.)

  d. Metabolism.
  (1) Limited hepatic function, owing to immaturity or illness state, may affect dosage regimen of some antibiotics, requiring smaller or less frequent doses of some antibiotics (e.g., nafcillin, erythromycin).

  e. Excretion.
  (1) Limited renal function with lower gestational age may prolong half-life of antimicrobials excreted by the kidneys (e.g., aminoglycosides, cephalosporins, penicillin).
  (a) This limited renal function (glomerular filtration rate and tubular secretion) commonly improves significantly in the first few days of life. For this reason, serum antibiotic levels must be monitored closely and dosage adjustments made accordingly.

DIURETICS

A. Introduction.
1. Commonly used in both acute and long-term neonatal intensive care to encourage the removal of excessive extracellular fluid.
2. Site of action of nearly all diuretic agents is the luminal surface of the renal tubular cell.

B. Basic principles of diuretic use.
1. Use must be based on good understanding of renal physiology and function of the various segments of the nephron in the neonatal population.
2. Diuretic drugs whose primary purpose is to cause the excretion of excess extracellular fluid commonly cause loss of electrolytes along with the water loss. Knowledge of specific action for each diuretic drug will assist the clinician in monitoring for undesirable electrolyte losses.
3. Pharmacological response is dependent on existing level of renal function and on the drug's ability to reach the target tissue in amounts adequate to produce a diuretic effect.
4. Any drug or other therapy that increases glomerular filtration rate may have an indirect diuretic effect. Therefore, some drugs that act on the cardiovascular system to increase cardiac output or increase renal blood flow through vasodilation may cause diuresis. Maximal water and electrolyte excretion usually occurs in the first days of use. Later, decreased glomerular filtration rate and hyperaldosteronism that result from diuretic-induced hypovolemia limit these losses.

C. Specific considerations in the newborn population.
1. Pharmacodynamics.
  a. Renal tubular function is relatively limited and tends to be more so with less mature neonates.
  b. Clinical response to diuretic agents is commonly affected because of existing poor renal tubular absorption.
  (1) Potentiates electrolyte loss with many diuretic agents (e.g., furosemide, chlorothiazide).
2. Pharmacokinetics.
  a. Absorption.
  (1) Oral absorption may be limited, requiring longer or a larger per kilogram

dose to achieve the desired effect (e.g., furosemide). Others are absorbed well orally (e.g., chlorothiazide).
  b. Distribution.
    (1) Some diuretic medications are strongly protein bound. Some concern has been raised over displacement of bilirubin from albumin (e.g., furosemide, spironolactone).
  c. Excretion.
    (1) Many diuretic drugs are dependent on reaching the lumen of the proximal tubule in order to achieve diuresis.
    (2) Low glomerular filtration rate with limited renal tubular function may delay excretion as well as limit effectiveness of the drug. (Example: plasma clearance of furosemide has been shown to be prolonged in prematures and newborns with renal failure.)

CARDIOVASCULAR AGENTS

A. Introduction.
1. A broad group of drugs that affect the regulation, inhibition, or stimulation of the cardiovascular system.
2. Increasing utilization in acute and long-term care of the neonatal intensive care patient.

B. Types of cardiovascular drugs.
1. Inotropic agents.
  a. Improve cardiac output by increasing the heart rate (chronotropic effect), increasing the force of myocardial contraction (inotropic effect), and increasing vascular tone.
  b. Most widely studied of cardiovascular drugs.
  c. Used most commonly in cardiovascular resuscitation and long-term support of the myocardium.
  d. Includes the following:
    (1) Digitalis glycosides (e.g., digoxin).
    (2) Sympathomimetic amines (e.g., epinephrine, dopamine, dobutamine, isoproterenol).
      (a) Clinical responses stimulated by this group of drugs are classified according to effects on "receptors" in the body. These receptors are categorized as either alpha or beta types and further subcategorized as alpha-1 or alpha-2 and beta-1 or beta-2.
        i. Alpha-1-adrenergic receptor response: constriction and contractions of vascular smooth muscle.
        ii. Alpha-2-adrenergic receptor response: decreased motility and tone of intestine and stomach.
        iii. Beta-1-adrenergic receptor response: increased strength and rate of myocardial contraction.
        iv. Beta-2-adrenergic receptor response: vascular smooth muscle dilation and bronchial muscle relaxation.
      (b) Response to each of these medications depends on relative amounts of alpha- and beta-effects.
      (c) Prolonged administration of sympathomimetic amines can cause a diminished response in alpha- and beta-receptors. Results in diminished clinical efficacy, referred to as tachyphylaxis.
2. Antihypertensives.
  a. Used to normalize blood pressure in patients with hypertension.
  b. May be used to inhibit pathophysiological changes that cause increased blood pressure (e.g., captopril), or directly reduce blood pressure through changes in intravascular volume (diuretic drugs) or resistance (e.g., diazoxide, hydralazine).

3. Vasodilators.
   a. May be used to acutely diminish blood pressure in hypertensive patients, alter vascular resistance or capacities in congestive heart failure, and reduce pulmonary vascular resistance in conditions that are associated with pulmonary hypertension.
   b. Includes drugs such as diazoxide, hydralazine, nitroprusside, tolazoline, and propranolol.
4. Antiarrhythmics.
   a. Used for drug therapy of cardiac arrhythmias causing adverse effects on cardiovascular stability.
   b. This group includes digoxin and lidocaine.

C. **Basic principles of cardiovascular drug use**.
1. Wide range of pharmacological action of this class of medications requires specific, in-depth knowledge about each drug prior to use.
2. In-depth knowledge of pathophysiological basis of neonatal cardiovascular disease is necessary to ensure proper application of this class of drugs.
3. Many of these drugs have overlapping effects. This overlap in clinical response makes optimal choice of drug difficult.
4. Extensive knowledge and application of invasive and noninvasive cardiovascular monitoring techniques in the neonatal population are necessary.

D. **Specific considerations in newborn population**.
1. Pharmacodynamics.
   a. Specific, in-depth knowledge about neonatal cardiovascular physiology and pathophysiology is required to determine need for these types of medications.
   b. Cardiovascular drugs are commonly used in conjunction with other medications that may affect the newborn's response to the drug regimen. (Example: digoxin/furosemide combination—electrolyte loss with diuretic may change toxic response to inotropic agent.)
2. Pharmacokinetics.
   a. Absorption.
      (1) Many cardiovascular drugs cannot be safely given through any absorptive barrier. This makes intravenous administration necessary in most cases.
   b. Distribution.
      (1) Poor cardiac output/shock states may affect distribution of drug to all tissues.
      (2) Drug administered for desired response to one target organ may cause undesirable systemic response. (Example: systemic hypotension following administration of tolazoline as a pulmonary vasodilator.)
      (3) Some cardiovascular drugs are highly albumin bound. Raises question of possibility of indirect bilirubin displacement from albumin.
   c. Metabolism.
      (1) Hepatic metabolic activity may markedly affect bioavailability of drug. (Example: high rate of first-pass clearance with oral hydralazine administration.)
      (2) Metabolites of drug may cause toxic response. (Example: cyanide liberation as a result of nitroprusside metabolism.)
      (3) Rapid metabolism and serum clearance may require constant intravenous infusion (e.g., dopamine, dobutamine).
   d. Excretion.
      (1) Impaired renal function will markedly affect excretion and bioavailability of some drugs.
         (a) Requires particular attention to careful monitoring of clinical response and serum drug levels.

CENTRAL NERVOUS SYSTEM DRUGS

A. Introduction.
1. In adult patients, the most widely used group of medications.
2. Value of pain control and mood alteration in the neonatal population has only recently been recognized.
3. Recent interest in CNS drugs in the newborn population leaves the body of knowledge about these drugs limited.
4. Use of these drugs is increasing as neurobehavioral assessment skills increase among neonatal caregivers.

B. Definitions.
1. Analgesic drug: a medication that provides diminished sensation of pain. Helps to promote diminished response to painful event (e.g., morphine, meperidine, acetaminophen).
2. Anesthetic drug: a medication that removes pain sensation either through peripheral nerve block (e.g., lidocaine) or through central nervous system effect (e.g., high-dosage fentanyl citrate).
3. Sedative/hypnotic drugs: medications that provide mood alteration in patients with anxiety. Divided into two groups: barbiturates (phenobarbital, secobarbital) and non-barbiturates (chloral hydrate, chlorpromazine, lorazepam). Do not provide relief from pain.
4. Addiction: a lifestyle change that occurs in a drug-dependent person. This lifestyle change involves a focus on drug use. Cannot occur in a neonate.
5. Tolerance: a condition that may occur with many types of drugs. Tolerance exists when larger doses and higher serum concentrations of the drug are required to achieve the desired response, and commonly occurs in conjunction with physical dependence.
6. Dependence: a physiological state in which the individual requires regular drug administration for continued physiological well-being. Can be easily remedied through a dosage tapering regimen.

C. General principles.
1. Mechanism of action of CNS drugs is frequently not clearly understood.
2. Assessment of need for these drugs must be carefully performed as an ongoing process.
   a. Careful attention must be paid to differentiation of need for sedation, pain relief, or both.
   b. These medications may cause the development of drug tolerance and/or dependence.
3. Consideration must be made for the risks/benefits of the medication in relation to potential side or toxic effects.
4. Much is not known about neonatal neurological development. The effect that CNS drugs may have on that development is largely unknown.

D. Specific considerations in the newborn population.
1. Pharmacodynamics.
   a. Limited knowledge of central nervous system development in premature and term neonates provides a special need for caution in the use of CNS-active medications.
   b. Specific physiological characteristics in the neonatal population requires careful observation for harmful side or toxic effects. (Example: blood pressure decreases with morphine administration.)
   c. Narcotic analgesics may cause respiratory depression and may precipitate respiratory failure in newborns.
2. Pharmacokinetics.
   a. Absorption.
      (1) Poor gastrointestinal motility and high first-pass clearance may make oral administration ineffective for many drugs (e.g., morphine, meperidine).

(2) Oral/rectal absorption of mild analgesics and sedatives is often adequate.

(3) Careful assessment of clinical response is necessary.

b. Metabolism.

(1) Slower hepatic metabolism may cause prolonged half-life and increase potential for toxic effect caused by metabolites (e.g., meperidine).

(2) Hepatic disease may markedly increase the risk of toxic effects (e.g., chloral hydrate).

c. Excretion.

(1) Limited renal function or failure may cause toxicity as a result of accumulation of drug or metabolites (e.g., meperidine, chloral hydrate).

(2) Drug may have direct effect on renal function.

(a) Diminished blood flow to kidney (e.g., morphine).

(b) Diminished urinary output. (Examples: morphine-caused changes in smooth muscle tone; chlorpromazine effect on renal tubular function.)

Specific Nursing Implications for Drug Administration in the Neonate

A. **Nurses' responsibility**. Primary moral, legal, and ethical duty for patient care places primary responsibility for providing safe drug administration on nursing in most cases.

B. **Specific, in-depth knowledge** about the pharmacodynamics and pharmacokinetics of drugs administered in the neonatal intensive care unit is absolutely necessary in the informed assessment of clinical response and potential for risk.

C. **Careful assessment of vital sign parameters and clinical responses** may assist in the evaluation of desirable or undesirable drug responses.

D. **Careful observation for therapeutic and toxic drug effects** will allow safe drug administration, minimizing toxic responses while achieving maximal desired response.

E. **Monitoring renal function through intake and output measurements** may alert care team to potential changes in drug metabolism and/or excretion.

F. **Meticulous drug dosing**. Giving the medication at the correct time and over the correct time interval is essential for many drugs to have maximal desired effect with minimal undesired effects.

G. **Facilitation of drug serum level monitoring with absolute accuracy** makes safe administration of drugs with a narrow margin between effective and toxic levels possible.

H. **Cross-checking**. Because of the very small volumes of medication commonly given to the neonatal intensive care patient, a system for regular cross-checking of drug volume accuracy prior to administration should be established when possible.

I. **Drugs known to have very specific recommendations for safe administration** should be given under a defined protocol for administration.

J. **Drug precautions**. Any drug or drug preparation known to have a high risk of adverse effect in the neonate should be removed from the patient care area or should be specifically labeled to avoid inadvertent administration.

K. **Facilitation of or participation in clinical trials** designed to evaluate a drug's efficacy does much to advance the body of knowledge related to neonatal pharmacology.

L. **Recognition of established clinical experience with individual drugs in the neonatal population is essential**. Some drugs are introduced into the clinical area after only minimal study of specific drug response in the neonate, and early observation of potential toxic effects may avert a later disaster.

Acknowledgments

The author would like to thank Helen Fiechtner, Pharm. D., for her thoughtful review of this manuscript; and Crystal Wolfe for assistance in manuscript preparation.

STUDY QUESTIONS

1. In the first days following birth, the volume of body water in the neonate normally:
   a. Decreases.
   b. Increases.
   c. Stays the same.

2. Tachyphylaxis to cardiovascular drugs may be caused by:
   a. Changes in drug absorption.
   b. Increased metabolism of the drug.
   c. Limited numbers of receptor molecules.

3. After the initial few days of diuretic therapy with some diuretic drugs, the quantity of diuresis:
   a. Decreases.
   b. Increases.
   c. Stays the same.

4. The effects that central nervous system medications have on neonatal neurodevelopment are:
   a. Generally predictable.
   b. Largely unknown.
   c. Well quantified.

5. Drugs bound to circulating plasma proteins:
   a. Are readily excreted.
   b. Cannot act on receptor molecules.
   c. Contribute to target organ response.

6. Transcutaneous drug absorption in the low birthweight neonate is aided by:
   a. High skin water content and decreased skin thickness.
   b. Increased subcutaneous blood flow and skin perfusion.
   c. Limited skin surface area in relation to body weight.

7. In the normal pre-term neonate, renal function in the first week of life improves as a function of:
   a. Birthweight.
   b. Chronological age.
   c. Gestational age.

8. Gastrointestinal pH is fully normalized to adult values by age:
   a. 2–3 months.
   b. 4–5 months.
   c. 6–8 months.

9. Some drug antagonists act by:
   a. Altering sites on the receptor molecules.
   b. Displacing active drug from plasma proteins.
   c. Speeding drug bio-transformation.

10. A drug's volume of distribution:
    a. Can charge markedly with physiological changes.
    b. Depends on the drug's route of administration.
    c. Is a fixed value over time.

11. The "first-pass" effect:
    a. Can limit bioavailability of oral medications.
    b. Is dependent on normal renal function.
    c. Occurs only with intravenous drug administration.

Answers to Study Questions

1. a	5. b	9. a
2. c	6. a	10. a
3. a	7. b	11. a
4. b	8. c	

BIBLIOGRAPHY

Aranda, J.V., Hales, B.F., Reider, M.F.: Developmental pharmacology. *In* Fanaroff, A.A., and Martin, R.J. (eds.): Neonatal-Perinatal Medicine — Diseases of the Fetus and Newborn, 5 ed. St. Louis, C.V. Mosby, 1992.

Benet, L.Z., Mitchell, J.R., and Sheiner, L.B.: Pharmacokinetics: The dynamics of drug absorption, distribution, and elimination. In Gilman, A., Rall, T.W., Nies, A.S., and Taylor, P. (eds.): The Pharmacological Basis of Therapeutics, New York, Pergamon Press, 1990.

Besunder, J.B., Reed, M.D., and Blumer, J.L.: Principles of drug disposition in the neonate: A critical evaluation of the pharmacokinetic-pharmacodynamic interface. Clin. Pharmacokinet., *14*:189–216, 1988.

Bhott, D.R., Fumon, G.I., Wirtschafter, D.O., et al.: Neonatal Drug Formulary. California Perinatal Association, 1988.

Bourne, H.R., and Roberts, J.M.: Drug receptors and pharmacodynamics. *In* Katzung, B.G. (ed.): Basic and Clinical Pharmacology. Norwalk, CT, Appleton & Lange, 1989, pp. 10–28.

Chen, M.S.: Special aspects of perinatal and pediatric pharmacology. *In* Katzung, B.G. (ed.): Basic and Clinical Pharmacology. Norwalk, CT, Appleton & Lange, 1989, pp. 763–769.

Clark, J.B., Queener, S.F., and Karb, V.B.: Pharmacological Basis of Nursing Practice. St. Louis, C.V. Mosby, 1990.

Giacoia, G.P., and Yaffe, S.V.: Drugs and the perinatal patient. *In* Avery, G.B. (ed.): Neonatology: Pathophysiology and Management of the Newborn, 3rd ed. Philadelphia, J.B. Lippincott, 1987, pp. 1317–1348.

Gynyon, G.: Pharmacokinetic considerations in neonatal drug therapy. Neonatal Network, 7(5):9–12, 1989.

Katzung, B.G.: Basic principles of pharmacology. *In* Katzung, B.G. (ed.): Basic and Clinical Pharmacology. Norwalk, CT, Appleton & Lange, 1989, pp. 1–9.

Martin, R.G.: Drug disposition in the neonate. Neonatal Network, 4(4):15–19, 1986.

Powlak, R.P., and Herfert, L.A.T. (eds.): Drug Administration in the NICU: A Handbook for Nurses. Petaluma, CA, Neonatal Network, 1988.

Reid, M.D., and Besunder, J.B.: Developmental pharmacology: Ontogenic basis of drug disposition. Pediatr. Clin. North Am., 36(5):1053–1073, 1989.

Roberts, R.J.: Drug Therapy in Infants: Pharmacologic Principles and Clinical Experience. Philadelphia, W.B. Saunders Co., 1984.

Romirez, A.: The neonate's unique response to drugs: Unraveling the causes of drug iatrogenesis. Neonatal Network, 7(5):45–49, 1989.

SOCIAL TRENDS AND FAMILY CARE

Bonny Sham

Perinatal Substance Abuse

Objectives

1. List three physiological or behavioral signs of an infant exposed to cocaine in utero.
2. Describe the effects of cocaine during pregnancy.
3. List three physiological characteristics of an infant diagnosed with fetal alcohol syndrome.
4. List three nursing interventions (non-pharmacological) appropriate for withdrawing infants.
5. List two psychological characteristics of women who abuse drugs and alcohol.
6. List two nursing interventions applicable when working with mothers who abuse drugs and alcohol.

The use of illicit drugs has exploded in the general population, in every group, in every age range. Cocaine use has reached epidemic proportions; methamphetamine is growing in availability and popularity. Polydrug use is often the norm. Among the many victims of this pervasive tragedy of substance abuse, a new victim emerges: the newborn infant, compromised before birth with often profound neurological and physical sequelae extending into childhood. This chapter explores the common compounds having an adverse effect on the developing fetus and newborn. Psychological and social profiles of drug-dependent mothers are outlined, and nursing interventions are suggested.

Cocaine

A. **Described as one of the most powerfully addicting substances** of human abuse.

B. **Highly addictive in nature**, resulting in a pattern of compulsive, repetitive behavior that can cause disruption in families, problems in daily functions, physical and mental deterioration, and even death.

C. Incidence.
1. In 1986, the National Institute on Drug Abuse estimated that 25 million people in the United States had tried cocaine at least once in the previous year and that 4–6 million use it regularly.

2. In 1988, a survey of 36 hospitals in the United States found that 11% of pregnant women delivering in those hospitals had used an illegal drug (Chasnoff, 1989).

D. Pharmacology.
1. An alkaloidal agent derived from leaves of the South and Central American plant *Erythroxylon coca*.
2. Imported as a salt and sold as an odorless, white, crystalline powder.
3. Actions are similar to amphetamines, providing a local anesthetic and a powerful, short-acting stimulant.
4. Reaches the brain and central nervous system (CNS) within 3 minutes of being snorted.
5. Reaches the brain and CNS within 7–30 seconds of being smoked (crack).

How Cocaine Works

A. Blocks the pre-synaptic re-uptake of norepinephrine and dopamine, producing an excess of neurotransmitters at the post-synaptic receptor sites.

B. Reduces the re-uptake of neurotransmitters in the cerebral cortex, hypothalamus, and cerebellum.

C. Produces a hyperaroused state that is experienced as extreme euphoria. Shortly afterward, the experience becomes one of dysphoria, irritability, impatience, pessimism, fatigue, and a strong desire for additional cocaine.

D. CNS effects include peripheral vasoconstriction, tachycardia, and hypertension, which may result in acute myocardial infarction, cerebral vascular accident, renal and bowel infarction, and pulmonary edema.

Cocaine in Pregnancy

A. Many cocaine users are actually polydrug users.

B. Cocaine is fat soluble and of relatively low molecular weight so it readily passes the blood-brain barrier as well as moves across the placenta by diffusion.

C. In pregnant women, the cocaine metabolite may persist for as long as 4–7 days after use, thereby increasing the exposure to the fetus.

D. Maternal effects.
1. Placental vasoconstriction is the most deleterious effect.
2. When placental vessels constrict, blood flow to the fetus is reduced, resulting in fetal hypoxia.
3. Use in the first trimester results in a high incidence of spontaneous abortions.
4. Women are often anorexic, resulting in fetal malnutrition.
5. Abruptio placentae with stillbirth is very common throughout pregnancy; this may be attributed to maternal hypertension.
6. Damage done to placental and uterine vessels in early gestation places the fetus at continued risk throughout pregnancy, even after usage ends (Chasnoff, 1988).
7. Third-trimester cocaine use can induce sudden onset of uterine contractions, fetal tachycardia, and increased fetal activity within minutes to hours of ingestion.
8. It is best for the fetus if maternal usage ceases at any time throughout gestation.

E. Fetal and newborn effects.
1. Fetal hypoxia.
2. Prematurity.
3. Growth retardation with decreased birth weight and head circumference, even microcephaly; six times more likely to be growth retarded.

4. Fetal disruption, secondary to intrauterine interruption of blood supply to developing or previously developed structures; defects of the forearm or amputation defects of the medial rays of the hands are the most common.
5. May present with CNS dysfunction, such as tremulousness, marked irritability, muscular rigidity, hypertension, and an exaggerated startle response.
6. Additional findings.
    a. Abnormal sleep patterns, poor feeding ability, vomiting, sneezing, high-pitched cry, frantic fist sucking, disorganized rooting, tachypnea, diarrhea, yawning, fever, hyper-reflexia, and abnormal electroencephalogram (EEG).
7. Renal anomalies are at a two to three times greater risk than average.
8. Genitourinary tract anomalies, including hydronephrosis and hypospadias. Prune belly syndrome has been reported.
9. Cranial defects and cardiac anomalies have been reported.
10. Ileal atresia with bowel infarction have been reported.
11. Frequencies of congenital malformations are not easy to substantiate because cause and effect are usually hypothesized, not proved. Also, they are known to vary according to maternal age, race, geographic location, and maternal health.
12. Behavioral effects based on the Brazelton Neonatal Behavioral Assessment Scale.
    a. Difficulty responding to the human voice and face.
    b. Exhibit depressed interactive behaviors and poor responses to environmental stimuli.
    c. Maintain alert states with difficulty, alternating between periods of sleep and agitation.
    d. Respond poorly to comforting by caregivers.
    e. Startle easily.
    f. Change states rapidly.
    g. By 1 month of age, state control abilities are improved but remain less competent than those of drug-free newborns.
    h. Become easily distressed as manifested by rapid respirations, frantic gaze aversion, color changes, and disorganized motor activity.
    i. These findings may be permanent, resulting in later difficulties in concentration, abnormal play patterns, and flat, apathetic moods (Hurt, 1990).

Methamphetamine

A. **A form of amphetamine:** a stimulant that affects the CNS by accelerating its activities.

B. **Can be inhaled**, injected, smoked, or taken orally.

C. **Pharmacology.**
1. Enhances the presynaptic release of norepinephrine.
2. Alters CNS neurotransmitters.
3. Effects are similar to cocaine.
4. A sense of intense physical and psychological exhilaration is produced, lasting from 2–14 hours, depending on the dosage.
5. Limited information exists regarding use during pregnancy.

D. **Newborn effects.**
1. Appear less impaired in the first year of life as compared to other substance-exposed infants.
2. Present with less lethargy, better feeding and state control.
3. Late outcome may be more severe than predicted by early signs. Oculomotor apraxia, pronounced intention tremors, severe active hypotonia, and hemiparesis have been described in children who had benign neonatal courses (Dixon,

1989). These abnormalities suggest frontal lobe dysfunction that may only be manifested at school age.

Fetal Alcohol Syndrome

A. History.
1. Jones and Smith described "fetal alcohol syndrome" (FAS) in 1973 (Jones, 1986).
   a. Defined FAS as a pattern of prenatal and postnatal growth deficiencies, developmental delay, and facial dysmorphology.
2. "Fetal alcohol exposure" (FAE) is a term applied to infants who were exposed to alcohol in utero but do not manifest the physical characteristics.

B. Incidence.
1. It is difficult to estimate accurately the occurrence of FAS.
2. FAS for the total population is reported to be 1.9:1000 live births (Weiner and Morse, 1988).
3. FAS is reported world-wide.
4. Occurs in all ethnic groups.
5. Occurs in all socioeconomic levels.
6. 8–11% of childbearing women are either problem drinkers or alcoholics (Abel, 1990).
7. Among alcoholic-dependent women, 30–40% produce FAS children.

C. Pharmacology of ethanol.
1. Ethanol and its metabolite, acetaldehyde, are critical components of alcohol.
2. It is absorbed rapidly from the stomach and the intestines.
3. Ethanol and acetaldehyde can alter fetal development by disrupting cell differentiation and growth.
4. Ethanol impairs normal placental function. It alters the transfer of essential nutrients to the fetus.
5. Ethanol reaches the fetus through diffusion across the placental membranes bidirectionally at a rate dependent on the concentration gradient.
6. Fetal ethanol concentration is eliminated by maternal hepatic biotransformation.
7. Variability in infants is related to factors such as dose levels, chronicity of alcohol use, gestational stage and duration of exposure, and sensitivity of fetal tissues.

D. Dosage of alcohol.
1. Risk is greatest with the consumption of more than 3 oz of absolute alcohol per day (which translates into six standard drinks).
2. At lower levels, the association is less clear.
3. Outcome is associated with chronicity as well as the amount. The most affected children are born to women in the chronic stages of alcoholism.

E. Birth order.
1. There is a significant risk of a sibling having FAS, given another case in the family.
2. Firstborn children appear less likely to present with FAS than subsequent offspring (Abel, 1990).

F. Gestational stage.
1. Exposure at critical developmental stages affects particular systems.
2. Exposure during the first trimester can disturb embryonic organization of tissues, resulting in morphologic abnormalities.
3. When heavy drinking ceases during pregnancy, abnormalities and growth retardation that develop in later stages will be prevented.

G. Effects during pregnancy.
1. Spontaneous abortion is increased approximately two- to four-fold in moderate and heavy drinkers.
2. Neural tube defects have been documented in offspring of heavy drinkers.
3. Prematurity has not been identified as direct result of alcohol consumption.
4. Growth retardation: the average birth weight for an infant with FAS is 2000 g as compared with the median birth weight of 3000 g for all infants.
5. Abruptio placentae: there is an increased risk with alcohol consumption.
6. Breech presentation: FAS is strongly associated with breech presentation for both moderate and heavy drinkers.

H. Diagnosis of FAS.
1. The diagnosis of FAS is made when there are clinical signs in each of the following categories:
    a. Pre-natal and/or post-natal growth retardation.
    b. Characteristic facial dysmorphology.
    c. CNS involvement.
2. These children have a higher frequency than average for possessing non-specific malformations. A careful history is important to differentiate alcohol-related birth defects from those due to other compounds.

I. FAS characteristics.
1. Growth disturbances.
    a. Decrease in weight, length, and head circumference in both the neonatal period and during childhood.
    b. Growth retardation persists even when nutrition is adequate in childhood.
2. Facial dysmorphology.
    a. These characteristics represent growth failure in the midface, which may reflect abnormal brain growth.
        (1) Eyes: epicanthal folds, strabismus, ptosis, hypoplastic retinal vessels.
        (2) Mouth: poor suck; cleft lip or palate; small teeth; long, thin and straight upper lip; poorly developed philtrum; area between the nose and the upper lip appears elongated.
        (3) Face: bulging forehead, under-developed mandible.
3. CNS abnormalities.
    a. Delays in mental and motor development.
    b. Hyperactivity.
    c. Altered sleep patterns.
    d. Feeding problems.
    e. Language dysfunction.
    f. Perceptual problems.
    g. Low muscle tone and slow reflexes within the first week of life. This improves over the first month.
    h. Brazelton findings: poor habituation, low arousal.
    i. IQ scores.
        (1) Measure between 70–89, with a range from 16–130. Retardation is greatest and the chance for improvement least in those children with the most dysmorphology and the lowest birth weight.
4. Non-specific abnormalities (Weiner and Morse, 1988).
    a. Skeleton: retarded bone growth, fusion of cervical vertebrae.
    b. Heart: atrial and ventricular septal defect, tetralogy of Fallot, patent ductus arteriosus.
    c. Kidney: renal hypoplasia, hydronephrosis.
    d. Immune system: increased infections, particularly otitis media.
    e. Tumors: non-specific neoplasms.
    f. Skin: abnormal palmar creases, irregular hair, whorls.

J. **Newborn withdrawal from alcohol**.
1. Withdrawal symptoms from alcohol are relatively mild in comparison with infant narcotic withdrawal.
2. Onset is between birth and 12 hours after birth.
3. Symptoms include the following:
   a. Hypertonia.
   b. Tremors.
   c. Opisthotonos.
4. Sleep little, cry more, and engage in exaggerated mouthing behavior.

K. **Nursing considerations** for FAS.
1. Careful assessment.
2. Documentation of growth parameters, including head circumference, length, and birth weight.
3. Careful examination of facial features.
4. Neurological assessment for symptoms of neonatal withdrawal patterns.
5. Genetics consultation is indicated if FAS is suspected.

Heroin and Methadone

A. **Many of the effects of opiate use** in pregnancy are correlated directly to the amount of prenatal care received and the maternal life style rather than to the drug itself.

B. **Morbidity and mortality** are less in infants born to methadone-dependent women who have adequate prenatal care.

C. **Pharmacology**.
1. Heroin is an opiate and acts as a CNS depressant.
2. Except for neonatal withdrawal syndrome, heroin is not believed to be teratogenic (Bingol, 1987).
3. Heroin produces a sense of euphoria within 10 seconds after injection.
4. Opiates interfere with the normal menstrual cycle, thereby reducing fertility. Many addicted women do not realize they are pregnant until between the fifth and seventh month.

D. **Effects on the pregnant woman**.
1. Toxemia in 10–15% of opiate-dependent women.
2. Miscarriages are common.
3. Multiple medical complications in 40–50% of pregnant addicts, including anemia, cardiac disease, hepatitis, urinary tract infections, and syphilis.
4. Other complications include hepatitis B, thrombosis, abscesses, and acquired immunodeficiency syndrome (AIDS).
5. Obstetrical complications.
   a. Toxemia.
   b. Abruptio placentae.
   c. Retained placenta.
   d. Post-partum hemorrhage.
   e. Premature delivery.
   f. Shorter than average labors.
   g. Precipitous deliveries.
   h. Breech deliveries.
6. Effects on the fetus.
   a. As a result of a reduction in placental blood flow, there is a higher incidence of stillbirth and fetal distress.
   b. Fetal infections.
   c. Fetal anemia.
   d. Fetal malnutrition and growth retardation, which may persist beyond the period of addiction.

e. Meconium staining.

f. Violent kicking of the fetus when narcotics are withheld.

7. Effects on the newborn.
   a. Post-natal complications result mainly from prematurity (nearly 50%) and symptoms of withdrawal (most estimates are 70–90%) (Finnegan, 1988).
   b. Hypoxia due to an unstable intrauterine environment and reduction in placental blood flow.
   c. Meconium aspiration and aspiration pneumonia.
   d. Increased incidence of SIDS.
   e. Lower Apgar scores with a need for resuscitation.
   f. Congenital infections.
   g. Lower incidence of respiratory distress syndrome.
   h. Lower degrees of physiological jaundice.
   i. Skin breakdown due to frequent and loose stools.

8. Comparison of methadone with heroin.
   a. With adequate prenatal care on a low-dose methadone program, perinatal outcome is improved in terms of prematurity, fetal loss, and medical complications.
   b. Infants still exhibit neonatal withdrawal symptoms similar to heroin-exposed infants.
   c. Both groups of infants present with low birth weight; however, methadone infants are larger.
   d. Methadone may be associated with a greater likelihood of neonatal seizures, more intense and longer withdrawal. However, these findings may be based on higher than now-recommended doses of methadone.

Neonatal Abstinence Syndrome (NAS)

A. **Over two-thirds of babies born to opiate-dependent women** will exhibit signs of NAS.

B. **Time of onset varies** from shortly after birth to 2 weeks of age.

C. **Symptoms appear** within 72 hours following birth in the majority of infants.

D. **Duration ranges** from 8–16 weeks or longer.

E. **Presentation of neonatal abstinence is variable**. It may be mild and transient, intermittent, delayed in onset or begin acutely, show improvement, and then revert to subacute withdrawal.

F. **Withdrawal is more severe** in infants whose mothers are chronic drug users.

G. **The closer to delivery a mother takes the drug**, the greater the delay of onset and the more severe the symptoms (Finnegan, 1990).

H. **Neonatal abstinence** is described as a generalized disorder characterized by 21 symptoms most commonly seen in withdrawing infants (Finnegan, 1990).

1. Neurological signs.
   a. Hypertonia.
   b. Tremors.
   c. Hyper-reflexia.
   d. Irritability and restlessness.
   e. High-pitched cry.
   f. Sleep disturbances.
   g. Seizures.

2. Autonomic system dysfunction.
   a. Yawning.
   b. Nasal stuffiness.
   c. Sweating.
   d. Sneezing.
   e. Low-grade fever.

f. Skin mottling.
3. Gastrointestinal abnormalities.
   a. Diarrhea.
   b. Vomiting.
   c. Poor feeding.
   d. Regurgitation.
   e. Dysmature swallowing.
   f. Failure to thrive.
4. Respiratory signs.
   a. Tachypnea.
   b. Increased apnea.
5. Miscellaneous.
   a. Skin excoriation.
   b. Behavioral irregularities.

I. Use of the Neonatal Abstinence Scoring System.
1. The Neonatal Abstinence Scoring System assists in the detection of the onset of withdrawal symptoms and charts the progression and response to therapeutic intervention (Finnegan, 1990).
2. Assess high-risk infants 2 hours after birth and then every 4 hours.
3. If, at any point, the score is 8 or greater, the scoring should be initiated every 2 hours and should be continued for at least 24 hours.
4. If pharmacotherapy is not needed by 72 hours of age, scoring may be discontinued and the infant can be discharged after 24 hours of observation.
5. If the infant scores ≥8 on three consecutive scoring times, the infant should be evaluated for pharmacotherapy.
6. Because NAS symptoms simulate common neonatal metabolic conditions such as hypoglycemia, hypocalcemia, sepsis, and meningitis, a complete blood count, calcium, and glucose levels should be obtained before therapy is initiated.
7. The recommended pharmacological agents are paregoric and phenobarbital.
   a. Paregoric is the drug of choice for infants exposed only to narcotics.
   b. Phenobarbital is effective for infants exposed to multiple drugs in utero.
8. Control is defined as meeting the following conditions:
   a. Scores ≤8.
   b. Infant is easily consolable.
   c. Rhythmic sleep and feeding cycle is achieved.
   d. Steady weight gain is achieved.

Marijuana Smoking

A. **The range of women reported** to use marijuana during pregnancy varies among reports from 5% to 34% (Zuckerman, 1988).

B. **Little is known about the effects on pregnancy** and the long-term consequences of prenatal exposure.

C. **Pharmacology.**
1. Marijuana comes from the plant *Cannabis sativa*.
2. The psychoactive ingredient is 1,9-tetrahydrocannabinol (9-THC).
3. 9-THC has a high affinity for lipids and accumulates in the fatty tissues throughout the body.
4. It produces an increased carbon monoxide blood level resulting in hypoxia.
5. Placental transfer is highest in the first trimester.

D. **Effects on the fetus.**
1. Findings are conflicting.
2. Marijuana users exhibit precipitous labor, and their infants are more likely to exhibit meconium staining (25% vs. 5%). These findings increase proportionally to the reported frequency of usage (Zuckerman, 1988).

3. No known chromosomal damage related to 9-THC.
4. Not associated with prematurity, decreased length, or congenital anomalies.
5. No association between marijuana use and Apgar scores or the need for neonatal medical interventions.
6. Lower birth weight is associated with marijuana use, although inconsistently.
7. There may be a synergistic effect of marijuana with other substances, specifically alcohol, which alters fetal growth and development.
8. Assumptions regarding marijuana use and pregnancy must be made cautiously due to the limited and inconsistent studies.

E. **Effects on the newborn**.
1. Data are limited regarding neurobehavioral functioning.
2. Brazelton findings suggest a poor response to a light stimulus or no habituation to it. Also, there are more tremors and startles and less success at self-quieting behaviors.
3. By 1 month of age, infants improve to the level of non-exposed newborns.

Cigarette Smoking

A. **Nicotine is the primary compound** of cigarette smoking.

B. **It is water and lipid soluble**.

C. **Nicotine crosses the placenta**; however, the greatest effects on the fetus are secondary to the placental vasoconstriction and reduced oxygen availability.

D. **Cigarette smoke contains carbon monoxide**, which combines with hemoglobin to form carboxyhemoglobin. This impairs oxygenation for both the mother and fetus, resulting in fetal hypoxia (Zuckerman, 1988).

E. **There is a dose-related response** between the number of cigarettes smoked and newborn effects.

F. **Effects during pregnancy** include increased spontaneous abortions.

G. **Effects on the newborn**.
1. Increase in intrauterine growth retardation.
   a. Decrease in birth weight.
   b. Decrease in head circumference.
   c. Decrease in length.
2. There is a small increased risk of congenital malformations, including CNS malformations, hypospadias, inguinal hernia, and eye and ear malformations.
3. It may be that cigarette smoking in combination with other variables contributes to this finding (Zuckerman, 1988).
4. Neurobehavioral effects suggest that children exposed to prenatal nicotine do less well on tests of cognitive, psychomotor, language, and general academic achievement.

Problems Associated with Maternal Drug Use

A. **General information** regarding drug-dependent women:
1. Drug-dependent women often have never experienced a positive relationship with their own parents.
2. They often come from dysfunctional families.
3. As children, the women were exposed to domestic violence, physical abuse, and sexual abuse.
4. As adults, they are often abused by their spouses.
5. Many have never observed positive parenting.
6. Many lack knowledge of normal child development and child care skills necessary for effective parenting.

B. **Psychological profile** of drug-dependent women.
1. Have multiple psychosocial problems.
2. Drug usage is usually an enduring pattern.
3. Demonstrate periods of serious depressions, a sense of powerlessness, and low self-esteem.
4. Often homeless with a lack of social supports.
5. Maintain satisfactory personal relationships with difficulty.
6. Are unable to modify their behavior from past experience.
7. Are unable to anticipate the consequences of their behavior.
8. Most women are single. The father is often drug dependent himself or not involved in parenting.
9. Living conditions are unstable, even dangerous environments.
10. With the birth of a sick infant, the drug-dependent mother lacks the coping mechanisms, skills, and support to assist her during this crisis.
11. These women experience intense guilt after the birth of their infant.

C. **Maternal-infant relationships**.
1. The attachment process between mother and infant, like all relationships, is one of reciprocity.
2. Factors in infants that contribute to poor parenting include behavior that is characteristic of prenatal drug exposure.
    a. Irritability.
    b. Neurologically disorganized.
    c. Rarely reach an alert state.
    d. Feed poorly.
    e. Have erratic sleep patterns.
    f. Resist comforting.
3. The drug-dependent mother is unskilled and lacks experience in mothering.
    a. A high-risk profile exists due to the severity of the mother's addiction coupled with her own psychological profile and life style, the infant's behavior, and the mother's lack of knowledge and experience in dealing with infants.

Management Recommendations

A. **Document maternal drug use patterns** and prenatal care.

B. **Obtain toxicology screening** for cocaine and its metabolites for all infants with a moderate index of suspicion. For urine, obtain the earliest urine possible.

C. **Consider human immunodeficiency virus (HIV) testing**, pending mother's consent and your hospital's policy.

D. **If a careful physical examination reveals any malformations**, growth retardation, or microcephaly, evaluate for etiology and consider screening for congenital infections.

E. **Obtain cranial ultrasound**, renal ultrasound, EEG, visual evoked response, and brainstem auditory response, based on clinical indications prior to discharge.

F. **Observe carefully** for signs of feeding intolerance.

G. **Evaluate for signs of withdrawal**, using an abstinence score (see earlier section on NAS).

H. **Counsel mother regarding breast-feeding**.

I. **Consult with social services**. A referral to agencies or for foster care as dictated by case (this includes FAS). The mother must be informed of all medical, social, and legal circumstances regarding the baby. This needs to be documented in the medical record.

J. **Initiate careful discharge planning** with attention to maintaining surveillance post-discharge, including evaluation of neurodevelopmental status.

Nursing Intervention

A. **The infant.**
1. Careful ongoing physical assessments, including the neonatal abstinence score.
2. Observe for seizure activity.
3. Assess the infant's tolerance of environmental stimuli.
4. Minimize environmental and physical stimulation.
   a. Provide dim lighting.
   b. Speak quietly around the baby.
   c. Consider bed placement to avoid high-traffic areas.
5. Provide pacifiers.
6. Swaddle tightly in a flexed position.
7. Provide gentle rocking in a vertical position to decrease irritability and restlessness.
8. Administer sedation as indicated.
9. Cluster activities to allow for extensive rest periods.
10. Consider gavage feeding without awakening occasionally for infants who have difficulties in sleeping.
11. Modulate sensory input as tolerated, e.g., feed in a quiet, dimly lit room without talking or looking at the infant.
12. For feeding difficulties, offer small, frequent feedings. High-caloric, low-volume feedings may be effective. However, diarrhea and general feeding intolerance may prohibit this approach.

B. **Mother-nurse interactions.**
1. The nurse must confront her own feelings regarding these issues.
2. Caretakers need to understand that "being addicted" means giving up control of one's life. Addiction is a disease, requiring treatment.
3. Develop a therapeutic relationship with the mother by establishing trust.
4. Provide consistency in caregivers, preferably with a primary nurse.
5. Provide clear information and specific guidelines for expected behavior.
6. Truthful information and education presented in a non-judgmental manner is the most effective.
7. Assist mothers to attach emotionally with their infants by encouraging touch and caretaking.
8. Provide positive reinforcement and immediate feedback for all caretaking activities.
9. Parent education should be goal directed. Outline clearly the caretaking and clinical milestones toward discharge.
10. Explain the infant's behavior. Discuss the baby's sensitivity to the environment and to excessive handling.
11. Explain to the mother that the infant's behavior is not a rejection of her.
12. Teach mothers to intervene *early* with a crying baby; explain that their response is not "spoiling" the infant but that the infant is not yet able to quiet himself or herself.
13. Provide kangaroo care opportunities whereby the infant is placed on the mother's chest skin-to-skin.
14. Acknowledge to oneself that these mothers and infants require flexibility, high energy, patience, and a non-judgmental attitude.

Breast-feeding and the Drug-dependent Woman

A. **Cocaine and methamphetamines**.
Breast-feeding is contraindicated. Cocaine remains for up to 60 hours after maternal ingestion.

B. **Alcohol**.
Moderate to heavy drinking has been shown to interfere with oxytocin release, causing inhibition of the letdown reflex. Alcohol may be consumed with caution during lactation.

C. **Heroin**.
Heroin-dependent women should not breast-feed.

D. **Smoking**.
The long-term effects of breast-feeding while smoking are unclear. If mothers smoke, it is recommended that they do not smoke at any time while actually nursing or in the infant's presence. If it is not possible to stop smoking, mothers should be encouraged to decrease the number of cigarettes and also consider low-nicotine cigarettes.

E. **Marijuana**.
Impairment of DNA and RNA formation and essential proteins has been reported (Lawrence, 1990). Breast-feeding is not recommended for these mothers.

F. **AIDS**.
The HIV antigen has been isolated in breast milk. It is recommended that every drug-dependent woman be screened for the HIV antibody and, if positive, be advised not to breast-feed (Wilton, 1988).

Ethical Considerations

A. **Problems of substance abuse** in pregnant women raises several ethical questions regarding rights of the mother and the rights of the fetus.
1. Who shares in the responsibility toward this issue?
   a. The health care system, the legal system, the public?
2. What are the rights of the pregnant woman who abuses drugs?
   a. Does she forfeit her autonomy and right to privacy because her choice will potentially do harm to the fetus?
3. Does the fetus have a greater need to be protected? Should the fetus be protected by law? (Becker and Burke, 1988)
4. What if the woman is unable to protect her fetus?

B. **The opinions of some legal writers** demonstrate a growing trend in the law that suggests that the child abuse and neglect statute be extended to include protection of the fetus.
1. The law courts have affirmed the view that "justice requires recognition that a child has a legal right to begin life with a sound mind and body" (Landwirth, 1987).
2. A woman's right to abuse her own body and threaten her own health should not extend to the body of the fetus.

C. **When the rights and the needs of the mother are separated** from the fetus, the resultant solutions appear adversarial. When the rights and needs of the mother and fetus are viewed as interrelated, solutions may be developed to support both.

D. **For clearly identified high-risk infants**, the greatest impact may only be possible by protecting the child. Sometimes, children need to be removed from an addicted family and an unstable home environment and placed in a protected environment until the mother can receive help with her addiction and lifestyle.

E. **Primary prevention is always suggested** to be the key in the health care framework, coupled with early intervention programs, prenatal care, education, and birth control information for young women (Becker and Burke, 1988). Basic life needs, such as shelter, financial and peer support, food, and adequate health care, are critical.

STUDY QUESTIONS

1. Which of the following is an effect of cocaine usage during pregnancy?
   a. Lower maternal heart rate.
   b. Placental vasoconstriction.
   c. Prolonged labor.

2. A pregnant woman who presents in labor with abruptio placentae and a history of drug use should be tested for:
   a. Chorioamnionitis.
   b. Polydrug use, especially cocaine.
   c. Rubella.

3. How is the diagnosis of FAS made?
   a. Constant, high-pitched crying in the infant.
   b. History of heavy alcohol use and characteristic signs in the baby.
   c. Toxicology screen in mother is positive.

4. An important nursing intervention when working with a drug-exposed infant is:
   a. Avoid swaddling.
   b. Minimize environmental stimuli.
   c. Provide ongoing stimulation to increase adaptation to environment.

5. An important nursing intervention when working with drug-dependent mothers is:
   a. Be direct, but not judgmental.
   b. Be distrustful of her family and friends.
   c. Leave her alone as much as possible.

Answers to Study Questions

1. b	3. b	5. a
2. b	4. b	

REFERENCES

Abel, E.L.: Fetal Alcohol Syndrome. Oradell, NJ, Medical Economic Books, 1990.

Becker, P., and Burke, S.: Neonatal drug addiction: An analysis from two moral orientations. Holist. Nurs. Prac., 2(4):20–27, 1988.

Bingol, N.: Teratogenicity of cocaine in humans. J. Pediatr., 110(1):93–96, 1987.

Chasnoff, I.J.: Drugs, Alcohol, Pregnancy and Parenting. Boston, Kluwer, 1988.

Finnegan, L.P.: Drug addiction and pregnancy. In Chasnoff, I. (ed.): The Newborn in Drugs, Alcohol, Pregnancy, and Parenting. Toronto, B.C. Decker, 1988, p. 314.

Finnegan, L.P.: Neonatal abstinence syndrome. In Nelson, N. (ed.): Current Therapy in Neonatal Perinatal Medicine. Toronto, B.C. Decker, 1990, p. 314.

Hurt, H.: Medical controversies in evaluation and management of cocaine-exposed infants. In Special Currents, May, 1990, M404. Columbus, Ohio, Ross Laboratories.

Jones, K.: Fetal alcohol syndrome. Pediatr. Rev., 8(4):122, 1986.

Landwirth, J.: Fetal abuse and neglect: An emerging controversy. Pediatrics, 79(4):508, 1987.

Lawrence, R.: Breastfeeding, 3rd ed. St. Louis, C.V. Mosby, 1989.

Weiner, L., and Morse, B.A.: FAS: Clinical perspective and prevention. In Chasnoff, I. (ed.): Drugs, Alcohol, Pregnancy and Parenting. Boston, Kluwer, 1988, p. 127.

Wilton, J.M.: Breastfeeding by the chemically dependent woman. In Chasnoff, I. (ed.): Drugs, Alcohol, Pregnancy and Parenting. Boston, Kluwer, 1988, p. 149.

Zuckerman, B.: Marijuana and cigarette smoking during pregnancy: Neonatal effects. In Chasnoff, I. (ed.): Drugs, Alcohol, Pregnancy and Parenting. Boston, Kluwer, 1988, p. 73.

BIBLIOGRAPHY

Adams, C., Eyler, F.D., and Behnke, M.: Nursing interventions with mothers who are substance abusers. J. Perinat./Neonat. Nurs., 3(4):43, 1990.

Alder, M.: Scientific perspectives on cocaine abuse. Pharmacology 29:20–27, 1987.

Atkins, W.: Cocaine: The drug of choice. In Chasnoff, I. (ed.): Drugs, Alcohol, Pregnancy and Parenting. Boston, Kluwer, 1988, p. 91.

Chasnoff, I.J., Hunt, C.E., Kletter, R., et al.: Prenatal cocaine exposure is associated with respiratory pattern abnormalities. Am. J. Dis. Child., 143:583–587, 1989.

Clarren, S.K., and Smith, D.W.: The fetal alcohol syndrome. N. Engl. J. Med., 298:1063–1067, 1978.

Coles, C.D., Smith, I., Fernhoff, P.M., et al.: Neonatal ethanol withdrawal: Characteristics in clinically normal, non-dysmorphic neonates. J. Pediatr., 105:445–450, 1984.

Deren, S.: Children of substance abusers: A review of literature. J. Substance Abuse Treat., 3:77–94, 1986.

Dixon, S.: Effects of transplacental exposure to cocaine and methamphetamine on the neonate. West. J. Med., 150:436–442, 1989.

Dixon, S., Bresnahan, K., and Zuckerman, B.: Cocaine babies: Meeting the challenge of management. Contemp. Pediatr., March, 1990.

Eliason, M., and Williams, J.: Fetal alcohol syndrome and the neonate. J. Perinat./Neonat. Nurs. 3(4):64, 1990.

Ernhart, C.B., Wolf, A.W., Linn, P.L., et al.: Alcohol-related birth defects: Syndromal anomalies, IUGR, and neonatal behavioral assessment. Alcoholism, 9(5):447–453, 1985.

Finnegan, L.P.: Substance abuse. Perinatol.-Neonatol. 6(4):17–23, 1982.

Flandermeyer, A.: A comparison of the effects of heroin and cocaine abuse upon the neonate. Neonatal Network, 42–48, Dec. 1987.

Fried, P.A.: Marijuana use by pregnant women: Neurobehavioral effects on neonates. Drug Alcohol Depend., 6:415, 1980.

Griffith, D.: The effects of perinatal cocaine exposure on infant neurobehavior and early maternal-infant interactions. In Chasnoff, I. (ed.): Drugs, Alcohol, Pregnancy and Parenting. Boston, Kluwer, 1988, p. 105.

Halliday, H.C., MacReid, M., and McClure, G.: Results of heavy drinking in pregnancy. Br. J. Obstet. Gynecol., 89:892–895, 1982.

Harrison, G.G., Branson, R.S., and Vaugher, Y.E.: Association of maternal smoking with body composition of the newborn. Am. J. Clin. Nutr., 38:757, 1983.

Hingson, R., Alpert, J., and Day, N.: Effects of maternal drinking and marijuana use on fetal growth and development. Pediatrics, 70:539, 1982.

Householder, J., Hatcher, R., Burns, W.M., et al.: Infants born to narcotic-addicted mothers. Psychol. Bull., 92:453, 1982.

Lynch, M., and McKeon, V.: Cocaine use during pregnancy: Research findings and clinical implications. JOGNN, 19(4): p. 285, 1990.

National Institute on Drug Abuse: Cocaine use in America. Prevention Networks, Department of Health and Human Services (Pub. No. ADM 86-1433). Washington, DC, US Government Printing Office, 1986.

Oro, A., and Dixon, S.: Perinatal cocaine and methamphetamine exposure: Maternal and neonatal correlates. J. Pediatr., 111:571–578, 1987.

Perinatal Advisory Council of Los Angeles: Perinatal protocol: Maternal substance use and neonatal drug withdrawal. J. Perinatol., 8(4):387–392, 1988.

Robe, L.B., Gromisch, D.S., and Iosub, S.: Symptoms of neonatal ethanol withdrawal. Curr. Alcohol., 8:485–493, 1981.

Russell, M.: The impact of alcohol-related birth defects in New York State. Neurobehav. Toxicol., 2:277–283, 1980.

Sokol, R.J., Miller, S.I., and Reed, G.: Alcohol abuse during pregnancy: An epidemiologic study. Alcoholism, 4:135–145, 1980.

Staisy, N., and Fried, P.: Relationships between moderate maternal alcohol consumption during pregnancy and infant neurological development. J. Studies Alcohol, 44:262–270, 1983.

Sullivan, K.: Maternal implications of cocaine use during pregnancy. J. Perinat./Neonat. Nurs. 3(4):12, 1990.

Ward, S., Schutz, S., and Kirshria, V.: Abnormal sleeping ventilatory patterns in infants of substance-abusing mothers. Am. J. Dis. Child, 140:1015, 1986.

Wegman, M.E.: Annual summary of vital statistics, 1986. Pediatrics, 80:817–827, 1987.

Weiss, R.: Subtypes of cocaine abuse. Psychiatr. Clin. North Am., 9:3–10, 1986.

Mary Ann Best

The Family in Crisis

Objectives

1. Define the concept of crisis.

2. Recognize the psychological tasks that the mother and family must accomplish to establish a healthy parent-child relationship following the crisis of a premature birth.

3. Describe assessment strategies for identifying a family in crisis.

4. Identify nursing interventions to support a family coping with stressful events surrounding the birth of their infant.

5. Evaluate maternal behaviors that have been found to be predictive of specific parenting outcomes.

6. Recognize emotional characteristics related to grief.

7. Describe nursing interventions to support the parents experiencing a perinatal loss.

8. Identify specific behaviors to be assessed in determining parental attachment to their infant.

9. Describe nursing strategies to promote parental acquaintance and attachment.

Impressive advances have been made in improving both the survival rate and quality of the survivors of neonatal intensive care units (NICUs) (Kennell and Klaus, 1982a).

When an infant requires medical care at birth due to prematurity, illness, or congenital malformations, or when an infant dies, the effect of these unexpected events on the parents can be overwhelming. The families of these infants may experience multiple crisis events during the infant's hospitalization (Johnson, 1986). Assessment skills are critical for the neonatal nurse who meets families at a period of crisis—usually when they are anxious, afraid and often experiencing circumstances of an emergency nature. It is the nurse who has a constant, ongoing interaction with the family and becomes the primary support for some families (Thornton et al., 1984). Nursing care is generally concerned with both the physiological and psychosocial needs of an individual and the family. However, the focus of this chapter is the psychosocial aspects of supporting parents who must cope with stressful events surrounding the birth of their infant.

Crisis and the Birth of the Less-Than-Perfect Infant

Pregnancy and transition to parenthood have been recognized as periods of stress and change during which mothers and fathers are attempting to master the normal developmental process of parenthood. These major life changes have been referred to as *developmental or maturational stressors*. In contrast, the birth of a premature or less-than-perfect infant and the death of an infant are situations that represent unexpected stressful life events for which a person or family is often physiologically unprepared. These situations are referred to as *situational or accidental stressors*. When such maturational and situational stressors occur simultaneously, the resulting pressure can overwhelm a person's usual coping resources and support systems. Ineffective coping causes personal and family psychological disequilibrium or crisis, until new ways of coping can be developed and maintained.

A. **Several psychological tasks** have been identified that the mother and family must accomplish to cope with the crisis of premature birth and to establish a basis for a healthy parent-child relationship (Kaplan and Mason, 1960; Siegel, 1982).
1. *Preparation for the possible loss of the infant:* they must consider the possibility of disability or death of the infant while simultaneously hoping for the infant's survival.
2. *Acknowledgement of failure to deliver a term infant:* the mother struggles with feelings of guilt and failure and searches for causes for the baby's condition.
3. *Adaptation to the intensive care environment:* they must be helped to develop secure relationships in an unfamiliar and stress-provoking setting.
4. *Resumption of interaction with the infant once the threat of loss has passed:* they must participate in the infant's care and gain confidence in their abilities.
5. *Preparation for taking the infant home:* they must understand the special needs and characteristics of the premature infant and the necessary precautions that must be taken yet maintain a positive relationship with the infant and realize that these needs are only temporary. Failure to resolve these tasks can contribute to such maladaptive parenting as overprotectiveness, resulting in the "vulnerable child syndrome" and negative child outcomes such as failure to thrive, emotional deprivation, and battering (Green and Solnit, 1964; Siegel, 1982).

B. **Definition.**
1. *Crisis:* a temporary disequilibrium that occurs when a people face an important problem or transitional phase that is so stressful that they are unable to cope using their customary problem-solving resources (Caplan, 1964; Penticuff, 1983).

C. **Discussion.**
1. During the period of disequilibrium early in the crisis situation, people are more willing to accept help and are more open to change (Caplan, 1964). Because nurses are often among the first members of the perinatal health care team to interact with the parents, they have an opportunity positively to influence the family's coping ability by recognizing signs of crisis and initiating the process of crisis resolution (Grant, 1978). Effective coping leads to successful resolution of the crisis and restoration of physiological equilibrium, which is necessary for establishment of a healthy parent-child relationship. Factors that influence a person's return to equilibrium include the following:
   a. Perception of the stressful event.
   b. Coping abilities.
   c. Available support system (Aguilera, 1990).

Identification of the Family in Crisis

Assessment

A. **Determine parents' understanding of the situation** (*i.e.*, realistic vs. distorted). The parents' ability to resolve the crisis depends on their realistic perception of the situation.

B. **Determine parents' adaptation and coping** with the stressful event.
1. Are the parents maintaining responsibilities related to activities of daily living (i.e., eating, personal grooming, etc.)?
2. To what degree has the family's normal lifestyle been affected by the crisis? (Are they able to return to work? keep house? care for other children in the household?)
3. Are the parents exhibiting coping skills?
4. To what extent has the financial status of the family been affected?

C. **Determine what support systems exist** for the parents and whether they are being used.
1. Who are the significant others in the lives of the parents?
    a. Biological kinship (family) and/or emotional kinship (friends).
2. What professional supports are available for the family?

Intervention

A. **Be present with the physician** at the initial meeting with the parents.

B. **Talk with the mother and father** together whenever possible.

C. **Determine and address the parents' perceptions** of the infant's condition (Taylor and Hall, 1980).

D. **Be consistent with information** given to parents by the staff. Conflicting information can result in misunderstanding, confusion, and mistrust (Oehler, 1981). It is helpful to have one person primarily responsible for synthesizing and communicating information to the parents (Kennell and Klaus, 1986).

E. **Do not overload parents with detailed information** about their infant during their initial visits to the NICU; provide basic facts and allow the parents time to process the information.

F. **Periodically assess the parents' understanding** of their infant's condition and their interpretation of the information that has been given to them (Taylor and Hall, 1980).

G. **Write notes from the infant to the parents** concerning current status (i.e., equipment, feedings, oxygen concentration, etc.) and take pictures of the infant periodically. A notebook containing the notes and pictures can be kept at the infant's bedside for the parents.

H. **Allow parents the freedom to express negative ideas without being judged.** Fear and frustration over inability to control their infant's circumstances are often the basis for parental anger displaced to staff.

I. **Determine parents' network of social support.**

J. **Encourage parents to share their concerns and fears** with each other.

K. **Assist parents in maintaining their relationship with the infant's siblings** by helping them to recognize the needs of the children and identify how the needs can be met.

L. **Encourage parents to attend a parents' support group.** Involvement in parental support groups has been demonstrated to facilitate parental grieving, reduce fears, and increase feelings of parental competence (Minde, 1980).

Evaluation

A. **Predictors of good maternal parenting outcomes** (Mason, 1963):
1. Anxiety level is moderate to high: she worries about the infant's chances of surviving, the possibility of abnormality, and her competence as a mother.

2. Seeks information about the infant.
3. Demonstrates warmth toward infant and in other relationships.
4. Has a support system (i.e., father of the infant, her mother, friends).
5. Has had a previous successful experience with a premature infant (i.e., previous child, a sibling, other relative), which enables her to feel more experienced and confident.
6. Recognizes positive attributes of the child (i.e., smiling) (Ventura, 1982).

B. **Predictors of poor maternal parenting outcomes** (Mason, 1963; Kennell and Klaus, 1986):
1. Exhibits an inappropriately low anxiety level.
2. Demonstrates passivity—does not actively seek out information related to infant's condition.
3. Has limited verbal interaction.
4. Visits infrequently and for short periods in the NICU.
5. Is unaware of the infant's needs.
6. During pregnancy, expressed little desire to have a child.
7. Is more likely to express disappointment about the sex of the infant.
8. Has no support system.

Grief and Loss

A. **Introduction**: Unfortunately, not all pregnancies result in a full-term, healthy infant. When adverse neonatal events occur, often the parents are overwhelmed by grief. As the parents realize that their newborn is "less than perfect" and not the infant of their fantasies, acute grief reactions occur. One of the early tasks of parenting is to resolve the discrepancy between the idealized infant and the real infant (Solnit and Stark, 1961). In the case of neonatal death, the parents also grieve for the lost opportunity to parent the child. To assist parents therapeutically in working through the feelings associated with loss, it is essential for nurses working with high-risk infants to understand the grief process, recognize typical parental behaviors associated with grief, and provide appropriate nursing interventions.

B. **Definitions**.
1. *Grief:* the response of sadness and sorrow to the loss of a valued object (Gardner and Merenstein, 1986).
2. *Anticipatory grief:* grieving that occurs before an actual loss. If the outcome for the infant is healthy, then anticipatory grieving can lead to difficulties in attachment and problems in the parent-infant relationship.
3. *Chronic grief:* unresolved or blocked grief; frequently seen in parents of a handicapped child in which there is a constant reminder of loss.

C. **Assessment:** A similar response occurs in the grief response to death, premature birth, or birth of an infant with a malformation. These responses do not necessarily occur in the same sequence for all people. In addition, the responses may overlap and recur.
1. Stages of grief (Drotar et al., 1975; Lancaster, 1986).
   a. Shock.
   b. Denial and/or panic: refuses to accept reality, may experience intense anxiety.
   c. Anger, guilt, and shame: awareness of loss suffered becomes acute.
   d. Acceptance, adaptation, and reorganization: grief continues but the individual is able to re-establish a state of equilibrium.

One of the goals of the staff working with parents is to encourage the development of attachment, or an affectional tie, between the parent and infant. However, because the birth of a premature or malformed infant creates a sense of loss, the parents must first resolve their grief before attachment can be fully achieved (Lancaster, 1986).

Interventions for Facilitating Grief

A. **Listen:** parents need to be given the opportunity to express their feelings.

B. **Acknowledge the pain of their loss:** gives the parents permission to talk about their loss and support for acknowledging and working through their grief (Garland, 1986).

C. **Convey an attitude of acceptance, openness, and availability to the family:** grieving people need permission to experience their feelings, regardless of how uncomfortable or unpleasant (Garland, 1986).

D. **Help the parents to understand the individuality of the grieving process.** Mothers and fathers usually have "incongruent grieving," i.e., they do not grieve at the same pace (Peppers and Knapp, 1980). This incongruence frequently leads to marital discord due to misconceptions about feelings and inability to communicate.

Interventions for Parents Experiencing a Perinatal Loss (Kleingbeil, 1986).

A. **Encourage the family to see, hold, and spend time with the infant** before and after death. Be sensitive to individual and cultural differences in rituals of saying "good-bye."
1. Physically bring the family together and offer them privacy. Some hospitals have a neonatal hospice program in which the family is involved with the infant's care (Butler, 1986; Landon-Malone et al., 1987; Siegel et al., 1985; Whitfield et al., 1982).

B. **Provide the parents with the following mementos:** photograph of the infant, identification bracelet, footprints, completed crib card, blanket, wisp of hair, birth certificate.
1. Keep these mementos in a file in the nursery for future retrieval should parents choose not to take the items at the time of the infant's death.

C. **Provide information about support groups and/or grief counseling.**

D. **Encourage the parents to name the infant.**

E. **Provide a booklet about perinatal loss for the parents.**

F. **Discuss options for autopsy, disposition of the body, and memorial or funeral service.**

G. **Offer option for the infant to be baptized.**

H. **Assist parents in understanding the importance of informing siblings about the death of the infant.** Suggest that they use simple statements based on the children's level of understanding (Gardner and Merenstein, 1985).

I. **Talk with parents about possible responses** from family and friends, who often minimize the infant's death in an attempt to offer comfort.

Interventions for Parents with a Pre-term or Malformed Infant

These interventions have been incorporated into the interventions listed in the previous section on the family in crisis and in the following section of family-infant bonding.

Family-Infant Bonding

Parents who have an infant who is born ill, prematurely, or malformed are potentially at risk for experiencing parenting difficulties. These stressful events around the time of the infant's birth generate feelings of anxiety, disappointment, and grief in the parents. Also, early disruptions in the acquaintance and attachment process between parent and infant place these parents in a state of increased vulnerability for establishing a nurturing relationship with their infant. Opportunities for parents to learn to interpret their infant's unique needs and develop reciprocal interaction through sensitivity to behavioral cues are also interrupted (Mercer, 1977). The relationship between parent-infant attachment and later parenting behaviors has been well established. In addition, the parent-infant attachment is the basis for all the infant's subsequent attachments and is the relationship through which a sense of self is developed (Kennell and Klaus, 1982a). Therefore, an important component of nursing care for the high-risk infant is facilitation of parent-infant interaction and attachment.

A. Definitions.
1. *Bonding:* is a gradual, reciprocal process that begins with acquaintance and attachment, is a unique and specific relationship between two people, and endures over time (Jenkins and Tock, 1986; Kennell and Klaus, 1982a). Bonding occurs on a different timetable for mothers than for fathers. Although mothers experience a sharp increase in bonding around the fifth month and experience an intensifying of these feelings throughout the pregnancy, the father's feelings usually tend to develop more slowly than the mother's and become congruent after birth when infant caretaking begins (Peppers and Knapp, 1980).
2. *Attachment:* refers to the quality of the bond or affectional tie between parents and their infant that begins early in the pre-natal period, appears to increase when fetal movement is felt, and is intensified with interaction between the parent and infant after birth (Lancaster, 1986).

C. Discussion. The development of a warm, nurturing, and reciprocal relationship between infant and parent is essential for a healthy physiological outcome to the crisis of the birth of a premature, sick, or malformed infant (Lancaster, 1986). "The parent 'at risk' cannot resolve a crisis surrounding birth of their infant and simultaneously establish warm attachment bonds while retaining his or her self-esteem without the support of others in the social system" (Mercer, 1977, p. 5). Neonatal nurses can provide this support by assessing the parents' responses to their infant and facilitating their acquaintance and attachment process with the infant.

D. Assessment.
1. Note pattern of parental visiting to the NICU and length of visits as well as frequency of phone calls — these activities have been predictive of mothers who are experiencing parenting difficulties (Kennell and Klaus, 1982a).
   a. If parents are not visiting frequently, be careful to determine the reasons (i.e., cultural practices following childbirth, conflicting obligations between work and family roles, or lack of transportation to hospital) before assuming the parents are unconcerned or that parenting difficulties exist.
2. Identify development of attachment behaviors. Mothers' activity with their infants has been found to be indicative of their initial adjustment to the infant, their important past and present interpersonal relationships, and their involvement in taking care of the infant (Minde, 1980). Examples of attachment behaviors include the following:
   a. Touching: typical maternal progression of touching the premature infant is

from fingertip touching of infant's extremities to palmar stroking of infant's trunk to holding and embracing the infant. This progression of touch usually occurs over a period of several visits to the NICU.

b. Looking "en face": aligning head with infant's head in the same plane to make eye-to-eye contact with the infant.

c. Talking to the infant, calling the infant by name.

d. Bringing pictures, toys, and/or clothes to the hospital.

Interventions to Encourage Family-Infant Bonding

A. **If at all possible, show the infant to the parents in the delivery room and allow them to touch the infant, if only for a few moments:** this helps to establish the reality of the infant for the parents (Kennell and Klaus, 1982 a,b; Litchfield, 1983).

B. **Encourage the parents to visit** their infant in the intensive care nursery as soon as possible.

1. Prior to visiting the nursery for the first time, prepare the parents for what to expect by giving them a booklet about the unit, describing the atmosphere of the nursery (i.e., noise, high activity level, infants attached to various kinds of equipment), and discussing the normal aspects of their infant as well as deviations.

2. If the mother is unable to visit due to conditions such as ordered bedrest or transport of the infant to another hospital, the father can be given pictures of the infant for the mother. Also, the mother should be given the phone number of the nursery and encouraged to call as often as desired.

3. For the parents of an infant born with a malformation, encourage the parents to see the infant together as soon as possible but do not force them to interact. Point out to the family the normal qualities of the infant as well as the abnormalities (Wallisch, 1983; Irvin, 1982).

C. **Ensure that the nurse assigned to the infant stays at the bedside during the family's first visit** to explain equipment and infant's condition, as well as to answer questions, provide emotional support, and encourage touching of the infant.

D. **Convey a positive, realistic attitude about the infant** rather than a negative or fatalistic viewpoint, which may alienate the parents and impair attachment (Ladewig et al., 1990).

E. **Assist the parents with holding** and cuddling their infant as soon as possible, based on the infant's condition and parent readiness (i.e., assist in managing respiratory and monitoring equipment, intravenous lines, etc.).

1. Some nurseries are implementing skin-to-skin care (also called "kangaroo care") by parents as an alternative to the traditional modes of providing care to stable, hospitalized premature infants. This care consists of positioning the infant, dressed only in diapers, upright and prone between the mother's breasts. This vertical position in skin-to-skin contact provides tactile stimulation and warmth from the mother, as well as opportunities for eye-to-eye contact, auditory stimulation, and breast-feeding. Mothers usually wear their own front-opening blouses or dresses that are loosely fitted. Fathers can also be encouraged to engage in kangaroo care (Affonso et al., 1989; Anderson, 1989; Luddington-Hoe, 1991).

F. **Encourage the parents to participate in caretaking activities** as warranted by the infant's condition and tolerance for input. Explain to parents of very premature infants the relationship between neurological maturity and capacity for handling stimulation (Als, 1979).

G. **Model nurturing parenting behavior** such as stroking, touching, and talking to the infant for parents who may need assistance in developing positive parenting behaviors.

H. **Give positive reinforcement** to parents as they interact with their infant. For example, "he seems to enjoy your holding him," or "she really eats well when you feed her" (Oehler, 1981).

1. Assisting parents to recognize positive changes in the infant in response to their caretaking has a strong impact on the parents and increases their feelings of success (Johnson, 1986).

I. **Suggest that the parents or siblings bring something** for the infant, such as a small toy, pictures of the family members to be taped on the infant's bed, and/or a tape recording of the parents' voices to be played to the infant.

1. Share personalized information about the infant with the parents, such as "she really enjoys sucking on her pacifier" or "she was really active while I was giving her a bath," to assist the parents in individualizing and accepting the infant.

J. **Allow sibling visitation** in the unit or window observation of the infant (Oehler, 1981).

K. **Following the mother's discharge from the hospital, maintain communication** with the parents by providing them with the phone number of the unit. For parents of transported infants, sending pictures and cards from their infant telling of current status, arranging for transportation assistance through social service agencies for parents who lack means for travel (Oehler, 1981), and maintaining frequent phone contact with parents can be helpful in promoting parent-infant attachment (Brown et al., 1989).

L. **Give the mother the opportunity to provide breast milk** for the baby should she so desire, and support her in this endeavor. However, be cautious not to over-emphasize the importance of this activity. Otherwise, if she should be unsuccessful or decide to stop breast-feeding for other reasons, feelings of guilt or disappointment may occur (Kennell and Klaus, 1982a).

M. **Provide a supportive environment** in which parents can gain confidence as they are becoming acquainted with their infant and are learning the skills needed to assume responsibility for the infant's care.

N. **Identify situations in which there are difficulties in parent-infant interaction or problems in the family's functioning** (Siegel, 1982).

O. **Be sensitive to cultural practices** that may influence parent-infant behaviors while bonding and attachment remain strong.

P. **Identify infants who are at risk for having developmental difficulties** (Siegel, 1982).

Evaluation of Parent-Infant Bonding

Evaluation of parental behaviors should be based on patterns over a period of time rather than on isolated incidents (Mercer, 1977).

A. **Positive attachment behaviors.** (Kennell and Klaus, 1982a).
1. Visits frequently.
2. Has named the infant.
3. Makes positive comments when talking to or about the infant.
4. Demonstrates increasing skill in holding the infant.
5. Displays increasing eye and bodily contact between parent and infant (i.e., kissing, fondling, stroking, nuzzling).

B. **Behaviors of concern** (Kennell and Klaus, 1982a).
1. Is overly optimistic.
2. Appears unconcerned about infant's condition.
3. Does not ask questions.

4. Is passive or indifferent.
5. Avoids close bodily contact by holding infant at a distance; props bottle whether or not infant is held; positions bottle such that milk is unable to flow from nipple.
6. Is unable to describe any physical or behavioral features unique to the infant.
7. Attributes inappropriate characteristics to the infant, such as "she's lazy and stubborn just like her father" (Wallisch, 1983).

Summary of Parental Needs to Be Met by NICU Staff
(Klaus and Kennell, 1982a)

A. **Help mother re-conceptualize image** of "ideal" infant to image of her premature, acutely ill, or malformed infant.

B. **Help mother deal with feelings of guilt**.

C. **Help parents to develop affectionate ties** with infant and learn to read infant's behavioral cues.

D. **Assist parents to gain confidence** in holding infant by encouraging them to participate in caretaking tasks.

E. **Promote communication** between the parents.

F. **Be sensitive to the unique needs** of the individual families.

G. **Assist families in preparing for the transition** to home care following discharge (Barnard, 1982; Cagan, 1988).

H. **Provide support for parents during the transition phase** following discharge of their infant (Brooten et al., 1986; Butts et al., 1988; Gennaro and Stringer, 1991).

I. **Assist parents to deal with neonatal death** in a personally meaningful way (Siegel, 1985).

STUDY QUESTIONS

1. Two days ago, Wendy Jones, age 33, gave birth by cesarean section to a premature infant of 26 weeks' gestation. During visits to the NICU, her husband, Fred, continued to insist that the infant will be "well enough" to be off the ventilator and be discharged with his wife in three more days. He is most likely experiencing which stage of the grief process?
   a. Anger
   b. Denial
   c. Depression

2. Mary Smith is visiting her premature infant in the NICU for the first time today. How can the infant's nurse provide a positive experience for her in the NICU environment?
   a. Convey a positive, realistic attitude about the infant
   b. Focus solely on the critical aspects of the infant's care
   c. Leave Mary alone at the bedside during most of the visit to provide her with some "private" time with her infant

3. What typical pattern of positive attachment behaviors would you expect Mary Smith to exhibit during visits with her infant?
   a. Embracing the infant while gazing at the infant "en face"
   b. Progression of fingertip touching of infant's extremities to palmar stroking of infant's trunk to embracing of the infant
   c. Progression of fingertip touching of infant's face to trunk to extremities to embracing the infant

4. Linda Cook, age 22, has delivered a stillborn infant at 30 weeks' gestation. Which nursing interventions would be most appropriate in supporting her and her family as they cope with the infant's death?
   a. Encourage the family to see, hold, and touch the infant
   b. Remove and discard the identification bracelet, crib card, and other mementos
   c. Suggest that the family keep busy at all times to "keep their mind occupied"

Answers to Study Questions

1. b
2. a
3. b
4. a

REFERENCES

Affonso, D.D., Wahlberg, V., and Persson, B.: Exploration of mothers' reactions to the kangaroo method of prematurity care. Neonatal Network, 7(6):43–51, 1989.

Aguilera, D.C.: Crisis intervention: Theory and methodology, 6th ed. St. Louis, C.V. Mosby, 1990.

Als, H., Lester, B. and Brazelton, T.B.: Dynamics of the behavioral organization of the premature infant: A theoretical perspective. *In* Field, T.M. (ed.): Infants Born at Risk. New York, SP Medical and Scientific Books, 1979.

Anderson, G.C.: Skin to skin: Kangaroo care in western Europe. Am. J. Nurs., 89:662–666, 1989.

Barnard, K.: Critical commentary. *In* Klaus, M.H. and Kennell, J.H. (eds.): Parent-Infant Bonding. St. Louis, C.V. Mosby, 1982, p. 194.

Brooten, D., Kumar, S., Brown, L., et al.: A randomized clinical trial of early discharge and home followup of very low birthweight infants. N. Engl. J. Med., 315:934–939, 1986.

Brown, L.P., York, R., Jacobsen, B., et al.: Very low birthweight infants: Parental visiting and telephoning during initial infant hospitalization. Nurs. Res. 38:233–236, 1989.

Butler, N.C.: The NICU culture versus the hospice culture: Can they mix? Neonatal Network, 5(2):35–42, 1986.

Butts, P.A., Brooten, D., Brown, L., et al.: Concerns of parents of low birthweight infants following hospital discharge: A report of parent-initiated telephone calls. Neonatal Network, 7(2):37–42, 1988.

Cagan, J.: Weaning parents from Intensive Care Unit care. MCN, 13(4):275–277, 1988.

Caplan, G.: Principles of Preventive Psychiatry. New York, Basic Books, 1964.

Drotar, D., Baskiewicz, A., Irvin, N., et al.: The adaptation of parents to the birth of an infant with a congenital malformation: A hypothetical model. Pediatrics, 56:710–717, 1975.

Gardner, S.L., and Merenstein, G.B.: Grief and perinatal loss. *In* Merenstein, G.B., and Gardner, S.L. (eds.): Handbook of Neonatal Intensive Care. St. Louis, C.V. Mosby, 1985, pp. 449–483.

Gardner, S.L., and Merenstein, G.B.: Perinatal grief and loss: An overview. Neonatal Network, 5(2):7–15, 1986.

Garland, K.R.: Unresolved grief. Neonatal Network, 5(3):29–37, 1986.

Gennaro, S., and Stringer, M.: Stress and health in low birthweight infants: A longitudinal study. Nurs. Res., 40(5), 1991.

Grant, P.: Psychosocial needs of families of high-risk infants. Family Commun. Health, 1(3):91–102, 1978.

Green, M., and Solnit, A.J.: Reactions to the threatened loss of a child: A vulnerable child syndrome. Pediatrics, 34:58–66, 1964.

Irvin, N.A., Kennell, J.H., and Klaus, M.H.: Caring for the parents of an infant with a congenital malformation. *In* Klaus, M.H., and Kennell, J.H. (eds.): Parent-Infant Bonding, 2nd ed. St. Louis, C.V. Mosby, 1982, pp. 227–258.

Jenkins, R.L., and Tock, M.K.S.: Helping parents bond to their premature infant. Am. J. Matern. Child Nurs., 11:32–34, 1986.

Johnson, S.H.: The premature infant. *In* Johnson, S.H. (ed.): Nursing Assessment and Strategies for the Family at Risk: High-Risk Parenting. Philadelphia, J.B. Lippincott, 1986, pp. 120–156.

Kaplan, D., and Mason, D.: Maternal reaction to premature birth viewed as an acute emotional disorder. Am. J. Orthopsychiat., 30:539–547, 1960.

Kennell, J.H., and Klaus, M.H.: Caring for the parents of premature or sick infants. *In* Klaus, M.H., and Kennell, J.H. (eds.): Parent-Infant Bonding, 2nd ed. St. Louis, C.V. Mosby, 1982a, pp. 151–226.

Kennell, J.H., and Klaus, M.H.: Caring for the parents of premature or sick infants. *In* Klaus, M.H., and Kennell, J.H. (eds.): Parent-Infant Bonding, 2nd ed. St. Louis, C.V. Mosby, 1982b, pp. 259–292.

Kennell, J.H., and Klaus, M.H.: Parent counseling. *In* Knuppel, R.A., and Drukker, J.E. (eds.): High-Risk Pregnancy: A Team Approach. Philadelphia, W.B. Saunders, 1986, pp. 551–560.

Kleingbeil, C.G.: Extended nursing care after a perinatal loss: Theoretical implications. Neonatal Network, 5(3):21–28, 1986.

Ladewig, P.W., London, M.L., and Olds, S.B.: Essentials of Maternal-Newborn Nursing, 2nd ed. Redwood City, CA, Addison-Wesley, 1990, pp. 818–836.

Lancaster, J.: Impact of intensive care on the parent-infant relationship. *In* Korones, S.B. (ed.): High Risk Newborn Infants: The Basis for Intensive Nursing Care, 4th ed. St. Louis, C.V. Mosby, 1986, pp. 407–417.

Landon-Malone, K.A., Kirkpatrick, J.M., and Stull, S.P.: Incorporating hospice care in a community hospital NICU. Neonatal Network, 6(1):13–19, 1987.

Litchfield, M.D.: Family-infant bonding. *In* Vestal, K.W., and Mackenzie, C.A.M. (eds.): High Risk Perinatal Nursing, Philadelphia, W.B. Saunders, 1983, pp. 64–79.

Luddington-Hoe, S.M., Hadeed, A.J., and Anderson, G.C.: Physiologic responses to skin-to-skin contact in hospitalized premature infants. J. Perinatol., 11(1):19–24, 1991.

Mason, E.A.: A method for predicting crisis outcome for mothers or premature babies. Public Health Rep., 78:1031–1035, 1963.

Mercer, R.T.: Nursing care for parents at risk. Thorofare, NJ, Charles B. Slack, 1977.

Minde, K.K.: Bonding of parents to premature infants: Theory and practice. In Taylor, P.M. (ed.): Parent-Infant Relationships, New York, Grune and Stratton, 1980, pp. 291–313.

Oehler, J.M.: Family-centered Neonatal Nursing Care. Philadelphia, J.B. Lippincott, 1981.

Penticuff, J.H.: Nursing assessment and management of the childbearing family in crisis. In Vestal, K.W., and McKenzie, C.A.M. (eds.): High Risk Perinatal Nursing. Philadelphia, W.B. Saunders, 1983, pp. 80–96.

Peppers, L.G., and Knapp, R.J.: Motherhood and Mourning: Perinatal Death. New York, Praeger, 1980.

Siegel, R.: A family-centered program of neonatal intensive care. Health Soc. Work, 7:50–58, 1982.

Siegel, R., Rudd, S.H., Cleveland, C., et al.: A hospice approach to neonatal care. In Corr, C.A., and Corr, D.M. (eds.): Hospice Approaches to Pediatric Care. New York, Springer, 1985, pp. 127–152.

Solnit, A.J., and Stark, M.H.: Mourning and the birth of a defective child. Psychoanalyt. Study Child, 16:523–537, 1961.

Taylor, P.M., and Hall, B.L.: Parent-infant bonding. In Taylor, P.M. (ed.): Parent-Infant Relationships. New York, Grune and Stratton, 1980, 315–334.

Thornton, J., Berry, J., and Dal Santo, J.: Neonatal intensive care: The nurse's role in supporting the family. Nurs. Clin. North Am., 19:125–137, 1984.

Ventura, J.N.: Parent coping behaviors, parent functioning, and infant temperament characteristics. Nurs. Res., 31:269–273, 1982.

Wallisch, S.: Stress: The infant, family and nurse. In Vestal, K.W., and McKenzie, C.A.N. (eds.): High Risk Perinatal Nursing. Philadelphia, W.B. Saunders, 1983, pp. 97–117.

Whitfield, J.M., Siegel, R.E., Glicken, A.D. et al.: The application of hospice concepts to neonatal care. Am. J. Dis. Child., 136:421–424, 1982.

Candice Cook Bowman

The Teenage Family

Objectives

1. Recognize the high probability that teenage parents with a sick infant will experience a crisis.

2. Identify the origins of the teenage parents' crisis as related to their individual situation, their stage of development, their role transition, and their sociocultural environment.

3. Identify aspects of their physical, physiological, and psychosocial development that form the basis of maturational crisis.

4. Indicate how the uneasy adjustment to the role of parent can adversely affect the teenager's relationships with family and peers.

5. Identify the risks of very young parental age for parenting in general and for morbidity outcomes of the neonate.

6. Describe likely crisis behaviors exhibited by the teenager that can be recognized and assessed by the nurse.

7. Identify likely outcomes of the teenager's situation, with and without nursing intervention.

8. Demonstrate how appropriate nursing diagnoses and associated interventions can be geared toward the preferred outcomes.

The admission of a newborn to a neonatal intensive care unit (NICU) is a destabilizing event for any parent. To a teenage parent, the effect is not just greater in magnitude but a wholly different experience. The developmental tasks of adolescence, compared with those of adulthood, highlight the well-known problems that teenagers have in parenting effectively. It has been said about females in this age group that "nine months is not enough for (their) development into the motherhood role" (Cram-Elsberry and Malley-Corrinet, 1986, p. 244). If nine months is not enough time for preparation, then certainly a premature birth, for which teenagers are at high risk, shortens the already inadequate amount of time for transition to parenthood. Add the crisis of bearing a sick newborn to this untimely passage into adult responsibility and it is easy to imagine how a teenage family can be ill equipped to manage such a situation. Insightful assessment and knowledgeable interventions by the NICU nursing staff can abate a potentially damaging set of circumstances.

The Teenage Parent in the NICU: Multiple Crises Needing Resolution

Hoff (1989) describes people in crisis as those who have suffered a sudden or threatened loss of anything they consider to be essential and important. For some, that loss may require a new mode of problem solving that they cannot accomplish with their present resources. Loss of an old role, and entry into a new and unknown one, leaves the teenager without adequate coping skills. Hoff's crisis model, which demonstrates the evolution of a crisis event from its origins to its resolution, is uniquely applicable to the adolescent who becomes a parent of a sick newborn. Figure 29–1 depicts the basic components of the model and serves as an organizing framework for this chapter. The following underlying assumptions of the model demonstrate why it can be a useful theoretical basis for working with these adolescent families who are, by definition, in crisis.

A. **People will resolve their crises with or without the aid of others, although the outcome may be detrimental.** Knowledge of this premise encourages the nurse to intervene, which increases the likelihood of a positive resolution.

B. **Positive resolution is seen as an opportunity for growth and development through creation of new resources and ways of problem solving.** This supposition promotes a more optimistic start for a working relationship between the nurse and the teenager. It also emphasizes the appropriateness of this paradigm for the transitional status of teenagers in general.

C. **The roots of crisis events are viewed as "origins" that can be generated from more than one source.** This allows the nurse to understand the probability of an event becoming a crisis and is an important assumption in working with teenagers who may be more at risk for ensuing problems than older parents of sick neonates.

D. **The likelihood of a crisis occurring is based on the following factors, as described by Schulberg and Sheldon (as used in Hoff):**
1. Probability of the distressing event occurring: emerging sexuality of adolescence makes teenage pregnancy an all-too-common occurrence.
2. Probability that a particular person will be exposed to the event: sexually active individuals are more likely to find themselves facing parenthood. Obstetrical risks specifically related to young maternal age have been documented for decades.
3. Vulnerability of a person to the event: the immature and dependent adolescent may adapt poorly to the stress of parenthood as well as to having a sick infant.

E. **Understanding the origins of crisis and their links with the normal "ups and downs" of life is crucial to successful assessment and intervention. Events that stimulate the occurrence of a crisis,** such as those of the teenage parent in the NICU, **can originate from:**
1. Being in a transitional state, such as:
   a. Adolescence to adulthood.

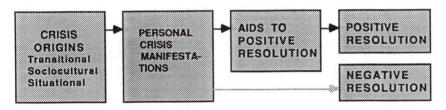

Figure 29–1
Hoff's crisis paradigm. The interactions between the components of the model provide a useful basis for assessing crisis behaviors and focusing interventions toward positive outcomes. (Modified from Hoff, L.: People in Crisis, 3rd ed. Menlo Park, CA, Addison-Wesley, 1989, p. 84.)

  b. Childhood to parenthood.
2. Being a part of a social-cultural structure and:
  a. Violating mores embedded in that structure, such as a teenager becoming pregnant and having a baby, *or*
  b. Behaving outside the accepted teenage social norms as the role of parent would demand (although these examples are culture specific).
  c. Being exposed to hazardous or disturbing situations, such as:
    (1) Birth of a first child.
    (2) Lack of experience with parenthood.
    (3) Bearing a sick newborn.

Regarding the circumstances of the teenage parent with a sick neonate through Hoff's paradigm gives the NICU nurse a special appreciation for the probability of the event reaching crisis proportions. It also can guide the nurse through relevant assessment and specialized interventions to promote these desired outcomes:
1. Assumption of the responsibilities characteristic of young adults.
2. Preparation of an effective parent.
3. Formation of a strong parent-infant bond.

Crisis Origins

TRANSITIONAL: THE ADOLESCENT

The turmoil of adolescence has been described in countless ways on a multitude of occasions by a myriad of observers. Parry-Jones (1985) summed up this period of altered patterns of precipitous growth as "a time of rapid physiological and psychological change, of intensive readjustment to the family, school, work, and social life, and of preparation for adult roles" (p. 584). The period of adolescence, generally accepted as the 10 or so years that follow the onset of puberty, has been viewed by all experts as a stepping stone of development in a lifespan perspective. The phase-specific tasks of psychosexual, cognitive, moral, and psychosocial development have been described by Freud, Piaget, Kohlberg, and Erikson, respectively. These classic theories have long been used by professionals in attempting to understand adolescents and their reactions to life events. This understanding must begin with an appreciation for the extreme bodily changes that precede displays of their often tumultuous psychosocial behavior.

Physical and Physiological Development

The bodily changes that occur during this period largely result from altered hormonal secretion and considerable skeletal growth, although the net results of both are mostly gender specific. Physical changes that occur are the following:

A. **For both** (although emphasized in males).
1. Increase in muscle bulk.
2. Widening and thickening of bones.
3. Increase in adrenal androgens.
4. Increase in skin thickness and oily secretions.
5. Increased libido.
B. **For females**
1. Large increase in hip width.
2. Steady rise in body fat as structural growth subsides.
3. Enlargement of breasts and appearance of pubic and axillary hair.
4. Onset of menarche between 12–16 years, although there is some variation between countries and cultures.

C. **For males**
1. Increase in shoulder breadth.
2. Overall increase in physical strength.
3. Loss of body fat.
4. Enlargement of penis and testes and appearance of pubic and body hair.
5. Thickened, darkened growth of facial hair.
6. Deepening of the voice (Cram-Elsberry and Malley-Corrinet, 1986; Graham and Rutter, 1985; and Lerner and Spanier, 1980).

The physical changes experienced in adolescence are generally welcomed by males because of the psychological advantages of increased strength, manliness, and athletic prowess. For females, the changes are less advantageous and are less likely to determine popularity with peers. Because of their greater sensitivity to social pressures, girls are more subject to distress if their physical development is not normally paced. Early and late maturation and development of an attractive body type have been repeatedly demonstrated to be related to subsequent psychosocial development. However, values dictated by the teenagers' social milieu seem to have a stronger influence on consequent sexual behavior than timing and degree of their sexual maturity (Graham and Rutter, 1985).

Psychosocial Changes

Development of the personality stems primarily from the adolescent's ability to redefine his or her sense of self, concurrent to changes in outward appearance. The formation of identity, according to Erikson, is based on future role attainment, which is prescribed by the social and cultural groups to which each teenager belongs (Lerner and Spanier, 1980). Teenagers must strive to achieve the role requirements of the young adult to transcend the adolescent stage. Those requirements include:

A. **Independence from adults.**
B. **Preparation for financial security.**
C. **Gender identification.**
D. **A stable, realistic, positive sense of self** (Yeaworth et al., 1980).

Reluctance to relinquish the security of dependent relationships can make transition to adulthood an unwanted step. Clinicians have found that the adolescent's task of identity definition versus rule confusion, described by Erikson, is a useful basis for understanding normal behavior (Parry-Jones, 1985). Committing one's self to attaining an adult role, then, is seen as a positive resolution of the adolescent's dilemma of "Who am I?" (Lerner and Spanier, 1980).

ADOLESCENCE AS A MATURATIONAL CRISIS

That adolescence is seen as maturational crisis is a widely held view that is incorporated into Hoff's paradigm (1989). She describes this transitional state, as with all developmental stages and social role changes, as a crisis source that has the following characteristics:

A. **Is earmarked by the experience of high anxiety.**
B. **Can be anticipated** and, therefore, prepared for.
C. **Requires normal social support** for a successful transition.
D. **Is relatively easy to resolve** because the individual's values usually do not conflict with societal expectations for the outcome, i.e., adult behavior.
E. **Is a period of vulnerability** to a crisis occurrence if a traumatic event is added to the transitional state.

F. **Aguilera and Messick** (1986) describe a number of stressful factors of normal adolescence that further emphasize a process of destabilization and impending crisis due to maturation, which include the following:
1. Conflict between self-perception and how others perceive him or her.
2. Dissatisfaction with body image.
3. Tentative seeking of freedom and rebellion against authority.
4. Desperate need to belong, to feel loved, wanted, and accepted.
5. Indecisive and confused pursuit of heterosexual involvement.

Adolescence alone is an unquestionable state of disequilibrium. Addition of further stressful factors puts the teenager at greater risk for a problematic outcome.

SOCIOCULTURAL: THE ADOLESCENT PARENT

In the adolescent's struggle for independence, associations with a peer group have mounting importance. In spite of the well-known strength of peer influence, the family remains the most important in determining attitudes, values, and beliefs (Lerner and Spanier, 1980). Teenage pregnancy and parenthood may be viewed as unacceptable behavior in both spheres of influence because the timing of such events is generally outside what is considered to be normal in most Western cultures. However, the well-reported high incidence of teenage pregnancy in low-income blacks may conflict with this view. It is quite possible that pregnancy and parenthood within the context of this sociocultural group could be regarded within their norm, although it has been noted by Phipps-Yonas (1980) that there are no data to suggest that adolescent parenthood is acceptable in any group in Western society. Nevertheless, the difficulties of continuing high school education for these young mothers attests to the degree of nonconformity that this breach of acceptable age-specific behavior represents, if viewed from the broader cultural perspective. Wise and Grossman (1980) reflected on the incipient effects of differences in evaluating findings of this nature. It may be prudent on the part of nurses, then, to be aware of their own perspectives when assessing teenagers' circumstances.

Violation of Conventions Dictated by Social Norms: Deviance

Childbearing, a result of personal action, does not become a crisis of sociocultural origin until judgment has been passed by other members of the social environment. In developing a Life Change Events Scale, Mendez et al. (1980) included "getting pregnant" with other extreme socially undesirable items, such as "being raped," "beating up someone," or "getting ready to kill oneself." (p. 387) They omitted these events from their questionnaire because they felt that it would be less threatening to the subjects, who were students in private college preparatory schools, and their parents. Even so, respondents rated "close girl friend pregnant" (Mendez et al., p. 386) as 15th out of 38 stressful items. These findings suggest the degree of stress that might result from such circumstances.

A. **Disruption to peer group relationships**.
1. In seeking the supportiveness of peer group associations, the pressures of conformity and popularity force teenagers into certain patterns of behavior that are dictated by the group. Teenage parents find that they suddenly have little in common with friendships formed prior to the pregnancy, and social isolation then becomes a problem as friends begin to disappear and, as a consequence, withdraw their support.
2. Wise and Grossman (1980) investigated a group of 30 predominately low-income, black adolescent mothers who felt neither isolated nor rejected by their families or friends, possibly due to the high incidence of pregnancy within their peer group. This finding may discount social deviance as a crisis origin for black teenagers, but it still emphasizes the importance of social support.

B. **Disruption to own family relationships**.
1. Garmezy and Rutter (1985) allude to the considerable psychiatric evidence that demonstrates the effect of family support in moderating the effects of stressful events experienced by children. Love and protection from the adolescent's own family is essential in avoiding feelings of ambivalence toward assuming the self-direction and independence required in his or her new role. Young maternal age has been demonstrated not to be a factor in development of weak affectional ties to the infant if an adequate support structure, such as a strong family bond, is in place (Koniak-Griffin, 1988).
2. Having a child during adolescence most likely will bring the teenager into direct conflict with his or her own parents because of the seemingly irresponsible sexual behavior that created the circumstance. Unmarried teenagers are more likely to remain under their parents' jurisdiction and, therefore, be prevented from making decisions concerning their infant's welfare. This effectively removes the stimulus for assuming a responsible parental role (Smith, 1984).

Mother's Profile

Much attention has been paid to the alarming epidemic of teenage motherhood in the United States. In surveying the literature for the consequences of bearing children during the teen-age years, Ruff (1987) found evidence for the following maternal factors:

A. **Potential health problems**.

B. **Emotional disturbance**.

C. **Interrupted education** leading to unemployment, poverty, and welfare dependence.

D. **Forced early marriage** and additional pregnancies.

E. **Characterizations of insensitivity** and impatience and tendency toward use of physical punishment, which may lead to abuse of their infants.

F. **Lack of knowledge** concerning normal infant development and how to stimulate it.

Phipps-Yonas (1980) concluded that there is no unique psychological profile that describes the type of adolescent girl who becomes pregnant, in spite of many investigations into a broad range of potential predictors. Wise and Grossman (1980) showed that correlates for easier adjustment to motherhood for their adolescent group were the following:
1. Greater independence from nuclear families.
2. Close relationship to baby's father during the post-partum period, although Ruff (1987) was surprised to find the opposite to be true in her group of 95 black adolescent mothers.
3. Planning and emotional involvement in the pregnancy.
4. "Less worrisome" neonatal behavior (Wise and Grossman, 1980).

Father's Profile

The adolescent father has been commonly portrayed as being involved only long enough to learn of the pregnancy before vanishing. Barret and Robinson (1986) discussed several of their own and others' findings in trying to gain insight into this group. They assert that adolescent fathers can be characterized by the following statements:

A. **In spite of more frequent sexual experiences**, did not know more about sexuality and reproduction than their peers who were not fathers.

B. **Were often viewed as having little control** over their circumstances or sexual urges but, in reality, were found to display as much self-control as their non-parent peers.

C. **Are psychologically healthy** and display normal adolescent behavior when facing less than optimal circumstances.

D. **Have less education**, unstable employment, and earn just above minimum wage.

E. **Feel helpless and alienated** by being excluded from decision making during the pregnancy and become more active in the new family, especially with financial support, when involved in that process.

F. **Have close, caring, and relatively long-lasting relationships** with their girlfriends in spite of wanting to remain unmarried.

G. **Continue to be attached** to the new family after the birth and express desires to participate in the lives of their children as they grow.

Risks to the Infant

Much of the health care literature suggests that teenagers are emotionally and intellectually ill-prepared for the role of parent. Phipps-Yonas (1980) summarized a huge body of evidence by concluding that children of adolescent parents are no more at risk for health problems than the general population, if good prenatal care and maternal nutrition are provided. She adds, though, that because these conditions are rarely met, young maternal age would have to remain a predictive factor for poor infant outcomes. Because childbearing seems to begin at an earlier age in lower socioeconomic groups, there exists an even more confusing picture of risk (Kinard and Klerman, 1980). Effects of young maternal age on offspring have been shown to be the following:

A. **Inaccurate assessment of infant development**: adolescent mothers inaccurately assessed the development of their infants more so than adult mothers. Overestimating or underestimating developmental progress is probably a result of the adolescent's immature cognitive processes and can place undue expectations on the infant (Becker, 1987).

B. **Reduced responsiveness in the infants**, which affects subsequent maternal-child interactions. Studies using the Brazelton Neonatal Behavioral Assessment Scale highlighted the following behavior often seen in these infants:
1. Abnormal arousal.
2. Poor response to stimuli.
3. Poor motor control.

C. **Poor physical health.**
1. Lower weight and stature up to 1 year of age.
2. High incidence of mortality and morbidity if the mother raises her child without a partner.

D. **Reduced cognitive development**: it is generally recognized that the older the mother at birth, the higher the intellectual functioning of the child (Lawrence and Merritt, 1981).

E. **Abuse and neglect**: several investigators found a higher incidence of abuse in adolescent families. However, when socioeconomic status was controlled for, maternal age was no longer a contributing factor. It is quite possible that abuse is a problem in all lower socioeconomic groups across the childbearing age range and, therefore, is a risk factor for this age group as well (Kinard and Klerman, 1980).

SITUATIONAL: THE ADOLESCENT PARENT OF A SICK NEWBORN

The literature is only weakly conclusive on the issue of increased likelihood of adolescent mothers to bear sick or premature infants. Two outcomes, though, prematurity and low birthweight (generally <2500 g), seem to have the most solid association with young maternal age, keeping in mind the irreducible correlate of low socioeconomic status.

Prematurity

Prematurity, birth between 20–37 weeks, is most significant in mothers under 15 years of age (Carey et al., 1981). Factors found by this group to be associated with teenage mothers who deliver prematurely were the following:

A. **Low weight** prior to the pregnancy.

B. **Low socioeconomic status**.

C. **Being single**.

D. **Smoker**.

E. **Narcotic usage**.

F. **Anemia** (hemoglobin <11 g).

G. **First child**.

H. **Poor prenatal care**.

Low Birthweight (LBW)

In contrast to previous data that demonstrated appropriate newborn weights for gestational age in under 18 year old mothers, Lawrence and Merritt (1981) found the following:

A. **The risk of delivering an infant under 2500 g** was six times greater for 14 year old and younger mothers.

B. **The 15–19 year old group** delivered LBW infants three times more frequently than 20–29 year old mothers.

C. **Adolescent black mothers** consistently had a higher frequency of infants under 1500 g when compared with 20–29 year old blacks. Brown et al. (1989) found a greater proportion of 72 mothers bearing LBW infants to be teenaged when compared with the national average for all births.

Other Possible Outcomes

A. **When adverse pregnancy outcomes were related to age**, Ventura and Hendershot (1984) found that very LBW and low 1-minute Apgar scores were attributed more often to mothers in their teens who were not married at, or soon after, conception and those who did not seek prenatal care in the first trimester of their pregnancy.

B. **Lawrence and Merritt** (1981) found the following more frequently in neonates of teenage black mothers compared with their older counterparts:
1. Hypoglycemia.
2. Respiratory distress syndrome.
3. Pneumonia.
4. Seizures and apnea.
5. Necrotizing enterocolitis.

Pneumonia was the only complication seen in a similar comparison of white newborns.

C. **Maternal behavioral factors** during pregnancy, listed above, were associated with 45–47% of black and white teenage mothers who gave birth to infants with complications.

D. **Length of hospital stay** was also found to be slightly longer for NICU infants of the younger mothers.

E. **Incidence of anomalies** was slightly higher in infants of adolescent mothers (Carey et al., 1981).

In spite of the liberalized views toward sexuality seen in this last postwar period, teenagers today, if they become parents, receive a confusing and distressing message concerning what is acceptable behavior within the confines of their social structure. Pressures such as these tend to compound the identity crisis of adolescence added to the likelihood of having a sick and/or premature newborn.

Personal Crisis Manifestations

Temperament, as well as developmental features, influence the way teenagers react to stressful events (Garmezy and Rutter, 1985). Transient periods of depression, anxiety, and mood fluctuations are characteristic of normal adolescent behavior, which makes detection of disturbed behavior difficult (Taylor, 1986). However, a close look at specific manifestations with associated nursing diagnoses may alert the NICU nurse to the adolescent in crisis.

INTERPERSONAL BEHAVIORS

With the Spouse or Partner: Ineffective Family Coping

Outcomes of the relationships of adolescent parents in general seem to vary considerably with marital status of the couple:

A. **Married**: fewer teenage parents are married now than ever before because of less restrictive views regarding illegitimacy. Marriage around the time of pregnancy or childbirth becomes far less frequent with younger maternal age, although on the average, about half do marry. Divorce rates for teenage marriages are twice as high as for couples in their early 20s. If the couple married:
1. Prior to conception, divorce is least likely.
2. Between conception and birth, the marriage probably had a hasty, unfavorable start and more than likely will have an unfavorable end (Lerner and Spanier, 1980).

B. **Not married but together:** When Ruff (1987) found that black adolescent mothers reacted poorly to their infants if they remained in contact with the father, she conjectured that teenage fathers may force their partners to divide their affection between them and the infants. As adolescents, they would insist that their needs be met first, which may put undue pressure on the mother of a sick infant.

Little evidence is available specifically regarding the outcomes of married or unmarried teenage couples whose infants spend time in the NICU. One must naturally conclude, though, that the added stress may cause irrevocable breakdown of their relationships.

With the Infant: Altered Role Performance and Parenting

Maternal-infant attachment and interactions have been observed, described, and measured by many. For the teenage group, the following summarizes those findings.

A. **Unmarried mothers and their infants** attached poorly when:
1. The mother's school grade level was lower, which was thought to be a result of less maturity and lack of exposure to childbearing curriculum taught in higher grades.

2. When the child's gender was male, possibly due to the mother's own struggle with male-female relationships (Ruff, 1987).

B. **Poorer interactions were also seen** when the neonate had mild to severe complications (Wise and Grossman, 1980).

With Own Family Members: Altered Family Processes

Some amount of intergenerational conflict is normal for teenagers, but some families cope with the ensuing turmoil more easily than others who may be facing a situational crisis as well. If the teenage parent is not yet emancipated from his or her own nuclear family, the evidence of conflict may be more obvious. Conflict with families stems from the teenager's fear, ambivalence, and confusion about adopting the next transitional role. Some behavioral manifestations of familial alienation are the following:

A. **Extreme rebelliousness**, i.e., delinquency, substance abuse, and running away (Taylor, 1986).

B. **Hostility toward own parents**, i.e., angry outbursts, temper tantrums, and withdrawal either alone or further into peer groups (Parry-Jones, 1985).

With NICU Staff: Personal Identity Disturbance, Impaired Social Interaction

Fajardo (1988) discussed her experiences with parents exhibiting dysfunctional behavior in the NICU. Parents, not necessarily adolescents, who perceive a deficit in themselves or in their relationships with others are unrealistic in their expectations for the infant to fill this gap, often display rage toward the NICU staff in the form of being:

A. Critical.

B. Challenging.

C. Openly hostile.

In trying to rectify the perceived deficiency, the teenager may then become overly reliant on staff members to help define his or her sense of self. This process is evidenced by the teenager becoming excessively:

1. Passive.
2. Compliant.
3. Conforming (Taylor, 1986).

INTRAPERSONAL BEHAVIORS

The point at which adolescent parents become incapable of withstanding stress through use of their own internal resources is when they show the following generalized symptoms of crisis:

A. Depression.

B. Anxiety.

C. Anger.

D. Denial.

E. Suspicion.

F. Excessive guilt.

G. Absence of affect.

H. Feeling of inadequacy and failure (Smith, 1984; Taylor, 1986).

How one perceives the degree of stress in a particular event is critical in resolving a crisis and is dependent on the cognitive style of the individual (Aguilera and Messick, 1986). The well-known incompetence of teenagers to think laterally and longitudinally restricts their ability to overcome destabilizing situations. Fajardo (1988) noted that teenagers are unrealistic about their abilities to perform as parents and tend to idealize their infants.

COPING METHODS: INEFFECTIVE INDIVIDUAL COPING

Coping is a tension-reducing mechanism used in an attempt to preserve psychological integrity in the face of adversity (Aguilera and Messick, 1986). Coping responses are highly individualistic and depend on cognitive styles that make dysfunctional coping in the teenager difficult to classify. Knowing the categories of problem-solving responses used by people of all ages in stressful circumstances may be useful to the NICU nurse. They are discussed below.

A. **Attempting to remove stressors**, either constructively or destructively. Examples of how the teenager might respond in this way are:
1. Denying the severity of the infant's condition (although, on a temporary basis, this may be a form of healing).
2. Placing blame for the infant's condition on the NICU staff.

B. **Removing oneself from exposure** to the event, such as:
1. Allowing own parents to take charge.
2. Not visiting the hospitalized infant.

C. **When the above fail, compromising expectations of the perceived outcomes by rationalizing, such as:**
1. Retaining the image of the idealized baby.
2. Having unreal notions about ease of parenting a high-risk infant (Aguilera and Messick, 1986).

Crisis Resolution

As in all interventions with patients and their families, it is useful to be cognizant of the objectives that drive those interventions, as well as the outcomes that may result when those objectives are not met. Crisis, by definition, is shortlived as individuals cannot exist indefinitely in such an anxious state. Hoff (1989) suggests that resolution, after several days or weeks, usually comes in one of three forms:

A. **Return to the pre-crisis state**, although nothing about the person changes, such as learning new ways of coping.

B. **Growth from the experience**, in that the person discovers new personal and external resources.

C. **Development of abnormal behavior patterns** that may be dangerous to the person and, in this instance, the infant.

POSITIVE RESOLUTION

Adult Role Attainment

Committing oneself to a role means assuming the socially prescribed attitudes, values, and beliefs that are assigned to that role. Lerner and Spanier (1980) characterized the adolescent who makes the successful transition as one who:

A. **Is capable of abstract thought processes.**

B. **Is morally principled.**

C. Views self positively.

D. Has a **centralized locus** of behavior control.

Effective Caretaking

Generally speaking, those who are content with their role will be effective at carrying out the tasks of that role. Teenagers who remain socially integrated and retain strong ties with their own families, in spite of problems, will be most successful as new parents.

Strong Parent-Infant Bond

A strong parental-infant tie ensures the survival of the infant. This is evidenced by the inordinate amount of sacrifices that parents seem to make in caring for their infants. The difficulty in attachment is a problem that both adolescent mothers whose own support is less than optimal and all mothers of NICU babies have in common. Immaturity and situational problems make the attachment process an especially difficult but necessary struggle for the adolescent to win (Fig. 29–2).

NEGATIVE RESOLUTION

Role Confusion

Those adolescents who refuse to make the commitment to the adult responsibilities associated with the parental role are at risk for poor ego development and, hence, will be kept from making their contribution to society, as Erikson suggested that all people must do.

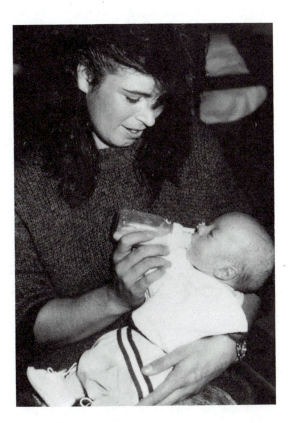

Figure 29–2
This teenage mother lovingly cares for her growing premature infant who had several months of intensive treatment in an NICU.

Separates and Isolates Self

Divorce and estrangement from former familial and peer relationships put the adolescent mother in a dangerous position. Isolation, added to a dim economic future, may severely threaten her ability to provide a secure, loving environment for her infant.

Neglects or Abuses Infant

Despite the difficulties in correlating abusing families with young maternal age, the risk for a teenage mother to bond poorly with an infant who has spent the majority of the critical bonding period in the NICU remains. The subsequent maladaptive maternal-infant interactions may increase the potential for abuse (Klaus and Kennell, 1982).

Aids to a Positive Resolution

Hoff (1980) appeals to health care providers to be sensitive to others' problems and lack of resources and do all that is possible to help individuals become stronger by developing more effective problem-solving skills. Parry-Jones (1985) approaches his adolescent clients with a broad contextual view of their environment and developmental status. He cites the most common difficulties he has found in working with teenagers as:

A. Establishing trust.
B. Talking about uncomfortable feelings.
C. Coping with help-rejecting behavior.

With this knowledge in mind, the NICU nurse can deftly plan her interventions along the avenues outlined in the following sections.

TRANSITIONAL: FACILITATION OF ADJUSTMENT TO THE NEW ROLE

Two approaches should be taken to promote an adaptive response to the new role, which, in this instance, means a commitment to parenting.

A. **Allowing a gradual return to a non-crisis state:** this will allow them to test the new role and ameliorate the sense of loss of the idealized baby. Golan (1980) notes that situational crises can often mask difficulties with a transitional phase. This knowledge can be used by the NICU nurse by frequently discussing teenagers' perceptions of their new role while retreating from the parents periodically to allow them to grieve for the well baby they thought they would have.

B. **Providing a healthy adult role model:** consistent caregivers will facilitate trusting relationships to develop outside the teenagers' social milieu and, thus, provide them with a broader exposure to other, perhaps healthier, adults.

SOCIOCULTURAL: ENHANCEMENT OF SUPPORT SYSTEMS

Without question, total functional support promotes better outcomes for both the adolescent parent and the infant. Phipps-Yonas (1980) suggests that it is futile to encourage the adolescent to become independent of her family because that scenario is known to lead to the most dismal results. Three approaches should be used to enhance supports.

A. **Build on strengths** inherent in the existing social network.
1. Encourage grandparents and other relatives to assist in the baby's care, but be careful to maintain the parent in the primary role.

2. Encourage the father to be involved in the baby's care, especially with decision making, but avoid encouraging the couple to marry in light of divorce statistics for this group.
3. Allow the mother to bring her close friends to visit the infant if unit policy permits. This will involve important members of the existing peer group.

B. **Introduce the adolescent to other mothers** with NICU babies: the success of parent support groups in the NICU is well known and may be essential for the teenager to try to understand her own feelings.

C. **Encourage the mother to begin investigating** a broader social network, because it will be difficult for her to imagine the problems of isolation.

SITUATIONAL: BETTER USE OF RESOURCES

When a nurse recognizes signs of crisis in the adolescent, a multidisciplinary approach should be taken. Kelting (1986) suggests that improving an NICU parent's self-concept is essential in overcoming a crisis through the following approaches:

A. **Counsel of social workers.**
B. **Involvement in a specialized support group.**
C. **Close rapport** with the nursing staff.

After some degree of stability has been reached, a small number of consistent nursing staff should be assigned to care for their adolescent's infant. When trust is established and the teenager is willing to accept help, nurses are valuable resources for teaching the teenage mother or father how to care for their infant. When teaching adolescent parents in the nursery, the nurse should:
1. As early as possible, begin to inform the parents of the infant's social capabilities and what they can do to stimulate such behavior. This was a very strong recommendation of Riesch and Munns (1984), who studied the effect of this intervention on mothers of both term and pre-term infants. Early social interaction between parent and infant promotes bonding.
2. Use the Brazelton Neonatal Behavioral Assessment Scale as an effective tool to demonstrate how poor alerting and attending behavior is typical of premature infants. Lack of this knowledge may adversely affect interactions with their own infant (Buckner, 1983).
3. Gradually help the parent to become aware of the "real" as opposed to the "ideal" child and his or her realistic potential for development (Fajardo, 1988).
4. Remain nonjudgmental regarding one's own opinions about teenage childbearing, because they are value laden, and any such transgression by the nurse will lead to mistrust.
5. Explore the mother's personal concerns as well as those regarding the infant. This will help meet the needs stemming from the teenager's egocentrism.
6. Teach general baby care on a one-to-one basis rather than sending the teenage mother to longer hospital classes. A teenager's somewhat reduced attention span and limited learning ability, especially if school performance was low, require that additional forms of teaching at the appropriate level be used, i.e., films and videos.
7. Always demonstrate handling and care of the infant first and use praise when the teenage parent attempts to perform the tasks. The adolescent is not likely to take the initiative to provide care for the infant in the nursery and so must be prompted.
8. Avoid power struggles, set and enforce limits, such as arrival in time for feedings, visiting on a regular basis (Fullar, 1986).

NICU nurses should be fully knowledgeable about a variety of community-based informational and educational, supportive, and financial services to facilitate con-

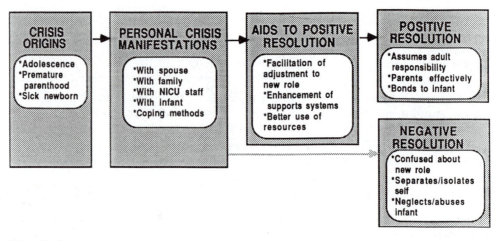

Figure 29–3
Hoff's crisis paradigm adapted for the adolescent parent in the NICU. Several origins increase the probability of a crisis occurring for this family. With the knowledgeable intervention of the NICU nurse, the desired outcomes as indicated can be achieved. (Modified from Hoff, L.: People in Crisis, 3rd ed. Menlo Park, CA, Addison-Wesley, 1989, p. 84.)

tact between the teenage parent and these organizations. A concise summary of available state and federal organizations has been outlined by Headlee (1988) and can be a useful directory for nursing staff.

Summary

Evaluating the adolescent parent of an NICU infant by using an adapted version of Hoff's crisis paradigm (Fig. 29–3) can highlight the increased probability of a crisis occurrence for these young mothers and fathers. It can also be a useful framework for designing a plan of care for parents in this age group.

To "walk a mile in another's shoes" is a way of appreciating vicariously how an experience may affect someone. Not many NICU nurses will have experienced the trauma of having their own newborn admitted to an NICU, but all NICU nurses will have endured the upheaval of adolescence. Realization of how these combined experiences can destabilize even the strongest of people will put every NICU practitioner in a far better position to work successfully with the teenage family toward promoting a better outcome.

STUDY QUESTIONS

1. The increased probability of crisis occurrence for the parent of a sick newborn who is adolescent, is mostly a result of the:
   a. Poor ability of the teenager to cope.
   b. Severity of the infant's condition.
   c. Unwanted role of parent.

2. A factor that assists the teenager in finding his or her identity is:
   a. Consistency between self-concept and how others view him or her.
   b. Late physical development, e.g., of breasts or musculature.

   c. Reluctance to relinquish dependent relationships.

3. A teenager's poor adjustment to the role of parent would most likely be due to:
   a. Continued contact with old friends.
   b. Marriage to the baby's father.
   c. Separation from the nuclear family.

4. The health problems of infants of adolescent parents are:
   a. The least when combined with low socioeconomic status.

b. Not commonly linked to abuse and neglect.

c. Still numerous even with good prenatal care and maternal nutrition.

5. The most widely accepted morbidity outcomes for infants of adolescent mothers are:

a. Birth defects and longer hospital stays.

b. Prematurity and low birthweight.

c. Still not known.

6. A teenage parent allows his or her own parents to take charge while the infant is in the NICU. This demonstrates:

a. A healthy response.

b. A realistic response.

c. Removal of oneself from the situation.

7. An all too familiar outcome of negative crisis resolution for the teenage parent with a sick newborn is:

a. Drug dependency.

b. Juvenile delinquency.

c. Social isolation.

8. Which of the following best describes the goals of nursing interventions for this situation?

a. Encouraging the grandparents to take over the primary task of child care.

b. Helping the teenage parent to feel confident in the new role.

c. Urging the teenage couple to see a marriage counselor.

9. The most fundamental aspect of nursing care uniquely designed for the adolescent parent in the NICU is:

a. Appreciating how their compounded circumstances can easily stimulate a crisis.

b. Remaining nonjudgmental about teenage childbearing.

c. Teaching baby care on a one-to-one basis.

Answers to Study Questions

1. a	4. b	7. c
2. a	5. b	8. b
3. c	6. c	9. a

REFERENCES

Aguilera, D.C., and Messick, J.M.: Crisis Intervention Theory and Methodology, 5th ed. St. Louis, C.V. Mosby, 1986.

Barret, R.L., and Robinson, B.E.: Adolescent fathers: Often forgotten parents. Pediatr. Nurs., 12(4):273–277, 1986.

Becker, P.T.: Sensitivity to infant development and behavior: A comparison of adolescent and adult single mothers. Res. Nurs. Health, 10:119–127, 1987.

Brown, L., Brooten, D., Kumar, S., et al.: A sociodemographic profile of families of low birthweight infants. West. J. Nurs. Res., 11(5):520–528, 1989.

Buckner, E.B.: Use of Brazelton Neonatal Behavioral Assessment in planning care for parents and newborns. JOGN Nurs., 12(1):26–30, 1983.

Carey, W.B., McCann-Sanford, T., and Davidson, E.C. Jr.: Adolescent age and obstetric risk. Semin. Perinatol., 5(1):9–25, 1981.

Cram-Elsberry, C., and Malley-Corrinet, A.: The adolescent parent. In Johnson, S.H. (ed.): Nursing Assessment and Strategies for the Family at Risk: High Risk Parenting, 2nd ed. Philadelphia, J.B. Lippincott, 1986, pp. 243–261.

Fajardo, B.: Brief intervention with parents in the special care nursery. Neonatal Network, 6(6):23–30, 1988.

Fullar, S.A.: Care of postpartum adolescents. MCN, 11:398–404, 1986.

Garmezy, N., and Rutter, M.: Acute reactions to stress. In Rutter, M., and Hersov, L. (eds.): Child and Adolescent Psychiatry: Modern Approaches. London, Blackwell, 1985, pp. 152–176.

Golan, N.: Using situational crises to ease transitions in the life cycle. Am. J. Orthopsychiatr., 50(3):542–550, 1980.

Graham, P., and Rutter, M.: Adolescent disorders. In Rutter, M., and Hersov, L. (eds.): Child and Adolescent Psychiatry: Modern Approaches. London, Blackwell, 1985, pp. 351–365.

Headlee, J.: Community and agency resources. In Ballard, R.A. (ed.): Pediatric Care of the ICN Graduate. Philadelphia, W.B. Saunders, 1988, pp. 329–330.

Hoff, L.: People in Crisis, 3rd ed. Menlo Park, CA, Addison-Wesley, 1989.

Kelting, S.: Supporting parents in the NICU. Neonatal Network, 4(6):14–18, 1986.

Kinard, E.M., and Klerman, L.V.: Teenage parenting and child abuse: Are they related? Am. J. Orthopsychiatr., 50(3):481–488, 1980.

Koniak-Griffin, D.: The relationship between social support, self-esteem, and maternal-fetal attachment in adolescents. Res. Nurs. Health, *11*:269–278, 1988.

Lawrence, R.A., and Merritt, T.A.: Infants of adolescent mothers: Perinatal, neonatal, and infancy outcome. Semin. Perinatol., *5*(1):19–32, 1981.

Lerner, R.M., and Spanier, G.B.: Adolescent development: A life-span perspective. New York, McGraw-Hill, 1980.

Mendez, L.K., Yeaworth, R.C., York, J.A., et al.: Factors influencing adolescents' perceptions of life change events. Nurs. Res., *29*(6):384–388, 1980.

Parry-Jones, W.L.L.: Adolescent disturbance. *In* Rutter, M., and Hersov, L. (eds.): Child and Adolescent Psychiatry: Modern Approaches. London, Blackwell, 1985, pp. 584–598.

Phipps-Yonas, S.: Teenage pregnancy and motherhood: A review of the literature. Am. J. Orthopsychiatr., *50*(3):403–431, 1980.

Riesch, S.K., and Munns, S.K.: Promoting awareness: The mother and her baby. Nurs. Res., *33*(5):271–276, 1984.

Ruff, C.C.: How well do adolescents mother? MCN, *12*:249–254, 1987.

Smith, D.L.: Meeting the psychosocial needs of teenage mothers and fathers. Nurs. Clin. North Am., *19*(2):369–379, 1984.

Taylor, C.M.: Mereness' Essentials of Psychiatric Nursing, 12th ed. St. Louis, C.V. Mosby, 1986.

Ventura, S.J., and Hendershot, G.E.: Infant health consequences of childbearing by teenagers and older mothers. Public Health Rep., *99*(2):138–146, 1984.

Wise, S., and Grossman, F.K.: Adolescent mothers and their infants: Psychological factors in early attachment and interaction. Am. J. Orthopsychiatr., *50*(3):454–468, 1980.

Yeaworth, R.C., York, J., Hussey, M.A., et al.: The development of an adolescent life change event scale. Adolescence, *15*:91–97, 1980.

Linda Henry Therrien

Discharge Planning for the High-Risk Neonate

Objectives

1. Outline the goals of the discharge planning process.

2. Discuss the challenges influencing discharge planning.

3. Describe the process of discharge planning.

4. Evaluate the quality of discharge planning.

Discharge planning is defined as a coordinated, collaborative, multidisciplinary process that ensures that all individuals and their families have a plan for continuity of care as they transfer from acute care in a hospital setting to care in their community (AHA, 1983). The process partners families with health professionals as they plan for safe, appropriate care at home. Discharge planning is a process that begins upon hospital admission and progresses in harmony with the family's level of readiness.

Goals and Objectives of Discharge Planning

A. **Quality outcomes for children and their families**, measured by stabilization or growth in physical, psychosocial, developmental, and spiritual arenas.

B. **Family growth and confidence gained** in their ability to independently care for their child, utilizing available community resources.

C. **Client advocacy** through enabling and empowering families with the knowledge and skills necessary for continued growth and community integration.

D. **Coordination of care** to decrease fragmentation.

E. **Maximizing reimbursement for care** that a child needs by efficient planning for care in the most appropriate settings.

F. **Active, multidisciplinary team participation** in the planning, implementation, and evaluation process.

G. **Decentralized, on-going support for communities** as they strive to provide quality, holistic care for children and families.

Challenges that Influence the Value of Discharge Planning

A. **Increasing numbers of children surviving with complex and often chronic conditions**. An estimated 10% of U.S. children are affected by chronic health problems, primarily of the respiratory system (Fox and Newacheck, 1990). More than 230,000 low birthweight infants are born each year in the United States, of whom 36,000 weigh less than 1500 g (Brooten, 1986).

B. **Awareness is growing of the potential negative effects of long-term hospitalization**, including the physical environment (Blackburn, 1982) and prolonged separation from the family (Jeffcoate et al., 1979).

C. **Advances in technology are occurring in the hospital setting** (such as extracorporeal membrane oxygenation) **and in the home care arena** with the advent of ventilators and computerized infusion pumps for home use.

D. **Rising health care costs and the need for creative cost-containment** (Goldsmith, 1989).

E. **Reimbursement sources are demanding cost-effective alternatives to lengthy hospitalization and participating in care delivery decisions**. Many insurance companies hire nurses as case managers, whose decisions may affect the length of hospital stay, the choice of home care providers, and the equipment and supplies that will be covered by insurance.

F. **Access to specialized pediatric home care services and supplies may be limited**, owing to resource availability and financial barriers.

G. **Legislative initiatives** will address long-term care innovations, access to care, and efficient use of resources on a state and national level.

Criteria for Consideration of Discharge Planning

A. **The family, nurse, physician or other health care team members** recognize a need for post-hospital services or equipment.

B. **The length of hospitalization could be shortened** with the provision of home care and/or other community services.

C. **The family has a need for psychosocial support and teaching** in preparation for discharge.

D. **There is a recognized history or potential for abuse or neglect,** or the child requires county Social Services involvement for transition to the community.

The Discharge Planning Process: The Nurse's Role

A. **Assumptions of planning**.
1. Although the complexity and individuality of needs vary, every child and his or her family has some particular needs after discharge that must be addressed.
2. Families need and deserve open, honest communication and accurate information (Stone, 1989).
3. Discharge planning is a continual, interdisciplinary process that begins upon admission. Nursing plays a critical role in coordination of all the disciplines and services involved.
4. Hospitalization is a crisis for families. The time of discharge creates another crisis.
5. Families may be overwhelmed and frightened at the prospect of caring for their child at home.
6. Parents forget or do not assimilate what is taught to them during hospitalization (Staggs, 1984).

7. Families need opportunities to succeed by participating in their child's care as early as possible, and increasing this participation as they are able.
8. Families will be in different stages of adjustment and different levels of readiness.
9. Community involvement in the planning of care and preparation for discharge is critical in the transition to home.

B. **Assessment**.
1. What are the identified physical, behavioral, and developmental needs of the infant?
   a. Oxygen and related equipment requirements.
   b. Medications and treatments.
   c. Nutritional status and dietary requirements: does the infant need any special formula, and is it available in the community?
   d. Behavior and sleep patterns.
   e. Neurological and developmental status.
2. What does the family perceive to be their strengths and needs (include siblings, grandparents, and significant others)?
   a. How would they prioritize their identified and anticipated concerns and needs?
   b. How would they describe their family, their roles, and their relationships? Have they changed?
   c. What is the level of their self-esteem and confidence?
   d. What knowledge and skills do they possess? What do they need? How do they learn best?
   e. What resources and supports do they need, and what is available?
   f. How do they ask for help?
   g. Are there any recognized barriers for safe care at home, such as finances, insurance, transportation, language, cultural orientation, motivation, and attitudes?
   h. Is the home environment safe and does it have adequate wiring, plumbing, and telephone availability?
   i. Describe a typical 24 hour day. What changes in the family schedule will need to occur as a result of caring for the child at home?
3. Describe the community and resources available.
   a. Geographical location: consider elevation, road accessibility, and climate factors.
   b. Accessibility to medical care and type available.
   c. Availability of nursing, therapy services, and equipment.
   d. What resources exist for emergency care?

C. **Development of the plan**.
1. Determination of the services needed, their frequency and duration, and the specific supplies and equipment requirements.
2. Determination of the specific provider requirements.
   a. Physician services: specialty requirements.
   b. Nursing services: can care be delivered on an intermittent basis, or does the baby need continuous nursing care? Can the care be provided by an RN or by an LPN? What experience and expertise are required? What orientation and training will the nurse need prior to discharge? What are their credentials, staff consistency, and 24 hour availability?
   c. Rehabilitative services: what credentialing, expertise, or experience are needed? What communication, orientation, and training will be needed?
   d. Laboratory and radiology services: can it be done locally, and what technical support is needed?
   e. Social work services: could the family benefit from on-going counseling and support or assistance in accessing resources?
   f. Nutritional support: specialized formulas, enteral or intravenous feeds, specialized equipment and supplies.

g. Equipment and supplies: what should be sent home from the hospital, and where will the family replenish their supplies once they are home?

3. Determination of the reimbursement resources to cover what will be needed (Fox and Newacheck, 1990). Seek social work assistance in this process.
   a. Delineate the charges for all supplies, equipment, and services.
   b. Determine the current daily hospital charges so that cost comparisons can be used for negotiation with the insurance company for coverage of home care needs (Kaufman et al., 1986).
   c. Encourage the family to review their health insurance policies to obtain information on specific policy inclusions and exclusions.
   d. Inquire with local community groups to determine what alternative resources exist for coverage of supplies, equipment, and services.
   e. Determine if the family is eligible for any state-funded programs such as Medicaid and handicapped children's programs.
4. Identify the vendors and providers for all post-discharge needs.
5. Arrange for a multidisciplinary discharge planning conference when discharge to home seems a realistic possibility; determine the composition and frequency of meetings for future planning.
6. Determine how the community and follow-up providers will be involved in the discharge planning process.
7. Develop a teaching plan with the family that incorporates specific learning strategies (Sowden and Kayuha, 1988).
8. Determine the orientation and training needs of the home care team.

D. Implementation of the plan.
1. Initiate the teaching plan, which includes increased opportunities for family involvement in care and their gradual assumption of responsibility for all care prior to discharge (McCarthy, 1986).
2. Utilize a checklist format to document progress and timelines for completion of requirements.
3. Determine the tentative date for discharge in collaboration with the physician, the family, and other members of the health care team.
4. Determine the reimbursement for all services and supplies (Galten, 1986).
5. Coordinate all case conferences.
6. Teach community providers specific procedures and orient them to the individual infant and his or her needs and responses.
7. Order equipment that will be needed so that the family can familiarize themselves with the equipment prior to discharge.
8. Teach equipment cleaning, safety, and repair.
9. Develop the emergency plan, including specific contact people and telephone numbers (Steele and Morgan, 1989).
10. Make arrangements with the local fire department, rescue squad, and utility companies for emergency situations, including power outages.
11. Change the infant's schedules for medications, feedings, and treatments to a home schedule.
12. Provide, if possible, a private place with a calm atmosphere, dim lights, and opportunities for the infant and family to interact and learn.
13. Complete all written instructions and home programs for transition to home.
14. Assist the family in scheduling all necessary follow-up appointments.

E. Evaluation of the plan: how do we define quality in the discharge planning process?
1. Were the goals and objectives met?
2. Did the family and community providers feel adequately prepared to care for the infant after hospital discharge?
3. Was communication effective?
4. Were resources utilized efficiently?
5. Was the length of hospitalization and costs of care decreased?

6. Are the family and the community successfully meeting the needs of the child at home?
7. Were any liabilities incurred?
8. How much satisfaction did the nurses receive from their participation in the discharge planning process?
9. What are the current studies and research findings on discharge planning for the high-risk neonate?
   a. A study of 15 ventilator-dependent children by D. Hazlett (1989) reported that home ventilator management is medically safe, with a significant reduction in costs, as compared with hospitalization. However, most parents felt overwhelmed by their child's care and felt unprepared for the reality of care at home.
   b. Dorothy Brooten's study in 1986 concluded that early discharge of low birthweight infants, with follow-up nursing care in the home, is safe and cost-effective.

STUDY QUESTIONS

1. Discharge planning for the high-risk neonate should begin:
   a. After stabilization of the child and in the early stages of hospitalization.
   b. When the date for discharge has been set.
   c. When the parents feel comfortable in all aspects of their child's care.

2. The nurse's role in the discharge planning process is:
   a. None, as it is the physician's responsibility.
   b. Only to teach the parents the care required.
   c. To coordinate the assessment, development, implementation, and evaluation of the plan.

3. The family's role in the discharge planning process is:

   a. None.
   b. To be a passive observer of the care, planning, and decision making.
   c. To participate in the plan development and evaluation; to participate in care and decisions regarding care.

4. Community participation in discharge planning occurs:
   a. Only if requested by the physician or family.
   b. Prior to discharge through participation in the planning and training.
   c. Upon discharge from the hospital.

5. Discharge planning is important because:
   a. Hospitals have a policy that mandates it.
   b. It is required by JCAHO.
   c. It promotes family empowerment, cost-efficient utilization of resources, and safe transitions to home and community-based care.

Answers to Study Questions

1. a	3. c	5. c
2. c	4. b	

REFERENCES

American Hospital Association (AHA): Introduction to Discharge Planning. Chicago, 1983.
Blackburn, S: The neonatal ICU: A high-risk environment. A. J. Nurs., *11*:1708–1712, 1982.
Brooten, D.: A randomized clinical trial of early hospital discharge and home follow-up of very-low-birth-weight infants. Med. Econom. Digest, Nov. 15, 1986, pp. 6–7.
Fox, H., and Newacheck, P.: Private health insurance of chronically ill children. Pediatrics, *85*(1):50–57, 1990.
Galten, R.: Funding pediatric home care. Caring, December 1986, pp. 43–51.
Goldsmith, J.: A radical prescription for hospitals. Harvard Bus. Rev., May–June 1989, pp. 104–111.

Hazlett, D.: A study of pediatric home ventilator management: Medical, psychosocial, and financial aspects. J. Pediatr. Nurs., 4(4):284–294, 1989.

Jeffcoate, J., Humphrey, M., and Lloyd, J.: Disturbance in parent-child relationship following pre-term delivery. Develop. Med. Child Neurol., 21:344–352, 1979.

Kaufman, J., Lichtenstein, K. and Rosenblatt, A.: Service coordination: A systems approach to medically fragile children. Caring, November 1986, pp. 42–48, 62.

McCarthy, S.: Discharge planning for medically fragile children. Caring, November 1986, pp. 38–41.

Sowden, L., and Kayuha, A.: Pediatric chronic illness: Making the move from hospital to home. Contin. Care, July 1988, pp. 18–19.

Staggs, K.: Pediatric discharge and home care planning. Coordinator, March 1984, pp. 21–22.

Steele, N., and Morgan, J.: Emergency planning for technology-assisted children. J. Pediatr. Nurs., 4(2):81–87, 1989.

Stone, D.: Professional perceptions of parental adaptation to a child with special needs. Children's Health Care, 18(3):174–177, 1989.

BIBLIOGRAPHY

Clements, D., Copeland, L., and Loftus, M.: Critical times for families with a chronically ill child. Pediatr. Nurs., 16(2):157–161, 1990.

Council on Scientific Affairs: Home care in the 1990s. JAMA, 263(9):1241–1243, 1990.

Hogue, E.: Liability for premature discharge: An update. Pediatr. Nurs., 17(1):76–78, 1991.

Kaufman, J., and Lichtenstein, K.: Children with catastrophic illness: Principles of care management. Case Manager, October 1990, pp. 12–20.

Kun, S., and Brennan K.: Pediatric discharge planning: Challenges and rewards. Caring, May 1985, p. 37.

Scharer, K., and Dixon, D.: Managing chronic illness: Parents with a ventilator-dependent child. J. Pediatr. Nurs., 4(4):236–247, 1989.

Thomas, K.: How the NICU environment sounds to a preterm infant. Maternal-Child Nurs., 14:240–251, 1989.

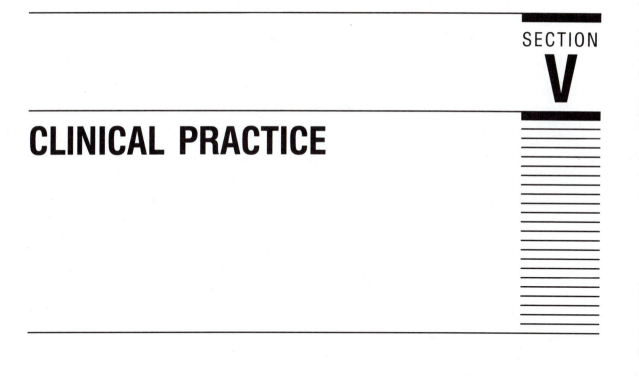

CLINICAL PRACTICE

Mary K. Buser

Neonatal Transport

Objectives

1. Identify the advantages and disadvantages of one-way versus two-way transport.

2. Discuss important considerations in the selection of transport vehicles.

3. Discuss the important factors to be considered in making a decision on team composition.

4. Describe the process of neonatal transport from referring call to discharge of patient to the receiving hospital.

5. Identify potential risks associated with the transport environment.

6. Discuss legal/ethical considerations relating to neonatal transport.

7. Develop a quality assurance plan for a neonatal transport team.

In the late 1950s and early 1960s, intensive care for newborns first became available. As the scope of care for these critically ill infants expanded, so did the number of hospitals offering this service. Unfortunately, owing to the uneven distribution of these services, many areas remained without available resources. In the early 1970s, the need to regionalize perinatal care was recognized by health care providers. In 1976, the National Foundation–March of Dimes released the report *Toward Improving the Outcome of Pregnancy*, which described regionalized care and identified criteria for level I, II, and III hospitals (Committee on Perinatal Health, 1976). This committee also recommended the establishment of formal relationships between hospitals delivering different levels of care within a region so that every baby could receive appropriate care. The concept of regionalization led naturally to the need for the development of neonatal transport. This chapter discusses many aspects of neonatal transport. Stabilization of the infant prior to transport is discussed in previous chapters.

Historical Aspects

A. **In 1899,** when most infants were born at home, the first ambulance incubator was developed to transport premature infants from home to Chicago's Lying-In Hospital (Cone, 1985).

B. In 1935, the Chicago Board of Health operated a special ambulance with incubator, oxygen, and humidity, staffed with public health nurses (Chou and MacDonald, 1989).

C. In 1948, the New York City Maternity and Newborn Division of the Department of Health established a well-organized transport service staffed with ambulance drivers, nurses, a pediatrician, and a transport clerk (Losty et al., 1950; Wallace et al., 1952).

D. In 1966, Dr. Sydney Segal published guidelines for neonatal transport (Segal, 1966), expanded in 1972 into a comprehensive transport manual (Segal, 1972).

Philosophy of Neonatal Transport

A. **Neonatal transport is one component of an organized approach to regionalized care**, including level I, II, and III nurseries; perinatal centers; maternal transport; and neonatal transport.

B. **Maternal transport results in improved neonatal outcomes when compared with neonatal transport** (Harris et al., 1981; Harris et al., 1978; Lamont et al., 1983; Levy et al., 1981; Miller et al., 1983).
1. Despite careful maternal screening, infants requiring intensive care will continue to be born in hospitals not equipped to provide that service.
2. Interfacility transport, such as neonatal transport, is inherently different than typical emergency medical services.
   a. Stabilization during interfacility transport is accomplished in the controlled setting of a medical facility, such as a hospital or medical clinic, as compared with stabilization performed at the scene of an accident with limited support services.
   b. Interfacility transport is done through moving a patient from a controlled setting to the uncontrolled setting of transport before arriving back at the controlled setting of the receiving center. Scene response systems move a patient from an uncontrolled setting to the controlled setting of a medical facility. The EMS focus is on immediate, short-term stabilization to sustain the patient to arrival at the medical facility. Interfacility transport systems focus on providing intensive care services from the referral facility throughout the transport, thus spending more time in stabilization at the point of origin.

C. **One-way versus two-way transport.**
1. One-way transport utilizes services of the transport team from the referral hospital to the receiving center. Two-way transport utilizes the services of the transport team originating at the receiving center traveling to the referral hospital and returning to the receiving center.
2. Advantages of one-way transport.
   a. Time savings in patient arrival at receiving center.
3. Disadvantages.
   a. Small numbers of transports make justification of expense and maintenance of experienced staff and equipment difficult.
   b. May deplete the limited resources of local EMS services for the duration of the transport.
4. Advantages of two-way transport.
   a. More cost-effective use of expensive equipment.
   b. More experienced transport staff.
   c. May make dedicated, and therefore more available, vehicles possible.
5. Disadvantages.
   a. Time delay in moving patient from referring facility.

D. **Neonatal back/return transport.**
1. Advantages.

a. More efficient use of beds at tertiary centers.
b. Improved relations between community hospitals and perinatal center.
c. Greater opportunity for parental involvement.
d. Familiarity of primary MD with infant prior to discharge home.
e. Decreased cost during convalescence.

2. Disadvantages.
a. Difficulty in acquiring third-party payment for return transport. Savings in daily charges in community hospital may justify the expense of the transport.
b. Potential need for transport back to tertiary center if patient deteriorates at community hospital.

Selection of Transport Vehicles

A. General considerations.
1. Appropriate vehicle selection will be dictated by cost, patient needs, and size and geographical characteristics of referral area.
2. Vehicles must be appropriately equipped, including power supplies, oxygen and compressed air supply, suction, lighting, altitude pressurization where appropriate, means for securing Isolettes and all equipment, and room for adequate personnel.
3. An integrated system utilizing multiple modes of transportation allows maximum flexibility to meet patient needs.
4. Decisions regarding appropriate vehicle for individual transport should be made by team member most familiar with the impact on patient care and outcome, advantages and disadvantages of each vehicle, and cost considerations.

B. Specific vehicle considerations.
1. Ambulance.
a. Advantages.
(1) Most cost-effective means of transport.
(2) Expenses of specially equipped dedicated ambulances can be covered by a smaller volume of trips.
(3) Ability to carry equipment and personnel for twins.
b. Disadvantages.
(1) Long response times as a result of distance, traffic, and geographical location.
2. Helicopters.
a. Advantages.
(1) Speed in response to calls and returning patient to the receiving center for distances under 100 miles (Thomas et al., 1990).
(2) Decreased response time useful as a marketing tool.
b. Disadvantages.
(1) Impact of noise and vibration on patient's stability and monitoring.
(2) Temperature control.
(3) Safety.
(a) Figures reveal an accident rate in helicopter aeromedical programs to be three times the rate of other commercial helicopter services (Collett, 1987).
(4) High operational costs.
3. Fixed-wing aircraft.
a. Advantages.
(1) Primarily beneficial for long-distance transports, usually greater than 100–150 miles.
b. Disadvantages.
(1) Without contractual agreements with aircraft vendors, inadequately equipped aircraft may be a problem.

(2) Requires coordination of ground transportation for both ends of the trip.

(3) Although fixed-wing transportation is expensive, costs may compare favorably over long distances when staff time is taken into consideration.

Transport Personnel

A. Composition among neonatal transport teams varies, using combinations of the following personnel.
1. Registered nurses/neonatal nurse practitioners.
2. Respiratory therapists.
3. Physicians.
4. Emergency medical technicians/paramedics.

B. Roles for transport personnel must be clearly outlined in job descriptions, including functions, responsibilities, and qualifications.

C. American Hospital Association Obstetric and Newborn Services Survey of 1989 reveals the following team compositions:
1. Nurses, 69%.
2. Respiratory therapists, 51%.
3. Neonatologists, 29%.
4. Residents, 18%.
5. Other, 17%.

D. Team composition considerations.
1. Physicians.
   a. Neonatologists provide highest level of clinical expertise. May strain resources available in a busy neonatal transport service. May provide increased public relations with community physicians.
   b. Residents may provide less consistency as a result of rotations and variable exposure to neonatal intensive care. May be less comfortable in public relations with community physicians.
   c. Fellows may provide more consistency and increasing levels of expertise as they move through their fellowship.
   d. In some systems, physicians may be used on an as-needed basis for the most critical patients.
2. Registered nurses.
   a. Require advanced knowledge and procedural skills. Have been shown to be highly effective with availability of phone consultation to physicians. Educational requirements range from in-service programs to neonatal nurse practitioner programs (Cook and Kattwinkel, 1983; Thompson, 1980).
3. Respiratory therapists.
   a. Frequent team members, owing to the overwhelming majority of neonates with a respiratory component to illness.
   b. May assist with nursing functions as the second member of a nurse/respiratory therapist team.
   c. Responsible for respiratory equipment, airway maintenance, participation in maintaining adequate oxygenation and ventilation during transport.
4. EMT/paramedics.
   a. Role varies, depending upon experience and education in neonatal care.
   b. Functions may include assisting with nursing and respiratory therapist responsibilities.

E. Considerations in selecting team composition.
1. Time and distance of transports in referral area.
2. Expertise of community hospitals and referring physicians and staff.
3. Availability of potential team members.
4. Volume of transports.

F. **Expertise required within the transport team.**
1. Assessment.
    a. History.
    b. Physical examination.
    c. Laboratory/x-ray interpretation.
2. Knowledge of physiology/pathophysiology.
3. Patient management.
4. Procedures.
    a. Endotracheal intubation.
    b. Arterial access (umbilical artery catheters, percutaneous indwelling catheters, arterial vessel sampling).
    c. Needle thoracentesis.
    d. Tube thoracostomy.
    e. Venous access.
5. Familiarity with characteristics of transport environment.

Transport Equipment

A. **Transport equipment must be checked on a regular basis** to ensure that it is adequately stocked, functioning properly, and ready for immediate transport.

B. **Recommended equipment operable on battery power.**
1. Portable incubator.
2. Cardiorespiratory monitor with pressure tracing.
3. Transcutaneous O_2/CO_2 monitor.
4. Pulse oximeter.
5. Infant ventilator.
6. Non-invasive blood pressure monitor.
7. IV pumps.

C. **Equipment kits** (Table 31–1).

Table 31–1
NEONATAL EQUIPMENT INVENTORY

This equipment list is designed for critical care interfacility neonatal transport.
Respiratory Equipment
Laryngoscope handle with blades size Miller 0 and Miller 1
Spare laryngoscope bulbs and batteries
ET tube stylette
Anesthesia bag (500 ml) with manometer/self-inflating bag with manometer
Face mask sizes 0 and 1
ET tubes sizes 2.5, 3.0, and 3.5
Suction catheter and glove sets, sizes 5/6 Fr, 8 Fr, and 10 Fr
Thoracentesis setups:
60 cc syringe
3-way stopcock
23 gauge butterfly
Alcohol and povidone-iodine (Betadine)
Heimlich valve set-ups
Argyle trocar cannula, 10 Fr and 12 Fr
Intravenous Therapy Equipment
250 cc bags of D_5W and $D_{10}W$
IV pump tubing
IV filters
Platelet and blood infusion sets

Continued

Table 31-1
NEONATAL EQUIPMENT INVENTORY (*Continued*)

UAC catheters sizes 3.5 and 5 Fr
IV extension tubing
T-connectors, multiport connectors
Steri drape
Syringes, sizes from 1 cc through 60 cc
Needles, assorted sizes 18 gauge through 25 gauge
3-way stopcock and stopcock plugs
Betadine and alcohol wipes
Scalp vein needles, sizes 23 and 25 gauge
Quick caths, sizes 22, 24 and 26 gauge
Medication additive labels
Disposable razors
Paper tape measure
Tongue blades
Armboards, sizes premature and infant
Assorted tape
Umbilical tape
Betadine and alcohol, one bottle each
4.0 silk suture with curved needle
Umbilical artery catheterization/thoracotomy set, including:
2 sterile drapes, iris forceps, needle holders, scissors, curved forceps, tongue tissue forceps, sterile 2 × 2s,
    umbilical tape, scalpel and blade
Blunt end adapters, sizes 17, 18, and 20 gauge

Thermoregulation and Monitoring Equipment

Stocking hat
Saran wrap/bubble wrap
Portawarm
Silver swaddler
Thermometers
Limb leads
Chest electrodes
Heart monitor lead wires
Capillary tubes
Glucose screening strips
Lancets
Arterial transducer tubing

Miscellaneous

Blood culture bottles
Scissors and hemostat
Flashlight
2 × 2s
Limb restraints
Safety pins
Rubber bands
Pacifier
Cotton balls
Benzoin/liquid adhesive tape
Xmas tree adapters
5 Fr and 8 Fr feeding tubes
Germicidal cleaning cloth
Salem sump tubes, 10 Fr, 12 Fr
Replogle tube, 10 Fr
Sterile glove packs
Sphygmomanometer with cuffs sizes premature, newborn, and infant
Neonatal stethoscope
Trash bag/needle disposal system

Medications

Epinephrine 1 : 10,000
$NaHCO_3$, 4.2%
$NaHCO_3$, 8.4%

Table 31-1
NEONATAL EQUIPMENT INVENTORY (*Continued*)

Naloxone hydrochloride (Narcan)
Atropine
Calcium gluconate 10%
Glass filter needles
Dopamine
Dobutamine
Isoproterenol (Isuprel)
Tolazoline (Priscoline)
Prostaglandin E_1
Phenobarbital
Phenytoin (Dilantin)
Diazepam (Valium)
Fentanyl
Pancuronium bromide (Pavulon)
Chloral hydrate
Morphine sulfate
Concentrated sodium chloride and potassium acetate
Lidocaine (Xylocaine) 1%
Heparin, 1000 U/ml
0.9% normal saline diluent
Sterile water dilutent
Flush solution
Antibiotics
5% albumin
$D_{50}W$
Hyaluronidase (Wyadase)

The Neonatal Transport Process

A. **The referral call**.
1. The referral call should be handled by a designated physician who is responsible for acquiring adequate information in order to make a provisional diagnosis, anticipate potential complications during transport, and provide consultation for care of the infant as needed until the transport team arrives.
2. Information to be obtained during the referral call includes the following:
    a. Time and date of referral call.
    b. Patient name.
    c. Referring physician.
    d. Referring institution, including city, state, and phone number.
    e. Maternal pre-natal, labor and delivery history.
    f. Date and time of birth.
    g. Gestational age and birthweight.
    h. Apgar scores.
    i. Details of delivery room stabilization.
    j. Subsequent neonatal course, including:
       (1) Significant findings of physical examination.
       (2) Laboratory data.
       (3) X-rays.
       (4) Vital signs.
       (5) Respiratory support.
       (6) Fluid management.
       (7) Other pertinent patient findings or medical management.
B. Selection and notification of team members.
C. Selection and dispatch of appropriate vehicles.
D. Selection of appropriate equipment and supplies.

E. Enroute to referring hospital.

1. Team members will discuss provisional diagnosis, proposed plan of care, and division of responsibilities.
2. RN:
   a. Calculates emergency and anticipated medication dosages and IV fluids based on birthweight.
   b. Develops differential diagnoses.
   c. Anticipates potential complications.
   d. Identifies history and diagnostic study results to be obtained at referring hospital.

F. Stabilization at referral hospital.

1. Introduce transport team members to referring physicians, staff, and family members.
2. Assess infant to determine need for any immediate interventions.
3. Obtain further details of history and current management.
4. Review x-rays.
5. Obtain vital signs, including glucose screening and blood pressure unless done recently by referring staff.
6. Perform physical assessment.
7. Initiate monitoring systems as appropriate, which may include direct arterial blood pressure monitoring, transcutaneous O_2 and CO_2, and pulse oximetry.
8. Begin switch to transport equipment, including ventilator and IV pumps, carefully monitoring changes in patient status.
9. Attempt to normalize or optimize blood gases, blood pressure, temperature, perfusion, serum glucose, and acid-base balance.
10. Consult with designated transport physician regarding management plan and anticipated complications enroute.
11. Notify receiving nursery of estimated time of arrival, current patient status, and anticipated patient needs on admission.
12. Speak with parents:
    a. Updating current patient status, anticipated complications during transport, and treatment plans.
    b. Assess their understanding of their infant's condition, plans for traveling to receiving center, and their needs for both physical and emotional support.
    c. Provide information about receiving center, including location, phone numbers, attending physician, primary/admitting nurse, visiting policy.
    d. Take Polaroid picture of infant and leave with parents.
    e. Obtain copies of pre-natal, labor and delivery, and neonatal records; x-rays; placenta; transport consent.
13. Enroute to receiving hospital.
    a. Continuous monitoring of temperature, pulse, respirations, blood pressure, oxygenation/ventilation status as indicated.
    b. Documentation at regular intervals as indicated by infant's condition.
       (1) Vital signs, blood pressure, color, tone.
       (2) Readings of oxygenation and ventilation monitors, respiratory support settings.
       (3) Serum glucose screenings.
       (4) Important documentation times include status of infant on arrival at referring hospital, on departure from referring hospital, and at time of transfer of care to receiving hospital staff.
14. Upon arrival at receiving center, notification of parents and referring staff of safe completion of transport. Ideally, frequent follow-up would be provided to parents, referring staff, and physicians during the infant's stay at the receiving center.

Documentation

A. Owing to the inherently unstable environment of transport, careful documentation of patient status and care provided must be maintained throughout transport.

B. Logistical documentation.
1. Time of transport call.
2. Time of departure enroute to referring hospital.
3. Time of arrival at referring hospital.
4. Time of departure from referring hospital.
5. Time of arrival at receiving hospital.
6. Transport delays.
7. Transport staff.
8. Mode of transportation.

C. Patient care documentation.
1. Significant maternal history, including previous medical history, pre-natal, labor and delivery.
2. Date and time of birth.
3. Gestational age.
4. Birthweight.
5. Delivery room resuscitation, including Apgar scores.
6. Subsequent neonatal course, including laboratory and x-ray findings.
7. Patient status on arrival of the transport team, including physical assessment and vital signs, and current patient management.
8. Problem list, including current and resolved problems.
9. Ongoing documentation of patient assessment; status, management, including rationale and patient response, consultations with designated transport physician.

Transport Environment

A. Altitude
1. Anticipate increased oxygen or ventilatory support at higher altitudes.
2. Avoid intubation enroute by anticipating need for intubation during transport based on diagnosis and expected clinical course.
3. Supplemental oxygen for staff above 10,000 feet.

B. Dysbarism.
1. Increased atmospheric pressure results in expansion of gases.
2. Anticipate expansion of "trapped" gases in body spaces.
    a. Gastrointestinal: insert orogastric tube and empty stomach of air.
    b. Pulmonary air leaks: consider needle thoracentesis or tube throacostomy for decompression.
    c. Middle ear: pacifier.

C. Effects of motion.
1. Staff discomfort and motion sickness. Stock appropriate medications for staff in transport kits.
2. Anticipate patient instability on ascent and descent.

D. Noise and vibration.
1. Encourage use of ear protection for staff.
2. Provide routine hearing screens for staff.
3. Anticipate patient instability.

Legal/Ethical Considerations

A. **Legal issues**.

1. Determination of level of responsibility of the receiving and referring staffs and institutions during the transport process has not been clearly established and is open to legal interpretations (Lazar, 1991).

   a. The referring institution's level of responsibility gradually decreases as the receiving physician and transport team assume increasing responsibility for the management and care of the infant.

   b. The receiving institution acquires increasing responsibility from the time of the transport call and initial consult, increasing to the time of admission to the receiving hospital (Fig. 31–1).

2. The transport team should ensure that the parents had adequate information regarding the infant's status and specific transport considerations at the time that informed consent was obtained.

3. Expanded responsibilities of transport team members should be clearly outlined in their job functions and responsibilities and compatible with practice acts.

4. The implications of health care professionals providing care across state lines needs to be investigated.

B. **Ethical issues**.

1. Dilemmas regarding the transport of neonates should be addressed by administrative, medical, and nursing staff and include the following:

   a. Infants with expected poor outcomes, including genetic disorders, severely asphyxiated infants, extremely immature infants, lethal anomalies.

   b. Cost constraints, particularly for back/return transports and/or experimental therapies such as heart and liver transplants.

Quality Assurance/Quality Control

A. **Quality control measures may include the following**:

1. Transport statistics.
2. Equipment failure.

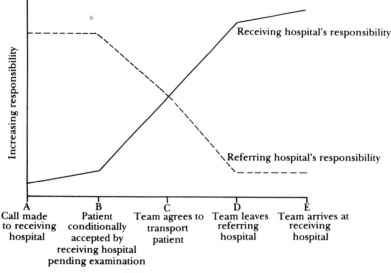

Figure 31–1
Changing levels of responsibility for patient care. (From Brimhall, DC: The hospital administrator's perspective. *In* MacDonald, M.G., and Miller, M.K.: Emergency Transport of the Perinatal Patient. Boston, Little, Brown, 1989.)

3. Transport delays.
4. Equipment checks.
5. Stabilization times.
6. Response times.
7. Completion of safety in-services.

B. **Quality assurance may be attained through a number of mechanisms.** A combination of these mechanisms is probably most effective.
1. Case review by the medical director and/or nursing director.
2. Use of peer review.
3. Regular staff meetings.
4. Case review with team members can be effectively accomplished by review of selected cases, including the following:
   a. Initial referral call.
   b. Transport logistics.
   c. Stabilization of the infant by the referring hospital as well as the transport team.
   d. Care provided during transport.
   e. Patient outcome.

C. **Peer review may be used to provide input to individuals.**
1. Appropriateness of care provided.
2. Clarity of treatment plan.
3. Treatment plan rationale and outcome.
4. Documentation.

D. **Issues identified through any of these mechanisms should be addressed with recommendations and plans for follow-up.**

STUDY QUESTIONS

1. The primary disadvantage of two-way neonatal transport is:
   a. Less cost-effective use of expensive equipment.
   b. Less experienced transport staff.
   c. Time delay in moving patient from the referring facility.

2. The primary disadvantage of ground vehicles (in comparison with rotor wing) for neonatal transport is:
   a. High operational costs.
   b. Impact of noise and vibration on patient stability and monitoring.
   c. Long response times, owing to distance, traffic, and geographical location.

3. The health care professionals used most frequently to staff a neonatal transport are:

   a. Nurses.
   b. Physicians.
   c. Respiratory therapists.

4. In anticipation of the effects of dysbarism, an appropriate measure to take would be:
   a. Supplemental oxygen for staff above 10,000 feet.
   b. Use of an orogastric tube to remove air from stomach.
   c. Use of ear plugs.

5. Responsibility of the receiving institution to the patient begins with:
   a. Arrival of the transport team at the referring hospital.
   b. Departure from the referring hospital.
   c. The referral call.

Answers to Study Questions

1. c
2. c

3. a
4. b

5. c

REFERENCES

Chou, M., and MacDonald, M.G.: Landmarks in the development of patient transport systems. *In* MacDonald, M.G. and Miller, M.K. (eds.): Emergency Transport of the Perinatal Patient. Boston, Little, Brown, 1989.

Collett, H.M.: Aeromedical accident trends. Hospital Aviation, 6:6, 1987.

Committee on Perinatal Health: Toward Improving the Outcome of Pregnancy. White Plains, NY, National Foundation–March of Dimes, 1976.

Cone, T.E.: History of the Care and Feeding of the Premature Infant. Boston, Little, Brown, 1985, p. 46.

Cook, L.J., and Kattwinkel, J.A.: A prospective study of nurse-supervised versus physician-supervised neonatal transports. J. Obstet. Gynecol. Neonatal Nurs., 12:371–376, 1983.

Harris, B.A., Jr., Wirtschafter, D.D., Huddleston, J.F., and Perlis, H.W.: In utero versus neonatal transportation of high-risk perinates: A comparison. Obstet. Gynecol., 57:496, 1981.

Harris, T.R., Isaman, J., and Giles, H.R.: Improved neonatal survival through maternal transport. Obstet. Gynecol., 52:294, 1978.

Lamont, R.F., Dunlop, P.D., Crowley, P., et al.: Comparative mortality and morbidity of infants transferred in utero or postnatally. J. Perinat. Med., 11:200, 1983.

Lazar, R.A.: Selecting an air ambulance service. Avoiding negligence in the air. Medic-Air, 10–11, March 1991.

Levy, D.L., Noelke, K., and Goldsmith, J.P.: Maternal and infant transport program in Louisiana. Obstet. Gynecol., 57:500, 1981.

Losty, M.S., Orlofsky, I., and Boles, T.: A transport service for premature babies. Am. J. Nurs., 50:10–12, 1950.

Miller, T.C., Densberger, M., and Krogman, J.: Maternal transport and the perinatal denominator. Am. J. Obstet. Gynecol., 147:19, 1983.

Segal, S.: Transfer of a premature or other high-risk newborn infant to a referral hospital. Pediatr. Clin. North Am., 13:1195–1205, 1966.

Segal, S. (ed.): Manual for the Transport of High-Risk Newborn Infants. Sherbrooke, Quebec, Canadian Pediatric Society, 1972.

Thomas, F.T., Wicham, J., Clemmer, T.P., et al.: Outcome, transport times and costs of patients evacuated by helicopter versus fixed-wing aircraft. West. J. Med., 153:40–43, 1990.

Thompson, T.R.: Neonatal transport nurses: An analysis of their role in the transport of newborn infants. Pediatrics, 64:887–892, 1980.

Wallace, H.M., Losty, M.A., and Baumgartner, L.: Report of two years experience in the transportation of premature infants in New York City. Pediatrics, 22:439–447, 1952.

BIBLIOGRAPHY

Bose, C.L., Jung, A.L., and Thornton, J.W.: Neonatal transport. The practical issues. Perinatology-Neonatology, 8(5):61–73, 1984.

Bose, C.L., LaPine, T.R., and Jung, A.L.: Neonatal back-transport. Cost effectiveness. Med. Care, 23:14–19, 1985.

Bowman, E., Doyle, L.W., Murton, L.J., et al.: Increased mortality of preterm infants transferred between tertiary perinatal centres. Br. Med. J., 297:1098–1100, 1988.

Budd, R.A., and Donlen, J.M.: Clinical evaluation of the neonatal transport team. Crit. Care Nurse, 4(5):24–28, 1984.

Campbell, A.N., Lightstone, A.D., Smith, J.M., et al.: Mechanical vibration and sound levels experienced in neonatal transport. Am. J. Dis. Child., 138:967–970, 1984.

Chan, L.S., Vogt, J.F., and Winters, L.: Comparison of neonatal mortality rates between transports to tertiary and intermediate neonatal intensive care units. J. Perinatol., 9(2):141–146, 1989.

Chance, G.W., Matthew, J.D., and Williams, G.: Neonatal transport: A controlled study of skilled assistance. J. Pediatr. 93:662–666, 1978.

Clarke, T.A., Zmora, E., Chen, J.H., et al.: Transcutaneous oxygen monitoring during neonatal transport. Pediatrics, 65:884–886, 1980.

Cook, L.J., and Kattwinkel, J.: A prospective study of nurse-supervised versus physician-supervised neonatal transports. J. Obst. Gynecol. Neonatal Nurs., 12:371–376, 1983.

Eastes, L.E.: Evaluating the clinical practice of flight nurses: Complexities and innovations. J. Nurs. Quality Assurance, 3(3):75–83, 1989.

Ferrara, A., and Harin, A.: Emergency Transfer of the High-Risk Neonate. St. Louis, C.V. Mosby, 1980.

Finsterwald, W.: Neonatal transport: Communication—the essential element. J. Perinatol., 8(4):358–360, 1988.

Greene, W.T.: Organization of neonatal transport service in support of a regional center. Clin. Perinatol., 7:187–195, 1980.

Guy, M.: Neonatal transport. Nurs. Clin. North Am., 13:3–11, 1978.

Hermansen, M.C., Hasan, S., Hoppin, J., and Cunningham, M.D.: A validation of a scoring system to evaluate the condition of transported very-low-birthweight neonates. Am. J. Perinatol., 5(1):74–78, 1988.

Hood, J.L., Cross, A., Hulka, B., and Lawson, E.E.: Effectiveness of the neonatal transport team. Crit. Care Med., 11:419–423, 1983.

Jung, A.L., and Bose, C.L.: Back tansport of neonates: Improved efficiency of tertiary nursery bed utilization. Pediatrics, *71*:918–922, 1983.

Kanter, R.K., and Tompkins, J.M.: Adverse events during interhospital transport: Physiologic deterioration associated with pretransport severity of illness. Pediatrics, *84*(1):43–48, 1989.

Lynch, T.M., Jung, A.L., and Bose, C.L.: Neonatal back transport: Clinical outcomes. Pediatrics, *82*(6):845–851, 1988.

MacDonald, M.G., and Miller, M.K., (eds.): Emergency Transport of the Perinatal Patient. Boston, Little, Brown, 1989.

Marlow, J., and Chiswick, M.L.: Neurodevelopmental outcome of babies weighing less than 2001 g at birth: Influence of perinatal transfer and mechanical ventilation. Arch. Dis. Child., *63*(9):1069–1074, 1988.

McBurney, B.H.: The role of the community hospital nurse in supporting parents of transported infants. Neonatal Network, *6*(4):60–63, 1988.

McClosley, K.A., King, W.D., and Byron, L.: Pediatric critical care transport: Is a physician always needed on the team? Ann. Emerg. Med., *18*(3):247–249, 1989.

Panneth, N., Kiely, J.L., and Susser, M.: Age at death used to assess the effect of interhospital transfer of newborns. Pediatrics, *73*:854–861, 1984.

Pettett, G., Merenstein, G.B., Battaglia, F.C., et al.: An analysis of air transport results in the sick newborn infant: Part I. The transport team. Pediatrics, *55*:774–782, 1975.

Roper, H.P., Chiswick, M.L., and Sims, D.G.: Referrals to a regional neonatal intensive care unit. Arch. Dis. Child., *63*(4):403–407, 1988.

Smith, D.F., and Hackel, A.: Selection criteria for pediatric critical care transport teams. Crit. Care Med., *11*:10–12, 1983.

Spitz, L., Wallis, M., and Graves, H.F.: Transport of the surgical neonate. Arch. Dis. Child., *59*:284–288, 1984.

Sukhani, R.: Anesthetic management of the newborn. Clin. Perinatol., *16*(1):43–60, 1989.

Sumners, J., Harris, H.B., Jones, B., et al.: Regional neonatal transport: Impact of an integrated community/center system. Pediatrics, *65*:910–916, 1980.

Tammelleo, A.D.: Nurse liability in patient transfer. Regan Report on Nursing Law, *29*(8):1, 1989.

Thompson, T.: Neonatal transport nurses: An analysis of their role in the transport of newborn infants. Pediatrics, *65*:887, 1980.

Verloove-Vanhorick, S.P., Verwey, R.A., Ebeling, M.C., et al.: Mortality in very preterm and very low birth weight infants according to place of birth and level of care: Results of a national collaborative survey of preterm and very low birth weight infants in The Netherlands. Pediatrics, *81*(3):404–411, 1988.

Weingarten, C.T.: Nursing interventions: Caring for parents of a newborn transferred to a regional intensive care nursery—a challenge for low risk obstetric specialists. J. Perinatol., *8*(3):271–275, 1988.

Willett, L.D., Leushcen, M.P., Nelson, L.S., and Nelson, R.M., Jr.: Ventilatory changes in convalescent infants positioned in car seats. J. Pediatr., *115*(3):451–455, 1989.

Janet Pinelli

Case Studies

Objectives

1. Identify risk factors associated with common disease states in neonates.

2. Identify common signs and symptoms associated with common disease states in neonates.

3. Identify the differential diagnoses associated with common diseases in newborns.

4. Identify nursing management issues associated with common diseases in neonates.

5. Identify the controversial issues in the medical management of common disease states in newborns.

6. Identify the short- and long-term complications associated with common disease states in neonates.

This chapter consists of eight case studies that reflect common disease states occurring in neonates. Each case begins with a description of the situation and is followed by the presentation and management of the disease.

At the end of each case are the study questions and answers. Readers are encouraged to work through the questions before referring to the answers.

The intent of this approach is to facilitate critical thinking and problem-solving through application of knowledge gained in the previous chapters. Although there are only eight case studies, their commonness and format are intended to provide a degree of generalizability.

CASE STUDY NO. 1

Baby S is a 3 day old male infant, born at 36 weeks' gestation, who was transferred to the regional NICU because of abdominal distention and feeding intolerance.

The maternal history indicated that the mother is a 27 year old, primiparous, married woman who had a non-complicated pregnancy.

The labor and delivery history included the following facts:

- Baby was born by vaginal vertex delivery following spontaneous onset of labor and rupture of membranes 8 hours prior to delivery.
- Apgar scores were 7 at one minute and 9 at five minutes; the baby responded quickly to suctioning and oxygen.
- Birthweight was 1950 g; head circumference was 31.5 cm; length was 46 cm.

The baby was admitted to the level II nursery because of his prematurity and small size for gestational age.

Presenting Problem

By Dubowitz examination, the baby's physical characteristics were consistent with dates at 36 weeks. There was no obvious etiology for the growth retardation, but a TORCH screen was sent with the initial work-up. This was later found to be negative.

At 2 hours of age, the baby was assessed as being "jittery." At that time, the heelstick blood work revealed a Chemstrip of 29 mg/dl (1.6 mmol/liter), hemoglobin of 23.5 mg/dl (235 g/liter), hematocrit of 73.6%, platelets of 191,000, and a WBC of 12,200 with no left shift in the differential count. The baby received a bolus of 10% dextrose in water intravenously and was started on feedings. The baby was breast-fed with formula supplements and had an intravenous infusion with 10% dextrose in water. His Chemstrips were 47 mg/dl (2.6 mmol/liter) after feeds and 32 mg/dl (1.8 mmol/liter) before feeds. He passed meconium at 9 hours of age and voided at 10 hours of age.

The intravenous was discontinued on the second day of life when the baby was breast-feeding well with stable Chemstrips.

On the evening of day 2, at approximately 55 hours of age, the baby was noted to be dusky in color and lethargic. He passed a bloody stool and had a tense abdomen with bowel sounds. His temperature was 36.4°C, respiratory rate 72, BP 75/58 mm Hg, and a Chemstrip of 144 mg/dl (8.0 mmol/liter). A blood culture was taken, and the baby was started on ampicillin, gentamicin and clindamycin. An abdominal x-ray at that time showed definite gross intramural air throughout the colon and air in the portal system, but no free air in the peritoneal cavity. Further heelstick blood work at that time showed hemoglobin 20.3 mg/dl (203 g/liter); hematocrit 43.3%; WBC 3900 with no left shift in the differential count; microfibrinogen 4.1 g/liter; Na 126 mEq (mmol)/liter; K 7.1 mEq (mmol)/liter; and Cl 96 mEq (mmol)/liter. The pediatric surgeon was consulted, and a nasogastric tube to low suction was initiated. The infant was transferred to the regional NICU early in the morning on the third day of life.

Management

The initial physical examination in the NICU revealed the following data:

- Cardiovascular/respiratory: normal heart sounds, no murmurs, equal air entry, pale color with poor perfusion, HR 120, RR 54, BP 81/45 mm Hg, T 36.3° C.
- Abdomen: soft, reddened skin color; tender with generalized guarding; slight distention; absent bowel sounds; frank bleeding per rectum.
- Chest/abdominal x-ray: lungs clear and well expanded, intramural air in colon with no free air or air in portal system.

The medical treatment at that time included the following orders: ampicillin and amikacin; NPO; intravenous Aminosyn solution; fresh-frozen plasma, nasogastric tube to low suction with replacement of losses with 0.45% NaCl solution and four hourly abdominal x-rays (anteroposterior and left lateral decubitus).

On the next day, the infant continued to drain green bile from the nasogastric tube, pass bloody stools, and have abnormal abdominal signs—i.e., erythema from the level of the umbilicus to the groin, distention, tenderness, and guarding. Bowel sounds had returned, however. The WBC on this day did show a left shift in the differential count. The abdominal x-rays showed continued pneumatosis with possible abdominal wall edema but no free air. Clindamycin was added to the antibiotic therapy.

The parents were very anxious about their son's illness. They asked numerous questions about the equipment, the treatments, and the baby's status.

Gradually, over the 14 day treatment regimen, the abnormal abdominal signs resolved and the x-ray and CBC normalized. The nasogastric drainage was clear, and the stools became guaiac-negative.

On the last day of the treatment regimen, the CBC showed a WBC of 26,100 with a left shift in the differential count. Clinical examination revealed a soft, non-tender abdomen with bowel sounds; scant nasogastric aspirates, no decreased joint movement or redness; no masses; and normal vital signs. The abdominal x-ray was unremarkable. An abdominal ultrasound performed on that day showed no masses. Specimens of blood, urine, and stool and a mouth swab were sent for culture.

The infant remained clinically stable the following day. The nasogastric tube was removed, and he was started on small feeds. Antibiotics were discontinued. During the next 24 hours, the infant manifested the following signs: T 38°C; skin pale and mottled; irritable with handling; cool peripherally with a capillary refill time greater than 5 seconds; passing loose, green mucous stool with no frank blood;

residuals with feeds; abdomen soft with no distention or masses but possible tenderness in the LLQ; chest clear; other vital signs stable.

The medical treatment at that time included a complete septic work-up, fresh-frozen plasma, and initiation of cloxacillin and amikacin.

One of the parents' major concerns was related to the cause of the disease; the mother thought that her breast milk might have caused the relapse. Their other concerns involved the infant's discomfort and protracted hospitalization.

The following day, abnormal abdominal signs increased to include distention and diffuse tenderness with guarding. The abdominal x-ray showed gaseous distention of the bowel loops but no intramural air. The CBC showed a WBC of 13,400 with 36% bands and 29% neutrophils.

This second course of intravenous antibiotic therapy (cloxacillin and amikacin) was continued for 7 days with no enteral feeds. Blood, urine, and CSF cultures were negative after 5 days. Stool cultures were positive for coagulase-negative staphylococci and gram-positive cocci.

The parents were naturally upset by the setback in their son's progress. They understood what had happened because of the on-going discussions they had with the staff regarding potential complications of this disease. They continued to visit on a daily basis and meet weekly with the social worker.

Study Questions

1. What are the risk factors for necrotizing enterocolitis (NEC) in this case study?

- Prematurity; small for gestational age; polycythemia-hyperviscosity; hypoglycemia.

2. What are other risk factors that are associated with NEC?

Although the exact cause of NEC remains undetermined, several factors have been associated with this disease. These factors include intestinal mucosal injury (due to pre-/post-natal ischemia/hypoxia, polycythemia/hyperviscosity, or suboptimal blood flow related to cardiac or respiratory dysfunction), bacterial colonization (primary or secondary), presence of substrate, low birthweight; prematurity, small for gestational age, exchange transfusions, maternal pre-eclampsia, umbilical catheters, immature immune system, hyperosmolar enteral solutions, hypothermia, hypoglycemia, and anemia (Am-

spacher, 1989; Cheromcha and Hyman, 1988; Wiswell et al., 1988; Kliegman and Fanaroff, 1984, 1981; Kliegman, 1979).

It should be noted, however, that a number of premature and term infants (10–13.6%) who have had no identifiable risk factors develop NEC (Kliegman and Fanaroff, 1981; Yu & Tudehope, 1977; O'Neill et al., 1975).

3. What signs and symptoms of illness did Baby S manifest initially?

- Lethargy, duskiness, bloody stools, tense abdomen, hypothermia, hyperglycemia, tachypnea, neutropenia, poor perfusion.

4. What are the differential diagnoses, and what additional investigations are indicated?

- Sepsis, NEC, intestinal obstruction, bowel perforation.
- CBC; blood, urine, stool, CSF for culture; chest and abdominal x-ray; serum for electrolytes.

5. What are the signs and symptoms associated with NEC, and what other diagnoses do they mimic?

The onset of NEC occurs most frequently on the third day of life, with a range of 1–10 days in over 90% of cases. The most common clinical sign is abdominal distention. Other common early signs may include gastric residuals, with or without bile; lethargy; and occult or frank blood in the stools. However, the infant may present with temperature instability; vomiting; apnea and/or bradycardia prior to the onset of GI signs. Later signs include erythema of the abdomen, palpable or visible loops of bowel, diarrhea, abdominal tenderness and/or rigidity, respiratory failure, cyanosis, mottling, jaundice, acidosis, decreased urine output, coagulopathy, hypotension, and shock. The onset of this disease may present over the course of a few hours or over 1–2 days. It may progress rapidly to a fatal outcome or resolve completely over time.

The diagnosis of NEC is confirmed by the radiographic demonstration of intramural air (pneumatosis intestinalis). Hepatic portal gas and free air (pneumoperitoneum) in the peritoneal cavity are indications of more serious disease.

The clinical presentation of NEC is consistent with neonatal sepsis, intestinal obstruction, or volvulus; the diagnosis may be delayed until GI symptoms are apparent. Blood cultures are positive in 29–37% of cases, with

Escherichia coli the preponderant organism found (Amspacher, 1989; Mollitt et al., 1988; Kliegman and Fanaroff, 1981, 1984; Kliegman, 1979).

6. What are the initial nursing management issues identified in this situation?

The nursing actions in this situation arise from the need to closely monitor the disease process and to anticipate possible complications. The major complication of NEC is bowel perforation and overwhelming septicemia. Other complications include fluid/electrolyte imbalance, anemia, respiratory distress, hypothermia, and hematological compromise. Nursing actions, therefore, would include the following: frequent monitoring of vital signs, color, and perfusion; frequent visual assessment of the abdomen; stool, gastric, and glucose testing; accurate intake and output; and maintenance of intravenous fluids and nasogastric tube patency. Nursing actions related to the infant's comfort would include minimal handling, nursing in supine or lateral positions, pain management, and mouth care. Care should also be taken to maintain a neutral thermal environment for the infant and prevent cross-contamination with other infants. Finally, nursing interventions for the parents should be directed toward provision of information about the infant's status, disease etiology, treatments, and equipment as well as allowing time for parents to verbalize fears and ask questions. Parents should also be encouraged to participate in their child's care as much as they are able (Amspacher, 1989; Gennaro, 1980; Pohodich, 1983; Meier and Paton, 1984).

7. What are the controversial issues in the prevention and treatment of NEC?

Prevention:

- Delayed oral feeding, use of breast milk, reduced feeding volumes, avoidance of hyperosmolar enteral solutions, prophylactic oral administration of antibiotics, avoidance of umbilical lines.

Treatment:

- Use of oral/nasogastric aminoglycosides; routine use of anaerobic antibiotic coverage —i.e., clindamycin, chloramphenicol; length of antibiotic treatment—i.e., 10 or 14 days; timing of initiation of feeds; routine barium contrast studies as follow-up (Faix et al., 1988; Mollitt et al., 1988; Kliegman and Fanaroff, 1981, 1984; Kosloske et al., 1981;

Schullinger et al., 1981; Gregory et al., 1981; Kliegman, 1979).

8. What are the potential short- and long-term complications of NEC?

Short/immediate:

- Shock, sepsis, acute tubular necrosis/oliguria, disseminated intravascular coagulation (DIC), gastrointestinal perforation or necrosis (10–69%), intra-abdominal abscess (2%), neutropenia-thrombocytopenia, acidosis.

Long/delayed:

- Stricture (3–22%), recurrent NEC (4%), short gut syndrome, malabsorption syndrome, cholestasis, atresia, aganglionosis, enterocolic fistula, polyposis, anastomotic stenosis or leak, chronic salt and water depletion.

Overall mortality is 20–40%. The mortality is higher in patients who developed overwhelming sepsis or DIC and who are of very low birthweight (Faix et al., 1988; Kliegman and Fanaroff, 1981, 1984; Kosloske et al., 1981; Schullinger et al., 1981; Gregory et al., 1981).

9. What is the differential diagnosis on day 14 in this case, and how could it be confirmed?

- Abscess, recurrence of NEC, secondary infection, perforation, osteomyelitis.
- Abdominal x-ray and ultrasound, positive culture(s), physical examination (Cheromcha and Hyman, 1988; Kliegman and Fanaroff, 1984; Kliegman, 1979).

CASE STUDY NO. 2

Baby B is a 29 weeks' gestation female infant, admitted to the NICU following an unexpected vaginal breech delivery in the family physician's office.

The maternal history indicated that the mother is 22 years old G5, T2, A3, P1.* Mrs. B had one visit to the physician's office at about 12 weeks' gestation to confirm the pregnancy but refused an examination. She sought no further prenatal care.

Mrs. B began to have cramping and spotting on the morning of delivery and went to her physician's office for an assessment. While in

---

*Gravida, Term, Abortions, Preterm.
    5   2   3   1

the office, she delivered her baby aided by the physician. The baby was quickly transported to the NICU.

Further discussion with the mother revealed that she had used intravenous cocaine the night before the delivery. She smoked about 7 cigarettes per day throughout the pregnancy but denied using other drugs or alcohol at any other time. Significant medical history included hepatitis at age 2½ years. At the present time, her husband is in prison and has a history of substance abuse.

Presenting Problem

By Dubowitz examination, the baby's physical characteristics were consistent with dates at 29 weeks' gestation. On admission to the NICU, the weight was 1200 g with a head circumference of 27 cm and a length of 39 cm.

On arrival to the unit, the baby's core temperature was 33.4°C, heart rate 136, respiratory rate 60, BP 42/22 mm Hg. Physical examination was unremarkable except for some hypertonia and frequent myoclonic jerking.

A few hours after admission, the baby began to have frequent episodes of apnea and bradycardia. The initial capillary blood work revealed Chemstrips 40–83 mg/dl (2.2 to 4.6 mmol/liter), Ca 3.8 mEq/liter (1.9 mmol/liter), hemoglobin 17.6 mg/dl (176 g/liter), WBC 31,700 with no left shift in the differential count, and platelets of 456,000. A capillary blood gas sample, with the baby in room air, was within acceptable limits.

Management

The medical treatment at that time included the following orders: NPO; intravenous 10% dextrose solution with calcium; serum for electrolytes; a complete septic work-up; aminophylline, ampicillin, and amikacin; urine for drug screen; serum for TORCH screen; EEG; and cranial ultrasound. The infant was treated with universal precautions.

In addition to the apneic and bradycardiac episodes, the baby was overly sensitive to stimulation. She was often irritable and crying. Sometimes she was difficult to settle and would only sleep for short periods.

Mrs. B visited her daughter frequently. She held her baby but asked few questions.

Gavage feedings were initiated on the fifth day of life. The baby frequently vomited during or after feeding, so that progress to full feeds was slow. Nutrition was supplemented with Aminosyn and lipids.

Antibiotics were discontinued after a 7 day course when all cultures were negative. A rubella titer, CMV and toxoplasmosis IgMs, radioimmunoassay screen for hepatitis (types A and B), and ELISA for HIV were all negative.

The initial cranial ultrasound at 1 week of age showed a small left subependymal hemorrhage. A repeat examination at 2 weeks and subsequent EEG were normal.

The infant was transferred to a community, level II unit at 2 weeks of age in order to be closer to her mother. At that time, she had no abnormal neurological signs, she was gaining weight, and her apnea and bradycardia were well controlled on theophylline.

Study Questions

1. **What factors in the maternal history in this case study are consistent with indicators of substance abuse in pregnant women?**

• Age; three previous spontaneous abortions; no pre-natal care; premature labor and spotting in current pregnancy; spouse with substance abuse problem.

2. **What are other risk factors associated with the substance abuser?**

Studies suggest that an increasing number of infants are born to women who are substance abusers. The prevalence in the U.S. ranges from 10 to 25% of all newborns (Lewis et al., 1989; Rodgers, 1989; Dixon, 1989; Chasnoff, 1987, 1989; Frank et al., 1988; Kennard, 1990).

The cocaine-addicted woman has a high incidence of pregnancy complications: premature labor, precipitous labor, abruptio placentae, fetal monitor abnormality, fetal death, meconium staining, low birthweight, or small for gestational age infants. She also has a high rate of infectious disease complications, especially hepatitis and venereal disease (Chasnoff, 1987, 1989; Frank et al., 1988; Rodgers, 1989; MacGregor et al., 1987; Chouteau et al., 1988). A Boston study demonstrated that cocaine users were less likely than non-users to be married; were usually Hispanic, black, or born outside the U.S.; and were less well nourished. Cocaine users demonstrated greater use of alcohol, cigarettes, marijuana, opiates, and other illicit drugs during pregnancy (Frank et al., 1988). Substance abuse in pregnancy is a growing problem in our society. Early detection can be enhanced through identification of possible risk factors and careful history taking (Sullivan, 1990).

3. What signs and symptoms did Baby B manifest that are consistent with in utero exposure to cocaine?

- Abnormal respiratory pattern—i.e., apnea and bradycardia; hypertonia; myoclonic jerking; hyperirritability; feeding intolerance; abnormal cranial ultrasound—i.e., subependymal hemorrhage; and a positive urine screen for cocaine.

Chasnoff and associates concluded that infants pre-natally exposed to cocaine have a significantly higher incidence of abnormal cardiorespiratory patterns than non-exposed infants. They also found that this was normalized with theophylline treatment without further problem (Chasnoff, 1989).

Neurobehavioral symptoms manifested by cocaine-exposed newborns have been well documented in recent literature. Although these infants do not usually exhibit the range of abstinence symptoms seen in narcotic-exposed infants, abnormal behaviors are still evident. These include alteration in visual processing, decreased quality of alertness, tremors, and exaggerated startle reflex. They may also include seizures, extreme irritability, hypertonia, diaphoresis, tachycardia, tachypnea, poor tolerance for oral feedings, disturbed sleep patterns, and diarrhea (Smith, 1988; Chasnoff et al., 1989; Dixon, 1989; Kennard, 1990).

A study by Dixon and Bejar compared the echoencephalographical results of drug-exposed term neonates with those of well infants and drug-free but ill, asphyxiated infants. The drug-exposed infants had a similar rate of abnormalities as the ill group but a significantly higher rate than the well group (Dixon and Bejar, 1989). In this case study, the minor subependymal hemorrhage could have also been related to the prematurity and/or traumatic birth and hypothermia and not necessarily to the cocaine exposure. The study by Dixon and Bejar (1989) suggests investigation for cerebral infarcts/hemorrhage in all drug-exposed neonates.

Toxicological evaluation of urine of neonates born to women using cocaine show evidence of its metabolite (benzoylecgonine) for as long as 4–6 days after delivery (Chasnoff, 1989; Osterloh and Lee, 1989; Rodgers, 1989). This analysis can be useful to confirm the suspicion of drug effect or withdrawal in the newborn.

4. What are the differential diagnoses and the additional investigations indicated?

As previously stated, the infant's prematurity could explain some of the signs and symptoms manifested by Baby B. These included respiratory distress, hypoglycemia, hypocalcemia, and hyperbilirubinemia. The occurrence of apneic and bradycardiac episodes is also consistent with sepsis and apnea of prematurity. In view of the potential for sepsis, in addition to the maternal and delivery history, a full septic work-up was completed and the baby received antibiotics on admission to the NICU. The TORCH screen was also ordered because of the maternal history but was negative. A bacterial or viral sepsis was never confirmed.

If this infant suffered a mild hypoxic-ischemic encephalopathy at birth, this could account for some of the initial neurological signs and symptoms noted. The small subependymal hemorrhage identified in Baby B is a common finding in premature infants as well as in infants who have suffered an ischemic insult.

Neurological, as well as growth and developmental, follow-up would be indicated, not only in view of the confirmed cocaine exposure, but also because of the prematurity.

5. What are the initial nursing management issues identified in this situation?

The nursing care included minimizing stimulation of the infant by placing her in a darkened, separate room in an incubator. Care activities were organized in order to minimize disturbances. Baby B was swaddled to prevent inadvertent startling. Opportunities for non-nutritive sucking were provided as a comfort measure and to facilitate sucking reflex coordination.

During visits by the mother, the nursing staff would encourage the mother to hold her baby. They offered information about the baby's clinical status and behavioral responses. The staff treated Mrs. B in a nonjudgmental fashion. A social work consult was requested because of the drug abuse and lack of support at home.

As stated previously, the behavior of cocaine-exposed neonates is often adversely affected. The effects of cocaine can be described for parents and compared with the behavior typical of any premature infant. Research findings suggest that these infants are unable to respond to their mothers or fathers in a reciprocal manner. They exhibit poorly organized behavior and can create parental feelings of frustration and inadequacy. Early intervention programs or parenting programs may be helpful in some cases. If mothers are feeling any guilt about their drug usage, this behavior may reinforce the guilt. The stress signals seen in drug-exposed infants are similar to those exhibited by premature infants. In Baby B's case, the explanation for many of her behaviors were incorporated into the usual teaching about premature infant development.

The ongoing care included close monitoring for signs of fluid and electrolyte imbalance; respiratory distress; sepsis; and neurological abnormalities, especially seizures. The response to feeding was carefully monitored and discussed with the medical staff. Small volume, every 2 hour gavage feedings of high-calorie premature formula provided adequate nutrition for Baby B. Intravenous Aminosyn and lipids provided supplemental nutrition until full enteral feedings were achieved (Lewis et al., 1989; Torrence and Horns, 1989; Sullivan, 1990).

6. What are the potential short- and long-term complications of the cocaine-exposed infant?

Short/immediate:

- Infants delivered to mothers who have used cocaine during their pregnancy tend to be premature, of low birthweight, and shorter and have a smaller head circumference. There is a difference of opinion as to whether or not cocaine exposure causes an increased incidence of congenital malformations (Chasnoff, 1987; Rodgers, 1989).
- The effects of pre-natal cocaine contribute to the increased incidence of meconium passage into the amniotic fluid and placental problems, which may place the infant at risk during the delivery.
- Infants may suffer effects of cocaine in their system for several days or weeks after birth; therefore, they may exhibit signs of intoxication or withdrawal.
- Cerebral infarctions and strokes have also been identified in cases of cocaine-exposed neonates.

Long/delayed:

- Children born to cocaine-addicted mothers have a three times greater risk of sudden infant death syndrome.
- There has also been an increased incidence of infections and hospitalization documented during the first year of life.
- Infants may experience secondary withdrawal symptoms of neurobehavioral disturbances at 2–8 weeks of age.
- Long-term outcome data are still largely unavailable, but these children should be considered at high risk for developmental and learning disabilities (Dixon, 1989; Lewis et al., 1989; Rodgers, 1989; Chasnoff, 1987, 1989; Anday et al., 1989).

CASE STUDY NO. 3

Baby C is a 3 day old male infant, born at 38 weeks' gestation, who was transferred from the level I nursery after a cyanotic episode.

The mother is a 24 year old primigravida who had a vaginal culture 3 weeks prior to delivery that was positive for group B streptococci. She received a 10 day course of antibiotics at that time, and then antibiotics 4 days prior to delivery.

Baby C was born by spontaneous vaginal delivery after 2 hours of ruptured membranes. The Apgar scores were 9 at one minute and 9 at five minutes. The birthweight was 2.45 kg.

The initial physical examination upon arrival in the level I nursery was unremarkable except for the presence of several pustules on both arms and the chest. These were swabbed, and the Gram stain for culture and sensitivity was negative. Swabs were also sent for virology investigation.

Presenting Problem

Baby C remained well until the evening of the third day of life, when he had a cyanotic episode lasting 5–10 minutes. Other symptoms at that time included jaundice, poor feeding, and pustules on the legs. Baby C was transferred to the level III nursery for investigation.

The physical examination revealed a jaundiced, mildly unwell looking infant, who was well perfused and not irritable. He was in no respiratory distress, had no hepatosplenomegaly, and had no dysmorphic features. Several scattered pinpoint scabs were noted on his arms and chest.

Shortly after admission to the NICU, Baby C had a series of apneic episodes that required the initiation of mechanical ventilatory support. A complete sepsis work-up was ordered, and the baby was started on antibiotics.

The parents were very concerned about their son's condition. The mother was weepy and overwhelmed with the situation. The parents asked many questions about the source of the suspected problem.

Management

Over the next 48 hours, Baby C experienced a gradual deterioration. He required increasing supplementary oxygen and mechanical ventilatory support. He was poorly perfused, with a decreased urine output and mottling of the extremities. Scattered crepitations were audible in both lung fields, the liver was palpable 1.5 cm below the right costal margin, and the spleen tip was palpable. Secretions from the endotracheal tube were thick, purulent, and contained fresh blood, but were negative to Gram's stain.

Hematological investigations revealed the following: hemoglobin of 18 mg/dl (180 g/liter); WBC 4500 with 13% myelocytes, 9% metamyelocytes, 20% bands, and 20% neutrophils; and platelets of 56,000. The coagulation profile was: INR 5.1, PTT 128 seconds, and fibrinogen 60 mg/dl (0.6 g/liter). The liver function tests were: GGT 142, ALK Phos 203, CK 93, and LDH 471. The chest x-ray showed coarse bilateral opacification.

Baby C was given transfusions of platelets and plasma as well as intravenous vitamin K. A third antibiotic was added despite the continued negative reports from the cultures. The infant became hypotensive, and dobutamine was commenced.

Baby C continued to deteriorate overnight. A follow-up chest x-ray showed a right pleural effusion, which required aspiration. The liver was now palpable 6 cm below the right costal margin and the spleen at about 3–4 cm. The WBC showed a progressive left shift, associated with leukopenia and thrombocytopenia. At this point, the infant was placed in isolation and acyclovir was commenced.

The parents, who had been aware of their son's changing status, realistically feared for his survival. They discussed their feelings with the nursing staff and the social worker.

The following day, Baby C continued to suffer from hypoxemia, hypotension, renal failure, hypoalbuminemia, hepatitis and disseminated intravascular coagulation. In spite of frequent blood product replacement, high-pressure ventilation, correction of metabolic acidosis, antibiotics, inotropic agents, and acyclovir, Baby C continued on a progressively deteriorating course. On the morning of his seventh day of life, he suffered a sudden deterioration, associated with bradycardia, from which he could not be resuscitated.

The post-mortem examination showed a diffuse hepatic, pulmonary, and splenic necrosis with features of herpes simplex virus infection. There was also growth of herpes simplex virus from the pleural fluid and autopsy samples (i.e., lung, spleen, liver). However, no virus was isolated from the cerebral spinal fluid or endotracheal tube aspirate.

Study Questions

1. What are the risk factors for infection in this case study?

• Maternal history of group B streptococcal infection.

2. What are other risk factors that are associated with infection?

Certain risk factors have been associated with neonatal infection. Some of these can be generalized to all infections, whereas others are specific to the organism—in this case, herpes simplex virus (HSV). With respect to infections, in general, the risk factors include pre-natal, intrapartum, or post-natal exposure to the pathogen; prematurity; prolonged rupture of membranes; and socioeconomic factors (Whitley, 1988; Feigin & Cherry, 1987). Risk factors specifically associated with HSV infections in neonates include socioeconomic factors, increasing maternal age, previous HSV infection, sexual partner with HSV infection, cervical versus other lesion locations, multiple versus single lesions, prolonged rupture of membranes, non-white versus white infants, maternal peripartum infection, and fetal scalp monitoring (Whitley, 1988; Freij and Sever, 1988; Feigin and Cherry, 1987; Hodgman, 1981).

It is important to note, however, that 60–80% of infants who develop HSV disease are born to women who are asymptomatic for genital infection at the time of delivery and have neither a past history of genital herpes or a sexual partner with the disease (Whitley, 1988; Feigin and Cherry, 1987; Klein and Remington, 1990). The rate of occurrence of neonatal HSV infection has been reported as 1–6 per 10,000 and in some areas 1 per 1500 live births (Whitley, 1988; Canadian Task Force, 1979; Freij and Sever, 1988; Klein & Remington, 1990).

The timing of the infection in the mother and whether the infection is recurrent or primary have specific consequences for the infant as well. Eighty per cent of all HSV neonatal infection is transmitted during the intrapartum period (Whitley, 1988). The risk of transmission to the newborn in cases of primary infection is 40–50% but is only 4–5% in recurrent disease (Canadian Task Force, 1979; Freij and Sever, 1988; Feigin and Cherry, 1987). There is a 30–40% risk of infection for infants delivered vaginally to mothers with the virus present in the birth canal at the time of delivery. However, virtually all cases of neonatal infection are acquired from mothers with active infection at the time of delivery (Feigin and Cherry, 1987). Herpes simplex virus can reach the fetus hematogenously via the placenta, by ascension from an infected cervix, or by contact between the infant and infected cervix during vaginal delivery (Freij & Sever, 1988). Natal infection, as in the case of Baby C, is most likely acquired secondary to aspiration of infected vaginal secretions into the upper respiratory tract of the infant (Feigin & Cherry, 1987).

3. What signs and symptoms of illness did Baby C manifest in the level I nursery?

- Pustules on arms and chest, poor feeding, lethargy, jaundice, cyanosis.

4. What additional signs and symptoms of illness did Baby C manifest initially in the level III unit?

- Severe apneic episodes, poor perfusion.

5. What are the differential diagnoses, and what additional investigations are indicated?

The differential diagnoses include necrotizing enterocolitis; bacterial sepsis (which may be concomitant as well, particularly group B *Streptococcus, Staphylococcus aureus, Listeria monocytogenes*, and other gram-negative bacteria), various cutaneous disorders (such as erythema toxicum, neonatal melanosis, acrodermitis enteropathica), vesicular rashes (such as varicella-zoster virus, enteroviral disease, disseminated cytomegalovirus infection), or congenital rubella infection (Whitley, 1988; Feigin and Cherry, 1987).

The diagnostic work-up should include virology and bacterial blood cultures (TORCH); CSF, stool, urine, throat, nasopharyngeal, and conjunctivae specimens for bacterial and virology culture; chest and abdominal x-rays; liver function tests; and complete blood count, coagulation screen, and blood gases (Whitley, 1988; Feigin and Cherry, 1987). An ophthalmology consult may also be included. Virus isolation is the definitive diagnostic test. However, as in the case of Baby C, viral culture growth may take several days, so that therapeutic decisions cannot await study results.

In the presence of central nervous system disorder, an electroencephalogram, cranial ultrasound, or computed tomography may be useful. Serological diagnosis of HSV is not of great clinical value (Whitley, 1988; Freij and Sever, 1988).

Approximately 67% of infants develop signs and symptoms within the first week of life. The average length of time between the onset of disease and the diagnosis is 5.0–6.5 days, regardless of whether or not vesicles are present (Freij and Sever, 1988).

6. What signs and symptoms of progressive or deteriorating infection did Baby C manifest?

- Increasing respiratory distress with copious, thick endotracheal secretions; mottling; hepatosplenomegaly; hypotension; bleeding diathesis; oliguria; leukopenia; thrombocytopenia; left shifted differential; abnormal liver function tests; abnormal coagulation profile; hypoalbuminemia.

7. What are the signs and symptoms associated with HSV infection, and what other diagnoses do they mimic?

The signs and symptoms of HSV infection range from mild to severe and generally fall into three categories: (1) localized disease (skin, eyes, mouth); (2) encephalitis, with or without skin, eye, or mouth involvement; (3) disseminated infection involving multiple organs (brain, lung, liver, adrenal, skin, eye, or mouth) (Whitley, 1988; Feigin and Cherry, 1987). Disseminated infection, with or without CNS involvement, accounts for about 49% of cases; CNS and skin/eyes/mouth cases account for about 51%; and about 1% are asymptomatic (Feigin and Cherry, 1987).

Encephalitis occurs in about 60–75% of cases (Whitley, 1988). In 20–40% of cases, the infants do not develop skin rash (Whitley, 1988; Canadian Task Force, 1979; Feigin and Cherry, 1987). In the absence of skin vesicles, the diagnosis is very difficult because the other clinical signs are often non-specific and are the same as any type of neonatal sepsis—i.e., temperature instability, lethargy, respiratory distress, anorexia, vomiting, cyanosis, mottling, hypotension, jaundice, and disseminated intravascular coagulation (Whitley, 1988; Feigin and Cherry, 1987; Prober, 1985; Paes, 1986; Klein and Remington, 1990).

8. What are the initial nursing management issues identified in this situation?

The nursing management of this infant related mainly to close monitoring of vital signs, color, perfusion, respiratory status, and maintenance of intravenous fluids. The initial diagnosis was sepsis, so that his response to treatment or any deterioration would also be important to note. Monitoring for development of drug side effects, especially with respect to renal and cardiovascular status, is important to consider. Because of the uncertainty of the diagnosis, the nurse should observe the infant for particular signs of infection that may be more specific (Haggerty, 1985; Devore et al., 1983).

As Baby C's condition worsened and the specific diagnosis became more evident, proper isolation technique became a major nursing issue. Extreme care must be taken to prevent cross-infection as well as to protect the caretakers (Haggerty, 1985; Devore et al., 1983).

On-going monitoring expanded to include neurological vital signs. The coagulopathy required careful evaluation of puncture sites and bleeding during procedures. The infant's deterioration on the last day required every skill of the intensive care nurse, with respect to assessing, decision making, and technical expertise. Proper support of the parents in this situation is important but difficult to achieve when the physical demands of the infant are so high. In this case, the team approach works well and can include the clinical nurse specialist, social worker, clergy, and other nurses in the support of the parents. Close communication among the medical staff and nurses responsible for the infant and parents will facilitate consistency of information and decision making. It is important to remember that women whose infants have contracted a congenital infection often experience a great deal of guilt, and they need the opportunity to express these feelings. Because of the infant's death, the nurse will also be involved in the grieving process (Devore et al., 1983).

9. What are the controversial issues in the prevention and treatment of HSV infection?
Prevention:

Because most women shedding HSV at delivery will be asymptomatic with no previous history, prevention is not easily achieved. Anticipatory antiviral treatment for HSV exposure is not warranted because most exposures result from maternal reactivation, in which the attack rate is less than 5%. Routine culture then becomes a research strategy of little clinical value (Prober, 1985). Serological determination has prognostic significance because a woman with a primary infection at delivery is 10–20 times more likely to infect her infant. However, at the present time, commercial assays are not available (Prober, 1985; Canadian Task Force, 1979).

For women with a history of genital herpes herself or in her partner, clinical examination at the time of delivery is recommended —i.e., no weekly screening in the last trimester. If there is evidence of active disease, a cesarean section is recommended (if membranes are ruptured less than 12 hours) (Canadian Task Force, 1979; Prober, 1985; Lissauer and Jefferies, 1989; Freij and Sever, 1988).

Treatment:
Acyclovir is the drug of choice in the treatment of neonatal HSV infection (Whitley, 1988; Whitley et al., 1988; Whitley, 1986).

Prophylactic treatment with acyclovir is not recommended for infants who are exposed to maternal HSV virus but who are asymptomatic with negative cultures (Prober, 1985; Lissauer and Jefferies, 1989; Freij and Sever, 1988). Feigin and Cherry recommend consideration of prophylactic treatment in high-risk situations—i.e., in which the risk of infection is 40–50%—but not in low-risk cases—i.e., in which the risk of infection is less than 4% (1987).

Use of fetal scalp electrodes is contraindicated in women with a history of recurrent genital herpes (Whitley, 1986).

10. What are the potential short- and long-term complications of neonatal HSV infection?

Short-term:
Mortality in the absence of treatment is 17–87%, depending on the extent of infection (Whitley, 1988; Canadian Task Force, 1979; Freij and Sever, 1988; Feigin and Cherry, 1987). The outcome with primary infection is likely to be more severe (Canadian Task Force, 1979). Mortality rate with treatment is reported at 15–20% (Freij and Sever, 1988). There is no difference in the severity of outcome for premature versus term infants or for HSV-1 versus HSV-2 infection (Feigin and Cherry, 1987).

Long-term:
From 20 to 90% of survivors are impaired; the worst prognosis is for infants with disseminated disease (Whitley, 1988; Feigin and Cherry, 1987). Major sequelae involve the central nervous system and include diffuse brain damage, seizures, microcephaly, spasticity, paralysis, growth retardation, and chorioretinitis with visual loss (Feigin and Cherry, 1987).

CASE STUDY NO. 4

Baby R is a term male infant, born by an uncomplicated vaginal delivery, to a 28 year old primipara woman. Four hours after transfer to the newborn nursery, Baby R was found to be tachypneic and pale. Further examination revealed heart sounds heard louder on the right side of the chest and diminished differential air entry to the lungs. Baby R was transferred to the NICU, in oxygen, with a nasogastric tube in place.

Study Questions

1. What are the differential diagnoses at this time?

- Sepsis/pneumonia; respiratory distress syndrome; spontaneous pneumothorax; congenital diaphragmatic hernia.

2. What investigations are indicated?

- Chest and abdominal x-rays; blood gas analysis; complete blood count; serum electrolytes.

The admission x-ray revealed a left diaphragmatic hernia. The CBC and serum electrolytes were within normal limits, but the capillary blood gas showed mixed respiratory and metabolic acidosis.

3. What are the signs and symptoms associated with congenital diaphragmatic hernia (CDH), and what other illness does it mimic?

Although polyhydramnios is a common pre-natal marker for CDH, 50–80% of cases do not present with this sign (Williams, 1982; Cullen et al., 1985).

The symptoms of CDH at birth range in severity from mild tachypnea to severe asphyxia with profound hypoxemia, hypercapnia, and acidosis (Bohn 1987). The picture of illness may resemble staphylococcal pneumonia, respiratory distress syndrome, or asphyxia.

Even with radiographical studies, CDH mimics space-occupying lesions in the chest, intrathoracic stomach, pleural effusion, adenomatoid malformation of the lung, and congenital lobar emphysema (Williams, 1982; Cullen et al., 1985; Schumacher and Farrell, 1985).

The physical findings diagnostic of CDH are present in 85% of affected infants (Schumacher and Farrell, 1985). These symptoms include cyanosis, dyspnea/respiratory distress, cardiac dextroposition, scaphoid abdomen, barrel-shaped chest, diminished breath sounds, distant heart sounds, bowel sounds in the chest, loss of abdominal tympany, and dullness to percussion and poor perfusion (Williams, 1982; Cullen et al., 1985; Schumacher and Farrell, 1985; Platzker, 1986).

The parents were in a state of shock and disbelief. They seemed to understand the diagnosis and the surgical repair that was necessary. They spent time with their son prior to surgery.

4. What are the preoperative nursing management issues?

Basic preoperative nursing care includes maintaining a neutral thermal environment, provision of fluids, decompression of the bowel through patent nasogastric tube, and placement in Fowler's position on the affected side to aid in bowel decompression and ventilation (Williams, 1982; Schumacher and Farrell, 1985). Attention to parental needs with respect to explanations of the condition, status, and treatments, as well as listening to questions and fears, is also an important part of the preoperative care (Williams, 1982).

Baby R went for surgical repair at 24 hours of age, after he was stabilized in the NICU. A left chest drain was inserted. Baby R had been intubated and was paralyzed upon return to the unit. He required moderate ventilatory support in 40% oxygen to remain well oxygenated and hyperventilated. Baby R had difficulties voiding postoperatively and required dopamine, albumin, and furosemide. He received fresh-frozen plasma for decreased perfusion, cool peripheries, and decreased urine output. A continuous morphine infusion was initiated for pain control.

5. What are the postoperative nursing management issues?

In addition to the basic care requirements, careful monitoring of the infant's status and response to treatment is essential. Third-space losses can be estimated by the degree of edema, weight gain, and urine output. Signs of persistent pulmonary hypertension of the newborn (PPHN) can be inferred by comparing pre-ductal and post-ductal $TcPO_2$ monitor values, which reflect the degree of right-to-left pulmonary cardiac shunting. The development of PPHN may be avoided by keeping the infant slightly hyperoxic and alkalotic (Cullen et al., 1985; Schumacher and Farrell, 1985).

Percussion and postural drainage, as the infant tolerates, will assist in the maintenance of alveolar expansion and function, as will maintaining patency of the chest drain (Williams, 1982; Schumacher and Farrell, 1985; Cullen et al., 1985). The paralyzed infant requires close observation for muscle movement or vital sign changes that indicate the need for more medication, regular position changes and passive range of motion, careful support when moving, mouth care, and artificial tears (Carter and Spence, 1984).

6. What are the controversial issues in the prevention and treatment of CDH?

Treatment:

The majority of infants with CDH require intubation immediately after birth. They should also have a nasogastric tube inserted at that time. Mask bagging and swallowing of air will result in distention of the bowel in the chest, which will further compress the lungs (Williams, 1982). Ventilatory support is usually best achieved with low pressures and a rapid rate. This pattern will aid in the prevention of overexpanding the lungs and possible rupture (Williams, 1982; Schumacher and Farrell, 1985).

Infants who cannot be stabilized preoperatively have a very high mortality rate. A method to predict outcome before and after surgical repair has been developed by Bohn (1987). This method is based on an analysis of blood gases, indexed to a measure of alveolar ventilation (Bohn, 1987). An ability to predict outcome would be helpful for determining which infants would benefit from conventional management versus more novel techniques (Bohn, 1987). The most recent techniques are high-frequency oscillation and extracorporeal membrane oxygenation (ECMO). In a study by Heaton and colleagues (1988), ECMO was given to patients with CDH who failed to respond to aggressive ventilatory and pharmacological management and whose condition was deteriorating. Seven of 12 infants survived long-term.

There has been increasing interest in the pharmacological treatment of pulmonary hypertension, which is a serious complication in the postoperative period. Currently, the most frequently used drugs are tolazoline, acetylcholine, phentoamine, and chlorpromazine (Williams, 1982; Cullen et al., 1985; Ein and Barker, 1987). Problems still exist with the use of pulmonary vasodilators because of their effect on the systemic circulation as well as the pulmonary vasculature (Ein and Barker, 1987).

Prevention:

The most recent and controversial issue related to the prevention of CDH is the development of fetal surgery (Harrison, 1988).

Use of pre-natal ultrasound to diagnose CDH may facilitate adequate preparation at the time of delivery and prevent delay in diagnosis and treatment.

7. What are the potential short- and long-term complications or outcomes of CDH?

Short-term:

In addition to the usual postoperative complications that occur with infants, the repair of a diaphragmatic hernia presents several specific problems. As previously stated, PPHN is a serious complication in this disorder, both pre- and postoperatively. Mortality in these patients may be as high as 80% (Cullen et al., 1985). There is no question that PPHN is an important determinant in survival, as are degree of lung hypoplasia, size of the infant, asphyxia, and pulmonary barotrauma (Williams, 1982; Cullen et al., 1985; Schumacher and Farrell, 1985; Bohn, 1987; Shochat, 1987).

Overall, the survival of infants with CDH has not changed significantly in the past 10 years and remains at about 50% (between 44 and 83%) (Platzker, 1986; Bohn, 1987; Ein and Barker, 1987; Heaton, 1988).

Long-term:

For those who survive the perioperative period, the long-term outcome is generally excellent. Although there appears to be a decrease in pulmonary function on testing, clinically these children function no differently than their peers (Williams, 1982; Cullen et al., 1985; Schumacher and Farrell, 1985). They also show no increased susceptibility to respiratory infections (Williams, 1982).

Baby R had a relatively smooth postoperative recovery. Apart from some initial perfusion problems, he progressed without any major complications. He was extubated 8 days after surgical repair and was started on enteral feeds on the twelfth day. Baby R was discharged home prior to the end of the third postoperative week. His parents remained actively involved in his care throughout his hospitalization.

CASE STUDY NO. 5

Baby D was a term male infant born by vaginal delivery, weighing 3.7 kg. Mrs. D was a 29 year old gravida 2 para 2 woman, whose first child was alive and well. Her pregnancy was uncomplicated except for a persistent cold and some spotting in the last trimester.

Baby D appeared to be progressing well until about 30 hours of age. At that time, he was noted to be mucousy and was not breast-feeding well. He then became pale, cyanotic, slightly tachypneic and lethargic. He was placed in oxygen and transferred to the level III nursery.

On admission to the NICU, Baby D's physical examination revealed the following additional information: poor perfusion, mottled skin, systolic murmur at the left lower sternal border with a gallop rhythm, and liver palpable 5 cm below the right costal margin.

1. What are the differential diagnoses, and what additional investigations are indicated?

The differential diagnoses would include congenital heart disease, sepsis, metabolic abnormality, PPHN, airway obstruction or abnormality, and lung disease or malformation.

Further investigations should include chest x-ray, echocardiogram, electrocardiogram, arterial blood gases, serum electrolytes, and complete blood count with differential (Hazinski, 1983, 1984; Clochesy et al., 1986).

The initial chest x-ray showed cardiomegaly with increased pulmonary vascular markings. The ECG showed sinus rhythm with right bundle branch block pattern and a paucity of left ventricular forces. Baby D's deteriorating condition required intubation and mechanical ventilation. Pulses were greatly diminished in all four limbs.

The parents were confused and shocked over the sudden illness of their son. They were so overwhelmed with the situation that they could only stay at the bedside for a short period of time. They spoke at length with the physicians and nursing staff and had a good understanding of the potential problems.

An echocardiogram revealed hypoplastic left heart syndrome and dysplastic tricuspid valve. A continuous intravenous infusion of prostaglandin E_1 was initiated, and the infant was supported with intravenous dextrose.

2. What are the initial nursing management issues in this situation?

The initial nursing care is directed toward four major goals: (1) preventing or detecting signs of deteriorating status, (2) performing diagnostic tests, (3) maximizing the infant's oxygenation, and (4) supporting the parents (Hazinski, 1983). Signs of deteriorating status in Baby D included respiratory distress related to cardiovascular insufficiency; and hypoxemia manifested by metabolic acidosis, decreased perfusion, pallor, mottling, cyanosis, and decreased skin temperature. Continuing signs of congestive heart failure would in-

clude pulse pressure differences, tachycardia, edema, abnormal weight gain, diaphoresis, hepatomegaly, oliguria, and peripheral hypotension (Hazinski, 1983, 1984; Clochesy, 1986; Bailey et al., 1986; Bailey and Lay, 1989).

Nursing actions directed toward maximizing the infant's oxygenation include maintaining a neutral thermal environment, minimizing exertion or agitation, and frequent observation of oxygen requirements via transcutaneous and saturation monitors (Hazinski, 1983, 1984; Clochesy, 1986). Scrupulous attention must be paid to the arterial and venous lines, especially with the prostaglandin infusion.

Parental support is directed toward their need for information and clarification as well as their emotional needs. Parents often feel responsible for the infant's illness. They are coping with the uncertainty of outcome as well as the impact of the diagnosis. It is important to determine the sources of support that the parents can utilize. This may include family, friends, clergy, and social worker (Hazinski, 1983, 1984; Clochesy, 1986).

3. What are the controversial issues in the treatment of hypoplastic left heart syndrome?

Short-term treatment for duct-dependent cardiac lesions would include the use of prostaglandins to maintain the patency of the ductus arteriosus. Because of their rapid clearance, prostaglandins are administered in a continuous parenteral infusion (Cohen, 1983; Hazinski, 1984). The extent of additional treatment would then depend upon the decision reached by the parents and medical team.

Many newborns with hypoplastic left heart syndrome will not survive long enough to make further treatment an option. Some parents do not choose aggressive management and want only palliative care provided for their infant. The remaining options for these infants are two-stage complex reconstructive surgery or cardiac transplantation.

Palliative surgery for this lesion is the procedure developed by Norwood and colleagues. Mortality for the procedure ranges from 44 to 90%, depending on the center. Long-term complications of the surgery include aortic arch obstruction (67 to 80%) and progressive hypoxemia (Pigott et al., 1988; Bailey et al., 1986; Gersony, 1990). The second stage, or corrective surgery, is the Fontan procedure, which is performed at 12–20 months of age. Survival for the second surgical procedure is approximately 50%, but the long-term outcomes are unknown. Its success depends mainly on the existence of near-normal growth and development of the branch pulmonary arteries (Pigott et al., 1988; Clochesy, 1986).

The final option is cardiac allotransplantation. Loma Linda University Medical Center has had the most experience with this procedure to date. Although their early success rate is 84–88%, 30–70% of infants die on the waiting list (Gersony, 1990; Bailey et al., 1986). For those infants who are eligible for transplant from a physiological perspective, their parents must assume a large financial burden as well as the responsibility and commitment to devote their entire energies to the care of the child. Long-term outcome statistics are not yet available, owing to the limited number of neonatal cardiac transplantations that have been performed.

For infants who will not receive surgical intervention, care is directed toward physical comfort. Parents are encouraged to be involved in all aspects of care. Infants may be taken home or transferred to their referring hospital, depending on the parents' wishes and the infant's stability. For the infants who will remain in hospital, the environment is normalized as much as possible. The survival of these infants beyond 1 month is rare, and the average age of death is 5 days (Bailey et al., 1986; Bailey and Lay, 1989).

In the case of Baby D, his parents were spared the agony of the decision making. On the third day of life, within a few hours of the confirmed diagnosis, Baby D deteriorated further. Attempts to stabilize him were unsuccessful, and he died of cardiac failure and hypoxia.

CASE STUDY NO. 6

Baby A was born at 25 weeks' gestation and weighed 620 g. His mother is 22 years old, and this was her first pregnancy. Her pregnancy was uncomplicated until 2 weeks prior to delivery, when she began having contractions. She was admitted to a perinatal center and was treated with bedrest, vasodilatin, and betamethasone (Celestone). Labor continued, and Baby A was delivered vaginally, 48 hours later. Membranes were ruptured at the time of delivery.

Initial Management

Baby A was intubated in the delivery room and then transferred to the NICU. The initial investigations included blood, swabs (from umbilicus and ears), and aspirates (from stomach and endotracheal tube) for culture and sensitivity; chest x-ray and cranial ultrasound; serum for glucose and calcium; blood gas; and complete blood count. The initial treatments included insertion of umbilical arterial and venous catheters, ampicillin and amikacin, 5% dextrose solution at 100 ml/kg/24 hours, radiant warmer, heat shield, and application of oxygen saturation monitor.

During the first 24 hours, Baby A was weaned to room air with ventilatory pressures of 12/3.

More complete electrolyte results revealed the need to add calcium to the dextrose solution. An initial cranial ultrasound showed no evidence of hemorrhage.

The parents visited within the first few hours after delivery. They had spoken to the neonatologist, prior to delivery, regarding the probable physical needs of their baby and the support measures that would be instituted. They had also discussed risk factors with respect to mortality and morbidity. Mr. and Mrs. A were overwhelmed with the NICU environment and the small size of their son. Baby A required minimal mechanical ventilation and no extraordinary cardiovascular support. The most difficult problem related to his care was maintaining fluid and electrolyte balance. The case study focuses primarily on this aspect of care. During the first day of life, the serum sodium level increased from 140 to 148 mEq/liter and the urine output was 0.8–1.0 ml/kg/hour. Total fluid intake was increased to 150 ml/kg/24 hours.

During the second day, the serum glucose, BUN, creatinine, potassium, and calcium levels remained fairly stable. However, the serum sodium concentration continued to rise to 150 mEq/liter. The serum bilirubin level rose to 6.0 mg/dl (103 μmol/liter), and phototherapy was commenced. Urine output had increased to 2.1–4.9 ml/kg/24 hours. Total fluid volume was increased to 250 ml/kg/24 hours to account for the effect of the phototherapy and to respond to the increasing serum sodium value.

By the third day, Baby A was experiencing a diuresis, with urine output reaching 8.5 ml/kg/hour and serum sodium dropping to 140 mEq/liter. His weight on that day was 560 grams, 11% below his birthweight.

The parenteral solution included the following constituents per kilogram in 24 hours: 0.5 g of protein, 3 mEq (mmol) of sodium, 1 mEq (mmol) of phosphorus, 2 mEq (mmol) each of potassium and calcium (1 mmol/L) , 0.2 mEq (mmol) of magnesium, MVI pediatric solution, and 0.6 ml of a trace element solution. The dextrose solution provided 4.0 mg/kg/minute of glucose and a total fluid volume of 300 ml/kg/24 hours.

Phototherapy was discontinued on day 4, and the fluid volume was decreased to 280 ml/kg/24 hours. Urine output remained elevated at 7 ml/kg/hour. There was a further decline in the serum Na to 135 mEq (mmol)/ liter, with increased urinary losses. Body weight decreased further to 14% below birthweight.

Over the next 3 days, Baby A's weight remained approximately the same. Urine output fluctuated between 4.1 and 8.0 ml/kg/hour, and intake was gradually decreased to 220 ml/kg/24 hours. Serum electrolytes remained stable, and intake was not altered. The protein was increased by 0.5 g/kg/day, and lipids were initiated on Day 7.

Small, bolus feedings of expressed breast milk were given by gavage tube. Increases were not well tolerated, so that Baby A's main nutritional requirements were met through the parenteral route.

During the eighth to tenth day of life, body weight increased by 20 g and the urine output stabilized at 4–5 ml/kg/hour. The total fluid volume was maintained over those 3 days at 200 ml/kg/24 hours. Protein intake was maintained at 3 g/kg/24 hours, and the lipids were increased slowly.

The total fluid volume was then decreased and maintained at 165 ml/kg/24 hours. Baby A's weight steadily increased to 660 g. Enteral feedings were better tolerated and were increased slowly. By the end of the third week of life, Baby A's weight was 730 g and he was tolerating full enteral feedings of expressed breast milk. He was receiving vitamin D, 400 IU, and Poly-Vi-Sol, 0.3 ml daily. His estimated caloric intake was 120 kcal/day.

Study Questions

1. What are the risk factors for premature birth in this case study or other factors that are associated with premature birth?

There did not appear to be any risk factors associated with this premature birth, as is the situation for over 60% of cases (Lee, 1988). Several authors have identified certain factors that have been associated with an increased risk for premature birth. These may relate to the mother's previous obstetrical history or current pregnancy and include low socioeconomic status, less than 20 or more than 40 years old, less than 5 feet (152 cm) in height, less than 100 pounds (45.5 kg) pre-pregnant weight, less than 7 pounds (3.3 kg) weight gain by 22 weeks, albuminuria, weight loss of 5 pounds (2.3 kg), head engaged at 32 weeks, placenta previa, cervical surgery, two or more children at home under 6 years old, single parent, less than 1 year since last birth, heavy work, long/tiring commute, fetal congenital anomalies, multiple gestations, maternal uterine anomalies, hypertension, bleeding, infection or febrile illness, previous pre-term labor and/or birth, diethylstilbestrol exposure, cone biopsy, three or more first-trimester abortions, two or more second-trimester abortions, fibroids, cigarette smoking (more than 10/day), street drug use, abdominal surgery after 18 weeks, uterine irritability, polyhydramnios, cerclage, and effaced and/or dilated cervix (Lee, 1988; Herron, 1988; Creasy and Herron, 1981). Although the current risk screening systems, which utilize many of these factors, do not have high predictive value, they are of particular importance when they involve multiple risk factors.

2. What are the initial nursing management issues identified in this situation?

Nursing management of the very low birthweight (VLBW) infant begins in the delivery room. With the establishment of a patent airway and adequate circulation, maintenance of normal body temperature is crucial for the infant (Bhat and Zikos-Labropoulou, 1986; Brueggemeyer, 1990). Heat losses from warm, wet skin should be minimized through placement on a radiant warmer; drying skin with a warm towel; and using warm, humidified oxygen (Bhat and Zikos-Labropoulou, 1986).

The ability to regulate thermoneutrality is very limited in the VLBW infant. The child can tolerate only very narrow ranges of ambient temperature fluctuation. Maintenance of a neutral thermal environment allows the infant to utilize energy necessary for vital functions, including growth (Brueggemeyer, 1990).

Continual assessment of oxygenation and ventilation is another important management issue. In this situation, Baby A was intubated and mechanically ventilated. Attention must be paid to the patency of the airway through assessment of breath sounds, suctioning, and physiotherapy. Careful monitoring of oxygen needs will prevent hypo- or hyperoxygenation (Southwell, 1990).

Care of the skin is one of the most challenging management issues, with prevention of lesions being the most effective treatment. Thirteen per cent of a pre-term infant's body weight is skin, compared with 3% in an adult. The major goals for skin care include avoiding exposure to harsh or sensitizing agents—i.e., isopropyl alcohol, soap; reducing contact with environmental irritants; considering quality and quantity of all substances applied to the skin; and reducing the risk of epidermal stripping by minimizing use of adhesives and removing tape slowly and carefully (Kuller and Tobin, 1990).

Other issues relate to the on-going assessment for signs of patent ductus arteriosus, intracranial hemorrhage, and sepsis.

The NICU as a source of iatrogenic stress for infants has been well documented (Vanden-Berg, 1990). In the VLBW infant, this environment can be even more detrimental because of the child's inability to tolerate either the incoming stimuli or his response. A single disturbance often results in complete disorganization, from which the baby has great difficulty recovering (Southwell, 1990). Protection of the VLBW infant from environmental stress becomes a major role for the nurse.

For Baby A, fluid and electrolyte balance was the major concern in his management. The key goals for care are (1) maintain normal body fluid composition and volume; (2) prevent dehydration or overhydration, and (3) replace on-going water losses (Turner, 1990). The maintenance requirement for fluid is to replace the normal physiological losses—i.e., insensible water loss, free renal water requirement, and water loss through the stool (Oh, 1988). The VLBW infant has a low glomerular filtration rate and limited concentrating and diluting capacity, which makes him relatively intolerant of fluid and electrolyte imbalance (Costarino and Baumgart, 1986; Oh, 1988).

Despite the mixed and confusing literature on the renal function of infants with respiratory distress syndrome, there appears to be agreement that the diuresis on the second or third day necessitates close monitoring of fluid therapy (Costarino & Baumgart, 1986; Oh, 1988). This was evident in Baby A's case, where his water losses and hypernatremia required an increase in fluid intake to 300 ml/kg/day.

Factors that affect fluid requirements include radiant warmers; single- and double-walled incubators; phototherapy; increased ambient temperature; respiratory distress; hypermetabolic problems; increased body temperature; furosemide therapy; diarrhea; glycosuria; ostomy or chest drain losses; intravenous alimentation; heat shields; thermal blankets; high humidity; warm, humidified endotracheal tube air; and renal oliguria/diuresis (Kerner, 1983; Turner, 1990). Knowledge of factors that affect fluid and electrolyte balance will help the nurse to minimize and account for fluid losses. Frequent monitoring of peripheral perfusion, edema, central venous pressure, urine output, osmolality/specific gravity, hematocrit, BUN, and serum and urine electrolytes and glucose, as well as changes in body weight, will provide the necessary data upon which to make individualized management decisions (Kerner, 1983; Costerino and Baumgart, 1986; Pildes and Pyati, 1986).

Readiness for enteral feeds can be determined by the presence of bowel sounds, absence of bile in stomach, passing of stool, and absence of abdominal distention. Once feeding is initiated, careful attention must be made to how well the infant tolerates feeds (Lefrak-Okikawa, 1988).

Lastly, the care of the parents is of great nursing importance. Parents require information, clarification, and emotional support. They need to feel that they have a place and a role in the care of their child. Opportunities for expression of fear, anger, and frustration should be provided. Parents without the support of family or friends may require extra input from social work, clergy, and nursing staff. Sensitivity to individual needs of mothers and fathers and to the changes from day to day will enhance the nurses' effectiveness in working with parents.

3. What are the controversial issues in the fluid and electrolyte management of VLBW infants?

Shaffer and Meade (1988) investigated sodium balance and extracellular volume regulation in VLBW infants. Their data, as well as that of others, indicated that administration of sodium is probably unnecessary during the first few days of life because of the infant's large extracellular volume (Schaffer and Meade, 1988; Oh, 1988). Some earlier work supported the practice of administering about 3 mEq/kg/day during the first 5 days of life in order to prevent late hyponatremia (Guignard and John, 1986). Other investigators, however, did not recommend additional sodium until the time of diuresis (Costerino and Baumgart, 1986).

Timing of enteral feeding in VLBW infants continues to generate much debate. The risks and benefits of early versus late feeding, in the more recent literature, seem to support earlier feeds (Lefrak-Okikawa, 1988). Also, the nutritional requirements of the VLBW infant and the best method to achieve that are also unresolved. The suitability of breast milk, fortifiers, and various formulas continues to be studied (Kerner, 1983; Adamkin, 1986; Lefrak-Okikawa, 1988; Turner, 1990).

4. What are the potential short- and long-term complications/outcomes of VLBW infants?

Short-term:

Survival rates for VLBW infants who weigh 500–1000 g range from 40 to 70% (Lawhon and Melzar, 1988).

The short-term complications of extreme prematurity can be related to the management issues previously discussed. Inappropriate fluid and electrolyte management can result in symptomatic patient ductus arteriosus; necrotizing enterocolitis; bronchopulmonary dysplasia; dehyration associated with hypernatremia, oliguria, and hyperglycemia; intracranial hemorrhage; pulmonary edema; and congestive heart failure (Kerner, 1983; Costarino and Baumgart, 1986; Pildes and Pyati, 1986; Oh, 1988).

Inadequate thermoregulation can result in cold stress and subsequent hypoxia, patent ductus arteriosus, increased energy expenditure and metabolism, overheating, and apnea (Brueggemeyer, 1990).

Long-term:

Of those infants weighing less than 1500 g, 30% will have moderate to major developmental delays. Of the infants less than 800 g, 50% will have similar delays (Lawhon and Melzar, 1988).

The long-term complications in these infants relate mainly to the consequences of their treatment. Long-term hyperalimentation has resulted in hyperlipidemia, cholestasis, demineralization of bone, and anemia (Turner, 1990; Adamkin, 1986).

Oxygen toxicity to lungs and eyes and barotrauma to lungs from mechanical ventilation have contributed to the incidence of retinopathy of prematurity and bronchopulmonary dysplasia (Southwell, 1990; VandenBerg, 1990; Leonard et al., 1990; Yu et al., 1983; Escobedo & Gonzalez, 1986).

Asphyxia and intracranial hemorrhage contribute to sensory, motor, and mental difficulties. The long-term outcome of 24–25 week infants will be questionable for years to come.

We know they are at risk for sensorineural hearing loss, visual impairment, mental retardation, language handicaps, poor school performance, and behavioral problems. They may also have emotional and social maladaptation, especially if they come from disadvantaged homes. The long-term effect on their parents has also yet to be determined (VandenBerg, 1990; Leonard et al., 1990).

CASE STUDY NO. 7

Baby C is a term male infant born to a 30 year old gravida 2 para 2 woman. The pregnancy was uneventful until the time of delivery, when there was a significant abruptio placentae. The infant was unresponsive at birth and was intubated immediately. He received a full resuscitation requiring epinephrine, cardiac compressions, and large quantities of volume expanders (including normal saline, fresh-frozen plasma and, packed red blood cells). Apgar scores where 2 at one minute, 2 at five minutes, and 5 at ten minutes. At ½ hour of age, the serum pH was 7.10 with a $PaCO_2$ of 14 and a PaO_2 of 191.

Initial Presentation

The initial physical examination revealed the following information: general hypertonia with cycling movements, tonguing, and lip smacking; normotensive anterior fontanel with equal and reacting pupils. Baby C was noted to be bleeding easily from puncture sites with fresh blood in the endotracheal tube secretions. He passed no urine but did pass a stool, which appeared to contain sloughed intestinal mucosa. The cord hemoglobin was 12.4 mg/dl (124 g/liter) with 295,000 platelets, and the baby's initial hemoglobin was 9.8 mg/dl (98 g/liter) with 219,000 platelets. The first chest x-ray showed a right pneumothorax.

Initial Management

Baby C was treated aggressively during the initial period. He developed major dysfunction of several organ systems.

Following insertion of a chest drain, he continued to be ventilated with high pressure and rate settings in order to maintain a state of hypocapnia.

Even though he had received a loading dose of phenytoin at birth, Baby C experienced a seizure within the first 24 hours of life. He required numerous doses of Valium as well as phenobarbital and additional phenytoin to control the seizures. He was fluid restricted to 35 ml/kg/day for both neurological as well as renal status. Dopamine and furosemide were used to improve perfusion and to stimulate the renal tubules. The associated consumptive coagulopathy and anemia also required aggressive treatment. Baby C received a transfusion of packed red blood cells after the initial blood work. A CBC performed 1½ hours after the transfusion showed a hemoglobin of 10.3 mg/dl (103 g/liter) with 82,000 platelets. Following a second red cell transfusion, the hemoglobin rose to 15.0 mg/dl (150 g/liter), but the platelets dropped to 72,000. A transfusion of platelets and a third transfusion of red cells resulted in a hemoglobin of 18.2 mg/dl (182 g/liter) with platelets of 148,000. The initial coagulation screen was normal, but subsequent screens were abnormal.

The gastric aspirate from the initial work-up was positive for group B *Streptococcus*; therefore, the baby was started on antibiotics.

With careful monitoring of serum and urine electrolytes, Baby C remained in a relatively balanced state.

On-going Management

Baby C was weaned to continuous positive airway pressure (CPAP) by day 4 and was extubated 2 days later. He required a small amount of supplemental oxygen until 2 weeks of age. His chest tube was removed on day 6.

The infant was seizure free after day 4 of life. The cranial ultrasound was normal, and the CT scan at 2 weeks of age showed cerebral edema but no atrophy. Within the first week, the clinical neurological examination demonstrated normal tone; strong suck; and an active, alert infant.

By day 2, Baby C had established a satisfactory urine output. The early serum creatinine concentration rose to 4.0 mg/dl (354 mmol/liter) but dropped to .38 mg/dl (33 mmol/liter) over a period of time. A subsequent renal ultrasound was normal.

This infant required twice-daily cryoprecipitate and fresh-frozen plasma transfusions over the first 3 days, as well as several platelet transfusions. By day 3 of life, the coagulation screen had returned to normal. The differential of the high white cell count was left shifted; therefore, antibiotics were continued.

Although the abdominal x-rays showed no definitive evidence of necrotizing enterocolitis (NEC), the intestinal sloughing indicated the likelihood of severe ischemic colitis with a strong potential for NEC. Baby C was kept NPO on parenteral fluids, in addition to the antibiotic therapy, with frequent abdominal x-rays in the early stages.

Mr. and Mrs. C. visited their son frequently. They were aware of the critical nature of his condition and the uncertainty of the short- and long-term outcome. Mr. C. asked many questions, whereas his wife was more quiet. Mrs. C. only began to visit the NICU by herself on day 3. The parents received information on their son's status by both nursing and medical staff. They also received support from the social worker.

Study Questions

1. What are the risk factors for asphyxia in this case study?

• Abruptio placentae.

2. What are other risk factors that are associated with perinatal asphyxia?

There is really no agreement about the most effective way to identify the fetus at risk for asphyxia. Only 20% of mothers will develop risk factors that will initiate fetal monitoring, and almost 50% of fetal deaths will occur in the low-risk group (Jacobs and Phibbs, 1989).

The literature cites a number of factors thought to place the fetus or neonate at risk for asphyxia. Risk factors related to the previous history include medical problems, low birthweight, stillbirth or neonatal death, toxemia, abruptio placentae, placenta previa, diabetes, pyelonephritis or chronic renal disease, low urinary estriol, anemia, and drug abuse (Phibbs, 1981; Jacobs and Phibbs, 1989). Antepartum factors include hypertensive disease, multiple gestation, intrauterine growth retardation (IUGR), decreased fetal movement, lupus anticoagulant, active medical problem occurring after 12 weeks' gestation, cholestasis, low maternal serum alpha-fetoprotein, blood type or group isoimmunization, older primigravida (>35 years old), drug abuse, and polyhydramnios (Phibbs, 1981; Jacobs and Phibbs, 1989; Hill and Volpe, 1989). Intrapartum factors include premature or postmature delivery, macrosomia, fetal malformations, abruptio placentae, placenta previa, trauma, undiagnosed vaginal bleeding, cord prolapse or compression, maternal hypotension, sedative or analgesic drugs given just prior to delivery, prolonged rupture of membranes, meconium in the amniotic fluid, fetal heart rate decelerations or acid-base disturbance, cesarean section, breech or other abnormal presentation and delivery, prolonged labor, and birth trauma (Phibbs, 1981; Jacobs and Phibbs, 1989; Hill and Volpe, 1989). Postnatal factors include severe pulmonary disease, congenital heart disease, large patent ductus arteriosus, severe recurrent apneic spells, and sepsis with cardiovascular collapse (Hill and Volpe, 1989).

3. What signs and symptoms of hypoxic-ischemic encephalopathy (HIE) did Baby C manifest initially?

• Hypertonia, seizures, oliguria, coagulopathy, intestinal mucosal sloughing, poor respiratory effort.

4. What are the signs and symptoms associated with HIE in the term infant?

The signs and symptoms can be categorized according to the severity of the insult: (1) mild: hyperalertness or irritability, poor suck, uninhibited reflexes and sympathetic overactivity with a duration less than 24 hours; (2) moderate: lethargy, stupor, hypotonia, or abnormal tone, suppressed primitive reflexes and seizures; (3) severe: coma, flaccid tone, suppressed brainstem function, seizures, and increased intracranial pressure (Hill and Volpe, 1989).

Perlman (1989) found that single- or multiple-organ injury occurred in about 35% of affected infants. The most frequently involved organ was the kidney (50%), followed by the central nervous system (33%) and cardiorespiratory system (25%) (Perlman, 1989). This organ injury manifests itself through oliguria, cardiomyopathy (left ventricular dilatation or dysfunction, or right ventricular dysfunction), hypovolemic shock, primary pulmonary hypertension or respiratory insufficiency requiring mechanical ventilation; loss of tone, fixed posturing, reduced oculovestibular response, abnormal pupillary response, and fullness of anterior fontanel (Perlman, 1989; Jacobs and Phibbs, 1989). If tone returns within 1–2 hours after birth, there is a good chance for intact survival. If hypotonia is replaced by hypertonia with increased activity within the first 24 hours, the chance of survival is high, but so is the incidence of cerebral damage (Fanaroff and Martin, 1987).

Disseminated intravascular coagulation is associated with situations causing cardiovascular collapse, such as asphyxia (Blanchette and Zipursky, 1981; Fanaroff and Martin, 1987). Also, necrotizing enterocolitis has been associated with asphyxial insults (Phibbs, 1981; Fanaroff and Martin, 1987).

5. What investigations are warranted with the presentation of HIE?

Although cranial ultrasound is more useful with pre-term infants, computed tomographic scanning is generally more useful for term infants (Hill and Volpe, 1989). Electroencephalography is helpful in identifying seizure activity and its resolution. Brainstem auditory-evoked responses may be valuable for assessment of brainstem injury (Hill and Volpe, 1989). Serial investigations may provide helpful information related to injury progression or resolution as well as for prognosis.

Chest and abdominal x-rays provide information relative to respiratory disease or complication and intestinal response to injury. Renal ultrasound is indicated with evidence of kidney involvement.

Regular monitoring should include tests that reflect hematological and metabolic status as well as fluid balance (Fanaroff and Martin, 1987).

6. What are the initial nursing management issues identified in this situation?

The nursing actions in this situation arise from the need to closely monitor the effects of the hypoxic-ischemic insult to the various organ systems. These actions would include frequent monitoring of vital and neurological signs, color, and tissue perfusion; prompt recognition of seizures; accurate intake and output; maintenance of intravenous fluids; and maintaining adequate ventilation and oxygenation. Nursing actions related to the infant's safety include appropriate care if paralyzed or heavily sedated. Care should also be taken to maintain a neutral thermal environment so as not to exacerbate the hypoxia with acidosis. Finally, nursing interventions for the parents should be directed toward provision of information about the infant's status, treatments, and equipment, as well as allowing time for parents to verbalize fears and ask questions.

7. What are the controversial issues related to the prevention and treatment of asphyxia in term infants?

Prevention:
There is currently no reliable method of diagnosing asphyxia in utero. The development and use of highly technological methods have not demonstrated an impact or cost-effectiveness (Nelson, 1989; Jacobs and Phibbs, 1989). Certainly, when a high-risk situation is identified, a skilled team present at the delivery will have an impact on the immediate management. Fetal monitoring and biophysi-

cal profiles are commonly used to follow situations that have been identified as high risk antenatally (Jacobs and Phibbs, 1989).

Treatment:

The treatment of frank seizures is not a contentious issue. The drug(s) of choice, prophylactic treatment, and the treatment of subtle seizures in the comatose, ventilated patient are debatable issues, however (Whitelaw, 1989; Mizrahi, 1989).

The control of raised intracranial pressure and cerebral edema is also not well established (Fanaroff and Martin, 1987; Hill and Volpe, 1989). The benefits of intravenous mannitol, dexamethasone or other brain-preserving drugs have not been demonstrated in controlled trials (Hill and Volpe, 1989). The practice of fluid restriction and relative hyperventilation has been more generally practiced but not well researched.

8. What are the potential long-term outcomes associated with HIE?

Hill and Volpe (1989) have identified several useful prognostic factors in hypoxic-ischemic cerebral injury. These include data from electronic fetal monitoring and blood gas sampling, Apgar scores, severity of neurological symptoms, onset/duration and ability to control seizures, increased intracranial pressure, imaging data, and biochemical markers. Perlman (1989) also notes that no constant relationship between measures of fetal distress, such as fetal heart rate abnormalities, abnormal cord blood gas values, and Apgar scores, and subsequent long-term neurological outcome has actually been demonstrated. He was able to demonstrate a strong association between persistent oliguria and poor outcome (Perlman, 1989).

Nelson (1989) investigated the relationship of intrapartum and delivery room events to long-term neurological outcome. She found that most survivors of birth asphyxia do not later demonstrate major neurological disabilities, and that most children with long-term neurological disabilities did not show evidence of serious asphyxia in the perinatal period.

Mild encephalopathy is not associated with long-term sequelae. With moderate encephalopathy, 20–40% develop neurological sequelae, particularly if the abnormal signs persist for longer than 1 week. Virtually all newborns with severe encephalopathy develop major neurological sequelae. These sequelae include microcephaly, mental retardation, cerebral palsy, and seizures (Hill and Volpe, 1989).

CASE STUDY NO. 8

Baby L is a 28 weeks' gestation male infant born to a 27 year old single mother. The mother has a 10 year history of hypertension, and this first pregnancy was complicated with pre-eclampsia. She was treated with atenolol and nifedipine (Adalat), but her hypertension was not controlled and she required a cesarean section. Ms. L was given a course of betamethasone (Celestone) prior to delivery.

Initial Management

Baby L was intubated in the delivery room and transferred to the NICU. The Apgar scores were 7 and one minute and 8 at five minutes. His birthweight was 930 g, and the length and head circumference were appropriate for his age.

Baby L required high ventilatory pressures and rates in 100% oxygen for adequate gas exchange. Early chest x-rays showed bilateral, diffuse granularity with air bronchograms and decreased lung volume. The infant received two doses of surfactant in the first 24 hours of life, which resulted in only slight improvement in his status.

The initial problems also included severe hypotension and acute renal failure requiring dopamine and dobutamine infusions as well as colloid boluses and furosemide. A cranial ultrasound on the third day of life showed small, bilateral subependymal hemorrhages.

Ms. L visited her son later on the first day of life. She was in her first year of nursing school and was living with her parents. Ms.. L had some understanding of her infant's condition, but her own physical and emotional stress limited her ability to discuss the situation at length. The major problem related to her son's care was his respiratory disease. The case study focuses primarily on this aspect of care.

On-going Management

By the end of the first week of life, chest x-rays showed early changes of chronic lung disease. This progressed to more advanced chronic lung disease by day 15. Attempts to make significant changes in the ventilatory parameters were unsuccessful.

Dopamine was discontinued on day 8 and dobutamine on day 10. The creatinine level peaked at 1.7 mg/dl (150 mmol/liter) but eventually decreased to normal limits. The hyponatremia required significant supplementation with sodium to maintain a level of about 127 mEq (mmol)/liter.

Ms. L visited her son daily. She discussed his status with the nursing and medical staff and met with the social worker on a regular basis. Ms. L wanted to participate in any aspect of care that she could and was encouraged to do so by the staff. She had good support from family and friends but was no longer involved with the baby's father.

Long-Term Management

After infection and patent ductus arteriosus were excluded as contributing factors, a course of dexamethasone was initiated because of the continued inability to extubate the infant. At 1 month of age, a second course was given, following extubation on day 19, in an attempt to wean the inspired oxygen concentration. Dexamethasone therapy was delayed initially because the infant's work-up revealed a *Staphylococcus aureus* infection requiring treatment. Baby L suffered from persistent, pronounced hyperglycemia and glycosuria while on the dexamethasone. This development resulted in a shortened course of therapy on both occasions.

Methylxanthines were administered for control of apneic episodes. Follow-up cranial ultrasounds demonstrated resolution of the subependymal hemorrhages. Ophthalmology examinations showed no retinopathy. Baby L was transferred to a community secondary level unit for continuing care after more than 2 months in the NICU.

Study Questions

1. What are the initial nursing management issues identified in this situation?

In addition to the issues previously identified in Case Study No. 6, the cardiovascular and respiratory instability was the major problem to be addressed. Complications related to respiratory problems contribute significantly to the morbidity of this group (Southwell, 1990). Monitoring, therefore, is an important part of nursing management. In premature infants in the 24–29 week group, high peak inspiratory pressures and long inspiratory times contribute to the development of pulmonary interstitial emphysema, which may lead to bronchopulmonary dyplasia (BPD), as well as to the development of intraventricular hemorrhage. Length of time and amount of oxygen also contribute to the risk of lung injury (Kling,

1986). High peak inspiratory and expiratory pressures and long inspiratory times may also affect cardiac output and cause hypotension.

Very low birthweight infants are also at increased risk for pulmonary edema. Immature lungs contain relatively large amounts of connective tissue, which increase the opportunity for pulmonary edema (Kling, 1986). The transudate in the air spaces is clinically manifested as fine rales heard on auscultation of the lung fields. Pulmonary edema causes decreased lung compliance and vital capacity, which can impair gas exchange. The judicious use of fluids and sodium and the provision of adequate protein intake will minimize the negative effects of edema. The administration of diuretics and closure of hemodynamically significant ductus arteriosus may also be required (Kling, 1986).

Durand and his colleagues (1989) demonstrated the negative effects of endotracheal suctioning on pre-term infants. They found that it significantly increased blood pressure, intracranial pressure, and cerebral perfusion pressure in the first month of life. These changes were independent of changes observed in oxygenation and ventilation. Endotracheal suctioning is important in maintaining tube patency but should be used with the risk and benefits in mind.

The importance of nursing care is also illustrated in the study by Fox and Molesky (1990). They studied the effects of supine and prone positioning on neonates with respiratory distress syndrome. Their results indicated that prone positioning significantly improved the PaO_2.

Positioning may also facilitate development in very low birthweight infants. Bozynski and coworkers (1988) studied the negative effects of lateral positioning and showed no deleterious effects on oxygenation and ventilation. Lateral positioning may encourage behavior at midline in these infants.

The effect of maternal beta-blocker medication on neonatal blood pressure should be anticipated (Briggs et al., 1986). The bradycardia and hypotension, although transient, may require treatment. In this case, the hypotension also had a dramatic effect on renal blood flow and caused acute renal failure.

The crisis of premature birth places great demands on the parent with respect to coping and adaptation. The adaptive process involves initial crisis reactions, grief work, efforts to attach to the infant, and information gathering. It also includes the revision of expectation and roles, utilization of various coping mechanisms and support systems, and attempts to adjust to internal and environmental/situational stressors (Steele, 1987). In this case, the maternal illness was an additional stressor to deal with in the beginning phase.

2. What nursing management issues arose later in the case?

A continuing problem for Baby L was ventilation and oxygenation. With the development of bronchopulmonary dysplasia (BPD), the use of supplemental oxygen, mechanical ventilation, and fluid and nutrition therapy is crucial to the long-term outcomes (Nickerson, 1990). Infants with BPD require regular monitoring of oxygenation. They are susceptible to hypoxia because of their compromised status, so that stressors should be anticipated and minimized or avoided (Scherf, 1990). Infants with compromised respiratory function who are exposed to long-term hospitalization are at high risk for pulmonary morbidity (Scherf, 1989). They should be monitored carefully for subtle signs of infection.

Steele (1987) identifies three major issues to help parents to redefine their roles within the limitations of the NICU. These are coping with loss, overcoming barriers to bonding, and obtaining adequate information about the infant's current and future needs. She supports the provision of breast milk and use of appropriate sensory stimulation in order to enhance attachment (Steele, 1987).

Although results differ with respect to an increased incidence of child abuse in premature infants, it is the nurse's role to promote attachment under these stressful conditions and to help the parent make compensatory adjustments and learn the baby's cues (Yoos, 1989).

3. What are the controversial issues in the prevention and treatment of hyaline membrane disease in premature infants?

The improved survival of very low birthweight infants can be attributed in part to improvements in ventilatory support, nutritional requirements, and better resuscitation in the delivery room (Bhat and Zikos-Labropoulou, 1986). The decrease in the incidence and severity of hyaline membrane disease is also attributed to the widespread use of surfactant, tocolysis, and glucocorticoids (Kwong and Egan, 1986; Doyle et al., 1986; Bhat and Zikos-Labropoulou, 1986; Richardson, 1988; Harkavy et al., 1989; Couser et al., 1990; Lang et al., 1990; Miller and Armstrong, 1990).

With respect to surfactant replacement therapy, controversy still exists regarding the best

type of surfactant, the timing, and the number of doses that are most beneficial (Miller and Armstrong, 1990).

Kao and colleagues (1988) studied the effects of theophylline and/or diuretics on the oxygen consumption in infants with BPD. They found that although pulmonary function improved significantly, oxygen consumption was not decreased. Their results suggest that the increased oxygen consumption in infants with BPD is not secondary to the increased mechanical work of breathing.

4. What are the potential short- and long-term complications of hyaline membrane disease (HMD)?

Short-term:

Approximately 30% of neonatal deaths are associated with HMD (Richardson, 1988). The incidence of HMD at 37–40 weeks' gestation is 0.9%, whereas at 29–30 weeks it is 64.3% (Richardson, 1988).

One of the most serious complications associated with mechanical ventilation is pulmonary interstitial emphysema (PIE). It occurs in about 20–42% of all infants with HMD, and only about half of those infants will survive (Bhat and Zikos-Labropoulous, 1986; Yu et al., 1986). The most frequent incidence of PIE occurs in the lowest birthweight infants. About 55% of cases occur in the first 24 hours, and 43% are associated with other air leaks (Yu et al., 1986). Pneumothorax occurs in 16–17% of infants with HMD, of whom half will survive (Bhat and Zikos-Labropoulou, 1986).

Other short-term complications, which can also become chronic conditions, that are associated with HMD include pulmonary hypertension, atelectasis, pulmonary edema, subglottic stenosis, and respiratory tract infections (Sherf and Park, 1990).

Long-term:

Probably the most consistently associated complication of HMD is BPD. In 54% of infants with BPD, HMD was the primary disease. BPD occurs in 15% of infants weighing less than 1000 g and in 3% of those more than 1000 g (Yu et al., 1983). Other investigators cite a 65% incidence of BPD (Bhat & Zikos-Labropoulou, 1986). Of those infants requiring mechanical ventilation, 10% will develop BPD (Yu et al., 1983). Most studies have shown a definite relationship between low gestational age and BPD. These infants are also more likely to have experienced intraventricular hemorrhage, retinopathy of prematurity, and nutritional difficulties (Saigal and O'Brodovich, 1987).

Infants with BPD continue to experience poor health following discharge, and a significant proportion require re-hospitalization, mainly for infection (Saigal and O'Brodovich, 1987). Infants with BPD may also have severe visual impairment, poor growth, neurodevelopmental disorders, and developmental delay. However, they do tend to improve after the first 2–3 years (Saigal and O'Brodovich, 1987). In contrast, uncomplicated HMD is not associated with significant impairment of lung function in childhood (Saigal and O'Brodovich, 1987).

Leonard and his colleagues (1990) followed infants less than 1250 g for 4.5 years to compare the effects of two medical risk factors (intracranial hemorrhage and severe chronic lung disease) and abuse/neglect on neurodevelopmental outcomes. They found that the greatest factor associated with later abnormality was the parenting risk factor (abuse/neglect). Infants with increasing severity of intracranial hemorrhage had increasingly worse neurological and cognitive impairment, whereas chronic lung disease (without intracranial hemorrhage) was not related to neurological outcome (Leonard et al., 1990).

Saigal and colleagues (1990) measured the intellectual and functional status of a regional cohort of infants born at birthweights of 501–1000 g at 5.5 years of age. Long-term survival was 49%. Seventy-eight per cent of these children were tested using standard psychometric tests (6% were blind and received alternate testing, and one child was untestable). Two-thirds of the children were performing adequately, and one-third were in the moderate to low range. Almost half of the children without neurosensory impairment and an IQ greater than or equal to 84 were identified to be at mild to high risk for future learning disabilities (Saigal et al., 1990).

REFERENCES

Adamkin, D.H.: Nutrition in very very low birth weight infants. Clin. Perinatol., 13(2):419–443, 1986.

Amspacher, K.A.: Necrotizing enterocolitis: The never-ending challenge. J. Perinat. Neonat. Nurs., 3(2):58–68, 1989.

Anday, E.K., Cohen, M.E., Kelley, N.E., and Leitner, D.S.: Effect of in utero cocaine exposure on startle and its modification. Devel. Pharmacol. Ther., 12:137–145, 1989.

Bailey, L.L., Nehlsen-Cannarella, S.L., Doroshow, R.W., et al.: Cardiac allotransplantation in newborns as therapy for hypoplastic left heart syndrome. N. Engl. J. Med., 315(15):949–951, 1986.

Bailey, N.A., Lay, P., and The Loma Linda University Infant Heart Transplant Group: New horizons: Infant cardiac transplantation. Heart & Lung, 18(2):172–177, 1989.

Bhat, R., and Zikos-Labropoulou, E: Resuscitation and respiratory management of infants weighing less than 1000 grams. Clin. Perinatol., 13(2):285–297, 1986.

Blanchette, V., and Zipursky, A.: Neonatal hematology. In Avery, G. (ed): Neonatology: Pathophysiology and Management of the Newborn (3rd ed.). Philadelphia, J.B. Lippincott, 1981, pp. 638–686.

Bohn, D.: Blood gas and ventilatory parameters in predicting survival in congenital diaphragmatic hernia. Pediatr. Surg. International, 2:336–340, 1987.

Bozynski, M.E.A., Naglie, R.A., Nicks, J.J., et al.: Lateral positioning of the stable ventilated very-low-birth-weight infant. Am. J. Dis. Child., 142:200–202, 1988.

Briggs, G., Freeman, R., and Yaff, S.: Drugs in Pregnancy and Lactation (2nd ed.). Baltimore, Williams & Wilkins, 1986, pp. 32a–33a.

Brueggemeyer, A.: Thermoregulation. In Gunderson L.P., and Kenner, C. (eds.): Care of the 24–25 Week Gestational Age Infant. Petaluma, CA, Neonatal Network, 1990, pp. 23–28.

Canadian Task Force on the Periodic Health Examination: The periodic health examination. CMJ 121:3–46, 1979.

Carter, K., and Spence, K.: Nursing of infants with pulmonary hypertension following repair of a diaphragmatic hernia. LAMP, 14(11):18–22, 1984.

Chasnoff, I.J.: Perinatal effects of cocaine. Contemp. Obstet./Gynecol., 25(5):163–179, 1987.

Chasnoff, I.J.: Cocaine, pregnancy, and the neonate. Women Health, 15(3):23–35, 1989.

Chasnoff, I.J., Hunt, C.E., Kletter, R., and Kaplan, D.: Prenatal cocaine exposure is associated with respiratory pattern abnormalities. Am. J. Dis. Child., 143:583–587, 1989.

Chasnoff, I.J., Lewis, D.E., Griffith, D.R., and Willey, S.: Cocaine and pregnancy: Clinical and toxicological implications for the neonate. Clin. Chem., 35(7):1276–1278, 1989.

Cheromcha, D.P., and Hyman, P.E.: Neonatal necrotizing enterocolitis: Inflammatory bowel disease of the newborn. Dig. Dis. Sci., 33(3):78s–84s, 1988.

Chouteau, M., Namerow, P.B., and Leppert, P.: The effect of cocaine abuse on birth weight and gestational age. Obstet. Gynecol., 72(3):351–354, 1988.

Clochesy, J.M., Whittaker, A.A., and Murdaugh, C.L.: Hypoplastic left heart syndrome: A review and the report of two cases. Heart & Lung, 15(1):23–28, 1986.

Cohen, M.A.: The use of prostaglandin and prostaglandin inhibitors in critically ill neonates. Maternal-Child Nurs., 8:194–199, 1983.

Costarino, A., and Baumgart, S.: Modern fluid and electrolyte management of the critically ill premature infant. Pediatr. Clin. North Am., 33(1):153–169, 1986.

Couser, R.J., Ferrara, T.B., Ebert, J., et al.: Effects of exogenous surfactant therapy on dynamic compliance during mechanical breathing in preterm infants with hyaline membrane disease. J. Pediatr., 116(1):119–124, 1990.

Creasy, R.K., and Herron, M.A.: Prevention of preterm birth. Semin. Perinatol., 5(3):295–302, 1981.

Cullen, M.L., Klein, M.D., and Philippart, A.I.: Congenital diaphragmatic hernia. Surg. Clin. North Am., 65(5):1115–1138, 1985.

Devore, N. Jackson, V., and Peining, S.: TORCH infections. Am. J. Nurs., 83:1660–1663, 1983.

Dixon, S.D.: Effects of transplacental exposure to cocaine and methamphetamine on the neonate. West. J. Med., 150(4):436–442, 1989.

Dixon, S.D., and Bejar, R.: Echoencephalographic findings in neonates associated with maternal cocaine and methamphetamine use: Incidence and clinical correlates. J. Pediatr. *115*:770–778, 1989.

Doyle, L.W., Kitchen, W.H., Ford, G.W., et al.: Effects of antenatal steroid therapy on mortality and morbidity in very low birth weight infants. J. Pediatr., *108*(2):287–292, 1986.

Durand, M., Sangha, B., Cabal, L.A., et al.: Cardiopulmonary and intracranial pressure changes related to endotracheal suctioning in preterm infants. Crit. Care Med., *17*(6):506–510, 1989.

Ein, S.H., and Barker, G.: The pharmacological treatment of newborn diaphragmatic hernia: Update Pediatr. Surg. Internat. 2:341–345, 1987.

Escobedo, M.B., and Gonzalez, A.: Bronchopulmonary dysplasia in the tiny infant. Clin. Perinatol., *13*(2):315–326, 1986.

Faix, R.G., Polley, T.Z., and Grasela, T.H.: A randomized, controlled trial of parenteral clindamycin in neonatal necrotizing enterocolitis. J. Pediatr., *112*(2):271–276, 1988.

Fanaroff, A., and Martin, R.: Neonatal/Perinatal Medicine (4th ed.). St. Louis, C.V. Mosby, 1987.

Feigin, N.D., and Cherry, J.D.: Textbook of Pediatric Infectious Diseases (2nd ed.). Philadelphia, W.B. Saunders Co., 1987.

Fox, M.D., and Molesky, M.G.: The effects of prone and supine positioning on arterial oxygen pressure. Neonatal Network, *8*(4):25–29, 1990.

Frank, D.A., Zuckerman, B., Amaro, H., et al.: Cocaine use during pregnancy: Prevalence and correlates. Pediatrics, *82*(6):888–895, 1988.

Freij, B., and Sever, J.: Herpesvirus infections in pregnancy: Risks to embryo, fetus, and neonate. Clin. Perinatol., *15*:203–231, 1988.

Gennaro, S.: Necrotizing enterocolitis: Detecting it and treating it. Nursing 80, *10*:52–55, 1980.

Gersony, W.M.: Cardiac transplantation in infants and children. J. Pediatr., *116*(2):266–268, 1990.

Gregory, J.R., Campbell, J.R., Harrison, M.H., and Campbell, T.J.: Neonatal necrotizing enterocolitis. Am. J. Surg., *141*:562–567, 1981.

Guignard, J., and John E.G.: Renal function in the tiny, premature infant. Clin. Perinatol., *13*(2):377–401, 1986.

Haggerty, L.: TORCH: A literature review and implications for practice. J. Obstet. Gynecol. Neonat. Nurs., 124–129, 1985.

Harkavy, K.L., Scanlon, J.W., Chowdhry, P.K., and Grylack, L.J.: Dexamethasone therapy for chronic lung disease in ventilator- and oxygen-dependent infants. A controlled trial. J. Pediatr., *115*:979–983, 1989.

Harrison, M.R.: The fetus with a diaphragmatic hernia. Pediatr. Surg., *3*:15–22, 1988.

Hazinski, M.F.: Congenital heart disease in the neonate. Part IV: Cyanotic heart disease. Neonatal Network, *2*(1):12–24, 1983.

Hazinski, M.F.: Congenital heart disease in the neonate. Part V: Admission of the neonate with heart disease. Neonatal Network, *2*(5):7–17, 1983.

Hazinski, M.F.: Congenital heart disease in the neonate. Part VII; Common congenital heart defects producing hypoxemia and cyanosis. Neonatal Network, *2*(6):36–51, 1984.

Hazinski, M.F.: Congenital heart disease in the neonate: Part VIII. Neonatal Network, *3*(2):7–19, 1984.

Heaton, J.F., Redmond, C.R., Graves, E.D., et al.: Congenital diaphragmatic hernia-improving survival with extracorporeal membrane oxygenation. Pediatr. Surg., *3*:6–10, 1988.

Herron, M.A.: One approach to preventing preterm birth. J. Perinat. Neonat. Nurs., *2*(1), 33, 1988.

Hill, A., and Volpe, J.J.: Perinatal asphyxia: Clinical aspects. Clin. Perinatol., *16*(2):435–457, 1989.

Hodgman, J.: Sepsis in the neonate. Perinatology-Neonatology, 45–50, 1981.

Jacobs, M.M., and Phibbs, R.H.: Prevention, recognition, and treatment of perinatal asphyxia. Clin. Perinatol., *16*(4):785–807, 1989.

Kao, L.C., Durand, D.J., and Nickerson, B.G.: Improving pulmonary function does not decrease oxygen consumption in infants with bronchopulmonary dysplasia. J. Pediatr., *112*(4):616–621, 1988.

Kennard, M.J.: Cocaine use during pregnancy: Fetal and neonatal effects. J. Perinat. Neonat. Nurs., *3*(4):53–63, 1990.

Kerner, J.A.: Manual of Pediatric Parental Nutrition. New York, John Wiley & Sons, 1983.

Klein, J., and Remington, J.: Current concepts of infections of the fetus and newborn infant. *In* Remington, J., and Klein, J. (eds.): Infectious Diseases of the Fetus and Newborn Infant (3rd ed.). Philadelphia, W.B. Saunders Co., 1990.

Kliegman, R.M.: Neonatal necrotizing enterocolitis: Implications for an infectious disease. Pediatr. Clin. North Am., *26*(2):327–343, 1979.

Kliegman, R.M., and Fanaroff, A.A.: Neonatal necrotizing enterocolitis: A nine-year experience. Am. J. Dis. Child, *135*:608–611, 1981.

Kliegman, R.M., and Fanaroff, A.A.: Medical progress. Necrotizing enterocolitis. N. Engl. J. Med., *310*(17):1093–1103, 1984.

Kling, P.: Respiratory distress syndrome in the tiny baby. Neonatal Network, *4*(5):7–13, 1986.

Kosloske, A.M., Burstein, J., and Bartow, S.A.: Intestinal obstruction due to colonic structure following neonatal necrotizing enterocolitis. Ann. Surg., *192*(2):202–207, 1981.

Kuller, J., and Tobin, C.: Skin care management of the low-birthweight infant. *In* Gunderson, L.P., and Kenner, C. (eds.): Care of the 24–25 Week Gestational Age Infant (Small Baby Protocol). Petaluma, CA, Neonatal Network, 1990.

Kwong, M.S., and Egan, E.A.: Reduced incidence of hyaline membrane disease in extremely premature infants following delay of delivery in mother with preterm labor: Use of ritodrine and betamethasone. Pediatrics, *78*(5):767–773, 1986.

Lang, M.J., Hall, R.T., Reddy, N.S., et al.: A controlled trial of human surfactant replacement therapy for severe respiratory distress syndrome in very low birth weight infants. J. Pediatr., *116*(2):295–300, 1990.

Lawhon, G., and Melzar, A.: Developmental care of the very low birth weight infant. J. Perinat. Neonata. Nurs., *2*(1):56, 1988.

Lee, M.L.: Infections and prematurity: Is there a relationship? J. Perinat. Neonat. Nurs., *2*(1):10, 1988.

Lefrak-Okikawa, L.: Nutritional management of the very low birth weight infant. J. Perinat. Neonat. Nurs., *2*(1):66, 1988.

Leonard, C.H., Clyman, R.I., Piecuch, R.E., et al.: Effect of medical and social risk factors on outcome of prematurity and very low birth weight. J. Pediatr.: *116*(4):620–626, 1990.

Lewis, K.D., Bennette, B., and Schmeder, N.H.: The care of infants menaced by cocaine abuse. Maternal-Child Nurs., *14*:324–329, 1989.

Lissaver, T., and Jeffries, D: Preventing neonatal herpes infection. Br. J. Obstet. Gynaecol., *96*(9):1015–1018, 1989.

MacGregor, S.N., Keith, L.G., Chasnoff, I.J., et al.: Cocaine use during pregnancy: Adverse perinatal outcome. Am. J. Obstet. Gynecol., *157*(3):686–690, 1987.

Meier, P., and Paton, J.B.: Clinical Decision Making in Neonatal Intensive Care. Orlando, Grune & Stratton, 1984.

Miller, E.P., and Armstrong, C.L.: Surfactant replacement therapy. Innovative care for the premature infant. J. Obste. Gynecol. Neon. Nurs., *19*(1):14–17, 1990.

Mizrahi, E.M.: Consensus and controversy in the clinical management of neonatal seizures. Clin. Perinatol., *16*(2):485, 1989.

Mollitt, D.L., Tepas, J.J., and Talbert, J.L.: The role of coagulase-negative Staphylococcus in neonatal necrotizing enterocolitis. J. Pediatr. Surg., *23*(1):60–63, 1988.

Nelson, K.B.: Relationship of intrapartum and delivery room events to long-term neurologic outcome. Clin. Perinatol., *16*(4):995–1007, 1989.

Nickerson, B.: An overview of bronchopulmonary dysplasia: Pathogenesis and current therapy. *In* Lund, C.H. (ed.): Bronchopulmonary Dysplasia—Strategies for Total Patient Care. Petaluma, CA, Neonatal Network, 1990.

Oh, W.: Renal function and fluid therapy in high risk infants. Perinat. Nephrol., *53*:230–236, 1986.

O'Neill, J.A., Stahlman, M.T., and Meng, H.C.: Necrotizing enterocolitis in the newborn: Operative indications. Ann. Surg., *182*:274, 1975.

Osterloh, J.D., and Lee, B.L.: Urine drug screening in mothers and newborns. Am. J. Dis. Child., *143*(7): 791–793, 1989.

Paes, B.: Group B streptococcal disease in mother and child: An approach to diagnosis and management. Mod. Med. Canada, *41*:134–142, 1986.

Perlman, J.M.: Systemic abnormalities in term infants following perinatal asphyxia: Relevance to long-term neurologic outcome. Clin. Perinatol., *16*(2):475–483, 1989.

Phibbs, R.: Delivery room management of the newborn. *In* Avery, G. (ed): Neonatology: Pathophysiology and Management of the Newborn. Philadelphia, J.B. Lippincott, 1981, pp. 212–231.

Pigott, J.D., Murphy, J.D., Barber, G., and Norwood, W.I.: Palliative reconstructive surgery for hypoplastic left heart syndrome. Ann. Thorac. Surg., *45*:122–128, 1988.

Pildes, R.S., and Pyati, S.P.: Hypoglycemia and hyperglycemia in tiny infants. Clin. Perinatol., *13*(2):351–375, 1986.

Platzker, A.: Congenital anomalies causing respiratory failure. *In* Thibeault, D., and Gregory, G. (eds): Neonatal Pulmonary Care (2nd ed.) Norwalk, CT, Appleton-Century-Crofts, 1986.

Pohodich, J.: Gastrointestinal crises: NEC. *In* Vestal, K., and McKenzie, C.H. (eds.): High Risk Perinatal Nursing. Philadelphia, W.B. Saunders Co., 1983, pp. 488–500.

Prober, C.: Treatment of bacterial infections in the neonate. Clin. Invest. Med., *8*:368–370, 1985.

Richardson, C.: Hyaline membrane disease: Future treatment modalities. J. Perina. Neonat. Nurs., *2*(1):78–88, 1988.

Rodgers, B.D.: Substance abuse in pregnancy. Med. Clin. North Am., *38*:6895–6901, 1989.

Saigal, S., Szatmari, P., Rosenbaum, P., et al.: Intellectual and functional status at school entry of children who weighed 1000 grams or less at birth: A regional perspective of births in the 1980s. J. Pediatr., *116* (3):409–416, 1990.

Saigal, S., and O'Brodovich, H.: Long-term outcome of preterm infants with respiratory disease. Clin. Perinatol., *14*(3):635–650, 1987.

Scherf, R.: Respiratory management of the infant with BPD. *In*: Lund, C.H. (ed.): Bronchopulmonary Dysplasia—Strategies for Total Patient Care. Petaluma, CA, Neonatal Network, 1990.

Scherf, R., and Park, S.A.: Complications in infants with bronchopulmonary dysplasia. *In*: Lund, C.H. (ed.): Bronchopulmonary Dysplasia—Strategies for Total Patient Care. Petaluma, CA, Neonatal Network, 1990.

Schullinger, J.N., Mollitt, D.L., Vinocur, C.D., et al.: Neonatal necrotizing enterocolitis. Am. J. Dis. Child., *135*:6121, 1981.

Schumacher, R.E., and Farrell, P.M.: Congenital diaphragmatic hernia. Major remaining challenge in neonatal respiratory care. Perinatology-Neonatology, July/Aug:29–44, 1985.

Shaffer, S.G., and Meade, V.M.: Sodium balance and extracellular volume regulation in very low birth weight infants. J. Pediatr., *115*(2):285–290, 1988.

Shochat, S.J.: Pulmonary vascular pathology in congenital diaphragmatic hernia. Pediatr. Surg. Internat., *2*:331–335, 1987.

Smith, J.E.: The dangers of prenatal cocaine use. Maternal-Child Nurs. J., *13*:174–179, 1988.

Southwell, S.M.: Respiratory management. *In* Porter Gunderson, L., and Kenner, C. (eds.): Care of the 24–25 Week Gestational Age Infant. Petaluma, CA, Neonatal Network, 1990, pp. 39–65.

Steele, K.H.: Caring for parents of critically ill neonates during hospitalization: Strategies for health care professionals. Maternal-Child Nurs. J., *16*(1):13–27, 1987.

Sullivan, K.R.: Maternal implications of cocaine use during pregnancy. J. Perinat. Neonat. Nurs., *3*(4):12–25, 1990.

Torrence, C.R., and Horns, K.M.: Appraisal and caregiving for the drug addicted infant. Neonatal Network, *8*(3):49–59, 1989.

Turner, J.C.: Nourishing the gestationally immature infant. *In* Porter Gunderson, L., and Kenner, C. (eds.): Care of the 24–25 Week Gestational Age Infant. Petaluma, CA, Neonatal Network, 1990, pp. 67–96.

VandenBerg, K.A.: Behaviorally supportive care for the extremely premature infant. *In* Porter Gunderson, L., and Kenner, C. (eds.): Care of the 24–25 Week Gestational Age Infant. Petaluma, CA, Neonatal Network, 1990, pp. 129–150.

Whitelaw, A.: Intervention after birth asphyxia. Arch. Dis. Child., *64*:66–68, 1989.

Whitley, R.: Natural history and pathogenesis of neonatal herpes simplex virus infections. Ann. Acad. Sci., *549*:103–117, 1988.

Whitley, R.: Neonatal herpes simplex virus infections. Clin. Perinatol., *15*:903–915, 1988.

Whitley, R.: Herpes simplex virus infections of the central nervous system. Am. J. Med., *85*:61–67, 1988.

Whitley, R., Alford, C., Hirsch, M., et al., and the NIAID Collaborative Antiviral Study Group: Vidarabine versus acyclovir therapy in herpes simplex encephalitis. N. Engl. J. Med., *314*:144–149, 1986.

Whitley, R., Corey, L., Arvin, A., et al., and the NIAID Collaborative Study Group: Changing presentation of herpes simplex virus infections in neonates. J. Infect. Dis., *158*:109–116, 1988.

Williams, R.: Congenital diaphragmatic hernia: A review. Heart & Lung, *11*(6):532–538, 1982.

Wiswell, T.E., Robertson, C.F., Jones, T.A., and Tuttle,

D.J.: Necrotizing enterocolitis in full-term infants. Am. J. Dis. Child., *142*:532–535, 1988.

Yoos, L.: Applying research in practice: Parenting the premature infant. Appl. Nurs. Res., 2(1):30–34, 1989.

Yu, V.Y.H., and Tudehope, D.I.: Neonatal necrotizing enterocolitis: 2. Perinatal risk factors. Med. J. Austral., *1*(19):688–693, 1977.

Yu, V.Y.H., Orgill, A.A., Lim, S.B., et al.: Bronchopulmonary dysplasia in very low birthweight infants. Austral. Paedi. J., *19*:233, 1983.

Yu, V.Y.H., Wong, P.Y., Bajuk, B., and Szymonowicz, W.: Pulmonary interstitial emphysema in infants less than 1000 g at birth. Austral. Paed. J. 22:189–192, 1986.

Jane Deacon

Radiological Evaluation of the Newborn

Objectives

1. Define common radiological terms used in describing an x-ray.

2. Differentiate the various densities that compose an x-ray.

3. Describe radiological findings that are commonly seen in newborn disease states.

4. Differentiate normal from abnormal findings on a chest x-ray.

5. Calculate a cardiothoracic ratio and discuss the significance.

6. Discuss common adjectives used in describing hyaline membrane disease, meconium aspiration syndrome, transient tachypnea of the newborn, and pneumonia.

7. Recognize findings on an x-ray that are consistent with congenital heart disease.

8. Describe an x-ray consistent with necrotizing enterocolitis.

9. Discuss congenital anomalies that are associated with specific radiographic findings.

10. Describe the appearance of bone fractures and conditions that predispose to fractures.

11. Identify correct x-ray positioning of umbilical lines and endotracheal tubes.

Radiographic evaluation of a sick newborn is an established part of the diagnostic process. This evaluation assists the clinician in determining a diagnosis or formulating a differential diagnosis upon which to treat the infant. Rarely is a newborn admitted to the NICU without having at least one x-ray, and frequently many are needed during the course of treatment. Nurses need to be familiar with common radiographic findings to add to the overall knowledge base for care of the infant. The purpose of this chapter is to review essentials of radiological evaluation through description and presentation of x-rays of various newborn disease states.

Basic Concepts

A. **Radiographs are composite shadowgrams** that represent the added varying densities (white through black) of many layers of tissues.

B. From these shadow forms, densities, and shapes, we can deduce or infer propositions concerning anatomy, pathology, and function.

Terminology

A. **Air bronchograms:** air outlining the bronchial tree.

B. **Artifact:** an unnaturally occurring silhouette that is artificially reproduced on the x-ray and is not a part of the patient.

C. **Cardiothoracic ratio:** a ratio computed by dividing the maximum cardiac width by the maximum thoracic width to determine the heart size.

D. **Expiratory film:** obtained when patient is in expiration. Appears to increase cardiac size, accentuate lung markings, and decrease normal rib expansion. Air bronchograms are not visible on expiratory films.

E. **Exposure:** amount of radiation used will produce a film ranging from light to dark. An underexposed film will be light, and an overexposed film will be dark.

F. **Hyperexpanded lungs:** lungs expanded greater than nine ribs.

G. **Hypoexpanded lungs:** lungs expanded less than seven ribs.

H. **Inspiratory film:** obtained when patient is in full inspiration. This is the most desirable for chest film interpretation.

I. **Interlobar fissure:** pleural space between lung lobes. Can be fluid filled and appear as a distinctive line.

J. **Lordotic film:** horizontal beam of the anteroposterior x-ray shot at an oblique angle. Anterior and posterior segments of the same ribs are superimposed. Clavicles are projected upwards. Can visualize lung tissue between ribs.

K. **Perihilar:** the radiographic area bordering mediastinal structures.

L. **Pleural effusion:** fluid in the pleural space.

M. **Radiolucent:** substances with varying degrees of transparency.

N. **Radiopaque:** substances that are dense and non-penetratable to x-ray.

O. **Rad:** fundamental unit of radiation measurement.

P. **Roentgen:** unit of exposure.

Q. **Rotation:** turned from the midline. Generally distorts chest structures. Heart and mediastinum are radiographed obliquely, and their shadows appear enlarged and distorted.

R. **Skinfold:** results from the folding of redundant skin. Manifests as a near-straight vertical line of variable length that generally extends beyond the chest and crosses body planes. The most common artifact seen in the newborn. Can mimic a pneumothorax or pleural effusion.

S. **Technique:** signifies correct exposure, positioning, timing in relation to inspiration, and proper labeling of a film.

T. **X-rays:** radiant energy of very short wavelength that penetrates substances opaque to light differently according to different wave lengths.

X-Ray Views Commonly Used in the Newborn (Fig. 33–1)

A. **Anteroposterior view** (plain film): x-ray passes through the patient from front to back. Most common view used in the newborn. Used for general assessment.

B. **Lateral:** x-ray beam passes horizontally through patient in the supine posi-

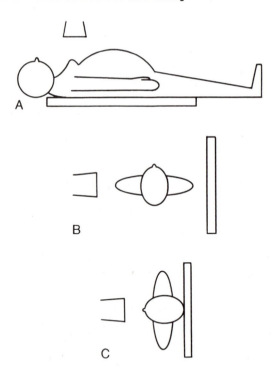

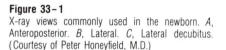

Figure 33-1
X-ray views commonly used in the newborn. *A*,
Anteroposterior. *B*, Lateral. *C*, Lateral decubitus.
(Courtesy of Peter Honeyfield, M.D.)

tion. Used to verify line placement, to check for free air in the chest and abdomen, and for general assessment.

C. **Lateral decubitus:** x-ray beam passes horizontally through the patient positioned right or left side down. Frequently used to check for free air or pleural effusions.

Radiographical Densities

A. **Radiodensities of various substances and tissues differ**, based on their composition.
1. The least dense substance (air) will radiograph black, since the sparse molecules offer no obstacle to the rays.
2. A very dense object such as lead or metal will radiograph white because no rays penetrate it and the film underneath remains unaltered.
3. Subcutaneous fat is very radiolucent. It is not homogeneous, as it contains circulating fluids and fibrous connective tissue, which radiographs dark gray.
4. Blood, muscle, and liver are of similar densities and will x-ray medium gray. Moist, solid, or fluid-filled organs and tissue masses have about the same radiodensity—greater than air but less than bone or metal.
5. Bone is composed of an organic matrix into which the complex bone mineral is precipitated. These organic substances will reduce the radiodensity of bone, and it will x-ray white with a tinge of gray.

B. **Differentiation of densities is the basis for interpretation of x-rays.**

Approach to Interpreting an X-Ray

A. **Develop a systematic approach and a definite order** for looking at a film.

B. **Labeling.** Note name or identification of the patient, date and time of film, and radiographic marking of right or left side of film.

C. **A comprehensive review of all systems** when evaluating an x-ray will train the reviewer to use a systematic approach, ensuring that no pathology is missed.

D. **Individually assess all anatomy and pathology on every film observed.**
1. Respiratory system.
   a. Rib expansion.
   b. Lung volume.
   c. Pulmonary vascular markings.
   d. Lung fields.
   e. Pathology.
   f. Presence of free air.
   g. Location of tubes.
2. Mediastinum.
   a. Heart.
      (1) Size.
      (2) Position of the apex.
      (3) Shape.
      (4) Pulmonary vascular markings.
      (5) Location, position of carina, air bronchograms.
   b. Trachea.
      (1) Location.
      (2) Presence/position of endotracheal tube.
   c. Thymus.
      (1) Size.
      (2) Presence or absence.
      (3) Sail sign.
   d. Diaphragms.
      (1) General contour.
      (2) Position.
      (3) Abdominal contents herniating through (diaphragmatic hernia).
      (4) Bulge of liver/bowel against elevated dome of diaphragm (eventration).
   e. Abdomen.
      (1) Passage of air throughout GI system.
      (2) Esophageal anomalies.
      (3) Location of gastric tubes.
      (4) Tracheoesophageal fistulas (air present in stomach with presence of proximal esophageal atresia with distal tracheoesophageal fistula).
      (5) Location of stomach.
      (6) Bowel gas pattern.
      (7) Presence of calcifications.
      (8) Presence of a bubbly pattern (pneumatosis intestinalis).
      (9) Free air.
      (10) Fluid/ascites/masses.
      (11) Dilated bowel loops.
   f. Skeletal system.
      (1) General skeletal appearance.
      (2) Fractures of long bones, clavicles, ribs, skull.
      (3) Number of rib pairs (normal = 12).
      (4) Rib appearance, density of mineralization.
   g. Tubes and catheters.
      (1) Endotracheal tube position.
      (2) Umbilical catheter placement.
      (3) Central venous catheters.
      (4) Chest tube location.
      (5) Gastric tubes.

The Respiratory System

A. The normal chest (Fig. 33–2).
1. Complete aeration of the chest occurs within a few breaths after delivery.
2. Residual fluid may be present in the alveoli after delivery. Early films (less than 6 hours) may show increased vascular markings as a result of this fluid.
3. Normal chest x-ray.
   a. Uniform radiolucent appearance.
   b. Lungs expanded between seven and nine ribs.
   c. Perihilar regions show some increased density as a result of vascular, bronchial, and hilar structures that produce some increase in density.
   d. The periphery shows few if any markings.
   e. Fluid in the various interlobar fissures represents a normal variation.

B. Thymus.
1. Appears as a smoothly rounded outline superior to the cardiac shadow that blends imperceptibly with the cardiac silhouette.
2. A definite notch can be seen at the junction of the cardiac silhouette and the thymus in some cases.
3. Generally more prominent on the right.
4. Shape may alter markedly with the degree of inspiration.
5. Involutes rapidly during times of stress.
6. Congenitally absent or aplastic in DiGeorge's syndrome.
7. Mediastinal air may lift thymus up, creating a "sail sign."

C. Trachea
1. Normally displaced slightly to the right by the left aortic arch.
2. A deviated trachea supports a mediastinal shift.
3. On inspiration, the trachea dilates and lengthens.
4. On expiration, the trachea constricts and shortens.
5. On deep inspiration, the trachea and major bronchi are distended and identifiable.

PULMONARY PARENCHYMAL DISEASE

A. Hyaline membrane disease (HMD) (Fig. 33–3).
1. Normal to underaerated appearance. Underaeration classically seen in the nonventilated patient.

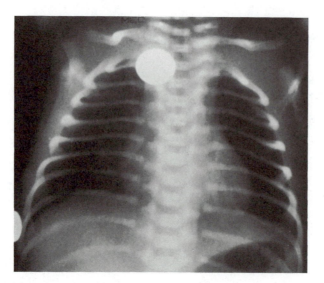

Figure 33–2
Normal chest appearance on an x-ray.

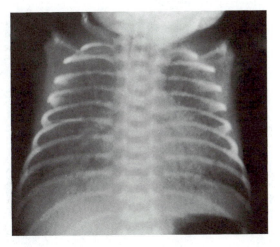

Figure 33-3
Hyaline membrane disease. Note reticulogranular lung pattern and air bronchograms.

2. Reticulogranular appearance bilaterally. This is a finely granular homogeneous pattern throughout both lung fields.
3. Air bronchograms with peripheral extension.
4. Generalized opacity or frank "whiteout" with severe disease (Fig. 33-4).
5. Similar pattern may be seen in group B streptococcal pneumonia and may be impossible to distinguish from hyaline membrane disease.

B. **Pulmonary interstitial emphysema (PIE)** (Fig. 33-5).
1. Hyperexpansion.
2. Pinpoint bubbles in the lung fields of infants with severe respiratory failure or pulmonary hypoplasia.
3. Bubbles are fixed in distention.
4. Often seen in association with pneumothorax or pneumomediastinum.

C. **Bronchopulmonary dysplasia (BPD)** (Fig. 33-6).
1. Pattern of ill-defined densities in both lung fields that progressively develops if acute respiratory disease fails to resolve and develops into chronic lung disease.
2. Small-cyst development follows.
3. Progressively larger, more irregular cyst development, frequently greater in the lung bases.
4. Generally, hyperexpanded lung fields (greater than nine ribs) with flattened diaphragms.

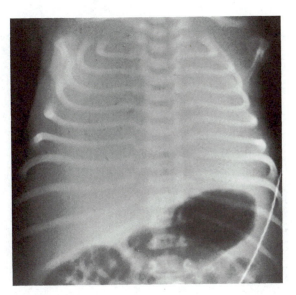

Figure 33-4
Severe hyaline membrane disease. Note a "white out" appearance bilaterally with faint air bronchograms visible.

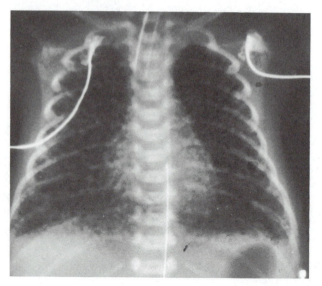

Figure 33–5
Pulmonary interstitial emphysema. Note hyperexpansion bilaterally and pinpoint dark bubbles throughout both lung fields.

D. **Transient tachypnea of the newborn (TTN)** (Fig. 33–7).
1. Pulmonary vascular congestion.
2. Symmetrical perihilar streakiness.
3. Mild to moderate hyperexpansion of lungs with flattened diaphragms.
4. Fluid in minor and major interlobar fissures.
5. Occasionally, mild to moderate cardiomegaly and pleural effusions (fluid accumulation in the pleural space).
6. Right side may be more affected than left.

E. **Meconium aspiration syndrome (MAS)** (Fig. 33–8).
1. History of meconium-stained fluid at delivery.
2. Mild cases may show a normal lung pattern to mild infiltrates with overexpanded lung.
3. Severe cases show extensive coarse, patchy infiltrates interspersed with radiolucence, which may represent overinflation in some areas.
4. General lung haziness superimposed over infiltrates.
5. Hyperexpanded lungs (greater than nine ribs).
6. High risk for air leaks.

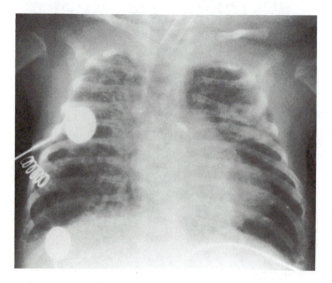

Figure 33–6
Bronchopulmonary dysplasia. Note ill-defined densities bilaterally. Also note fractured rib in the upper left chest and pale-appearing ribs.

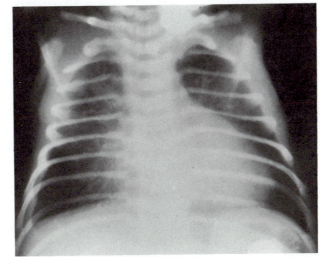

Figure 33–7
Transient tachypnea of the newborn. Note mild hyperexpansion and perihilar streakiness. A small pleural effusion is also present on the right side.

F. Pneumonia (Fig. 33–9).
1. Pulmonary infiltrates with varying patterns.
   a. Small, diffuse patches.
   b. Coarse, patchy infiltrates.
   c. Diffuse, hazy lung.
   d. Perihilar, interstitial streaking.
2. Reticulogranular pattern similar to that of hyaline membrane disease and often indistinguishable with group B streptococcal pneumonia.
3. Overinflation commonly present.

PULMONARY AIR LEAKS

A. Pneumothorax (Fig. 33–10).
1. Air accumulation in the intrapleural space.
2. Mediastinal shift of structures away from the affected side as air accumulates (tension pneumothorax).

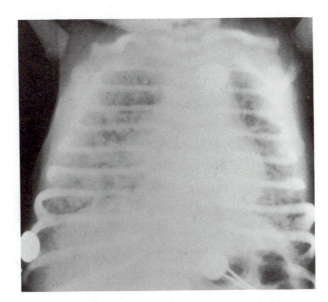

Figure 33–8
Meconium aspiration syndrome. Note the coarse, patchy infiltrates bilaterally.

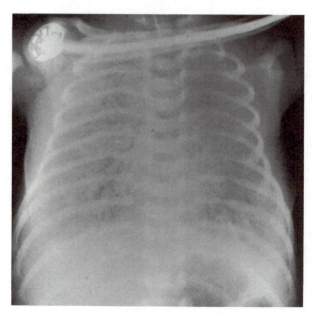

Figure 33–9
Group B streptococcal pneumonia. Note the reticulogranular appearance seen with hyaline membrane disease.

3. A pneumothorax not under tension may not exhibit a mediastinal shift.
4. Outline of the collapsed lung frequently evident.
5. Diaphragm on affected side will be flattened, owing to tension from air accumulation superior to it.

B. **Pneumomediastinum** (Fig. 33–11).
1. Air collection in the center of the chest.
2. Outlines and/or elevates the lobes of the thymus, creating a "sail sign" appearance.
3. On lateral film, there is an area of hyperlucency in the superior retrosternal space.
4. Mediastinal air can track into the subpleural space and result in a hyperlucent crescent of air just over the diaphragmatic leaflet. A larger collection of air over the diaphragmatic leaflet will represent a pneumothorax.

C. **Pneumopericardium** (Fig. 33–12).
1. Radiolucent halo of free air of varying width surrounding the heart.

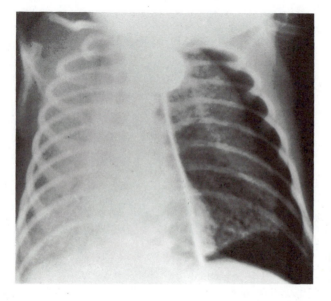

Figure 33–10
Left tension pneumothorax. Note the mediastinal shift toward the right side.

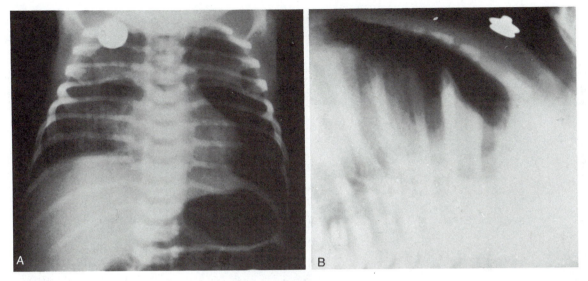

Figure 33-11
A, Pneumomediastinum with thymus lifted demonstrating the "sail sign." B, Pneumomediastinum on lateral view. Note that the air in the anterior chest outlines the thymus.

2. Width of air around the heart is proportional to the amount of air present.
3. Decreased cardiac size may indicate cardiac tamponade.
4. Other pulmonary air leaks and/or PIE are generally present.
5. Infant is usually receiving positive-pressure ventilation.

MISCELLANEOUS CAUSES OF RESPIRATORY DISTRESS

A. **Diaphragmatic paralysis** (phrenic nerve injury) (Fig. 33-13).
1. Elevation and fixation of a diaphragmatic leaflet.
2. Paralysis of the right diaphragmatic leaflet is more common than the left.
3. Mediastinum may be shifted away from the affected side.

B. **Eventration of the diaphragm** (Fig. 33-14).
1. Elevation of diaphragmatic dome into the thorax.
2. May occur unilaterally or bilaterally.
3. Smooth bulge blending with the diaphragmatic leaflet.
4. Abdominal organs may push up against the diaphragm but do not enter the chest because no opening exists.

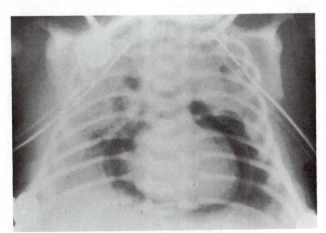

Figure 33-12
Pneumopericardium. Note that air completely encircles the heart. Bilateral chest tubes are also in place.

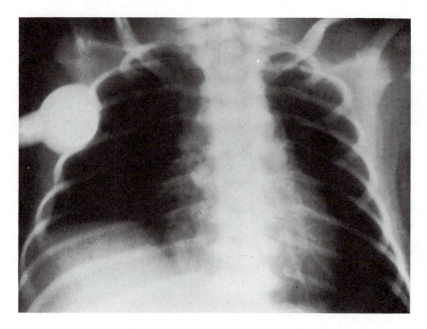

Figure 33–13
Paralysis of the right diaphragm. Note that the right diaphragm is markedly elevated in comparison with the left diaphragm.

C. **Pulmonary edema** (Fig. 33–15).
1. Common with patent ductus arteriosus, cardiac abnormalities, and chronic lung disease.
2. Interstitial fluid accumulation with diffuse haziness of the lungs.
3. May appear as a "white out" in severe pulmonary edema.

Thoracic Surgical Problems

A. **Congenital diaphragmatic hernia** (Fig. 33–16).
1. Herniation of abdominal contents through various portions of the diaphragm into the thoracic cavity.

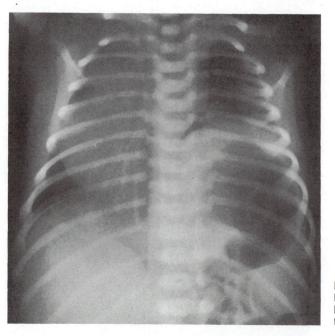

Figure 33–14
Eventration of the diaphragm. Note the left diaphragm bulging upward with the stomach pushing up against it.

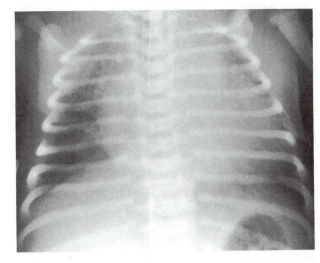

Figure 33-15
Pulmonary edema. Note congested lung
fields and cardiomegaly.

2. Eighty-five per cent occur on the left side through the foramen of Bochdalek.
3. Left hemithorax is filled with loops of bowel (which are usually expanded with
   air), stomach, and often liver.
4. Mediastinum is shifted away from the affected side.
5. Abdomen is relatively gasless and may be scaphoid on the lateral view.
6. A contralateral pneumothorax may be present with assisted ventilation.

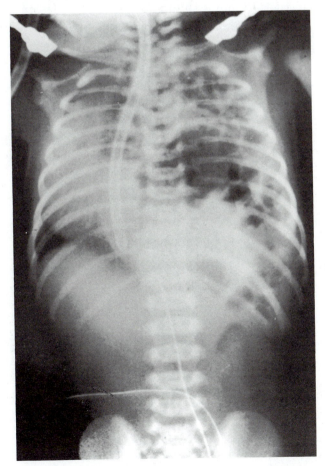

Figure 33-16
Left diaphragmatic hernia. Note the presence of bowel in the left side of the chest,
a mediastinal shift to the right, and a
lack of bowel in the abdomen.

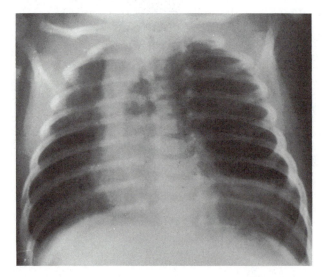

Figure 33–17
Congenital lobar emphysema. Note hyperlucency of the left upper lung lobe with a mediastinal shift toward the right.

7. If an x-ray is obtained before the bowel is expanded with gas, the involved hemithorax may appear entirely opacified with the mediastinal structures shifted to the opposite side.

B. **Congenital lobar emphysema** (Fig. 33–17).
1. Upper lobes are most commonly affected with the left lobe predominating.
2. Affected lobe is overdistended and hyperlucent but may also be opaque, secondary to fluid accumulation distal to the obstruction.
3. Mediastinum is shifted toward the unaffected side.
4. Herniation of lung across the anterior and superior mediastinum occurs with profound emphysema.

Cardiovascular System

A. **The heart.**
1. Size.
   a. Cardiothoracic ratio greater than 60% suggests cardiomegaly (Fig. 33–18).
   b. Incorrect positioning, poor inspiration, and lordotic positioning can falsely increase cardiac size.

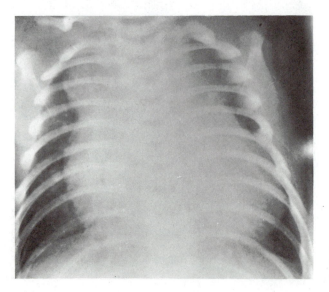

Figure 33–18
Cardiomegaly. Note that the enlarged heart occupies the majority of the thorax.

c. Rotation will distort cardiac silhouette.

d. Transient enlargement may exist as a result of polycythemia, perinatal anoxia, or normally increased fluid present at birth.

2. Position.

a. The cardiac apex normally points to the left.

b. Determination of the sites of the abdominal organs.

(1) Situs solitus (normal abdominal organ position).

(2) Situs inversus (inverted abdominal organs).

(3) Situs intermedius (midline liver/stomach).

c. "Mirror image" dextrocardia with situs inversus is the most common form of malposition. There is no increased risk of congenital heart disease with this type (Fig. 33–19).

d. Dextroversion is extreme right-sided rotation of the heart with no ventricular inversion and without great vessel transposition. Situs solitus is the rule. Cyanotic heart disease is often present.

3. Pulmonary vascularity.

a. Normal (Fig. 33–20).

b. Decreased vascularity manifests as hyperlucency in both lung fields (Fig. 33–21).

c. Congestion manifests as increased streakiness, hazy lung fields, and increased densities as condition worsens (see Fig. 33–15).

B. **Lesions with congested vascularity.**

1. Left-to-right shunt or intracardiac mixing.

a. Transposition of the great vessels: plain film shows egg-shaped cardiomegaly with congested lung fields or may be normal.

b. Total anomalous pulmonary venous return: cardiomegaly; increased pulmonary vascularity; and enlargement of the right atrium, right ventricle, and pulmonary artery. "Snowman" configuration of the heart is not generally

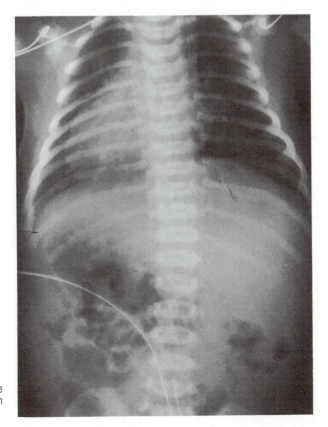

Figure 33–19
"Mirror image" dextrocardia. Note the apex pointing to the right with the stomach located on the right and liver on the left.

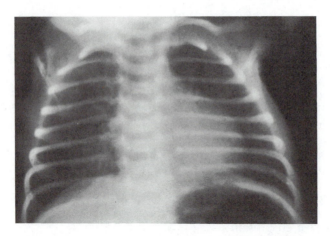

Figure 33–20
Normal pulmonary vascularity. Note the presence of vascularity radiating from the perihilar region.

seen in the newborn, owing to slow development of excessive pulmonary blood flow.

c. Atrioventricular (A-V) canal: pulmonary vascular resistance usually remains high enough to delay the onset of congestive heart failure until after the first 1–2 weeks, after which marked cardiomegaly and vascular congestion are evident.

d. Truncus arteriosus: the right ventricle is enlarged. Pulmonary vascularity will be increased or decreased, depending on which arteries, pulmonary or bronchial, supply the lungs.

e. Atrial septal defect (ASD): enlarged heart with a bulging pulmonary artery and pulmonary venous congestion.

f. Ventricular septal defect (VSD): cardiomegaly with venous congestion.

g. Patent ductus arteriosus (PDA): hazy pattern of pulmonary edema and cardiomegaly.

2. Left-sided obstruction: obstruction to the outflow of blood from the left side of the heart or obstruction to the return of blood from the lungs will eventually cause congestive heart failure.

a. Hypoplastic left heart syndrome (HPLHS): pulmonary vascularity may appear normal until significant cardiac decompensation is present, then cardiomegaly and congestive heart failure (CHF) become evident. Right atrial enlargement may also be seen. HPLHS is the most common cause of CHF in the first few days of life.

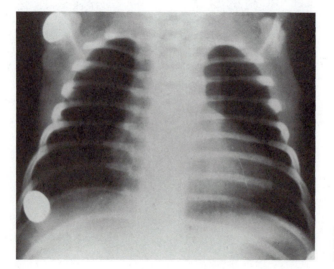

Figure 33–21
Hyperlucent lung fields from decreased blood flow to the lungs.

   b. Coarctation of the aorta: cardiomegaly and vascular congestion with a somewhat globular cardiac configuration. A bulging of the left cardiac border may be seen on plain film.

   c. Aortic stenosis: cardiomegaly and venous congestion are present on plain film.

C. **Lesions with decreased pulmonary vascularity**. All of these conditions have some form of right outflow tract obstruction. They can be located anywhere from the tricuspid valve to the pulmonary artery.

1. Hypoplastic right heart syndrome (HPRHS): stenosis or atresia of one of the right-sided valves.

   a. Pulmonary atresia is the most common form of HPRHS. Plain chest films show decreased pulmonary vascularity, cardiomegaly, and a small concave main pulmonary artery.

   b. Tricuspid atresia: complete atresia of the tricuspid valve and underdevelopment of the right ventricle and right outflow tract. Chest x-ray shows cardiac enlargement. The left ventricle is enlarged. The pulmonary artery is small and concave, and pulmonary vascularity is decreased.

2. Tetralogy of Fallot: the critical lesion in Tetralogy of Fallot is pulmonary stenosis. Chest x-ray findings consist of decreased pulmonary vascularity; a small, concave pulmonary artery; mild or no cardiomegaly; and a prominent cardiac apex as a result of right ventricular hypertrophy.

3. Pulmonary stenosis: severe cases of pulmonary valvular stenosis present in early infancy. This is referred to as critical pulmonary stenosis. Chest x-rays are normal in the neonate, but cardiomegaly with predominant right atrium and right ventricle, decreased pulmonary vascularity, and dilation of the pulmonary artery are eventually seen.

D. **Persistent pulmonary hypertension**.

1. Primary form (idiopathic): clear lungs, normal or slightly decreased pulmonary vascularity, and cardiomegaly with both right atrial and right ventricular enlargement.

2. Secondary form (aspiration syndromes, congenital diaphragmatic hernia, hypoplastic lung, myocardial dysfunction): lungs may not be clear, owing to the right-to-left ductal shunting present in these conditions and the underlying pathology present.

Gastrointestinal System

A. **Characteristics of the normal abdomen** (Fig. 33–22).

1. Bowel gas is present within 10–15 minutes of life.

2. By 12–24 hours, gas should have progressed throughout the entire GI tract.

3. Infants with respiratory distress frequently swallow large volumes of air, which will overdistend the intestinal loops.

4. A gasless abdomen can be seen in infants with decreased swallowing, decreased gut motility, vomiting, gastric decompression from suction, esophageal atresia without tracheoesophageal fistula, or intestinal obstruction, and in those chemically paralyzed.

B. **Abnormal gas patterns**.

1. Paralytic ileus versus mechanical ileus.

   a. With a paralytic ileus, large and small bowel become generally distended proportionate to their anatomical size. Multiple air-fluid levels exist. Isolated loops are hard to identify.

   b. With a mechanical ileus, differential distention of loops is present, which imply an obstruction. Bowel proximal to the obstruction is distended and that distal to the obstruction contains little or no air.

2. Level of obstruction.

   a. More loops are visualized with low obstructions.

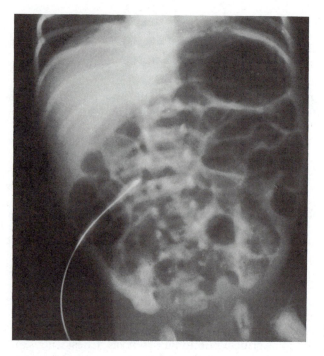

Figure 33–22
Normal bowel gas pattern. Note the presence of stomach bubble and air through the entire abdomen to the rectum.

    b. A large distended colon in normal position indicates an obstruction low in the colon.

    c. It is often difficult to differentiate between distended small intestine and the colon.

C. **The esophagus**.

1. May show indentations near the aortic arch and left mainstem bronchus.
2. May assume various configurations as a result of its flexibility during the respiratory cycle.
3. Air in the esophagus on a plain chest film is a normal finding.

D. **Esophageal abnormalities**.

1. Esophageal atresia (Fig. 33–23): a portion of the esophagus is absent, and both the distal and proximal portions of the esophagus end in blind pouches.

    a. Commonly associated with other anomalies of the GI tract, including imperforate anus and duodenal atresia or stenosis. Cardiac and renal anomalies may also be present (VACTERL/VATER association).

    b. Vertebral and rib anomalies are present in 25% of cases of esophageal abnormalities.

    c. On x-ray, a radiolucent, air-filled, distended proximal esophageal pouch is present. The abdomen is gasless, since no air enters. The proximal pouch can be further delineated by passing a radiopaque orogastric tube and obtaining a chest film to show the tube stopping at the level of the esophageal obstruction and not passing into the stomach.

    d. Aspiration pneumonitis of the upper lobes, especially of the right upper lobe, is also a common finding.

2. Esophageal atresia with tracheoesophageal fistula (Fig. 33–24).

    a. Esophageal atresia with fistulous connection of the distal esophagus to the trachea is the most common esophageal anomaly.

    b. A fistula from the upper pouch may also be present on rare occasion.

    c. Chest film demonstrates a dilated esophageal pouch with air present in the gastrointestinal tract.

3. Tracheoesophageal fistula with no esophageal atresia (H-type fistula).

    a. Difficult to identify without a barium study.

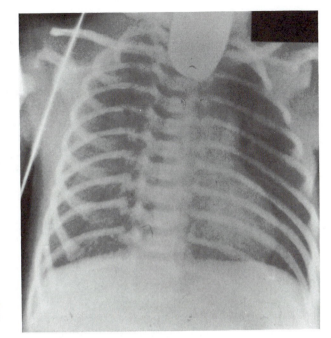

Figure 33-23
Esophageal atresia. Contrast medium outlines esophagus, which ends in a blind pouch.

    b. The fistula characteristically assumes an upwardly oblique configuration from esophagus to trachea on barium study.

    c. Pulmonary infiltrates may be present, owing to aspiration through the fistula into the lungs.

E. Stomach.

1. Often appears large in the newborn as a result of dilation with air.

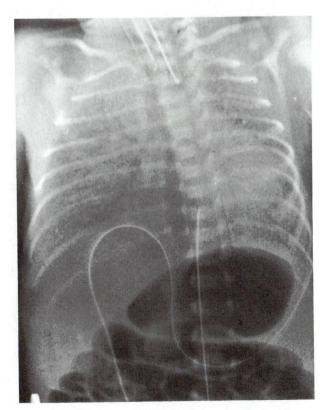

Figure 33-24
Esophageal atresia with tracheoesophageal fistula. An endotracheal tube is present with a gastric tube, which is unable to advance as a result of an esophageal atresia. Air is present in the abdomen, confirming the presence of a tracheoesophageal fistula.

2. Mucosal folds are absent in the newborn's stomach, so that the wall appears smooth.
3. The stomach begins to empty moments after it is filled.

F. **Abnormalities of the stomach.**
1. Pyloric stenosis.
   a. Symptoms develop 2–8 weeks after birth. Some infants may present with this abnormality in the first week of life.
   b. Plain films may be normal or demonstrate a distended stomach and disproportionately less gas in the small bowel.
2. Gastric perforation.
   a. Uncommon, but may occur secondary to gastric ulcers, hypoxia-induced focal necrosis, or gastric tubes.
   b. Overdistention as a result of distal obstruction with mechanical ventilation can also occur.
   c. Indomethacin therapy for ductal closure has been associated with gastric perforation.
   d. Free air (pneumoperitoneum) with absence of gastric gas is a common finding on x-ray.

G. **Duodenal abnormalities** (Fig. 33–25).
1. Duodenal atresia and stenosis.
   a. Infants with duodenal atresia present with vomiting in the first few hours of life. Those with stenosis present at variable times, depending on the degree of stenosis.
   b. Duodenal atresia and stenosis are a common finding in Down syndrome (trisomy 21).
   c. X-ray demonstrates dilation of the stomach and proximal duodenum producing the characteristic "double bubble" pattern. No air is present distal to the duodenum.
2. Annular pancreas.
   a. Pancreas grows in the form of an encircling ring around the duodenum. Intrinsic duodenal atresia or stenosis is commonly found.
   b. Presentation is similar to that of duodenal atresia or stenosis.
   c. X-ray findings are generally indistinguishable from that of duodenal atresia or stenosis.

H. **Abnormalities of the small bowel.**
1. Small bowel atresia and stenosis.

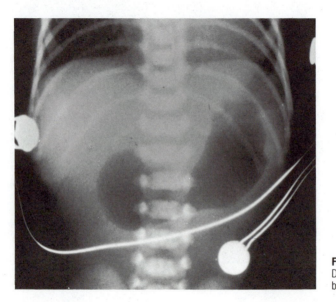

Figure 33–25
Duodenal atresia with characteristic double bubble pattern.

    a. Single or multiple areas of atresia or stenosis may exist.

    b. Clinically, abdominal distention and bile-stained emesis are apparent early on.

    c. Types of small bowel atresias.

        (1) High jejunal obstruction: stomach bubble and one or two loops of bowel are visible on x-ray.

        (2) Midjejunal obstruction: more dilated loops are visible on x-ray.

        (3) Distal ileal atresia: many dilated loops are visible on x-ray.

    d. Intramural calcifications may be present with perforation of the small bowel.

2. Meconium ileus (Fig. 33–26).

    a. Associated with cystic fibrosis.

    b. Obstruction results from impaction of thick, tenacious meconium in the distal small bowel. Ileal atresia or stenosis, ileal perforation, meconium peritonitis, and volvulus are common complications.

    c. Clinical presentation includes bile-stained emesis, abdominal distention, and failure to pass meconium.

    d. X-ray shows a low, small bowel obstruction with numerous air-filled loops of bowel. Air-fluid levels may be present, especially with complications such as volvulus and atresia or stenosis. Soap bubble effect as a result of trapping of air in meconium may be present.

    e. A contrast enema study is required once the diagnosis is made if peritonitis is not found. This will demonstrate a microcolon. The high osmolality of the water-soluble contrast agent will draw large amounts of fluid into the intestine and lubricate the meconium, allowing it to pass without surgical intervention. This technique is successful 25–40% of the time.

3. Midgut volvulus.

    a. The most common form of small bowel volvulus.

    b. The entire gut twists and spirals around the superior mesenteric artery and vein, resulting in vascular compromise, necrosis, and perforation.

    c. Presents with bilious vomiting.

    d. May be difficult to determine on x-ray. Findings vary from a normal abdo-

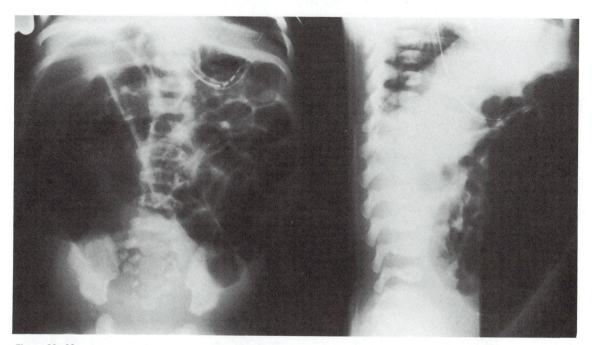

Figure 33–26
Meconium ileus with perforation and free air visible on lateral film.

men to one suggesting a gastric outlet obstruction or small bowel obstruction. Air arrested in the third portion of the duodenum is highly suspect.

e. The upper GI is the contrast study of choice. A barium enema may or may not reveal a displaced cecum.

I. **Abnormalities of the colon.**

1. Hirschsprung's disease (aganglionosis of the colon) (Fig. 33–27).
   a. Typical presentation is vomiting, abdominal distention, and failure to pass meconium within the first 24–36 hours of life.
   b. Commonly involves the distal colonic segment—the rectal and rectosigmoid areas.
   c. Plain films show some degree of low small bowel or colonic obstruction. Rectal gas may be absent or sparse. Numerous air-fluid levels may be present on upright view.
   d. A barium enema will support the findings, and a rectal biopsy will be confirmative.

2. Meconium plug syndrome, small left colon syndrome.
   a. Functional immaturity of the colon.
   b. Presents within the first 24–36 hours of age with abdominal distention, bilious vomiting, and failure to pass meconium.
   c. Diagnosis confirmed by contrast barium enema. Examination may also be therapeutic in dislodgement of the meconium.
   d. Plain films are non-specific and usually show a low small bowel obstruction. Air-fluid levels may be seen on the upright view with no gas in the colon.
   e. 15% of patients with meconium plug have associated Hirschsprung's disease and may require further radiographic examination.

J. **Necrotizing enterocolitis (NEC)** (Fig. 33–28).

1. Initial x-ray findings include generalized distention secondary to a paralytic ileus. Localized distention of loops may also be seen.
2. Subsequently, individual loops may become tubular with thickened bowel walls.
3. A persistent dilated loop may be evident on consecutive films.
4. At any point (stomach to rectum), pneumotosis cystoides intestinalis can be seen. This represents bacterial gas formation in the intestinal wall. The early

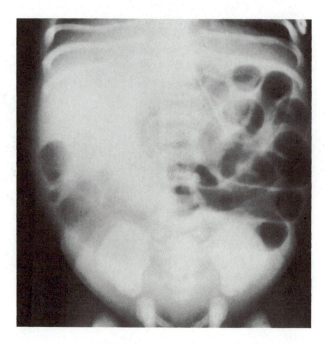

Figure 33–27
Hirschsprung's Disease. Note abdominal distention with dilated loops of bowel and lack of air present in the distal bowel.

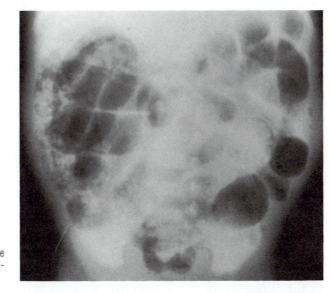

Figure 33–28
Necrotizing enterocolitis. Note presence of distended bowel loops and pneumatosis intestinalis.

x-ray includes a bubbly or foamy appearance in one or more areas of the bowel followed by concentric or linear air outlining the bowel lumen.
5. As NEC progresses, air may be seen in the portal venous system of the liver or as free air in the abdomen with perforation.

K. **Gastrointestinal air leaks.**
1. Pneumoperitoneum (see Fig. 34–26).
   a. Most commonly results from perforation of the GI tract and may be associated with the use of assisted ventilation.
   b. Most perforations occur secondary to NEC.
   c. Gastric perforations usually occur secondary to acute gastric ulceration, to focal necrosis owing to perinatal hypoxia, or as a result of gastric overdistention.
   d. Perforations may also be due to intestinal atresia and/or volvulus.
   e. Air may also dissect from the chest of neonates on high-pressure ventilation.
   f. Presents with abdominal distention and respiratory distress, or abdominal wall erythema.
   g. Plain film may not reveal free air. If pneumoperitoperitoneum is suspect, a lateral decubitus or cross-table view should also be obtained.
   h. On x-ray, the abdomen is distended and appears radiolucent. Individual loops of bowel are visible, owing to air inside and outside of the bowel wall. The falciform ligament (an opaque stripe) may be visualized in the right upper quadrant.
2. Portal venous air.
   a. Occurs secondary to bacteria-produced gas extending into the portal venous system. This is most commonly associated with pneumatosis intestinalis and NEC.
   b. May also occur as a complication of air iatrogenically introduced during catheterization of the umbilical vein.

L. **Peritonitis, ascites.**
1. Meconium peritonitis.
   a. Results from intrauterine GI perforation secondary to obstruction (atresia, stenosis, imperforate anus) and/or volvulus associated with meconium ileus.
   b. Calcifications are easily identifiable on x-ray and assume a patchy, irregular pattern. Multiple white speckled areas may be seen in one area or throughout the abdomen and may be present in the scrotum.

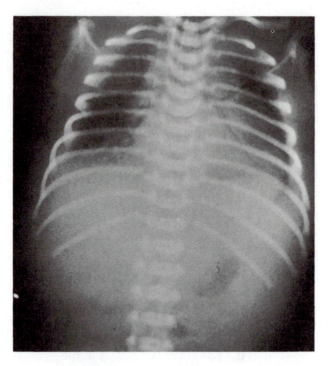

Figure 33–29
Abdominal ascites with bilateral pleural effusions.

     c. Calcifications will slowly disappear.
2. Ascites (Fig. 33–29).
     a. May result from urinary tract obstruction and is associated with fetal hydrops.
     b. Abdomen is distended with a uniform density surrounding a constricted, centralized bowel gas pattern.

Skeletal System

A. **Fractures:** occur most often during delivery with an increased incidence during breech deliveries. In breech deliveries, fractures can occur in both upper and lower extremities.
1. Clavicle: the bone most frequently fractured during delivery (Fig. 33–30). Fractures usually occur at the midclavicle. Common in large infants during a difficult vaginal delivery.

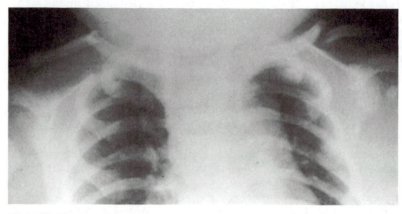

Figure 33–30
Fractured left clavicle.

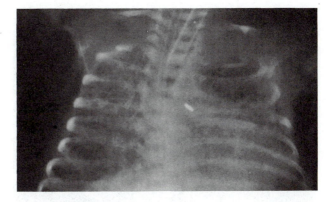

Figure 33-31
Fractured rib is present on the left with pale, "washed out" ribs.

2. Rib fractures: may occur at delivery and be asymptomatic. If many are fractured, the infant may show signs of respiratory distress and pain. Premature infants may develop rib fractures as a result of rickets 8–16 weeks or longer after birth (Fig. 33–31). These bones are fragile and may fracture with handling and chest physiotherapy. Fractures may be preceded by a thin, "washed out" appearance to the ribs.
3. Long bone fractures.
   a. Can occur through the diaphysis or at the epiphyseal-metaphyseal junction, and commonly occur at either end of the humerus and proximal femur.
   b. When these fractures heal, callus and subperiosteal new bone deposition are often quite marked.
4. Skull fractures.
   a. Can be linear, buckled, or frankly depressed.
   b. Linear and buckling fractures most often occur in the parietal bone and may be suspected in the presence of cephalohematoma or other skull trauma.
   c. CT scan are more helpful than plain films for evaluation of skull fractures.

B. **Bony dysplasias**.
1. Osteogenesis imperfecta.
   a. Tarda (type I): may or may not present in the neonatal period. On x-ray, there is thinning of the long bones, ribs, and clavicles. The ribs also show flaring at the costochrondral junctions. Fractures are variable but occur through the shafts of the long bones. As fractures heal, callus formation is evident with residual curvature deformities.
   b. Osteogenesis imperfecta congenita (type II): every long bone, rib, and clavicle shows numerous fractures, with the long bones being very ballooned. Infants die shortly after birth of a restricted thorax and hypoplastic lungs.
2. Dwarfism (Common types).
   a. Achondroplasia: short extremities and marked flaring of the metaphyses. Spinal curvature and narrowed spinal canal; short, squared-off iliac wings; deep-set sacrum; flat acetabular roofs; and bulky proximal femurs are classic signs.
   b. Thanatophoric dwarfism (type I) (Fig. 33–32): marked underdevelopment of the skeleton; extremely short, bent, or curved long bones and flaring of the metaphyses. Vertebral bodies are very flat and underdeveloped. Small, narrow thorax with pulmonary hypoplasia. Cloverleaf skull may be present. Uniformly fatal in the perinatal period.

Indwelling Lines and Tubes

A. **Endotracheal tubes:**
1. Optimal placement is 1.0–1.5 cm above the carina and below the level of the clavicles.

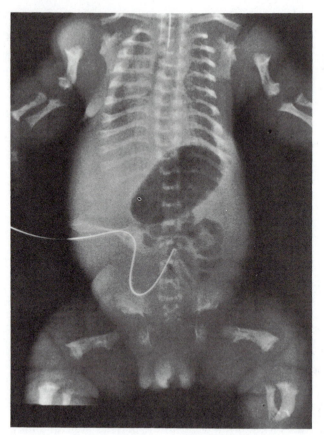

Figure 33–32
Thanatophoric dwarf. Note the small, narrow thorax and the shortness of the long bones.

2. Placement beyond the carina results in occlusion of one or the other bronchus (usually right mainstem) with subsequent atelectasis and clinical deterioration (Fig. 33–33). May also result in hyperinflation of the intubated lung.

B. **Umbilical arterial catheters** proceed from the umbilicus down toward the pelvis, make an acute turn into the internal iliac artery, continue toward the head into the bifurcation of the aorta, and move up the aorta slightly to the left of the vertebral column (Fig. 33–34, "A").

1. Low placement: L-3–L-4.
2. High placement: T-6–T-9.

C. **Umbilical venous catheters** proceed directly toward the head without making the downward loop. On lateral view, the catheter is directly distal to the abdominal wall until it passes through the ductus venosus. Correct placement is

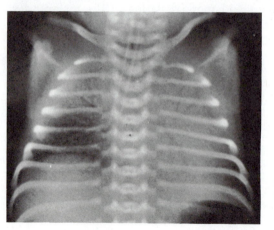

Figure 33–33
Endotracheal tube is down the right mainstem bronchus, causing atelectasis of the right upper lobe and entire left lung.

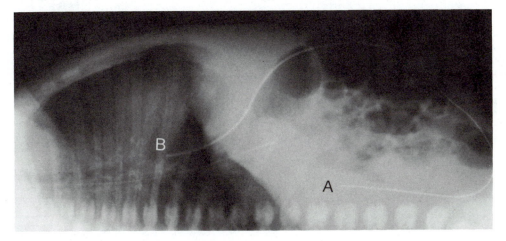

Figure 33–34
Umbilical arterial catheter **(A)** enters abdomen and proceeds distally as it enters the aorta. Umbilical venous catheter **(B)** proceeds toward the head, passes through the ductus venosus, and lies in the inferior vena cava.

above the diaphragm in the inferior vena cava and outside the right atrium (Fig. 33–34 "B").

D. Chest tubes (see Fig. 33–12).
1. X-rays are obtained to determine placement and effectiveness in reinflating the lung.
2. A lateral chest x-ray will determine if the tube is anteriorly or posteriorly placed. For air evacuation, anterior placement is desirable. For fluid evacuation, posterior placement is the general rule.
3. Correct placement will show the tube in the midclavicular line with the distal chest tube hole inside the thoracic space.

BIBLIOGRAPHY

Altman, A.R., Ball, W.S., and Kosloske, A.M.: Radiographic evaluation of the postoperative neonatal chest. Curr. Prob. Diagn. Radiol., *13*(1):1–40, 1984.
Brown Gregory, S.E.: Air leak syndromes. Neonatal Network, *5*(5):40–46, 1987.
Carty, H. and Brereton, R.J.: The distended neonate. Clin. Radiol., *34*(4):367–380, 1983.
Dillard, R.G., Crowe, J.E., and Sumner, T.E.: Pancuronium and abnormal abdominal roentgenograms. Am. J. Dis. Child., *134*(9):821–823, 1980.
Dunbar, J.S.: Nonpulmonary abnormalities recognizable in pediatric chest radiographs (review article). Radiol. Clin. North Am., *22*(3):723–740, 1984.
Edwards, D.K., Higging, C.B., and Gilpin, E.A.: The cardiothoracic ratio in newborn infants. Am. J. Roentgenol., *136*(5):907–913, 1981.
Gfeller-Varga D.A., and Felman, A.H.: Pneumoperitoneum: Diagnosis from chest radiographs. Clin. Pediatr., *19*(11):761–767, 1980.
Hilton, S.V.W., Edwards, D.K., and Hilton, J.W.: Practical Pediatric Radiology. Philadelphia; W.B. Saunders Co., 1984.
Koo, W.W.K., et al.: Radiological case of the month: Osteopenia, rickets, and fractures in preterm infants. Am. J. Dis. Child., *139*(10):1045–1046, 1985.
Miller, J.P., et al.: Neonatal abdominal calcification: Is it always meconium peritonitis? J. Pediatr. Surg., *23*(6):555–556, 1988.
Oliphant, M., et al.: Pulmonary parenchymal patterns at one month as a prognostic indicator in neonatal chronic lung disease. Perinatology-Neonatology, *11*(5):21–45, 1987.
Reingertz, H.G.: Normal radiographic heart volume in the neonate. Pediatr. Radiol., *13*(4):195–198, 1983.
Schreiner, R.L., and Bradburn, N.C. (eds.): Care of the Newborn, 2nd ed. New York, Raven Press, 1988.
Squire, L.F., and Novelline, R.A.: Fundamentals of Radiology, 4th ed. Cambridge, MA, Harvard University Press, 1988.
Swischuk, L.E.: Imaging of the Newborn, Infant, and Young Child, 3rd ed. Baltimore, Williams & Wilkins, 1989.
Vanderzalm, T.: The x-ray diagnosis. Emerg. Med., *15*(17):78–91, 1983.

Cindy Davis

Common Technical Procedures

Objectives

1. Explain the indications for various common technical procedures.

2. List the equipment and supplies necessary for performing common technical procedures.

3. Describe care and support needed for each patient undergoing technical procedures.

4. Identify anatomical landmarks for determining placement of needles or catheters for various technical procedures.

5. Describe the precautions to be familiar with for various technical procedures.

6. Describe common complications of various technical procedures.

Procedures common to the neonatal intensive care setting were once performed only by the physician. Today, the bedside nurse as well as the nurse in an expanded role performs a variety of procedures frequently and proficiently. Hospital protocols determine qualifications necessary for nurses performing these procedures.

However vital a procedure might be, the potential for complications must be considered. The patient's ability to tolerate the procedure must be weighed against the necessity of the procedure. The patient must be monitored closely during any procedure, and optimal care and support must not be compromised. Provisions must always be made for thermal support and adequate oxygenation. Documentation of the procedure and the patient's tolerance of the procedure on the patient's chart is also necessary. Informed consent may be necessary for some procedures. The nurse should be familiar with hospital protocol for obtaining informed consent. Discussing procedures with parents is important even if consent is not necessary.

For every procedure, care must be taken to adhere to universal precautions and aseptic technique, and these basic procedures should be adapted as necessary to conform to institutional and unit protocols and procedures.

Capillary Blood Sampling

A. Indications.
1. Small blood sample needed.
2. Arterial sample not necessary or possible.
3. Venous sample not necessary or possible.

B. Precautions.
1. Infection near selected puncture site.
2. Loss of skin integrity at the selected puncture site.
3. Coagulation defects.
4. Inadequate or impaired circulation in selected limb.
5. Inaccurate laboratory values may result from the following:
    a. Contamination of specimen with skin prep solution.
    b. Contamination of specimen with tissue fluid.
    c. Poor circulation at the puncture site.
    d. Hemolysis of specimen.

C. Equipment/supplies.
1. Supplies to prep for capillary blood sampling per hospital policy.
2. Lancet, tip not longer than 2.5 mm.
3. Container(s) for specimen(s).
4. Sterile gauze pad.
5. Warm (not more than 40° C) compress.

D. Technique.
1. Select puncture site on lateral or medial aspect of the heel (Fig. 34–1).
2. Warm heel.
3. Prep area selected for skin puncture per hospital policy.
4. Puncture heel perpendicular to skin.
5. Wipe away first drop of blood with sterile gauze pad.
6. Collect specimen as drops form at the puncture site.
    a. Blood flow is increased if the puncture site is dependent relative to the extremity.
    b. *Gentle* "milking" of extremity above puncture site may encourage blood flow.
    c. Squeezing and pinching at puncture site may cause hemolysis of specimen, contamination of specimen with tissue fluid, and/or bruising of extremity.

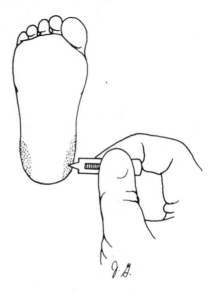

Figure 34–1
Capillary blood sampling from the heel. (From Fletcher, M.A., Mac-Donald, M.G., and Avery, G.B. (eds.): Atlas of Procedures in Neonatology. Philadelphia, J.B. Lippincott, 1983.)

7. After the specimen is collected, apply pressure with sterile gauze pad until hemostasis is ensured.

E. Complications.
1. Bruising.
2. Loss of skin integrity.
3. Infection.
4. Scarring.
5. Calcified nodules.

Venipuncture

A. Indications.
1. Arterial sample not necessary or possible.
2. Capillary sample not satisfactory or possible.

B. Precautions.
1. Infection near selected puncture site.
2. Loss of skin integrity near puncture site.
3. Coagulation defects.
4. Need to preserve venous site for possible cannulation.
5. Inadequate or impaired circulation in selected limb.

C. Equipment/supplies.
1. Supplies to prep for venipuncture per hospital policy.
2. Scalp-vein set.
3. Syringe(s) to collect specimen(s).
4. Sterile gauze pad.

D. Procedure.
1. Select vein.
   a. A gently applied tourniquet or direct pressure proximal to the potential puncture site may help by distending the vessel(s).
2. Position and stabilize area of puncture site to allow puncture in the direction of blood flow.
3. Prep area selected for puncture site.
4. Puncture skin at 15–45 degree angle just distal to planned site of vessel puncture, using shallower angle for smaller infants or for superficial vessels.
5. Advance needle slowly to puncture vessel.
   a. If resistance is met or vessel is not punctured, withdraw needle slowly to just below the level of the skin, locate vessel, and advance the needle again.
   b. If hematoma develops or bleeding occurs, occlude the vessel with pressure just proximal to the puncture site, withdraw needle, and apply pressure until hemostasis is ensured.
6. Upon entrance of blood into tubing, attach syringe and gently aspirate to obtain specimen.
7. After specimen is collected, occlude vessel with pressure just proximal to puncture site and withdraw needle.
8. Apply pressure to site until hemostasis is obtained.

E. Complications.
1. Hemorrhage.
2. Hematoma.
3. Infection.
4. Needle injury to adjacent structures.

Radial Artery Puncture

A. Indications.
1. Capillary and venous sites not satisfactory.

2. Capillary and venous samples not satisfactory.
3. Arterial line not available.

B. Precautions.
1. Infection near the selected puncture site.
2. Loss of skin integrity at the puncture site.
3. Coagulation defects.
4. Need to preserve arterial site for possible cannulation.
5. Inadequate or impaired circulation in the selected limb.
6. Inadequate collateral circulation distal to the selected puncture site.

C. Equipment/supplies.
1. Supplies to prep for arterial puncture per hospital policy.
2. Scalp-vein set.
3. Syringe(s) to collect specimen.
4. Sterile gauze pad.

D. Technique.
1. Select puncture site.
   a. Extend wrist.
   b. Palpate artery at distal wrist crease.
2. Assess collateral circulation by modified Allen's test.
   a. Elevate the hand.
   b. Apply pressure to occlude both radial and ulnar arteries.
   c. Milk hand from fingers to wrist to blanch the hand.
   d. Release pressure on ulnar artery.
   e. Adequate collateral circulation is indicated if color returns to the hand in less than 10 seconds.
3. Position and stabilize extended wrist to allow puncture against direction of arterial flow.
4. Prep area for skin puncture.
5. Puncture skin with needle at 15–45 degree angle, using shallower angle for smaller infants or more superficial arteries.
6. Advance needle slowly to puncture artery.
   a. If resistance is met, withdraw needle slowly to just below the level of the skin, palpate artery, and advance the needle again.
   b. If hematoma or bleeding develops, occlude artery with pressure just proximal to the puncture site, withdraw needle, and apply pressure until hemostasis is ensured.
7. Upon entrance of blood into tubing, attach syringe and aspirate gently to collect sample.
8. Occlude artery with pressure just proximal to puncture site and withdraw needle.
9. Apply pressure to site until hemostasis is ensured.

E. Complications.
1. Hemorrhage.
2. Hematoma.
3. Infection.
4. Distal ischemia.
   a. Arteriospasm.
   b. Hematoma.
   c. Thrombosis.
5. Needle injury to adjacent structures.

Peripheral Intravenous Line Placement

A. Indications.
1. Administration of IV fluids.

2. Administration of medications.

B. **Precautions**.

1. Infection near selected puncture site.
2. Loss of skin integrity near selected puncture site.
3. Coagulation defects.
4. Need to preserve venous site for possible cannulation.

C. **Equipment/supplies.**

1. Supplies to prep for peripheral IV placement per hospital policy.
2. Supplies for IV dressing per hospital policy.
3. Supplies for restraint, if used.
4. Scalp-vein needle or angiocatheter.
5. Sterile flush solution in small syringe.

D. **Procedure**.

1. Flush needle and tubing with flush solution. Flushing the angiocatheter is optional.
2. Select vein (Fig. 34–2).
   a. A gently applied tourniquet or pressure proximal to the intended puncture site may help distend vessel.

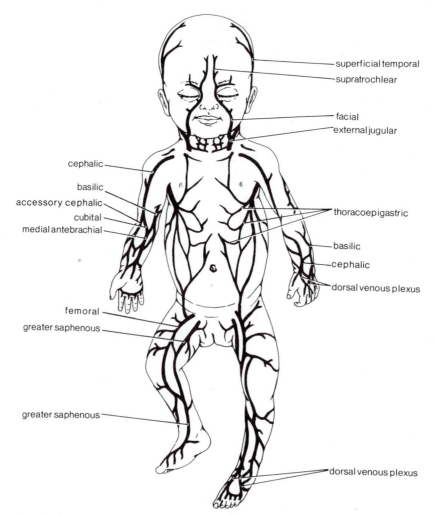

Figure 34–2
Peripheral veins. (From Fletcher, M.A., MacDonald, M.G., and Avery, G.B. (eds.): Atlas of Procedures in Neonatology. Philadelphia, J.B. Lippincott, 1983.)

3. Position and stabilize area of puncture site to allow puncture in direction of blood flow.
4. Prep area of puncture site.
5. Puncture skin at 15–45 degree angle just distal to planned site of vessel puncture, using shallower angle for smaller infants or for superficial vessels.
6. Advance needle slowly to puncture vessel.
   a. If resistance is met or vessel is not punctured, withdraw needle slowly to just below the level of the skin, locate vessel, and advance needle again.
   b. If a hematoma develops or bleeding occurs, occlude vessel with pressure just proximal to the puncture site, withdraw the needle/angiocatheter, and apply pressure until hemostasis is ensured.
7. Upon entrance of blood into the needle or tubing, remove stylet (if using angiocatheter), attach flush syringe, and flush gently to ensure position of the needle or cannula in vessel. If flush infiltrates the tissues surrounding the needle or catheter tip, occlude the vessel with pressure just proximal to the puncture site, withdraw the needle/angiocatheter, and apply pressure until hemostasis is ensured.
8. The needle or cannula may be carefully advanced in vessel while gently injecting a small amount of flush.
9. Secure and dress IV per hospital policy. Tape, dressing, and restraint must allow for easy inspection of the puncture site and circulation of the distal extremity, as well as evaluation of patency of the IV.

E. **Complications.**
1. Hemorrhage.
2. Hematoma.
3. Infection.
4. Air or clot embolus.
5. Tissue injury and possible necrosis after infiltration with infused solution and/or medication.
6. Needle injury to adjacent structures.
7. Injury to extremity from restraint.
   a. Compromised distal circulation.
   b. Pressure necrosis of tissues over bony areas.
   c. Pressure damage to peripheral nerves.
   d. Limb deformity after prolonged immobilization.
8. Inadvertent arterial line placement.

Thoracentesis

A. **Indication.**
1. Emergency evacuation of pneumothorax.

B. **Precautions.**
1. Infection near the selected puncture site.
2. Loss of skin integrity at the selected puncture site.

C. **Equipment/supplies.**
1. Supplies to prep for thoracentesis per hospital policy.
2. 23 g × ¾ inch scalp-vein set.
3. Three-way stopcock.
4. 20 ml syringe.

D. **Technique.**
1. Connect scalp-vein tubing and syringe to stopcock. The stopcock allows for aspiration of free air into the syringe and emptying of the syringe while maintaining a closed system.
2. Position infant on back, restrain if necessary.
3. Identify puncture site.

    a. Second or third intercostal space in midclavicular line.

    b. Identify and avoid breast tissue.

4. Prep area of puncture site.

5. Puncture skin at 45 degree angle just above third or fourth rib and advance needle at 90 degree angle while assistant aspirates gently.

6. When free air is obtained, stabilize the needle and continue aspiration until preparations for chest tube insertion are complete, or until the air leak is evacuated.

E. Complications.

1. Hemorrhage.

2. Infection.

3. Needle injury to lung or adjacent structures.

4. Damage to breast tissue.

Endotracheal Intubation

A. Indications.

1. Bag and mask ventilation is ineffective or undesirable.

2. Ongoing mechanical ventilation is required.

3. Tracheal suctioning is required.

B. Precautions.

1. The patient's heart rate must be monitored during the procedure, and monitoring of oxygen saturation is optimal.

2. Hypoxia during the procedure should be minimized.

    a. Free-flowing oxygen should be held near the nose and mouth of any infant with a respiratory effort to maximize oxygenation during the procedure.

    b. An intubation attempt should be stopped after 20 seconds so that the infant may be stabilized with bag and mask ventilation.

C. Equipment/supplies.

1. Laryngoscope.

2. Laryngoscope blade.

    a. Size 0 for pre-term or less than 3.5 kg infant.

    b. Size 1 for term or over 3.5 kg infant.

3. Endotracheal tube.

    a. 2.5 mm internal diameter (ID) for infants less than 1.0 kg.

    b. 3.0 mm ID for 1.0–2.0 kg infant.

    c. 3.5 mm ID for 2.0–4.0 kg infant.

    d. 4.0 mm ID may be necessary for infants over 4.0 kg.

4. Stylet, if desired.

5. Suction source and suction catheter.

6. Resuscitation bag and mask.

7. Oxygen source.

8. Supplies to secure endotracheal tube per hospital policy.

D. Procedure.

1. Select the appropriate sized endotracheal tube.

2. Insert the stylet, if used, and shape the endotracheal tube as desired. The stylet must be secured so that it does not protrude beyond the end of the endotracheal tube and cannot advance during the procedure.

3. Prepare the resuscitation bag so that the infant may be given bag and mask ventilation during the procedure, and can be hand ventilated when intubation is completed.

4. Aspirate gastric contents and suction the oropharynx.

5. Position the patient on a flat surface with the head midline and the neck slightly extended. The person performing the procedure must have easy access to the airway and equipment while positioned at the patient's head.

6. Hold the laryngoscope between the thumb and first three fingers of the left hand with the blade pointing away.
7. Open the patient's mouth with the fingers of the right hand and gently introduce the blade into the right side of the mouth.
8. Stabilizing the left hand against the left side of the patient's face, advance the blade tip to the base of the tongue and move the blade to the midline, pushing the tongue out of the way to the left.
9. Expose the pharynx by lifting the entire blade up in the direction the handle is pointing. Do not rock the tip of the blade up, using the upper gum as a fulcrum.
10. Gentle pressure applied over the trachea with the fifth finger of the left hand may help bring the glottis into view.
11. Any secretions interfering with good visualization should be removed with suctioning. Direct suctioning under laryngoscopy is ideal.
12. Identify anatomical landmarks (Fig. 34–3).
    a. The epiglottis is uppermost.
    b. The glottis is anterior, with vocal cords closing from side to side.
    c. The esophagus is posterior.
13. With vocal cords clearly identified, introduce the endotracheal tube into the right side of the patient's mouth with the right hand. Do not interfere with visualization by threading the tube through the curved laryngoscope blade.
14. Keeping the cords clearly in view, pass the endotracheal tube between the cords to the level of the vocal cord guide mark on the endotracheal tube. This will position the tip of the tube approximately midway between the vocal cords and the carina.
15. With a firm grasp on the endotracheal tube at the level of the patient's lip and stabilizing the right hand against the patient's face, carefully remove the laryngoscope with the left hand.
16. Carefully remove the stylet, if used, from the endotracheal tube.
17. Attach the resuscitation bag to the endotracheal tube and deliver manual breaths.
18. Assess tube placement.
    a. Both sides of the chest are auscultated for presence and intensity of breath sounds.
    b. Chest movement with manual breaths is assessed.
    c. The stomach is auscultated and assessed for distention.
19. If the tube is in too far and placed in a mainstem bronchus.
    a. Auscultation may reveal unilateral or unequal breath sounds.
    b. The tube should be withdrawn 0.5–1.0 cm and placement reassessed.
20. If the tube is in the esophagus.
    a. Air may be heard entering the stomach with manual breaths.
    b. The stomach may become distended.
    c. No breath sounds will be heard on auscultation of the chest during manual breaths, though air movement may be heard, especially over the lower chest.
    d. The endotracheal tube should be removed and discarded.

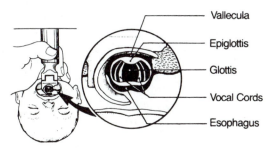

Figure 34–3
Anatomical landmarks for endotracheal intubation. (Reproduced with permission © *Textbook of Neonatal Resuscitation*, 1987. Copyright American Heart Association.)

Vallecula

Epiglottis

Glottis

Vocal Cords

Esophagus

21. When the tube is assessed to be in good position, its markings relative to the upper gum are noted, and the tube is secured per hospital policy.
22. Position of the tube must be confirmed by x-ray.
23. After tube placement is ensured by x-ray, any length of endotracheal tube that extends more than 4 cm beyond the lip should be cut off to limit dead space and the possibility of kinking.

E. Complications.
1. Hypoxia.
   a. During the procedure.
   b. Due to misplaced tube.
2. Bradycardia.
   a. Due to hypoxia.
   b. Due to vagal stimulus from laryngoscope, endotracheal tube, or suction catheter.
3. Trauma to oropharyngeal tissues.
4. Perforation of esophagus or trachea.
5. Infection.
6. Pulmonary air leak, especially with the endotracheal tube misplaced to a mainstem bronchus.
7. Loss of the endotracheal tube into esophagus or stomach after misplacement into the esophagus and disconnection from the endotracheal tube adapter.

Umbilical Artery Catheterization

A. Indications.
1. Frequent arterial blood sampling.
2. Continuous arterial blood pressure monitoring.
3. Vascular access when other sites not available or suitable.

B. Precautions.
1. Vascular compromise below level of umbilicus.
2. Abdominal wall defects.
3. Necrotizing enterocolitis.
4. Omphalitis.

C. Equipment/supplies.
1. Sterile instrument tray for umbilical catheterization.
   a. Drapes.
   b. Gauze pads.
   c. Small container for prep solution.
   d. Umbilical catheter of appropriate size.
      (1) 3.5 Fr for infants less than 1250–1500 g.
      (2) 5.0 Fr for infants over 1250–1500 g.
   e. Blunt needle adapter if catheter not designed with minimal dead space at hub.
   f. Scissor.
   g. Three-way stopcock.
   h. 10 ml syringe.
   i. Umbilical tape.
   j. No. 11 scalpel.
   k. 2 mosquito hemostats.
   l. Curved, non-toothed iris forceps.
   m. Needle holder.
   n. 4-0 silk suture with curved needle.
2. Sterile IV flush solution.
3. Sterile prep solution.

D. **Procedure.**
1. Place infant in supine position and restrain limbs if necessary.
2. Measure shoulder-umbilical distance and determine length of catheter to be inserted (Fig. 34–4).
   a. "Low position" requires catheter tip to be placed between L-3 and L-4.
   b. "High position" requires catheter tip to be placed between T-6 and T-10.
3. Prepare catheter.
   a. If not designed with minimal dead space hub, trim flared end and securely insert blunt-end needle adapter.
   b. Connect catheter or adapter to stopcock.
   c. Connect flush-filled syringe to stopcock.
   d. Fill stopcock and catheter with flush solution.
   e. Turn stopcock off to catheter.
4. Prep umbilical cord and surrounding abdomen, with assistant holding umbilical cord up out of procedure area.
5. Drape area.
6. Tie umbilical tape loosely at base of umbilical cord, to be tightened in case of bleeding.
7. Cut through umbilical cord 1.0–1.5 cm from skin.
8. Identify cord vessels.
   a. Vein is single, large, thin-walled vessel, often open.
   b. Arteries are two small, thick-walled constricted vessels.
9. Stabilize umbilical cord stump to best expose selected artery.
   a. Grasp portion of cut edge of cord with hemostat and apply gentle traction.
   b. Apply hemostats to opposite sides of the cut cord and roll them away from each other, causing the arteries to protrude from the cut surface of the cord.
10. Dilate artery.
    a. Insert one tip of curved iris forceps into selected artery and probe gently to depth of about 0.5 cm.
    b. With tips of forceps together, gently probe artery to depth of about 0.5 cm.
    c. Allow tips of forceps to gently spring apart, then slowly withdraw forceps from artery, dilating lumen as forceps is withdrawn.
    d. Continue to dilate lumen until forceps can easily be inserted about 1.0 cm into artery and catheter can be inserted into the vessel.
11. Insert catheter.
    a. With gentle traction on the cord stump toward the patient's head, insert catheter into the dilated vessel.

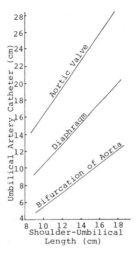

Figure 34–4
Umbilical artery catheter insertion length for shoulder-umbilical length. (Adapted from Dunn, P.M.: Arch. Dis. Child, *41*:69, 1966; *in* Cole, C.H. (ed.): The Harriet Lane Handbook, 10th ed. Chicago, Year Book Medical Publishers, 1984, p. 278.)

b. Advance catheter predetermined distance.
   (1) If resistance is met, *do not force catheter.* Apply steady, gentle pressure to catheter, with gentle traction on the cord.
   (2) If catheter cannot be advanced desired distance, discontinue attempts and catheterize second artery.
12. Aspirate blood to ensure catheter's presence in vessel. If blood cannot be aspirated, remove catheter and attempt catheterization of second artery.
13. Secure catheter.
    a. Place purse-string suture around the cord. Avoid piercing the vessels and the skin.
    b. Knot suture securely in cord close to catheter, then loop suture around catheter and secure additional knots.
    c. Suture around catheter must be tight enough to prevent catheter from sliding, but not so tight that flow through the catheter is obstructed.
14. Remove umbilical tape.
15. Temporarily tape flat loop of catheter to abdomen.
16. Confirm catheter position by x-ray.
    a. If catheter tip is too high, securing suture is removed and catheter is pulled back necessary distance and re-sutured.
    b. If catheter tip is too low for "high position" placement, it may be pulled back to "low position."
    c. If catheter tip is too low for "low position" placement, it must be removed.
    d. A catheter that is no longer sterile may not be advanced into the patient to adjust placement.
17. Tape catheter to abdomen using "bridge" or "goalpost" taping technique (Fig. 34–5).

E. **Complications.**
1. Mechanical.
   a. Perforation of vessels.
   b. Perforation of peritoneum.
   c. False aneurysm.
   d. Knot in catheter.
2. Vasospasm/embolism.
   a. Blanching/cyanosis/mottling of skin.
   b. Sloughing of skin.
   c. Necrosis of extremities.
   d. Intestinal necrosis and perforation.
   e. Necrotizing enterocolitis.
   f. Hypertension.
   g. Paraplegia.
3. Infection.
   a. Septicemia.

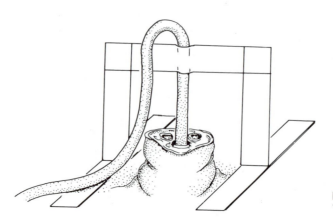

Figure 34–5
"Bridge" or "goalpost" taping technique.

   b. Septic arthritis.

   c. Osteomyelitis.

BIBLIOGRAPHY

American Heart Association: Textbook of Neonatal Resuscitation. Dallas, 1987.

Fletcher, M.A., MacDonald, M.G., and Avery, G.B. (eds.): Atlas of Procedures in Neonatology. Philadelphia, J.B. Lippincott, 1983.

Klaus, M.H., and Fanaroff, A.A.: Appendix I–2: Umbilical vessel catheterization. In Klaus, M.H., and Fanaroff, A.A. (eds.).: Care of the High-Risk Neonate, 3rd ed. Philadelphia, W.B. Saunders Co., 1986.

Stavis, R.L., and Krauss, A.N.: Complications of neonatal intensive care. Clin. Perinatol., 7(1):107–124, 1980.

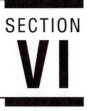
CURRENT ISSUES AND TRENDS IN NEONATAL CARE

Wendy Cornell

CHAPTER

35

Research

Objectives

1. Stimulate interest of RNs in neonatal intensive care units (NICUs) in becoming involved with research projects that can improve the quality of neonatal care.

2. Provide basic information regarding the research process to guide understanding of avenues for nursing staff application.

3. Encourage appropriate utilization of research findings in daily practice.

4. Examine issues of patient advocacy in neonatal research participation.

5. Promote creative thinking regarding ideas that can become the basis for neonatal nursing research.

Neonatal care environments are ripe for nursing research. The situations that the nurse in the NICU encounters daily can provide the basis for a myriad of nursing studies. Through research, effective care practices can be demonstrated, the impact of nursing care on patient outcomes can be studied, and elimination of unnecessary interventions can be facilitated. This chapter is designed to provide the bedside practitioner with some basic research knowledge to stimulate creative ideas and critical thinking. Initiating research takes commitment and awareness of the research process but is within the realm of the practicing nurse. Those who do not actively participate in research studies can evaluate the results of other practitioners to determine whether changes in practice are appropriate. Although our neonatal patients are entered into many medical research studies, our nursing-focused studies can have a different impact. Competition for neonatal research subjects in the NICU has not yet become an issue for nursing in most hospitals, but it may be indicative of our undertaking the challenge of neonatal nursing research in the future. Thoughtful consideration of our nursing research priorities, and the benefit of this work to our patients, needs to be articulated.

Basic Principles of Research

A. **Purposes of nursing research.**
1. Contributes to nursing science through:

a. Generation of information that improves understanding of human health-related experiences.

b. Re-affirmation of knowledge.

c. Expansion of existing nursing knowledge.

2. Facilitates nursing practice improvement by:

a. The discovery and/or verification of information that develops the scientific knowledge base of the nursing process (rather than relying on ritual as the determiner of practice).

b. Identification of models for care delivery that enhance efficient use of available resources while ensuring quality care.

3. Determines cost effectiveness in care delivery to:

a. Document the value of nursing care.

b. Demonstrate the cost savings of nursing interventions.

c. Examine the practices that may lead to more efficient patterns of caregiving.

4. Identifies the impact of nursing care on patient outcomes in:

a. Assessing alterations in length of stay related to nursing interventions.

b. Demonstrating use of interventions that promote health.

c. Promoting use of anticipatory nursing practices in various situations.

B. **Methods of nursing research.**

1. Study designs include a variety of ways to collect, analyze, and evaluate data to answer specific research questions.

a. Laboratory studies create a special environment for study subjects.

b. Field studies are conducted in real-life surroundings.

c. Retrospective studies examine phenomena of current interest via searching information available from the past. In contrast, prospective studies involve a future-oriented approach to data gathering.

d. Experimental studies manipulate or control the independent variable and then observe effects.

e. Non-experimental studies (descriptive and correlational research) do not include manipulation or control of the independent variable. The status of phenomena is summarized (or relationships are studied as they naturally occur).

f. Longitudinal studies involve long-term study of subjects (ex post facto) versus cross-sectional studies, which study one point in time.

g. Qualitative studies (phenomenological or grounded theory) uses descriptions of events or people to determine themes or patterns versus quantitative studies, which involve numerical data collections and statistical analysis to determine relationships among variables.

2. The most appropriate means of answering the research questions or testing the research hypothesis influences decisions in study methodology, including:

a. Target population identification.

b. Reliable and valid measurement of the variables.

c. Sample size and method of selection.

d. Data analysis methods.

C. **Research ethics.**

1. The rights of study subjects are incorporated in the researcher's fundamental responsibilities to safeguard the individual subject and are concerned with the welfare and societal value of humans.

a. parental consent is required for unemancipated minors.

b. Informed consent: provision of sufficient information (with a measure of assurance that individual understanding of what is expected is present) to provide non-coercive participation.

c. Confidentiality ensures that individual information shared will not be made public or available to others to maintain the privacy and dignity of the subject.

d. Anonymity assures that information shared cannot be linked with a particular subject, even by the researcher.

e. Subjects have a right to refuse to participate (or drop out of the study at any time) and still receive standard quality care.
2. Study benefit.
   a. Physical and psychological risks must be avoided; the scientific merit of the information gained must be worth the effort, cost, and potential risk and/or discomfort.
   b. Usefulness of results (the merit of knowledge enhancement) must be weighed against the potential impact on a greater population (the risk of the study).
   c. Avoidance of harm to subjects addresses the issues of vulnerability of study subjects, including:
      (1) Subjection to additional tests or procedures.
      (2) Temporary discomfort versus permanent damage.
      (3) Loss of privacy or confidentiality.
3. Responsibilities of researcher include:
   a. Scientific objectivity, truthfulness, and integrity; impeccable care of data gathered; honest disclosure of findings; and clarification and communication of results.
      (1) Competence of research denotes the ability of researcher to successfully complete the study, through understanding the complexities of the process and the potential risks and benefits to the study population.
      (2) An institutional review board approves the study process to ensure appropriate consent procedures and protection measures (to prevent undue risk or loss of personal rights and dignity).

Identifying Research Questions

A. **Clinical patient care experience** can provide curiosities, special interests, misconceptions, and insights that generate questions related to nursing care that are fruitful sources of research problems.
1. Topics may provide ideas and limitless questions regarding why practices and observations are as they are; how trends and patterns emerge and relate; what research has been done; and when enough knowledge is gathered to justify changes or continuation of current practices.
   a. Issues related to differences in treatment determine if relationships between different practices can be demonstrated and replicated (to provide generalizability to additional situations or populations).
   b. Creative ideas related to unresolved patient concerns use hunches and strong suspicions that can be studied (to provide solutions to nagging questions or bothersome problems).
   c. Patterns noted over time that are non-published phenomena can transform multiple individual experiences into a logical pattern.
2. Problems previously researched may provide suggestions for additional study and can indicate findings that are not working as predicted (or do not make sense). May note discrepancies that need further review or describe alternative explanations for findings that need to be tested.
   a. Inconclusive or contradictory results identify inconsistent findings or variations from anticipated results in practical application, which suggest a need for further research.
   b. Generalizability of results to other populations of patients relates the application of findings to a larger or different population, which bears exploration.

B. **Nursing practice questions** can assist in the development of a scientific base for clinical practice to advance nursing knowledge.
1. Systematic inquiry into the nursing care practices that influence patient care

outcomes will verify care practices and test interventions to improve patient care and promote effective use of time and resources.

2. Intellectual interests stimulate personal motivation and spur the continued interest and tenacity that are required to complete research projects.

3. Theory generation involves the development and testing of existing theories to generate knowledge and guide practice.

C. **Study feasibility** denotes a responsible assurance that the study can be carried out.

1. Measurability of the variables must validly reflect the concepts being studied.

2. Assessment of study subject access includes the availability of sufficient numbers of subjects who are willing and able to participate and an appraisal of concurrent studies that may conflict with accessibility.

3. Time, money, equipment, and personnel issues include:
   a. Time needed for development and completion of the study as well as the involvement of the participants.
   b. Expenses for printing, testing, participating, facilities, and computation of results.
   c. Research support for methodological review, statistical analysis, budget and financial administration.
   d. Availability of clinical experts and support staff.

Steps in the Research Process

A. **Problem identification** provides detail regarding the phenomena to be studied.

1. Narrowing the topic involves the selection of a few high-priority (very specific) variables that are measurable and may have potential for generalizability of the findings.

2. Formulating the question provides a statement of what provided the impetus for the study, the scope of the problem, the significance of the research, and the questions to be answered by the study.

3. Study variables are comprised of independent variables (that define the intervention or relationship that is manipulated or observed by the investigator) and have an effect on the dependent or outcome variables.

B. **Definition** of the study purpose and significance to nursing.

1. Justification for study specifies the value of the results to nursing practice and who will benefit from the information (generalizability of the knowledge to others).

2. Expectation for use of results may include:
   a. Validation of existing knowledge.
   b. Exploration of new ideas.
   c. Definition of patterns or concept interrelationships.
   d. Documentation of outcomes.

C. **Review of the literature** incorporates a search for a broader perspective of the problem or question to be studied.

1. Methods used in organizing and approaching an analysis of existing literature.
   a. Computer searches involve selection of key words of research question (may use headings from literature indices); reference librarian assistance is most helpful.
   b. Indices and abstracts that have reference listings and overviews of that content in published literature are available in most medical or nursing libraries.
   c. A variety of literature sources may provide valuable information on nursing and other related topics.
      (1) Nursing research is shared through journals, abstracts, books, bibliogra-

phies, unpublished theses, published reports of presentations at professional conferences, and personal communication with other researchers.

(2) Medical research is communicated through medical professional literature and may contain some related nursing content.

(3) Theoretical knowledge pursuits involve review of nursing and other discipline's frameworks (to determine what knowledge has been gained); stimulation of new practice ideas; and recommendations or directions for appropriate methods to answer research questions.

(4) Methodological reports provide studies of the development, evaluation, and testing of various research methods and instruments.

(5) Other research studies impart pertinent findings from other disciplines that may contain applicable content for nursing.

(6) Popular books, articles, and lay literature can produce ideas and approaches to conceptualizing research questions.

2. Note taking facilitates a critical analysis of results and exploration of the effectiveness of previous methods.

a. Examining knowns, versus unknowns involves contemplating the adequacy of research to the present.

(1) The extent of knowledge currently available supplies parameters of known information to define direction for additional study.

(2) Support for previous results may be verified with additional research (by demonstrating consistent findings) or rebutted through different results (outcomes).

(3) Identification of conceptual or theoretical frameworks that have guided study of the research question may be provided.

b. Methods used in previous studies should indicate the reliability, validity, and effectiveness attained.

(1) Study design includes a definition of participants, observations of variables, setting, time, and the role of the researcher.

(2) Sample size considers calculated adequacy to maximize the validity of the results.

(3) Results support or dispute the framework of study, note limitations, and describe the significance.

(4) Conclusions incorporate a demonstration of the meaning and worth of the research and can provide data-based generalizations.

c. Preparing the text includes summarization of significant earlier work with interpretations and their relationship to the present study.

3. Compilation of individual reports provides documentation of citations in a consistent, approved format and organizes the information in logical sequences.

a. Analysis of content contains an outline of reviews with concepts relating to current study and notations of consistencies and inconsistencies that underscore the importance of the proposed study.

D. **Development** of a conceptual or theoretical framework integrates diverse information to clarify assumptions, define variables, and provide direction for the conduct of the research.

1. Clarification of concepts involves communication of the focus of the study to aid understanding of the abstract ideas and phenomena under investigation.

2. Assumptions denote statements that are accepted as true for the purposes of the study.

3. Definitions of relationships among concepts provide the blueprint of how the generalizations in the study fit together.

E. **Limitations** of the study indicate the effects of additional variables that need to be factored into the study.

1. Other relevant variables that may confuse interpretation of the results are defined as uncontrolled variables.

2. Generalizability of findings to other populations and settings increases with attainment of a representative sample.

F. **Hypothesis formation** and research questions describe the prediction of relationships between variables.
1. Independent variables are naturally occurring or can be manipulated or controlled to have an effect on the outcome variable.
2. Dependent variables describe the effect (outcome) that is contingent on another variable.

G. **Study terms** and variable definition specify the terminology to assure clarity of meaning for readers.
1. Operational definitions convey an explanation of how the variables will be measured or observed.
2. Specification of population defines to whom the study results apply.
   a. Inclusion criteria designate guidelines for characteristics required to participate in the study.
   b. Exclusion criteria eliminate some participants who may confound the interpretation of the results.
   c. Study setting considerations include the availability of relevant subjects in a feasible population and location to assure a representative sample.

H. **Selection of research design** involves a determination of the most workable plan to answer the research question.
1. Types (different approaches to data gathering and analysis).
   a. Descriptive designs are used to identify or describe concepts.
   b. Comparative designs explore the contrasts between two or more groups.
   c. Experimental designs integrate scientific inquiry into the study of cause-and-effect relationships.
2. Data collection approaches include observation, recording of available data, and administration of standardized or developed instruments.
   a. Interviews facilitate the study process in gaining understanding of participants' perceptions through verbal questioning.
   b. Participant observation involves researcher interaction with subjects and observations of behaviors that can be covert or overt.
   c. Document analysis includes examination of records for analysis relating to research question (whether the data source was developed for that specific purpose).
   d. Correlation surveys examine the strength of the relationship between or among variables.
   e. Comparative surveys involve a retrospective look at relationships between what is existing and something that occurred in the past.
   f. Case studies employ an intensive investigation of people, groups, or situations that usually are naturally occurring.
   g. Prospective studies plan a futuristic approach to the study of the effect that an intervention or event will have on outcome variables.
   h. Retrospective studies provide a historical review of known effects and their potential causes.

I. **Sample selection** incorporates decisions regarding whom to study to assure systematic and representative selection from the larger population.
1. Probability sampling.
   a. Random sampling connotes that every element of the population has an equal chance to be a participant.
   b. Systematic sampling defines a preset strategy of selection from the population (e.g., every third person).
   c. Stratified sampling divides the population into stratified subsets and randomly selects a proportionate number of subjects from the subsets.
   d. Cluster sampling includes successive random sampling that breaks down the population into smaller and smaller units, in stages.
2. Non-probability sampling is non-random selection, which can decrease the chance of attaining a representative sample.

    a. Convenience sampling uses a relevant, available subject group.

    b. Expert sampling employs a choice of samples from experts in the area of the research question.

    c. Quota sampling involves dividing the population into stratified subsets, then selecting the sample in a non-random fashion that may be representative.

3. Sample size calculations take into consideration the variance error, anticipated effect size, and type of design planned (number of variables being studied).

    a. Homogeneity versus heterogeneity of study phenomena is postulated (smaller samples can be used for homogeneous populations).

    b. Achievement of statistical significance requires adequate sample size to note that a significant relationship exists.

    c. Effect size connotes the expected degree of magnitude of findings in the population studied.

    d. Study participation expectations acknowledge reluctance to participate, usual response rates for different methodologies, and availability of subjects.

J. **Data measurement planning** outlines a systematic process for gathering information from sources, for ease of analysis.

1. Organization of data is formulated prior to implementation of the study and provides a logical summarization framework.

    a. Instrument development and evaluation specify data to be measured and how the information will be recorded.

    b. Computer program development for the coding, entry, and analysis of data.

    c. Promotion of legibility and completeness (which influences the usefulness of data) and a standard approach to interpretation and methods of collection.

       (1) Plan for how incomplete data will be used and analyzed.

       (2) Interim analysis can allow for additional clarification of incomplete or questionably interpretable data.

2. Statistical analysis provides systematic interpretation of findings (in relation to the study problem) and is influenced by the type of data collected (use of statistician advice is recommended).

    a. Descriptive statistics organize and summarize information.

       (1) Frequency distribution arranges number values from lowest to highest.

       (2) Measures of central tendency describe the middle, general trend of the number findings (mean, median, and mode).

       (3) Measures of variability define ways that measure groups together (range, interquartile range, standard deviation, confidence intervals, standard error).

       (4) Measures of correlation denote the extent to which variables are related to each other (correlation coefficients).

    b. Inferential statistics assist in generalization of the sample characteristics to the larger population but cannot be used with all types of data.

       (1) The null hypothesis is a statement that no relationship exists between variables being considered, and differences can only be due to chance.

       (2) A defined level of significance denotes the probability that differences between sets of data are due to chance (acceptable levels are usually 0.01 or 0.05).

K. **Interpretation** of findings describes the search for the meaning and implication of the results.

1. Substantiation of the research hypothesis or question and affirmation of the conceptual framework of the study warrant pursuit of broader meaning of the results.

2. Analysis of the study design ascertains that the validity of the results is considered in light of the methods used and that plausible alternative explanations are examined.

3. Comparison with previous studies explores the relationship of new results to earlier study and theory.

4. The implications for nursing incorporate an assessment of what changes may be needed in practice, education, and research based on study findings.

L. **Dissemination** of research findings promotes communication of results, provides suggested changes in approaches for practice, and supplies ideas for concentration of research efforts.
1. Submission of articles and/or abstracts to journals, books, and other publications provides opportunities to discuss the study and findings.
2. Poster sessions involve preparation of abstracts and poster presentations regarding the study results for conferences, in hospitals and public displays.
3. Oral presentations contain concise, descriptive study reviews that are audience focused and communicate findings to others.

The Role of Research in Neonatal Nursing

A. **Quality of care issues** have heightened concern regarding quality improvement and consumer advocacy and provide new impetus to review practice.
1. Systematic evaluation of care focuses efforts (documenting the value of nursing care practices) in light of patient outcomes and nursing time economies.
   a. Efficiencies in practice versus routine (historical) methods of care provision require exploration to determine their effectiveness, cost, and impact on neonates.
      (1) Development of standards of care provides expected outcome measures (which need to be defined and tested in the hospital setting) to promote the standardization of practice through consistent knowledge bases of neonatal nursing care providers.
      (2) Exploration of the long-term effects of neonatal practice, practice implications for morbidity and mortality, and mechanisms to promote staff satisfaction through professional practice are needed.
   b. Avoidance of the "cookbook method" of caregiving (total reliance on strict adherence to policies and procedures) promotes attention to assessment of the individual infant and the integration of new research findings, as well as a willingness to explore new methods of caregiving in the dynamic environment of the NICU.
      (1) Research result critiques evaluate the validity of findings and determine if sufficient reliability exists to justify acceptance and changes in practice.
      (2) Credibility that findings may be replicated and demonstrated (for more than just the study situation) allows for incorporation into individual practice patterns.
2. The communication and value of the research to the practitioner impacts the use of study findings.
   a. Progressive change involves frequent review of new information that has been introduced in a manner that is perceived as useful and timely.
      (1) Critical analysis of new data (by those with neonatal expertise who have an awareness of practice standards) is valuable in consideration of nursing care changes based on study results. New material is better accepted when the practice framework of the unit is understood and patient advocacy guides caregiving.
      (2) Consideration of the impact of relinquishing old beliefs (when the mastery of old practices had enhanced self-esteem) affects the introduction of changes. Subtle outcomes may be more difficult to see, thereby reducing the visibility of the reinforcement for practice changes.
   b. Technology versus common sense and caring denotes the balance that needs to be maintained between the value of nursing (intuitive, sensible caregiving) with the development of high-technology tools in neonatal practice.
      (1) Because of rapid changes in caregiving (with limited supporting evidence), studies of the impact of recent advances are needed to provide

the reassurance that approaches to care have been productive and cost effective. Some resistance to change is inherent in rapid technological development with limited time for testing and gaining of expertise.

(2) Substantiating clinical observations in day-to-day practice provides fruitful ground for questions that need to be studied and verified. Caregivers have the expertise in observing patterns and suggesting relationships between variables.

B. **Specialists** in neonatal nursing care need continued opportunities for intellectual stimulation and demonstration of their value to practice to promote their full professional growth.

1. Establishment of a specific interest area (through familiarization with a body of specialized knowledge and advanced nursing care) is useful in professional presentations and for consultation with other, less expert staff.
    a. Creating experts among neonatal nurses involves:
        (1) Development of a particular area of interest, concern, or growth.
        (2) Utilization of opportunities for exploration and advanced knowledge development (which is then acknowledged and valued by colleagues).
    b. Conquering concerns through acceptance of a life-long need to continue learning includes:
        (1) Acknowledgement of the limitations of experts.
        (2) Ability to stand out and take risks, which enables the development and practical use of specialized knowledge.
2. Recognition of diversity in practice and rewards for advanced knowledge are personally valuable and marketable.
    a. Personal growth with the accumulation of knowledge through research and critical thinking promotes advanced practice and respect among interdisciplinary team members.
    b. Expansion of goals to include the versatility and accomplishment of research improves marketability and provides additional career opportunities.
3. Peer support and education can be provided through thoughtful, rational explanation of study results and nursing implications and can assist in the introduction of change and enhancement of patient care.
    a. Appropriate evaluation of the nursing implications by bedside care providers increases the likelihood of improved patient care through use of new knowledge.
    b. Encouraging staff participation through use of peers in unit-based research increases involvement, commitment to the process, and interest in the outcomes.
4. Much opportunity exists for developing the unique knowledge base of neonatal nursing through nursing research, and many people will be needed to fill the gaps in what is beneficial practice versus historical routine.

Interdisciplinary Research: Implications for Nursing

A. **Participation prerogatives** involve assessment of the level of commitment to research to determine the extent to which participation is a priority.

1. The study benefit must be considered in regard to the time expenditure (nursing investment) in the study process because more resources may be required than are available.
    a. Proposal development feasibility considerations include the anticipated workload for all participating (assuring that the most efficient use of time is promoted and agreed to by subjects and staff).
    b. Coordinating research and caregiving studies that require interventions with infants necessitates consideration of:
        (1) The care patterns and unique patient needs (to avoid interference or additional stress).

      (2) Needs that staff have in determining methods to incorporate study requirement into their care delivery process (to assure adherence to study procedures while maintaining care standards).

    c. Unit nurse managers and clinical specialists must be supportive and approving of all clinical studies that involve patients and staff.

2. Ethical considerations incorporate patient advocacy (the hallmark of NICU nursing and a major factor in the acceptance and involvement of staff in research studies), because these fundamental concepts must be considered, to avoid dilemmas for staff between personal values and plans for study.

    a. The intensity of nursing involvement with infants and families provides a strong basis for individual beliefs about the benefits of interventions. The ramifications of a particular study must be perceived to have a definite, beneficial impact without jeopardizing an already stressed family and staff unit.

    b. Support of studies is remarkably strong when staff can appreciate the value of the results to their patients or practice (even when the time requirements may seem excessive).

    c. Nursing leadership support and encouragement are essential to the progress and promotion of research efforts.

3. Juggling studies on tiny infants can become an issue in any NICU, when multiple research protocols are concurrently being conducted (and can impact on the availability of subjects and the possible interference in the progress of any particular study).

    a. Awareness of the contents of ongoing research can assist in assuring that infants are not overwhelmed by study interventions yet receive the benefit of experimental therapies that promote improved health and development.

    b. Data collection chaos can be minimized by coordination of study paperwork (an imperative when multiple trials are ongoing) to eliminate confusion with staff and increase the reliability of the results achieved.

4. The dynamic nature and seemingly constant change that are inherent in the NICU environment necessitate an ability of nursing staff to continually update and communicate their knowledge and skills.

    a. Organizing for efficiency involves establishing networks or communication pathways among staff than can assist in maintaining awareness of changes and advances.

    b. Critical analysis of studies, through journal review forums and community meetings with other care providers, can provide opportunities for discussion of new information and plans for additional research questions.

B. **In addition to participating directly** in research, nurses can provide research questions and concerns for others to consider.

1. Clinical insights regarding the patterns and potential relationships noted in caregiving can provide fertile topics for practical research.

2. Advances in caregiving skills and assessments may elicit nagging concerns that can be addressed through research.

C. **Promoting acceptance** of research with families and/or staff needs to be incorporated into the repertoire of staff practice because research is a fundamental component of many NICUs.

1. Acceptance of participation in study protocols is balanced with the caregiving needs and the ethical concerns that research elicits. Staff members need orientation to the studies and research milieu of the unit, with appropriate opportunities to discuss their concerns and suggestions.

2. Nursing leadership's provision of a welcoming environment for expression of feelings and concerns relating to research will enhance the ability of staff to participate in studies and may allow for development of a more efficient research process.

D. **Mechanisms for assuring** that staff are informed of research outcomes can provide positive feedback for involvement as well as enhance knowledge.

1. Reviewing results through expert staff analysis of new information in discussion with staff nurses is helpful in assuring that research is evaluated for merit.
2. Integration of findings and suggestions for change require attention to staff acceptance (and acknowledgment of the benefit of the changes to their practice). Effective change strategies need to be employed.
3. The great amount of neonatal information can be overwhelming to staff, and finding creative methods to promote continued attention to new ideas is imperative.

STUDY QUESTIONS

1. NICU nursing staff have an obligation to participate in research when:
   a. Families know nothing about the study.
   b. Nursing staff members have not been fully briefed on the study.
   c. Patient care will not be compromised.

2. A consideration that is essential to the critique of research findings is:
   a. A consistent, thorough approach to review of the components of reported studies.
   b. Expert knowledge of statistical analyses to assure accuracy in reporting of results.
   c. Reader familiarity with research designs and methodology.

3. The feasibility of a study depends on:
   a. Availability of an attending physician.
   b. Number of staff in the unit.
   c. Opportunity for commitment of staff time and energy as agreed by nursing leadership.

4. The decision to effect changes in neonatal practice based on study results depends on:
   a. How long the current practice has been in place.
   b. Participation in data collection by all staff.
   c. Thorough review of findings, discussion of implications for care and care providers, and a plan to evaluate the impact of the change on the patient, unit, and staff.

5. The responsibility of determining whether the benefit of a study is sufficient to encourage the participation of NICU staff, patients, and families rests with whom?
   a. Leadership staff and attending physicians.
   b. The bedside nurse and patient's family.
   c. The hospital review board.

6. Which of the following can facilitate the integration of research into NICU nursing practice?
   a. Availability of books about research on the unit.
   b. How many years of college the staff nurses have completed.
   c. Leadership support in creating forums for dissemination of research findings.

7. The first, basic step of the research process includes:
   a. Securing grants.
   b. Obtaining parental consents.
   c. Defining the study questions or hypotheses.

Answers to Study Questions

1. c	4. c	6. c
2. a	5. c	7. c
3. c		

REFERENCES

Donabedian, A.: Criteria and standards for quality assessment and monitoring. Quality Review Bulletin 12(3):99–108, 1986.

Goodwin, L.D., and Goodwin, W.L.: Qualitative vs. quantitative research or qualitative and quantitative research. Nurs. Res., 33(6):378–380, 1984.

Lieske, A.M. (ed.): Clinical Nursing Research. Rockville, MD, Aspen, 1986.

Meier, P.: Research methodologies in neonatal nursing. Neonatal Network, 2(2):16–22, 1983.

Nieswiadomy, R.M.: Foundations of Nursing Research. Norwalk, CT, Appleton & Lange, 1987.

Penticuff, J.H.: Neonatal nursing ethics: Toward a consensus. Neonatal Network, 5(6):7–16, 1987.

Polit, D.F., and Hungler, B.P.: Nursing Research: Principles and Practice, 3rd ed. Philadelphia, JB Lippincott, 1987.

Sexton, D.L.: Presentation of research findings: The poster session. Nurs. Res. 33(6):374–375, 1984.

Tanner, C.A., and Lindeman, C.A.: Using Nursing Research. National League for Nursing, 1989.

Ward, M.J., and Fetler, M.E.: What guidelines should be followed in critically evaluating research reports? Nurs. Res., 28(2):120–125, 1979.

Wilson, H.S. (ed.): Introducing Research in Nursing. Menlo Park, CA, Addison-Wesley, 1987.

Wilson, H.S.: Research in Nursing, 2nd ed. Redwood City, CA, Addison-Wesley, 1989.

Woods, N.F., and Catanzaro, M.: Nursing Research Theory and Practice. St. Louis, C.V. Mosby, 1988.

Joy Hinson Penticuff

Ethical Issues

Objectives

1. Describe ethical principles that guide practice in high-risk neonatal nursing.

2. Evaluate ethical decision making in neonatal intensive care.

3. Analyze key elements that result in ethical dilemmas in high-risk neonatal nursing.

4. Discuss resources for resolving ethical dilemmas, including institutional ethics committees.

This chapter deals with the ethical aspects of high-risk neonatal nursing. It is important to recognize that although ethics is being dealt with in a separate chapter, in fact, the ethical foundations presented here underlie the entirety of the nurse's practice. This is because nursing ethics has to do with our obligation to do good and to avoid doing harm to those in our care. Thus, when we strive to refine our clinical skills and to become more expert in carrying out complex humanistic and technical care, we are acting ethically. On the other hand, if we accept an assignment for which we are not clinically competent, we are acting unethically just as surely as if we tell an untruth. Unfortunately, the standard approach in many articles and books on nursing ethics has been to compartmentalize nursing ethics as though it deals only with ethical dilemmas. In reality, ethics is a part of every nursing action, because in each action we potentially do either good or harm to the patient. With this broad approach to nursing ethics, we now turn to a discussion of major ethical principles that guide nursing practice, ethical decision making, and prevention and resolution of ethical dilemmas in high-risk neonatal nursing.

Definitions

A. **Nursing ethics:** moral evaluation of behavior as good or harmful and moral duty and obligation in the practice of nursing.

B. **Principle of beneficence:** a rule of conduct that emphasizes the obligation to do good to others.

C. **Principle of non-maleficence:** a rule of conduct that emphasizes the obligation to avoid doing harm to others.

D. **Principle of respect for autonomy:** a rule of conduct that emphasizes the obligation to respect the fundamental right of the adult person to live according to his or her own values and goals. Inherent in the idea of autonomy is the notion of the person as a moral agent who is capable of understanding options, of reflecting on his or her values and life goals and making a decision, and of communicating decisions to others. Because of these competency issues, autonomy is usually viewed as the rational adult's right to self-determination. Infants and children are not considered autonomous because of their limited ability to comprehend, decide, and communicate.

E. **Principle of justice:** a doctrine that emphasizes the obligation to treat persons fairly, especially in the allocation of scarce health care resources.

F. **Ethic of care:** a doctrine that emphasizes the obligation to deal with patients and families in ways that consistently express a genuine sense of concern for their well being, an intention to help, and a recognition of each individual as a whole person, with values and life goals worthy of our respect.

G. **Ethical dilemma:** a situation in which a patient experiences or might experience harm because of violation of ethical principles, obligations, or values; or a situation in which it is difficult to determine what is morally right because ethical principles, obligations, or values are in conflict. In an ethical dilemma, there is no clear, morally right answer. Careful identification, consideration, and evaluation of the morally relevant aspects of the situation can assist in reaching a reasoned conclusion.

Principles of Ethics

The ethical principles defined in the previous section provide a basic foundation for nursing. But putting these principles into effect in daily practice is a challenging and difficult endeavor. The principles are actually ideals, and they reflect the ethical traditions of nursing through the centuries. Although nursing practice has changed remarkably over the past hundred years, the principles of doing good for others, avoiding doing harm, respecting the rights of others to live according to their own goals, and treating people fairly continue to be the essential reasons for everything we do in nursing.

Because each principle embodies a part of nursing's ethical tradition, it is important to understand that many ethical dilemmas are actually situations in which principles, values, or obligations come into conflict. Ethical practice requires that we go beyond a simple applying of ethical principles or a straightforward recognition of obligations, values, and goals. Ethical practice requires an evaluation of what the principles mean and which principles and obligations take precedence in each situation. Ethical practice requires not only our cognitive knowledge of the principle of beneficence, for example, but also an examination of what is good for a particular infant in our care. For one infant, doing good is to honor the parents' request to terminate life-sustaining

treatment. For another infant, doing good is to obtain a court order to institute life-sustaining treatment. How are we to decide the bewildering ethical decisions that confront us?

Ethical Decision Making

Ethical decision making is the process of coming to a conclusion about what is morally right to do in an ethical dilemma. This process is similar in some respects to the nursing process, with which many nurses are familiar. However, ethical decision making may seem different from nursing process because our feelings about the dilemma are often intense. Nurses may experience "ethical anguish" and even "ethical outrage" when they are confronted with dilemmas in clinical practice. In perinatal nursing, deeply held values about the sanctity of human life and the realization that our technology cannot promise intact survival can result in many mixed feelings as we attempt to do what is best for infants and childbearing families.

Thompson and Thompson (1985) and Pellegrino (1987) provide a flexible guide for the processes by which nurses make ethical decisions in perinatal care. The procedures include the following:

A. **Establish** the facts (as best can be determined) about diagnosis, condition, and prognosis.

B. **Determine** the parents' (or guardian's) view of what is best for the infant.

C. **Consider** the ethical principles and identify value conflicts in the situation.

D. **Identify** your own moral position.

E. **Communicate** your moral position with other members of the health care team.

F. **Identify** moral positions of key people involved.

G. **Determine** who should have the most decision-making authority; this is usually the parents, unless they are irrational or unable to grasp the infant's situation.

H. **Participate in** thorough discussion of all alternatives and the ethical principles and values inherent in choosing each alternative. All persons affected by the decision (including health care staff) should participate.

I. **Arrive at** a decision and implement it.

J. **Evaluate** and review results of the decision and action.

The first step in the process is the recognition that you are in an ethical dilemma. As noted in the earlier discussion, many situations can be categorized as ethical dilemmas. One example of an ethical dilemma is the question of whether aggressive treatment of the extremely premature infant is morally right. The possibility that the infant's life will be saved but that the child will suffer profound neurological deficit produces the ethical dilemma of whether life-sustaining treatment is ultimately a benefit for the child. The dilemma hinges on the conflict of two deeply held values: on the one hand, life is a cherished value, and all infants deserve a chance at life; on the other hand, for some infants, the amount of pain or air hunger to be endured makes life only a tortured existence. It may be morally wrong to prolong such existence. We can see in this example that values are in conflict, yet we do not know what the morally right decision should be.

An example from obstetrical nursing is the ethical dilemma of whether women should be forced by court order to remain on bedrest when pre-term labor threatens. Does the nurse caring for such a woman have an ethical obligation to assist the physician in carrying out a court order? Does the nurse have an obligation to the unborn fetus, which may be harmed if the pregnant woman does not remain in the hospital? Does the nurse have an ethical obligation to respect the autonomy of the obstetrical patient who wishes to leave the hospital for reasons that seem well thought out and rational? Should the nurse try to protect the fetus by persuading the pregnant woman to remain in the hospital? Or should the nurse respect the pregnant woman's right to make her own determination about what is best, given her life circumstances and her own values and goals? Should the nurse report the situation to nursing administration to try to prevent the physician from seeking a court order?

As you can see from these two examples, the nurse must choose among a number of alternative actions, not one of which seems clearly ethically correct, and the nurse's actions have the potential to either help or exacerbate the situation of infants and pregnant women and their fetuses. Because of this potential for the nurse's actions to result in good or harm to the patient, because of the many questions about which principles, obligations, and values should take priority in a situation, and because of the lack of a clearly right answer, we can identify these neonatal and obstetrical situations as instances of ethical dilemmas.

The process of ethical decision making proceeds from initial recognition that you are in the midst of an ethical dilemma to the second step: collecting all the available, morally relevant facts about the situation. These include the medical condition of the patient and prognosis and whether the condition and prognosis are known with certainty or whether there is a high degree of uncertainty or conflicting medical opinion. The amount of burden (invasive, painful procedures; long-term dependence on life support or artificial nutrition that severely limits mobility, affectionate, intimate human relationships, cognitive growth and satisfying personal development) presented by the therapy is also a morally relevant piece of information, because it addresses human suffering. Is this burden of short or long duration? What is the ratio of benefit to burden in the long-term prognosis? How certain is the benefit of the therapy, or is it experimental therapy, used only on a few patients, with inconsistent results?

The desires and values of the patient are extremely important pieces of information for the nurse confronted with an ethical dilemma. In nursing, our ethical code places great significance on the patient's right to make her own choices in health care. When the patient is unable to make decisions, we usually turn to the family, who decides what is best for the incompetent patient. In the neonatal intensive care unit (NICU), we usually look to the parents for consent for medical therapies. However, family autonomy does not mean that the family can make capricious decisions. Those members who would decide about life-sustaining treatment for the infant must meet three important criteria: the surrogate decision maker must put the infant's welfare above all other considerations, the surrogate must be able to make a rational decision, and the surrogate must be able to communicate that decision to others.

In most instances in the NICU, it is clear that therapy is in the infant's best interest; that is, the therapy does not itself produce undue pain, it is not experimental therapy with unknown outcomes, and it is likely that the infant will have normal developmental outcomes. In some instances, such as the infant with anencephaly, there is no effective treatment and, therefore, aggressive therapy would only prolong dying. But in other instances, such as with the extremely premature infant (birth weight less than 1000 g), treatment outcomes are uncertain and the therapy itself can be painful and of long duration. In these instances, it is morally correct to seek the input of the parents about how aggressive therapy should be (Penticuff, 1988). When the parents meet the three criteria listed earlier, their decision about treatment of their infant should be respected.

Of course, even when the infant's chances for intact survival are slim, most parents want aggressive therapies to be continued. However, there may come a point in therapy when the prognosis becomes bleak and further aggressive measures to save the infant's life seem cruel. Nurses, being in direct contact with the infant for prolonged periods, often feel conflict about whether what is being done for the baby is morally right. At this point, the nurse must take some action to resolve the ethical dilemma because a sense of ethical anguish may set in. Ethical anguish is emotionally costly, because it evokes high levels of anxiety, frustration, and a sense of helplessness. Nurses who experience ethical anguish are vulnerable to burn-out and erosion of their sense of personal ethical integrity. For these reasons, it is important to take an ethical stand when you are confronted with an ethical dilemma rather than passively letting the situation develop without your active input toward a resolution.

The third step in ethical decision making is to weigh the moral implications of each option and arrive at a conclusion. When the patient is clear about which option is most consistent with her own values, and she fully understands the situation and can make a decision, then we should be reluctant to over-ride the patient's wishes. When the patient is pregnant, however, the situation is less easily resolved. This is because the pregnant woman's actions and decisions about treatment affect the fetus, so that the decision is not only about the pregnant woman's life but it also affects the life and well-being of the fetus. Ethical dilemmas that involve the pregnant woman *and* the fetus are among the most complex of all the ethical problems in medicine and nursing practice.

Creation of Ethical Dilemmas in High-Risk Neonatal Nursing

Whenever health care can offer powerful therapies to prolong life, ethical dilemmas arise about whether it is morally right to prolong all life. When health care technology is powerless to save life, there is usually little conflict of ethical principles and values. But in neonatal intensive care, technology is powerful in that

many infants' lives can be prolonged. The question becomes one of whether the infant is better off because his or her life is prolonged. To practice nursing ethically, we must address issues of quality of life, considered from the standpoint of the infants' experience of benefit and burden in their lives. In considering these issues, we quickly find that we must identify and weigh our values and act in a manner that affirms our personal and professional morality. Some of the ethical dimensions of neonatal nursing are discussed in the following paragraphs.

The newborn infant with life-threatening illness admitted to the NICU presents many ethical dimensions as a patient. The infant cannot speak and has neither the intellectual capability to decide among available alternatives nor the life experiences from which to derive values that would guide moral choices. But decisions are required, because although the lives of some infants undergoing neonatal intensive care can be prolonged through aggressive and experimental therapies, the burden of therapy may outweigh the benefit to the infant, and prolongation of life may be futile and inhumane. Such a case is cited by Weir (1984):

> Mignon was an extremely premature infant. Born after only 19 weeks' gestation, she weighed 482 grams at birth. After seven months in the NICU, she was described by her physician in the following manner: she has been plagued with frequent kidney failures, liver problems that defy textbook description, and the usual lung problems . . . At seven months after delivery she is hanging in there. We have kept the [umbilical artery] catheter in her aorta all the way, so her hyperalimentation has been intraarterial . . . She can't suck because of the endotracheal tube. Of course, she has been constantly on positive pressure ventilation. But with no spontaneous breathing, all mechanical ventilation, her lungs are pretty damaged now" (p. 52).

A surrogate decision maker must take responsibility for choosing whether to permit or to forego aggressive, life-prolonging diagnostic and therapeutic interventions for such an infant in the NICU. Parents are usually presumed to be in the best position to decide these ethical questions, with input from nurses and physicians who serve in an advisory and information-sharing role (American Academy of Pediatrics, 1984; Caplan and Cohen, 1987; Penticuff, 1988). However, as one parent of an infant in the NICU noted, "For parents to have any role in ethical decision making they must know as much as possible about their child's current condition, treatments, and probable outcome . . . (yet) unless parents know enough to ask the right questions, they are rarely informed about the dangers or uncertainties of their child's condition and treatment" (Harrison, 1986, p. 172). There is increasing sentiment that parents should have prerogative in ethical decisions made on behalf of infants and children (Benefield et al, 1978; Caplan and Cohen, 1987; Duff, 1981; Penticuff, 1988; Stinson and Stinson, 1983; Veatch, 1984). To complicate matters further, in neonatal care there is much uncertainty of prognosis because of the developmental plasticity of the neonate. Although predictions for general categories of infants may be statistically valid, outcomes for a particular infant may be either much better or much worse than those for groups of infants.

Because of the problem in predicting outcome for any particular infant, a fundamental ethical issue in neonatal intensive care is the management of uncertainty (Caplan and Cohen, 1987). One approach is to initiate treatment for every infant and to continue aggressive treatment until it is certain that an infant will either die or be so severely impaired that, under any substantive standard, parents could be justified in withdrawing all except palliative therapies. This approach in which therapies continue until prognosis is nearly certain is currently the trend in many NICUs in the United States. The drawback is that some infants are kept alive, like Mignon, who might have experienced an early death as the lesser of two evils. Another, more individualized approach is that in which therapies are initiated and the infant's response and prognosis are periodically re-assessed. This approach considers such factors as severe neurological impairment and allows parents the option of withdrawing aggressive therapies before it is absolutely certain that an infant will either die or be profoundly impaired in capacity to relate to others or to the environment. The individualized approach requires that ethical dilemmas be faced before medical certainty is achieved.

In obstetrical nursing, many ethical dilemmas arise because the pregnant woman is held morally accountable for the well-being of the fetus in a pregnancy for which abortion has been rejected by the gravida. Because the pregnant woman and fetus are physically in-separable, diagnosis and treatment of one must affect the other. Indeed, as Murray (1987) points out, much medical treatment is administered to pregnant women to benefit the not-yet-born child. This ranges from non-invasive, non-experimental treatments that clearly benefit the fetus (education about appropriate nutrition, for example) to technologically sophisticated, invasive, and experimental treatments of uncertain fetal benefit (for example, fetal surgery). A central question remains: What ethical obligations are owed to the fetus as a patient, in light of the reality that the fetus's existence and the condition in which it exists are predicated on the choices of the pregnant woman? The question of ethical obligations to the fetus is complicated by the fact that the pregnant woman's liberty and physical integrity may necessarily be compromised to decrease risk of harm to the fetus. If such compromise of liberty or physical integrity is made through coercion, significant ethical issues are raised.

Some bioethics theorists (Annas, 1982; Murray, 1987; Engelhardt, 1985; Robertson, 1985) have raised questions about how far those in authority ought to intervene coercively in the life of a woman to benefit her fetus. Kolder and associates (1987) found that approximately 50% of medical directors of obstetrical residency programs thought that court orders should be obtained to compel unconsenting pregnant woman to undergo treatment, including surgery, thought to be life-saving or life-beneficial to the fetus. To date, court orders over-riding pregnant women's refusals have been obtained for cesarean sections in 11 states, for hospital detentions in 2 states, and for intrauterine transfusions in 1 state. Interestingly, 81% of the women involved were black, Asian, or Hispanic; 44% were unmarried; and 24% did not speak English as their primary language (Kolder et al, 1987).

Murray and Caplan (1985), Annas (1982, 1987), Kolder and associates (1987), Nelson and Milliken (1988), and others object to violations of the pregnant woman's autonomy through forced obstetrical interventions, arguing that the pregnant woman's obligations to the fetus she plans to carry to term can be no greater than her obligations to her already-born children. For this reason, for example, she cannot be compelled morally to undergo surgery such as cesarean section to save the fetus's life, just as a mother cannot be compelled to donate a kidney to save the life of her dying child. But persuasive arguments can be made that a pregnant woman who does not intend to have an abortion has an ethical obligation to accept reasonable, non-experimental medical treatment and to make lifestyle choices that will benefit and not harm her fetus. Nevertheless, as Nelson and Milliken (1988) point out, "It is quite another matter to transform [her] ethical obligation into a legal duty by enforcing it with the coercive power of the law." But the possibility for conflict between gravida and fetus emerges not only with the specter of court-ordered medical interventions. Other means of persuasions and manipulation of pregnant women are frequently employed when the fetus is seen as a patient.

Another reason that ethical dilemmas arise in neonatal intensive care and highly sophisticated and technical obstetrical care has to do with the organization's focus on provision of life-saving or life-prolonging technology. More humanistically oriented care may be perceived as lower in priority than care that saves life. In such environments, when life-prolonging therapy is questioned, conflicts can arise between those people who see the unit's mission as the saving of all life and those who see the mission as providing human care that considers quality of life as an important value. Although more intensive, highly technical care occurs in the NICU than in obstetrical units, as obstetrical technology increases, these climate aspects will become increasingly critical in ante-partum, intra-partum, and post-partum units as well.

Resources for Resolving Ethical Dilemmas

Probably the most important organizational characteristic relevant to nurses' involvement in resolution of ethical dilemmas is the overall effectiveness of the neonatal nursing staff in monitoring and influencing nursing and medical protocol in the unit. Associated with this factor are nursing administration's influence and control of resources within the overall hospital administrative structure. Where nursing maintains an influential position within the hospital and the NICU, neonatal nurses are more likely to influence overall infant care. This comprehensive influence of care includes, for example, requests for medication to alleviate infant pain and air hunger and changes in unit routine to allow for more involvement of families and more periods of undisturbed in-

fant rest. Where nursing is truly valued and influential, nurses frequently request team conferences that include the attending neonatologist for the purpose of reviewing an infant's responses to therapy and questioning whether additional aggressive therapies will be good for the infant.

The personnel resources of the unit can influence whether nurses are involved in resolution of ethical dilemmas. This is because when pool personnel frequently supplement neonatal nursing staff, or when many of the staff are part-time, consistent communication and cohesive action on behalf of infants and families may be impaired. Additionally, if there is high turnover of nursing staff, the overall level of nursing expertise in the unit will be diluted. If residents, medical students, and attending neonatologists rotate frequently, this may seriously hinder the process by which nursing input can influence medical planning. On the other hand, in some units that experience frequent resident rotations but have a stable nursing staff, there is much nursing influence because nursing expertise may be more developed than medical expertise.

Another aspect of the practice climate that influences nurses' involvement in the resolution of ethical dilemmas is the communication style of the unit. As can be seen in the steps of ethical decision making described earlier, communication is an essential element, and nurses must express themselves and be heard for ethical nursing practice to be possible. Communication style is powerfully affected by the patterns of relationships between nurses and physicians in the unit and the expertise and credibility of the nursing staff. Where nurses are highly expert and their communications are technically credible, relationships are more positive than in units where nurses are less expert. Expertise and credibility increase the influence of nurses, and their increased influence enhances the likelihood that they will be able to take part in resolution of ethical dilemmas in the NICU. If nurses are left out of the resolution process, then the unique perspective and traditional values of nursing may not be represented in decisions that will affect the lives and quality of life of infants and families in the unit. Another important negative factor when nurses are not involved in resolution of ethical dilemmas in the NICU is that the nurses then are likely to experience ethical anguish and ethical outrage (American Hospital Association, 1987), both of which can affect burn-out and turnover (Cameron, 1986).

Nursing credibility is important in light of research by Anspach (1987), which indicated that nurses and physicians communicate different observations about infant response to treatment and infant prognosis. Physicians, whose contact with infants is briefer and more technologically focused, were found to assess condition and prognosis largely on the basis of diagnostic technology (laboratory data, vital signs, respirator settings, and radiological evidence). Nurses, who are involved in close, continuous contact with infants, were found to assess condition and prognosis on the basis not only of diagnostic technology but also on cues gleaned from interactions with infants. Anspach (1987) concluded that medical practice is characterized by a diminishing attention to patients' subjective symptoms and that the difference in perspective between nurses and physicians can result in different views about what is best for some infants.

Whether there are shared values about the purpose of nursing care is also an important aspect of the practice climate that can affect nurses' involvement in resolution processes. Although nurses may not often discuss their views about what they think is best for some infants, a philosophy of caring does evolve when nursing staffs do not experience high rates of turnover and proportions of part-time personnel. This philosophy is institutionalized when nurses meet together to develop care plans. The attention given in care plans to alleviation of infant discomfort and to systematic inclusion of parents in the planning of infants' care may be a key indicator of nurses' ability to practice ethically in a unit.

The policies of the hospital and the NICU and whether nursing is well represented on an infant ethics committee can have an important impact on nurses' involvement in resolution of ethical dilemmas. Policies regarding who can call a meeting of the hospital infant ethics committee, indeed, the existence of such a committee and who may attend, are highly significant to resolution of dilemmas. The extent to which parents are included in frequent discussions of their infants' conditions, and the willingness of the medical and nursing staff to initiate conversations in which aggressive therapies are seen as optional rather than as imperative, all will have a bearing on both prevention and resolution of dilemmas. In general, the more open the communication pattern in the unit, the more respected nurses are, and the more involved parents are in daily decisions about their infants, the less likely ethical dilemmas are to arise and the more easily they are resolved.

Each nurse who is concerned about ethical aspects of practice should become more familiar with the policies and resources of the hospital (ability of nurses to call team meetings attended by physicians, to call and be thoroughly represented in ethics committee meetings, or, with the cooperation of medical administration, to initiate an infant ethics committee within the hospital if one does not already exist). The most comprehensive book on the structure and function of infant ethics committees is *Institutional Ethics Committees and Health Care Decision Making* (1984), edited by R. E. Cranford and A. E. Doudera.

As important as institutional policies and procedures are, the communication among nurses and physicians about the care of infants and families in the NICU should consist of on-going conversation about what each nurse and physician believes is morally right as well as the gradual evolution of a philosophy of care in the unit that can be supported by both nursing and medicine. How much families are to be involved in decisions, how much effort is to be spent in keeping infants free of pain and discomfort, and how much quality of life considerations will count in decisions to employ life-prolonging therapies are all important ethical issues about which there should be striving for agreement. Nursing should be represented on ethics committees, and those nurses who attend should accurately represent the views of all nurses participating in the care of the infant and family.

Finally, each nurse owes it to her or his own sense of ethical integrity to reflect seriously on values and personal philosophy of nursing care and to participate in communication and available unit and hospital processes toward resolution of ethical dilemmas encountered in practice. It is only when we are a part of resolution processes that we can know and authenticate that our practice of nursing is a significant moral force for the good of infants and families.

REFERENCES

American Academy of Pediatrics: Guidelines for Infant Bioethics Committees. American Academy of Pediatrics, 1984.

American Hospital Association: Moral distress in nursing. Hosp. Ethics, 3(4):1–4, 1987.

Annas, G.J.: Forced cesareans: The most unkindest cut of all. Hastings Cent. Rep., 12:16–17, 1982.

Annas, G.J.: Protecting the liberty of pregnant patients. N. Engl. J. Med., 316:1213–1214, 1987.

Anspach, R.R.: Prognostic conflict in life-and-death decisions: The organization as an ecology of knowledge. J. Health Soc. Behav., 28:215–231, 1987.

Benefield, D.G., Leibs, S.A., and Vollman, J.H.: Grief response of parents to neonatal death and parent participation in deciding care. Pediatrics, 62:171–177, 1978.

Cameron, M.: The moral and ethical component of nurse burn-out. Crit. Care Manag. Ed., 17(4):42B–42E, 1986.

Caplan, A., and Cohen, C.: Imperiled newborns. Hastings Cent. Rep., 17(6):7–32, 1987.

Cranford, R.E., and Doudera, A.E.: Institutional Ethics Committees and Health Care Decision Making. Ann Arbor, Health Administration Press, 1984.

Duff, R.S.: "Close-up" versus "distant" ethics: Deciding the care of infants with poor prognosis. Semin. Perinatol., 11(3):244–253, 1987

Duff, R.S.: Counseling families and deciding care of severely defective children: A way of coping with medical Vietnam. Pediatrics, 67(3):315–320, 1981.

Englehardt, H.T., Jr.: Current controversies in obstetrics: Wrongful life and forced fetal surgical procedures. Am. J. Obstet. Gynecol., 151:313–318, 1985.

Harrison, H.: Neonatal intensive care: Parents' role in ethical decision making. Birth, 13(3):165–175, 1986.

Kolder, V.E.B., Gallagher, J., Parsons, J.D., et al.: Court-ordered obstetrical interventions. N. Engl. J. Med., 316:1192–1196, 1987.

Murray, T.H., and Caplan, A.L. (eds.): Which Babies Shall Live? Clifton, NY: Humana Press, 1985.

Murray, T.H.: Moral obligations to the not-yet born: The fetus as patient. Ethic. Leg. Iss. Perinatol., 14(2):329–344, 1987.

Nelson, L.J., and Milliken, N.: Compelled medical treatment of pregnant women. JAMA, 259(7):1060–1066, 1988.

Pellegrino, E.D.: The anatomy of clinical-ethical judgements in perinatology and neonatology: A substantive and procedural framework. Semin. Perinatol., 11(3):202–210, 1987.

Penticuff, J.H.: Neonatal nursing ethics: Toward a consensus. Neonatal Network, 5:7–16, 1987.

Penticuff, J.H.: Infant suffering and nurse advocacy in neonatal intensive care. Nurs. Clin. North Am., 24(4):987–997, 1989.

Penticuff, J.H.: Neonatal intensive care: Parental prerogatives. J. Perinat. Neonat. Nurs., 1(3):77–86, 1988.

Robertson, J.A.: Legal issues in fetal therapy. Semin. Perinatol., 9:136–142, 1985.

Stinson, R., and Stinson, P.: The Long Dying of Baby Andrew. Boston, Little, Brown, 1983.

Thompson J.E., and Thompson, H.O.: Bioethical Decision Making for Nurses. Norwalk, CT, Appleton-Century-Crofts, 1985.

Veatch, R.M.: Limits of guardian treatment refusal: A reasonableness standard. Am. J. Law Med., 9(4):427–468, 1984.

Weir, R.F.: Selective Nontreatment of Handicapped Newborns. New York, Oxford University Press, 1984.

M. Terese Verklan

CHAPTER
37

Legal Issues in the NICU

Objectives

1. Define standards of care and guidelines for establishing the standard of care.

2. Define concepts of liability and negligence.

3. Discuss the importance of documentation in the patient's record and guidelines for charting.

4. Discuss the nurse's role in informed consent.

5. Identify scope of practice issues in providing patient care functions.

6. Define malpractice and the conditions that constitute malpractice.

In the not too distant past, obstetrics was the clinical area beset by fear of lawyers, malpractice suits, and loss of licensure. Today, litigation is becoming more common in our own area of specialization. Neonatal nurses must become cognizant of the minimum standards of professional conduct that they, as health care providers, must adhere to. Inherent in this role is the implication of legal accountability for one's actions (Kozier and Erb, 1988). The purpose of this chapter is to familiarize the nurse with the concepts and ramifications of legal concerns as they pertain to the realm of neonatal intensive care nursing. Topics to be discussed include standards of care, liability, documentation, informed consent, and scope of practice and malpractice issues.

Standard of Care

We must first define the term "standard of care" because its definition rests in the context in which is being used.

A. **Standard of care**, as used by professional associations, usually refers to a goal or guideline for excellence (Murphy, 1987). For example, NAACOG, the organization for obstetrical, gynecological, and neonatal nurses, publishes *Standards of Obstetric, Gynecologic and Neonatal Nursing*. These standards, together with the Standards of Practice and the Code for Nurses published by the American Nurses'

Association (ANA) frequently provide the criteria by which performance in our specialty is appraised.

B. **In the legal system**, standard of care is what a reasonable and prudent nurse would have done in similar circumstances (Murphy, 1987). The issue of excellence in practice or quality of care given does not pertain to the argument—what is being sought is reasonableness and prudence. A reasonable and prudent nurse is a nurse with like education, background, and experience who would behave in a corresponding manner, given a parallel set of events. Nurses' actions are judged by what another nurse would do in similar circumstances (Flynn and Heffron, 1988).

C. **Five basic types of evidence** are used to establish the legal standard of care.
1. Testimony from expert witnesses: expert witness testimony is essential to the understanding of the intricacies of a malpractice suit. The judge and jury are uneducated with regard to neonatal health care and therefore need assistance in understanding just what a reasonable and prudent nurse would have done in the given circumstances. (Did the nurse meet the accepted standard of care?) Professional nursing philosophies dictate that nurses be the only witnesses permitted to testify as experts in a nursing malpractice suit (Dyke, 1989).
2. Policies and procedures of the institution: the policy and procedure manual of the local institution is persuasive evidence of the standard of care in that setting (Murphy, 1987). In general, this manual is written by that institution's nurses or quality assurance committee to define what minimal criteria must be met with regard to that community's specific standard of care for its own practice setting. Being unaware of the policy and procedure for the standard clinical practice at your establishment is not an acceptable excuse for not being able to be held accountable for your realm of practice. Because the statutes of limitations endure for 18–21 years and standard care practices change dramatically over the years, keeping the policy and procedure manual will also help to determine what the standard of care was at the time the infant was hospitalized.
3. State and federal regulations: statutes and administrative codes, such as the rules of the state board of nursing, can be used to establish the standards of care (Murphy, 1987). Agencies that receive federal funding are subject to the code of federal regulations. These rules may require certain criteria be used in the delivery of health care, thereby establishing standards of care. The Joint Commission on Accreditation of Health-Care Organizations has also set out guidelines for the minimum level of practice deemed acceptable to enable that institution to receive its accreditation. However, these national standards vary in their usefulness to determine the legal standard of care in a particular situation, because they tend to be written in broad language that lacks sufficient specificity to prescribe activities for many situations (Murphy, 1987). The institution's own policy and procedure manual would then be closely examined.
4. Standards of professional organizations: professional associations such as the National Perinatal Association, the National Association of Neonatal Nurses, and those mentioned earlier have delineated nationally recognized standards of care.
5. Current professional literature: current texts and journal articles, although technically hearsay, aid in establishing the legal standard of care. Keeping theory and clinical practice on par with the literature and remaining current with regard to continuing education will assist nurses in ensuring that their professional standards are in keeping with their peers.

Liability

Until recently, nurses were viewed as non-professionals incapable of committing malpractice because they exercised no discretion—they merely followed instructions. Therefore, because the nurse was not responsible for diagnosis or treatment, malpractice was legally impossible (King and Sagan, 1989). The threat of professional liability claims has influenced obstetrical, gynecological, and neonatal nursing practice, both indirectly, through changes in the way many physicians (obstetricians and gynecologists in particular) practice medicine, and directly, through an increase in the number and severity of claims against nurses (Cohn, 1986). As most states now recognize the nurse, and especially the nurse practitioner, as a health care professional, the nurse will no longer be held merely to a negligence standard but will also be held to a professional standard (King and Sagan, 1989). For example, by analogy, a neonatal nurse practitioner can be held to the standard of a neonatologist.

With the rest of the health care system, nursing is constantly re-evaluating old roles and expanding innovative functions. The traditional principles of health care provider liability, such as respondent superior (defined below), premises liability, and negligence continues to be applicable.

One of the most fundamental concepts of liability facing both the professional and non-professional is negligence, which evaluates a person's actions or failure to act against what a responsible and prudent person would have done under the same or similar circumstances (Schanz, 1987). This is not the same as carelessness, because a nurse's careful conduct may still constitute legal negligence if what he or she does is not what other nurses would have done, given the same situation. Harm must result from the act, because without damage, no legal wrong has been committed. The four primary components of negligence on which a finding of culpable liability is premised are the following (Schanz, 1987):

A. **Duty of some type** owed from one person to another.

B. **A breach** of that particular duty.

C. **Injury and/or damage** being suffered by a party.

D. **A causal connection** between the breach of the duty owed and the injury or damage suffered by the plaintiff (referred to as proximal cause).

E. **A concept that nurse executives should be familiar with** is respondent superior which, in essence, stands for "let your superior respond" (Schanz, 1987). This doctrine:
1. Holds an employer legally liable for the negligent acts of employees that arise in the course of the employment, i.e., employers are held responsible for the acts of those whom they have a right to supervise or control (Bernzweig, 1981).
2. Has incredible liability implications for the health care institution, because any employee could potentially subject the employer to litigation due to acts of negligence.
3. Does not necessarily absolve or relieve the negligent employee from liability but rather permits both the employer and employee to be sued, with the potential for joint and several liabilities against both (Schanz, 1987).
4. Holds that negligent employees are always liable for their own conduct.

F. **An area of considerable controversy** in the liability arena is the quality assurance department:
1. Their task is to determine the standard of care for their institution.
2. It may be that they have provided the ammunition for the plaintiff's malpractice case. For that reason, many jurisdictions have provided a protective shield for quality assurance and risk management activity, which renders the materials generated and the thought processes engaged in during those activities "privileged" or otherwise non-discoverable and non-admissible in a litigation setting (Carr, 1989). The question of insurance for nurses is frequently discussed. Some people believe that nurses should not carry insurance, because this only provides them with "deep pockets," making them more attractive to the plaintiff. Others insist that being well insured will serve as good protection. And how much insurance is enough? Is the insurance coverage provided by the employer enough, or should we also invest in a personal policy for additional protection. Many nurses who practice in non-traditional settings cannot find an

insurance company who will underwrite their risks. The record claims losses experienced by professional inability insurers have caused record growth in the premiums that nurses, hospitals, physicians, and others must pay and has made professional liability insurance difficult, if not impossible, to obtain for some groups of health care providers (Cohn, 1986).

G. The costs of liability when a neonate is involved are high for three reasons (Cohn, 1986):
1. The cost of caring for a damaged infant with a normal life expectancy is high.
2. With the longer statute of limitations for minors, charges may be made years later, applicable to other medical malpractice actions.
3. There is sympathy toward the family, who may not be able to afford the needed care the child requires, as opposed to the "cold corporation with ample insurance coverage who will not really miss the money anyway."

Documentation

One of the nurse's fundamental responsibilities is to keep accurate records of the patient's physical and mental condition (Bernzweig, 1981). Charting documents (Ohio Nurses Association, 1979) include:

A. Professional surveillance of the patient.

B. Nursing action taken in the patient's behalf.

C. Patient's progress with regard to illness (Ohio Nurses Association, 1979). It also serves as a tool for evaluating the quality of care and providing evidence in any subsequent legal proceeding (Chez and Verklan, 1987). Whether the patient's medical record is an ally or enemy depends on how the nurse uses it (Schaefer, 1981). Thus, the prudent nurse will avoid the temptation to include in the chart remarks concerning:
1. The patient's or family's personality traits or idiosyncrasies (unless such remarks are relevant to the infant's treatment).
2. Personal views to the effect that the patient or family is a potential litigant.
3. Gratuitous admissions of legal liability with respect to untoward medical or nursing events (Bernzweig, 1981).

Accurate and concise charting is imperative as any omission is presumed not to have taken place. In a malpractice action the burden of proof rests with the plaintiff. In the case of *Coleman vs. Touro Infirmary of New Orleans* (506 So.2d 571 — LA), the plaintiff alleged that the defendants had been negligent by failing to treat an abruptio placentae prior to the premature delivery of the infant and that the defendants' actions or inaction had caused the child's death. There were several discrepancies between the patient's recollection of events and the medical record. The court consulted the chart, determined the nurses' notes stated another set of events, and concluded that the plaintiff failed to prove any act or omission by the obstetrician or hospital that resulted in the wrongful death of the Coleman infant.

D. Chart objectively.
1. The phrases, "appears to be" and "seems to be," which nurses were routinely taught 30 or 40 years ago (when nurses supposedly were not making a judgment or decision about what was happening to the patient) are out of place in today's nurses' charting (Creighton, 1987).
2. Careful documentation is a response to the theorem that the greatest liability is not in what is documented, but rather in what is not (Chez and Verklan, 1987).

E. Chart promptly.
1. Any significant changes in the patient's status.

2. The nursing actions undertaken to intercede in the situation, including notifying the physician of the concern.

In *Goff vs. Doctors General Hospital* (Cal. 1958), a case in which a woman suffered a post-partal hemorrhage, the evening nurse did not take vital signs and failed to notify the physician when she assessed the woman as going into shock. The physician was not informed until the night shift; the woman subsequently died, and the nurse and the hospital were held liable in damages (Creighton, 1987).

A medical record is no place for reference to an incident report having taken place. What should be documented is a factual account of what transpired and what was done. Incident reports enable the hospital or agency to make necessary investigations of untoward events to protect patients from any preventable consequences and the hospital or agency and its employees from potential liability (Creighton, 1987).

Sign and date every entry, ensuring that no vacant lines are left. An empty space may later prompt someone to fill in a "missing" piece of information. If a late notation must be made, chart the actual time you are making the notation and stipulate that it is for an earlier time, e.g., "1414 for 1300 Occupational therapy protocol completed with infant showing increased tolerance to activity by sitting upright in infant seat with no episodes of bradycardia." Keep in mind late entries are always viewed with a suspicious eye.

Even records of "routine care" must be documented. As negligence could be proven if this information is found wanting, appropriate flow sheets that list these routines along with times, dates, patient and caregiver identification, and nursing care outcomes are valuable in providing a means of documenting repetitious nursing activities.

F. **Errors** should be charted by:
1. Drawing a single line through what is in error.
2. Dating and signing the error.
3. Entering the correct notation. What if you are instructed not to *chart* an error by the attending physician? Nurses who accede to the demands of a physician to cover up the true facts of an unusual clinical episode by deliberately not mentioning it in the patient's chart not only may be subject to possible loss of licensure, but, in flagrant circumstances, they may even subject themselves to criminal action, leading to a fine or jail sentence (Bernzweig, 1981).
4. A common practice in teaching hospitals is "countersigning" nursing notes written by nursing students and licensed nurses. When you co-sign another's entry you are legally saying that you have, in effect, performed the procedure or similarly assessed the situation, and can be held jointly liable with that caregiver for any legal ramifications that may come about from that notation. Nurses who are required by hospital policy routinely to countersign documents or information in the patient's chart should protect themselves in one of two ways:
   a. By personally verifying the information being recorded.
   b. By noting in the record that the signature is included in accordance with hospital policy and is not based on personal knowledge of the information in question (Bernzweig, 1981).

Medical records are crucial in a court case as they provide the sequence of events, the time frame in which they occurred, and the participants in the care of the patient. If a nurse is named in a suit or is called to testify with regard to what took place, sometimes many years later, the chart serves as a memory aid. Statements contained in the medical record are not, in themselves, admitted into evidence; but rather, the testimony of the witness concerning the particular event —as reinforced by the medical record—becomes the direct evidence given under oath (Bernzweig, 1981). "A chart is a witness that never dies and never lies.

Careful, defensive charting is the only evidence that a nurse provided quality care" (Chagnon and Easterwood, 1986).

Informed Consent

According to the Iowa Supreme Court, the doctrine of informed consent arises out of the unquestioned principle that a patient has the right to exercise control over his or her own body in making an informed decision concerning whether to submit to a particular medical procedure (Murphy, 1988a,b). Section 1.1 of the ANA Code for Nurses states, "Clients have the moral right to determine what will be done with their own person; to be given accurate information, and all the information necessary for making informed judgments. . . . Each nurse has an obligation to . . . support those rights. In situations in which the client lacks the capacity to make a decision, a surrogate decision maker should be designated" (ANA, 1985).

A. **The patient and/or family must be given sufficient information** to enable them rationally to make an informed decision. Two legal standards measure the adequacy of this disclosure (Murphy, 1988).
1. The professional standard (physician standard); the physician must disclose the information that a responsible physician would disclose under the same or similar circumstances.
2. The lay standard (patient standard); the physician's duty to disclose is measured by the need of the patient and/or family to have access to all information material to make a truly informed and intelligent decision regarding the proposed medical procedure.

B. **It is outside the boundaries of nursing practice** to provide the patient and/or family with information regarding medical-surgical risks or benefits of treatment or suggesting alternate medical-surgical therapies. It would be appropriate for the nurse to inform the physician that the family has further need of clarification to enable them to comfortably come to a decision. If nurses are required to obtain patient and/or family signatures on consent forms, they should limit their inequity of patient and/or family understanding to two questions, as follows:
1. Has your physician discussed your surgery with you?
2. Are you ready to sign this consent form that indicates your consent to the procedure?

C. **To be able legally to give informed consent**, the person must have the capability of "capacity." Two aspects of capacity are crucial to consent (Hogue, 1989).
1. The patient must have attained a certain chronological age, most often 18 or 21.
2. The patient must be able to understand information related to the treatment, risks, etc.

D. **Neonatal patients clearly** do not meet the requisite criteria to be considered legally able to make an informed consent. Therefore, parents or the legal guardian need to receive and understand the necessary information to enable them to make an informed consent on behalf of the infant. When an infant requires medical treatment, it is customary to explain the procedures to, and ask consent from, the child's parents or guardian.

E. **What if the parents or guardian will not give consent?**
1. If physicians heed the parents' wishes and do not treat the infant, they may be guilty of child abuse or neglect, because laws stipulate that parents must provide needed medical care. Denial of this care can constitute a form of child neglect or abuse.
2. If physicians proceed to treat the infant, ignoring the parental objections, they

could be liable for battery, as their touching was intentional and there was a lack of consent.

3. The physician may petition the court for an authorization to provide the infant with the necessary treatment (i.e., obtain a court order).

F. **The most common example** of physicians' seeking court orders to intervene in treatment is that of refused consent for blood transfusions based on religious beliefs. This request is almost always granted, certainly in emergency situations. When parents refuse treatment for other reasons, the court will base its decision on several factors (Rhodes, 1987).

1. The infant's overall health and development.
2. The immediacy of danger to the infant if treatment is withheld.
3. The risks and benefits of the proposed treatment.

Scope of Practice

Each state possesses its own Nurse Practice Act, composed of statutes passed by its legislature defining the boundaries of nursing practice. These laws vary from state to state in their demarcation of nursing practice. In contrast with state medical practice acts, these statutes delineate nursing responsibilities in broad, universal nomenclature that generally must be examined with reference to the pertinent local law. The fundamental issue underlying the scope of practice questions is whether a particular act or procedure carried out by nurses is legally within or beyond the scope of their license to practice (Bernzweig, 1981).

There are numerous areas of medical and nursing practice that overlap one another; therefore, the same act may be considered the practice of medicine when performed by a physician and the practice of nursing when performed by a nurse (Bernzweig, 1981). These are the "gray areas" that have evolved partly in response to the nurse's increased level of preparation and partly due to the "high-tech" environment encouraged by many institutions and specialty units. Critical legal liability and scope of practice problems arise whenever the nurse assumes patient care functions of an independent nature that:

A. **Have long been held to be solely within the province** of physicians.

B. **Are not the subject** of standing orders.

C. **Have no support** in nursing practice acts.

D. **Are not generally recognized** as legitimate nursing functions by accredited professional organizations.

1. Between the 1940s and 1970s, advanced nursing practice was synonymous with specialization, which required a master's degree (Peplau, 1985). With the addition of nurse practitioners of various educational backgrounds, advanced nursing practice came to mean the practice of nurses in expanded roles, e.g., nurse midwives, nurse anesthetists, clinical nurse specialists, and nurse practitioners (Dunn, 1985). The ANA revised its principles in the early 1980s to aid the state licensing agencies in the development of nurse practice acts (ANA, 1985). However, these statutes were broad and inexplicit. In today's legal climate, what is wanted is specific reference to what exactly constitutes advanced nursing practice. Fewer than seven states do not have specific reference to advanced nursing practice in their nurse practice act. The predominant method used to authorize advanced nursing practice is state certification; second in frequency is licensure (Dunn, 1985).

   a. There is little structural autonomy for nurses relative to prescriptive authority (LeBar, 1984). The legal capacity to prescribe medications was not an early concern of those who were attempting to expand definitions of nursing in state nurse practice acts (Bullough, 1983). In most states, prescribing privileges were authorized subsequent to additional acts' clause amendments to the definition of nursing, with prescribing considered an "additional act" (Dunn, 1985). The legal authority for this expanded function, medications that may be prescribed, is in the statutes of the Nurse Practice Act or board of nursing rules.

b. As advanced nursing practice roles continue to expand, and as a surplus of physicians continues to grow, there will be further debates on what constitutes nursing functions. In 1983, the Missouri Supreme Court in *Sermchief vs. Gonzales*, the first judicial interpretation of advanced nursing practice, indicated that new functions for nurses may evolve without statutory constraints and that the nurses may diagnose and treat in accordance with standing orders and protocols (Dunn, 1985; MO, 1983). When nurses are involved in advanced practice, the issue is not whether they are competent to act but whether they are authorized to act (Greenlaw, 1984). State statutes and regulations grant authority to practice, but authority to act is given by administrative rules or regulatory references. Questions have been raised in those states that have broad statutory regulations with regard to the advanced practice nurse's authority to act: Are they legally empowered to perform the functions they render? Physicians on the executive committee of the medical society in Maryland have filed suit to challenge the authority of nurse practitioners to prescribe (*Drinkard et al. vs. Maryland Department of Health and Mental Hygiene, et al.*; Dunn, 1985).

Malpractice

A. **The term "malpractice"** means negligence on the part of the professional person, usually taking the form of a careless or imprudent act that results in injury to a client (Boullough, 1987). According to Hemelt and Mackert (1978), to prove successfully that malpractice has taken place, the plaintiff who brings the suit must demonstrate that the following conditions were met:
1. The defendant had a legal duty to the plaintiff.
2. The duty was breached.
3. The plaintiff actually suffered damage.
4. The defendant was the one who caused the damage.

Standard of care and the definition of what constitutes a reasonable and prudent nurse have been previously discussed. Legal cases can be cited that indicate that the standard of care for nurse practitioners is the same standard of care as would be expected of physicians (Boullough, 1987).

For a nurse, the risk of being sued is still relatively low. In any given year over the past 11 years, only 0.1% (on average) of nurse practitioners were sued (Pearson, 1987). As with physicians, the majority were nurse practitioners with obstetrical responsibilities. We can expect the number of suits against nurses to increase as incomes increase, as nurses move into advanced specialties that carry greater responsibility for decision making, and as they buy more malpractice insurance and are thus able to pay large damage claims (Boullough, 1987).

The federal government has initiated a national practitioner data bank that will maintain records of disciplinary action taken on licenses, hospital privileges, and payment in conjunction with malpractice suits. The idea developed as a solution to the growing problem of incompetent health care providers. The rules of Section 5 of Public Law 100-93, as it affects nurses, are unpublished (Bodenhorn and Hardy-Havens, 1989). There are many who will have to access to this bank; hospitals must check with the bank before granting privileges, state licensing boards to verify credentials, etc. Each nurse practitioner will need to become knowledgeable regarding the data base and periodically ascertain that the information regarding himself or herself is correct (Bodenhorn and Hardy-Havens, 1989).

B. **How can all nurses** practice preventive legal maintenance? Three general areas in which to focus prevention and defensive nursing practice are the following (Feutz, 1987):

1. Patient rights: this situation refers more to the parents or guardians of neonatal intensive care unit (NICU) infants. The NICU is a busy, noisy, frightening place to be suddenly thrown into. We are being trusted with the one possession most parents would rather die than part with—their newborn. And they have little or no control over what is happening to this tiny innocent they love so much. By keeping them informed of what is being done, who is performing the function, and the reason for the procedure, parents will not feel left out of the care of their infant. Familiarize them with the NICU by orienting them to equipment, staff, and family areas. Listen to their concerns and encourage their participation to build a relationship of trust. Congratulate them on the birth of their child. Sometimes we are so busy trying to save the life of the newborn that no one grants the status of "parent" to the parents. The infant dies, and they never are sure if they were ever parents. They are unhappy and frustrated, and then they sue.

2. Nursing skills: keeping your clinical skills and knowledge level current will foster competent nursing care. Attending inservice programs, national conferences, and continuing formal education will ensure that information is up to date. Many institutions have certification tests that nurses must pass annually to be considered competent with the unit's relevant clinical skills. Maintaining standards of care as promoted by our specialty organizations, such as NAACOG, the National Association of Neonatal Nurses, the American Association of Critical-Care Nurses (AACN), and the National Association of Pediatric Nurses Associates and Practitioners (NAPNAP), will provide the guidelines for what are considered minimum standards of nursing practice. Subscribing to and reading relevant professional journals will aid in informing you of the latest issues. For example, the technology that can diagnose genetic or congenital disorders during a pregnancy can lead to a lawsuit based on wrongful birth and wrongful life. Although this is relatively new ground, such lawsuits present risks for nurses and physicians engaged in genetic counseling and prenatal diagnosis, because the assertion in these cases is that the negligent counseling or inadequate information provided by the caregiver resulted in the birth of a defective child (Rhodes, 1989).

3. Documentation: although previously addressed at length, a few points bear repeating because this is the major shortcoming that accounts for the bulk of liability. Every staff member will tell you they know the importance of proper documentation, but they will also tell you there is inadequate time to do so and so it is given low priority. But on the chance that you will be named in a legal action, whether you were a practitioner or a primary nurse, or gave care for only one shift, that chart remains your best defense and should contain all pertinent activities and observations your nursing care encompassed. The typical deficiencies repeatedly seen in nursing documentation include the following (Feutz, 1987):
    a. Deliberate inaccuracies.
    b. Alterations in or destruction of records.
    c. Inconsistencies and contradictions.
    d. Unexplained time gaps in providing care.
    e. Subjective statements, opinions, and conclusions.
    f. Non-standard abbreviations.

Ensuring that your charting contains none of these inadequacies will go far in assuring that it will not become an enemy if scrutinized under close examination.

STUDY QUESTIONS

1. "Standard of care" usually refers to:
   a. A goal or guideline for excellence.
   b. What the insurance company requires.
   c. What a neighboring hospital does.

2. A charge of negligence usually assumes there was a breach of:
   a. Contract.
   b. Physician/patient confidentiality.
   c. Duty of some type owed the patients.

3. Charting documents refers to:
   a. Professional surveillance of the patient.
   b. The opinions of the caregivers.
   c. Whether or not the nurse/patient relationship was good.

4. Errors in the chart should be corrected by:
   a. Drawing a single line through the error.
   b. Starting a new chart.
   c. Using correction fluid so the error can be written over.

5. The correct person to obtain informed consent from a patient is:
   a. A bedside/primary nurse.
   b. The hospital attorney.
   c. The person performing the procedure.

6. The chart is your best defense when you are accused of malpractice as long as it does not contain:
   a. Abbreviations.
   b. Alterations in or destruction of records.
   c. Military time frequencies.

Answers to Study Questions

1. a   3. a   5. c
2. c   4. a   6. b

REFERENCES

American Nurses' Association: Code for Nurses with Interpretive Statements. Kansas City, MO, American Nurses' Association, 1985.

American Nurses' Association: Standards of Practice. Kansas City, MO, American Nurses' Association, 1973.

Bernzweig, E.P.: The Nurse's Liability for Malpractice: A Programmed Course, 3rd ed. New York, McGraw-Hill, 1981.

Bodenhorn, K., and Hardy-Havens, D.: Federal government initiates national practitioner data bank. J. Pediatr. Health Care, 3:160–162, 1989.

Boullough, A.: Malpractice insurance. J. Pediatr. Health Care, 1:1–7, 1987.

Bullough, B.: Prescribing authority for nurses. Nurs. Econom., 1:122–125, 1983.

Carr, M.J.: Legal aspects of standards of practice. DCCN, 8:111–112, 1989.

Chez, B.F., and Verklan, M.T.: Documentation and electronic fetal monitoring: How, where and what? J. Perinat. Neonat. Nurs., 1:22–28, 1987.

Chagnon, L., and Easterwood, B.: Managing the risks of obstetrical nursing. Am. J. Matern. Child Nurs., 11:303–310, 1986.

Cohn, S.: Trends in professional liability for OGN nurses (NAACOG Update Services, vol. 4, lesson 11). Princeton, Continuing Professional Education Center, 1986.

Coleman vs. Touro Infirmary of New Orleans, 506 So.2d 571—LA.

Creighton, J.: Legal significance of charting: I. Nurs. Manage., 18:17, 20, 22, 1987.

Drinkard et al. vs. Maryland Department of Health and Mental Hygiene et al.

Dunn, B.H.: Legal regulation of advanced nursing practice (NAACOG Update Series, vol. 4, lesson 8). Princeton, Continuing Professional Education Center, 1985.

Dyke, R.M.: The nurse expert witness: Professional implications. Neonatal Network, 8:35–39, 1989.

Feutz, S.A.: Preventive legal maintenance. J. Nurs. Admin., 17:8–10, 1987.

Flynn, J.M., and Heffron, P.B.: Nursing From Concept to Practice, 2nd ed. Norwalk, CT: Appleton & Lange, 1988.

Goff vs. Doctor's General Hospital, Cal. 1958.

Greenlaw, J.: Sermchief vs. Gonzales and the debate over advanced nursing practice legislation. Law Med. Health Care, 12:30–31, 36, 1984.

Hogue, E.E.: Consent for Minors. Pediatr. Nurs., 15:404, 1989.

Hemelt, M.D., and MacKert, M.E. Dynamics of Law in Nursing and Health Care. Reston, VA: Reston Publishing Co., Inc., 1978.

King, E.W., and Sagan,, P.R.: Nurse practitioner liability and authority. Nurs. Admin. Q., 13:57–60, 1989.

Kozier, B., and Erb, G.: Concepts and Issues in Nursing Practice. Menlo Park, CA: Addison-Wesley, 1988.

LeBar, C.: Prescribing privileges for nurses: A review of current law. (Publication no. D80). Kansas City, American Nurses' Association, 1984.

Murphy, E.K.: Establishing the legal standard of care. Assoc. Operat. Room Nurs. J., 46:188, 190, 192, 1987.

Murphy, E.K.: Informed consent: I. Assoc. Operat. Room Nurs. J., 47(4):1009–1016, 1988a.

Murphy, E.K.: Informed consent: II. Assoc. Operat. Room Nurs. J., 47(5):1294–1298, 1988b.

NAACOG: Standards of Obstetric, Gynecologic, and Neonatal Nursing, Washington, DC, NAACOG, 1991.

Ohio Nurses Association: Documenting home care. Columbus, OH, Ohio Nurses Association, 1979.

Pearson, L.J.: Comprehensive actuarial data on nurse practitioners . . . at long last. Nurs. Practit. 12:8–9, 1987.

Peplau, H.: Is nursing's self-regulatory power being eroded? Am. J. Nurs., 85:141–134, 1985.

Rhodes, A.M.: When parents refuse to consent. Matern. Child Nurs., 12:289, 1987.

Rhodes, A.M.: Wrongful birth and wrongful life. Matern. Child Nurs., 14:171, 1989.

Schaefer, M.S.: To avoid a lawsuit, keep the record straight. RN, 44:81–84, 1981.

Schanz, S.J.: Health-care provider liability: Traditional principles. Nurs. Econom., 5:311–316, 1987.

Sermchief vs. Gonzales, 600 S.W. 2nd 683 (MO, 1983).

Diane Gilchriest

Quality Assurance

Objectives

1. Define quality assurance.

2. Compare and contrast standards of care and standards of practice.

3. State one disadvantage to retrospective reviews.

4. Discuss two types of nursing quality assurance monitors.

5. Describe how the effectiveness of the quality assurance evaluation process is determined.

6. List three positive outcomes of interdisciplinary quality assurance activities.

Quality assurance activities are an important part of neonatal nursing care. Many nurses are aware of the term "quality assurance," but they experience it as little more than data gathering and documentation to meet an accreditation review. Health care consumers are also aware of quality. As more third-party payers reimburse at fixed rates, consumers will look to which health care institutions have the best "quality" reputation.

Excellence in neonatal nursing care means optimal, consistent care of patients' and families' physiological, psychological, sociocultural, and spiritual needs. Quality cannot be assured unless we can consistently document *what* we are doing, *why* we are doing it (scientific principles), and *how* our interventions have improved patient and family outcomes. Nurses, as professionals, are accountable for monitoring and improving their practice.

Quality Assurance

A. **Definition:** quality assurance in nursing is a planned, continuous, evaluative process to assure excellence of patient care.
1. Discussion.
   a. Assuring the quality of nursing care delivered to patients is the obligation of professional nurses.
   b. Quality assurance activities need to address the efficiency, cost, and effectiveness of care.

   c. Knowledge, skill, and caring attitude of the person delivering care are the keys to quality.

   d. Quality assurance should be integrated into every nurse's practice.

   e. Nurses at the bedside actually providing the patient care are in the best position to evaluate and document that quality care is being given.

   f. Accrediting bodies, such as the Joint Commission on Accreditation of Health Care Organizations, require that care be systematically and objectively monitored to evaluate the quality and appropriateness of patient care, problems identified and resolved, and that this process be documented.

   g. Components of an overall plan for quality assurance should include the following:

     (1) Identification of important aspects of care, potential or actual problems of care.

     (2) Objective assessment, using data collection tools, to delineate the cause and scope of the issue or care problem.

     (3) Implementation of actions to resolve problems or validate quality.

     (4) Periodic monitoring activities designed to assure that a desired level of quality is achieved and sustained.

     (5) Documentation of quality assurance activities.

     (6) Review of the nursing quality assurance plan as part of the hospital quality assurance plan.

     (7) The director of the nursing division has the ultimate responsibility for implementation of the nursing quality assurance process.

Assessment

A. **Standards are essential** to evaluation of nursing care. Standards define, qualitatively and quantitatively, the level of care the patient or client can reasonably and consistently expect to receive.

1. Standards of care: the type and scope of care the neonate and family can expect to receive, e.g., the neonatal nurse monitors the neonate's physiological responses to invasive procedures.

2. Standards of practice: the process of neonatal care delivered by nursing, e.g., the neonatal nurse provides opportunities for the parents to participate in their infant's care.

3. Criteria: specific, measurable statements that reflect attainment of the standard, e.g., all neonates have arterial blood gases drawn within 20 minutes of each change in oxygen concentration.

B. **Quality assurance evaluates** nursing care from the perspectives of structure, process, or outcomes of care.

1. Structure components: these are characteristics of the care delivery setting that indirectly influence care. They describe the environment and resources in it (i.e., physical unit and equipment, credentialing of staff).

   a. Criteria based on structure components identify conditions under which it is likely that quality nursing care will take place.

   b. Example: medication and emergency carts are checked and locked consistently.

2. Process components: these are aspects of direct nursing care as well as what constitutes that care (i.e., procedures, job descriptions, standards of care).

   a. Criteria based on process components identify how accurately a nursing action is performed.

   b. Example: within 24 hours of admission, the nurse writes a nursing care plan based on assessment data.

3. Outcome components describe health characteristics, behaviors, or status of the patient as the result of the nursing care provided (i.e., absence of complications, family knowledge of neonate's care).

a. Criteria based on outcomes are presumed to result from nursing interventions, but other factors operating in the patient, family, or environment can influence outcomes.

b. Example: parent is able to administer medication correctly to infant by discharge.

C. Quality assurance monitoring.

1. Retrospective review: comparison of predetermined criteria against documentation in the patient chart. The chart is reviewed after the patient is discharged.

   a. Advantages include convenient data source and ability to review large number of charts so patterns can be identified and effects of care monitored.

   b. A major disadvantage is dependence on the quality and accuracy of documentation to validate care given.

2. Concurrent review: comparison of predetermined criteria against documentation in the patient chart while care is in progress.

   a. Advantages include immediate feedback about patient processes and outcomes and the opportunity for immediate resolution of problems. This is often an effective method of review in the neonatal intensive care unit (NICU), where length of stay may be a week or longer.

   b. Disadvantages include difficulty in obtaining random samples for unbiased results and cost and time involved in this data retrieval method.

3. Prospective review: generally refers to case identification from a point in time forward. From that point, care may be evaluated either retrospectively or concurrently.

4. Nursing quality assurance monitors.

   a. Some topics of focus for monitoring include those that affect the greatest number of patients and tend to produce the most problems (e.g., spontaneous neonatal extubation).

   b. Other topics include major clinical functions of nursing (i.e., use of the nursing process and discharge planning).

   c. Generic monitors include those topics that are common to all hospital nursing units (e.g., intravenous therapy and medication administration).

Evaluation

A. Data analysis.

1. At specified intervals data that have been collected are tabulated and analyzed. Quality can be measured, in part, by a numerical ratio or pre-determined degree of compliance to the standards.

2. The results of monitoring may show that standards are consistently met or point to an area of concern or actual problem.

3. Trends can be identified by comparing current compliance rates with those from previous reports.

B. Taking action to resolve identified problems.

1. Common causes of problems.

   a. Lack of knowledge.

   b. Defects in the system (structure components).

   c. Performance problems (process components).

2. Plan of action includes the following:

   a. Who or what is expected to change.

   b. Who is responsible for implementing action.

   c. What action is appropriate in view of the cause, scope, and severity of the problem.

   d. When change is expected to occur.

   e. When follow-up will be re-evaluated.

3. The effectiveness of an evaluation process is determined by whether identified problems have been resolved and care has been improved and maintained.

4. Communicating: results of nursing monitoring and evaluation activities need to be shared with all members of the nursing department staff and through all other departments as established by hospital protocols. Written reports are generally required quarterly or semi-annually to the hospital quality assurance committee.

C. **Interdisciplinary quality assurance.**
1. The focus of quality assurance is quality patient care. Nursing plays a vital role in the holistic care of neonates and their families, but this care is a shared function of many disciplines. By incorporating the expertise of other disciplines (physicians, laboratory personnel, physical and respiratory therapy, social work), a more complete assessment of neonates' needs and care can be determined.
2. Coordination among the disciplines for the detection and resolution of problems has many advantages.
   a. Increasing awareness of each other's role. This understanding can lead to improved working relationships.
   b. Increasing ability to evaluate the entire scope of a problem by approaching it from different perspectives.
   c. Facilitating better communication of complex patient problems (those with multiple intervening structure or process variables).
   d. Decreasing duplication of data collected to promote more effective group problem solving.
   e. Discovering more effective methods of care.
3. With the rapid changes and increasing sophistication of care modalities in neonatal care comes the responsibility of assuring high quality of that care.

D. **Trends in quality assurance.**
1. Unit-based quality assurance.
   a. The trend in nursing quality assurance is now a more participative, decentralized approach. Nurses at the bedside, involved in direct patient care, are identifying care priorities and problems. More importantly, nurses are identifying patient care solutions that can have immediate results in terms of quality.
   b. Quality assurance and research.
      (1) Quality assurance and research differ in their scope and intent. Quality assurance intends to improve patient care in a particular practice setting, whereas research intends to be generalizable to multiple practice settings. Nursing research can enhance quality assurance by:
         (a) Testing the reliability and validity of measurement tools and methods.
         (b) Developing measurement tools that can differentiate between the technical and affective aspects of nursing care.
         (c) Validating criteria and standards of practice and care.
         (d) Incorporating more qualitative approaches to data collection and interpretation.
         (e) Suggesting priority areas for research.
         (f) Establishing, through studies, whether patient outcomes actually meet the established standards.
   c. Quality assurance and computers.
      (1) Identifying and resolving practice problems must be efficient and effective, especially in light of limited resources. Using computers in quality assurance programs can enhance information retrieval by:
         (a) Building a data base for ongoing tracking and trading of hospital-wide (generic) data, or for selecting practice monitors that require continuous or ongoing data collection.
         (b) Allowing the sharing of data among institutions with similar patient populations.

STUDY QUESTIONS

1. A method of proving that quality assurance activities are improving patient care is:
   a. Documentation of the effectiveness of care.
   b. Identification of care problems.
   c. Monitoring care activities.

2. In order for quality assurance activities to be successful, they must:
   a. Be complex and involve many variables and nursing concepts.
   b. Be conducted by graduate level practitioners.
   c. Be useful to nurses in clinical settings.

3. Standards of practice are an example of:
   a. Outcome components.
   b. Process components.
   c. Structure components.

4. The nurse is reviewing a neonate's chart for accuracy of assessment documentation. The neonate is still a patient in the unit. This type of review is called:
   a. Concurrent.
   b. Prospective.
   c. Retrospective.

Answers to Study Questions

1. a   3. b
2. c   4. a

REFERENCES

Aduddell, P.A., and Weeks, L.C.: A cost-effective approach to quality assurance. Nurs. Econom., 1:279–282, 1984.

Beyerman, K.: Developing a unit-based nursing quality assurance program: From concept to practice. J. Nurs. Qual. Assur., 2(1):1–11, 1987.

Block, D.: Quality assurance and evaluation research: A researcher's perspective. Nurs. Res., 29(2):68–73, 1980.

Burda, D.: Hospitals anxious over payment denials for quality. Hospitals, 61(12):48–53, 1987.

Carron, M.K.: Comprehensive quality assurance: Inception through evaluation. Caring, 1:17–19, 1988.

Decker, C.M.: Quality assurance: Accent on monitoring. Nurs. Manage., 16(11):20–24, 1985.

Driever, M.J.: Interpretation: A critical component of the quality assurance process. J. Nurs. Qual. Assur., 2(2):55–58, 1988.

Esper, P.S.: Discharge planning: A quality assurance approach. Nurs. Manage., 19(10):66–68, 1988.

Finley-Cottone, D., and Link, M.K.: Quality assurance in critical care. Crit. Care Nurse, 5(2):46–49, 1985.

Harrington, P., and Kaniecki, N.: Standards and quality assurance: A common sense approach. Nurs. Manage., 20(2):80–84, 1988.

Inzinga, M.: Legislative issues and health care trends: Quality assurance. Nurs. Admin. Q., 2:80–84, 1984.

Kelly, P.: Differentiating roles in quality assurance. DCCN, 3(2):104–109, 1984.

Kovner, C.: Using computerized databases for nursing research and quality assurance. Comput. Nurs., 7(5):228–231, 1989.

Larson, E.: Combining nursing quality assurance and research programs. J. Nurs. Admin., 11:32–35, 1983.

McGee, K.B.: Quality assurance can be more than just an exercise on paper. Focus Crit. Care, 15(2):27–30, 1988.

Megel, M.E., and Barna-Elrod, M.E.: Quality assurance: Taking a new look at collaboration between education and service. J. Nurs. Qual. Assur., 2(1):65–73, 1987.

Miller-Bader, M.M.: Nursing care behaviors that predict patient satisfaction. J. Nurs. Qual. Assur., 2(3):11–17, 1988.

Milton, D.: Challenges of quality assurance program evaluation in a practice setting. J. Nurs. Qual. Assur., 2(4):25–34, 1988.

New, N.A.: Quality measurement: Quick, easy and unit-based. Nurs. Manage., 20(10):50–51, 1989.

Patterson, C.H.: Standards of patient care: The Joint Commission focus on nursing quality assurance. Nurs. Clin. North Am., 23(3):625–637, 1988.

Pelletier, L.R., and Poster, E.C.: An overview of evaluation methodology for nursing quality assurance programs: I. J. Nurs. Qual. Assur., 2(4):55–62, 1988.

Poe, S.S., and Will, J.C.: Quality nurse-patient outcomes: A framework for nursing practice. J. Nurs. Qual. Assur., 2:29–37, 1987.

Porter, A.L.: Assuring quality through staff nurse performance. Nurs. Clin. North Am., 23(3):649–655, 1988.

Puta, D.F.: Nurse-physician collaboration toward quality. J. Nurs. Qual. Assur., *3*(2):11–18, 1989.

Saum, M.F.: Evaluation: A vital component of the quality assurance program. J. Nurs. Qual. Assur., *2*(4):17–24, 1988.

Schifiliti, C., Bonasoro, C.L., and Thompson, M.: Lotus 1-2-3: A quality assurance application for nursing practice, administration and staff development. Comput. Nurs., *4*(5):205–211, 1986.

Schroeder, P.: Directions and dilemmas in nursing quality assurance. Nurs. Clin. North Am., *23*(3):657–664, 1988.

Smelter, C.: Organizing the search for excellence. Nurs. Manage., *14*(6):19–21, 1983.

Wagner, D.N.: Who defines quality—Consumers or professionals? Caring, *10*:26–28, 1988.

Whittaker, A., and McCanless, L.: Nursing peer review: Monitoring the appropriateness and outcome of nursing care. J. Nurs. Qual. Assur., *2*(2):24–31, 1988.

Newborn Metric Conversion Tables

Table A-1
TEMPERATURE

Fahrenheit (F) to Centigrade (C)							
°F	°C	°F	°C	°F	°C	°F	°C
95.0	35.0	98.0	36.7	101.0	38.3	104.0	40.0
95.2	35.1	98.2	36.8	101.2	38.4	104.2	40.1
95.4	35.2	98.4	36.9	101.4	38.6	104.4	40.2
95.6	35.3	**98.6**	**37.0**	101.6	38.7	104.6	40.3
95.8	35.4	98.8	37.1	101.8	38.8	104.8	40.4
96.0	35.6	99.0	37.2	102.0	38.9	105.0	40.6
96.2	35.7	99.2	37.3	102.2	39.0	105.2	40.7
96.4	35.8	99.4	37.4	102.4	39.1	105.4	40.8
96.6	35.9	99.6	37.6	102.6	39.2	105.6	40.9
96.8	36.0	99.8	37.7	102.8	39.3	105.8	41.0
97.0	36.1	100.0	37.8	103.0	39.4	106.0	41.1
97.2	36.2	100.2	37.9	103.2	39.6	106.2	41.2
97.4	36.3	100.4	38.0	103.4	39.7	106.4	41.3
97.6	36.4	100.6	38.1	103.6	39.8	106.6	41.4
97.8	36.6	100.8	38.2	103.8	39.9	106.8	41.6

Note: $°C = (°F - 32) \times \frac{5}{9}$. Centigrade temperature equivalents rounded to one decimal place by adding 0.1 when second decimal place is 5 or greater.
The metric system replaces the term "Centigrade" with "Celsius" (the inventor of the scale).
Reprinted with permission of Ross Laboratories, Columbus, OH, 43216, © Ross Laboratories

Table A–2
LENGTH

Inches to centimeters

1 inch increments Example: To obtain centimeters equivalent to 22 inches, read "20" on top scale, "2" on side scale; equivalent is 55.9 centimeters.

Inches	0	10	20	30	40
0	0	25.4	50.8	76.2	101.6
1	2.5	27.9	53.3	78.7	104.1
2	5.1	30.5	55.9	81.3	106.7
3	7.6	33.0	58.4	83.8	109.2
4	10.2	35.6	61.0	86.4	111.8
5	12.7	38.1	63.5	88.9	114.3
6	15.2	40.6	66.0	91.4	116.8
7	17.8	48.2	68.6	94.0	119.4
8	20.3	45.7	71.1	96.5	121.9
9	22.9	48.3	73.7	99.1	124.5

One-Quarter (¼) inch increments Example: To obtain centimeters equivalent to 14¾ inches, read "14" on top scale, "¾" on side scale; equivalent is 37.5 centimeters.

10–15 Inches

	10	11	12	13	14	15
0	25.4	27.9	30.5	33.0	35.6	38.1
¼	26.0	28.6	31.1	33.7	36.2	38.7
½	26.7	29.2	31.8	34.3	36.8	39.4
¾	27.3	29.8	32.4	34.9	37.5	40.0

16–21 Inches

	16	17	18	19	20	21
0	40.6	43.2	45.7	48.3	50.8	53.3
¼	41.3	43.8	46.4	48.9	51.4	54.0
½	41.9	44.5	47.0	49.5	52.1	54.6
¾	42.5	45.1	47.6	50.2	52.7	55.2

Note: 1 inch = 2.540 centimeters. Centimeter equivalents rounded one decimal place by adding 0.1 when second decimal place is 5 or greater; for example, 33.48 becomes 33.5.
Reprinted with permission of Ross Laboratories, Columbus, OH, 43216, © Ross Laboratories.

Table A-3
WEIGHT (MASS)

Pounds and Ounces to Grams

Example: To obtain grams equivalent to 6 pounds, 8 ounces, read "6" on top scale, "8" on side scale; equivalent is 2948 grams.

OUNCES \ POUNDS	0	1	2	3	4	5	6	7	8	9	10	11	12	13	14
0	0	454	907	1361	1814	2268	2722	3175	3629	4082	4536	4990	5443	5897	6350
1	28	482	936	1389	1843	2296	2750	3203	3657	4111	4564	5018	5471	5925	6379
2	57	510	964	1417	1871	2325	2778	3232	3685	4139	4593	5046	5500	5953	6407
3	85	539	992	1446	1899	2353	2807	3260	3714	4167	4621	5075	5528	5982	6435
4	113	567	1021	1474	1928	2381	2835	3289	3742	4196	4649	5103	5557	6010	6464
5	142	595	1049	1503	1956	2410	2863	3317	3770	4224	4678	5131	5585	6038	6492
6	170	624	1077	1531	1984	2438	2892	3345	3799	4252	4706	5160	5613	6067	6520
7	198	652	1106	1559	2013	2466	2920	3374	3827	4281	4734	5188	5642	6095	6549
8	227	680	1134	1588	2041	2495	2948	3402	3856	4309	4763	5216	5670	6123	6577
9	255	709	1162	1616	2070	2523	2977	3430	3884	4337	4791	5245	5698	6152	6605
10	283	737	1191	1644	2098	2551	3005	3459	3912	4366	4819	5273	5727	6180	6634
11	312	765	1219	1673	2126	2580	3033	3487	3941	4394	4848	5301	5755	6209	6662
12	340	794	1247	1701	2155	2608	3062	3515	3969	4423	4876	5330	5783	6237	6690
13	369	822	1276	1729	2183	2637	3090	3544	3997	4451	4904	5358	5812	6265	6719
14	397	850	1304	1758	2211	2665	3118	3572	4026	4479	4933	5386	5840	6294	6747
15	425	879	1332	1786	2240	2693	3147	3600	4054	4508	4961	5415	5868	6322	6776

Note: 1 pound = 453.59237 grams; 1 ounce = 28.349523 grams; 1000 grams = 1 kilogram. Gram equivalents have been rounded to whole numbers by adding one when the first decimal place is 5 or greater.

Reprinted with permission of Ross Laboratories, Columbus, OH, 43216, © Ross Laboratories.

Recommended Schedule for Hepatitis B Vaccine

Infants of*	Dose†	Age
HBsAg–positive mothers	HB Vaccine 1	Birth–within 12 hr
	HBIG (0.5 ml IM)	Birth–within 12 h
	HB Vaccine 2	1 mo
	HB Vaccine 3	6 mo
HBsAg-unknown mothers	HB Vaccine 1	Birth–within 12 h
	HBIG	If mother HBsAg–positive, give 0.5 ml IM as soon as possible, *not* later than 1 wk after birth
	HB Vaccine 2	1–2 mo
	HB Vaccine 3	6 mo
HBsAg-negative mothers‡	HB Vaccine 1	Birth–within 12 h
	HB Vaccine 2	1–2 mo
	HB Vaccine 3	6–18 mo

*HBsAg, Hepatitis B surface antigen.
†HB, Hepatitis B; HBIG, hepatitis B immune globulin; IM, intramuscularly.
‡A second option is to administer HBV at 2-month intervals to conform to the schedules of other childhood vaccines, which can be administered concurrently.
Table modified from Centers for Disease Control: Hepatitis B virus: A comprehensive strategy for eliminating transmission in the United States through universal childhood vaccination: Recommendations of the Immunization Practices Advisory Committee (ACIP). MMWR *40*:(RR-13): 1–25, 1991; used with the permission of the American Academy of Pediatrics and The American College of Obstetricians and Gynecologists. *Guidelines for Perinatal Care,* © 1992.

Sharon M. Glass

Neonatal Pain Management

A. **Nervous system development pertaining to pain transmission.** (Anand, 1990; Anand and Hickey, 1987; Owens, 1984).

1. Interacting components of the nervous system.
   a. Central nervous system (CNS)/peripheral nervous system (PNS).
   b. Pain perception begins with stimulation of PNS.
      (1) Skin surface nerve endings carry impulses.
      (2) Sensory fiber development begins at approximately 7 weeks' gestation.
      (3) All cutaneous surfaces covered by approximately 20 weeks' gestation (density ≥ adult).
   c. Stimulus is transmitted and processed by CNS.
      (1) Nerve fibers enter the spinal cord through the dorsal roots.
      (2) Synapse in the dorsal horns and travel along the spinothalamic tract.
      (3) Development begins at approximately 13–14 weeks'/complete by 30 weeks' gestation.
2. Nerve fiber myelination.
   a. Impulse velocity depends on size of the nerve fiber and presence of myelin.
      (1) Myelinated (A-delta) fibers.
      (2) Unmyelinated (C-polymodal) fibers.
   b. Most nociceptive impulses travel on thinly myelinated or unmyelinated fibers.
   c. Myelination (and nerve function) begins at approximately 16 weeks' gestation.
   d. Infant's small size yields shorter intraneuronal distance, compensates for incomplete myelin development.
3. Thalamocortical pain fibers/hypothalamus.
   a. Thalamus is the relay station.
   b. Synapses sensory fibers and cortex—crucial for cortical pain perception.
      (1) Connections complete by approximately 20–24 weeks' gestation.
   c. Hypothalamic stimulation = adrenal stimulation/physiological response.
      (1) Adrenal secretion of cortisol, epinephrine, norepinephrine.
      (2) Increased levels detected in stressed fetus at approximately 16–21 weeks' gestation.
4. Cortical maturity.
   a. Development of cortex begins at approximately 8 weeks' gestation.
   b. Full complement of neurons (10^9) by approximately 20 weeks' gestation.

    c. Adequacy of integration/perception by immature cortex documented by EEG studies, which establish functional maturity.

       (1) Bursts first seen at approximately 20 weeks' gestation; synchronous by approximately 26–27 weeks.

       (2) Patterns of sleep/wakefulness by 30 weeks' gestation.

       (3) Visual and auditory-evoked potentials recorded <30 weeks' gestation.

    d. Increased glucose utilization by sensory areas suggests cortical activity.

B. **Attenuation of the stress response improves outcome.**

1. Surgical intervention (Anand et al., 1987; Troug and Anand, 1989).

    a. Physical and biochemical responses are attenuated with anesthesia.

    b. Level of response reflects invasiveness/duration of pain.

    c. Decreased mortality, morbidity, recovery time, costs, long-term consequences.

2. Environmental modulation (Als et al., 1986).

    a. Shorter duration of ventilator/oxygen therapy.

    b. Earlier normalized feeding behaviors.

    c. Decreased hospital costs, improved behavioral and developmental outcome.

3. Circumcision studies (Gunnar et al., 1981; Stang et al., 1988; Masciello, 1990).

    a. Without anesthesia: increased cortisol, reduction in REM sleep, altered behavior for 24–48 hours.

    b. Penile nerve block and local infiltration of prepuce show attenuation of stress responses.

C. **Infant pain responses.**

1. Responses modulated by infant state and individualized reaction.

2. Physiological.

    a. Increased heart rate, BP, RR (above baseline for individual infant).

    b. Others including shallow respirations, desaturation, pallor, flushing, palmar sweating, diaphoresis, dilated pupils.

3. Behavioral.

    a. Vocalizations: cry, whimper.

    b. Facial expressions: "cry face."

    c. Body movements: thrashing, tremulousness, limb withdrawal/flexion, legs bicycling, excessive reactivity.

    d. State changes.

       (1) Decreased sleep periods.

       (2) Rapid alteration sleep/awake cycles.

4. Biochemical.

    a. Increased stress hormones: glucocorticoids, catecholamines, glucagon.

       (1) Influence metabolic regulation, response to injury, stress adaptation.

       (2) Cascade of metabolic changes causes substrate mobilization and breakdown of protein, fat, and carbohydrate stores, glucocorticoids, catecholamines, glucagon.

    b. Increased metabolites: glucose, lactate, pyruvate, non-esterified fatty acids.

       (1) "Fight/flight" response for quick energy.

D. **Interventions.**

1. Nonpharmacological.

    a. Comfort measures, including pacifier, swaddling/boundaries, rocking, soothing verbalizations, positioning.

    b. Alternative procedures, including smallest needle gauge, automatic heel lance, monitor technician competence, maintain central venous access to minimize peripheral punctures when possible.

2. Pharmacologic: opioids. (See Chapters 6, 9, and 26 for non-opioid pharmacological interventions.)

    a. Morphine (Bhat et al., 1990; Maguire and Maloney, 1988; Seltin et al, 1989).

   (1) Bolus dose: 0.1 mg/kg every 8 hours in infants $\leq$ 30 weeks' gestation, 0.1 mg/kg every 4 hours in infants >30 weeks' gestation.
   (2) Continuous: load with 0.1 mg/kg and then begin with 0.01 mg/kg/hour.
   (3) Complications: respiratory depression, hypotension, bronchoconstriction, decreased GI motility/constipation, urinary retention.
   (4) Weaning—prolonged use: decrease dose 10%/day.
 b. Fentanyl (Koehntop et al., 1986; Maguire and Maloney, 1988).
   (1) Bolus dose: 2–5 μg/kg every 2–4 hours.
   (2) Continuous: load with 5 μg/kg and then begin with 2 μg/kg/hour.
   (3) Complications: respiratory depression, bradycardia, feeding intolerance, diminished clearance with increased intra-abdominal pressure.
   (4) Weaning: decrease by 10% every 6 hours.

REFERENCES

Als, H., Lawhon, G., Brown, E., et al.: Individualized behavioral and environmental care for the very low birth weight preterm infant at high risk for bronchopulmonary dysplasia: Neonatal intensive care unit and developmental outcome. *Pediatrics, 78*:1123–1132, 1986.

Anand, K. J. S.: The biology of pain perception in newborn infants. *Adv. Pain Res. Ther., 15*:113, 1990.

Anand, K. J. S., and Hickey, P. R.: Pain and its effects in the human neonate and fetus. *N. Engl. J. Med., 317*:1321–1329, 1987.

Anand, K. J. S., Sippell, W., and Aynsley-Green, A.: Randomized trial of fentanyl anesthesia in preterm babies undergoing surgery: Effects on the stress response. *Lancet, 1*:62–66, 1987.

Bhat, R., Chari, G., Gulati, A., et al.: Pharmacokinetics of a single dose of morphine in preterm infants during the first week of life. *J. Pediatr., 117*:477–481, 1990.

Gunnar, M. R., Fisch, R. O., Korsvik, S., et al.: The effects of circumcision on cortisol and behavior. *Psychoneuroendocrinology, 6*:269–275, 1986.

Koehntop, D. E., Rodman, J. H., Brundage, D. M., et al.: Pharmacokinetics of fentanyl in neonates. *Anesth. Analog, 65*:227–232, 1986.

Maguire, D., and Maloney, P.: A comparison of fentanyl and morphine use in neonates. *Neonatal Network, 7*(1):27–32, 1988.

Masciello, A. L.: Anesthesia for neonatal circumcision. *Obstet. Gynecol., 75*:834–838, 1990.

Owens, M. E.: Pain in infancy: Conceptual and methodological issues. *Pain, 20*:213–230, 1984.

Seltin, D. J., Lawlor-Klean, P., and Racoma, P. G.: Administration of continuous intravenous morphine infusion for the neonate. *Neonatal Network, 8*(2):60–62, 1989.

Stang, H. J., Gunnar, M., Snellman, L., et al.: Local anesthesia for neonatal circumcision: Effects on distress and cortisol response. *JAMA, 259*:1507–1511, 1988.

Truog, R., and Anand, K. J. S.: Management of pain in the postoperative neonate. *Neonatal Surg., 16*:61–78, 1989.

Apgar Score

The Apgar Score is a method of evaluating the newborn's condition at birth based on five characteristics: heart rate, respiratory effort, muscle tone, reflex irritability, and color. For each parameter, the infant receives a score of 0 if it is absent, 1 if it is present but abnormal, and 2 if it is normal. Traditionally a score is assigned at 1 and 5 minutes but in a prolonged resuscitation it can be assigned at any time to reflect the condition of the infant and the response to resuscitative efforts. With asphyxia, the Apgar characteristics generally disappear in a predictable manner: First, the pink coloration is lost; next respiratory effort; then tone followed by reflex irritability and, finally, heart rate.

Sign	Score 0	Score 1	Score 2
Heart rate	Absent	Below 100	Over 100
Respiratory effort	Absent	Weak, irregular	Good, crying
Muscle tone	Flaccid	Some flexion of extremities	Well flexed
Reflex irritability (Catheter in nose)	No response	Grimace	Cough or sneeze
Color	Blue, pale	Body pink extremities blue	Completely pink

Index

Note: Page numbers in *italics* refer to illustrations; page numbers followed by t refer to tables.

A

Abdomen, gas patterns of, abnormal, 627–628
  normal, 627, *628*
ABO incompatibility, 330, 330t
Abruptio placentae, 22–23
  clinical presentation of, 22–23
    fetal signs in, 23
    maternal signs and symptoms in, 22
    types of, 22
  potential complications of, 23
    fetal/newborn, 23
    maternal, 23
Acetaminophen, 161
Achondroplasia, 635
Acidosis, metabolic, 297–298
  excess acid load in, 297
  loss of bicarbonate in, 297
  underexcretion of acid in, 297
Acquired immunodeficiency syndrome (AIDS),
    breast-feeding and, 534
Acrocyanosis, 66
Adolescence, 550–552
  as maturational crisis, 551–552
  physical and physiological development in,
    550–551
    for both, 550
    for females, 550
    for males, 551
  psychosocial changes in, 551
Adolescent parent, 548–563. See also under
    Crisis.
  sick newborn and, 554–556
    low birthweight in, 555
    possible adverse outcomes and, 555–556
    prematurity in, 555
  sociocultural crisis and, 552–554
    family relationships disruption in, 553
    father's profile in, 553–554
    mother's profile in, 553
    peer group relationships disruption in, 552
    risks to infant in, 554
Adrenal gland, 311–314
  anatomy of, 311
  hormones of, 311
  hypofunction of, 311
  physiology of, at birth, 311
Adrenal hyperplasia, congenital, 311–314
  assessment in, 312–313
  clinical presentation of, 312

Adrenal hyperplasia (*Continued*)
    compensated/non-salt-losing disease in,
      312
    uncompensated/salt-losing disease in,
  complications of, 314
  definition of, 311
  diagnosis of, 313
    differential, 313
    newborn screening in, 313
    tests in, 313
  genitalia appearance in, 313
  outcome of, 314
  pathophysiology of, 311–312, *312*
  patient care management in, 313–314
  signs and symptoms of, 312–313
Air bronchograms, 613
Air leaks, 117–119
  clinical presentation/diagnosis of, 117–118
    pneumomediastinum in, 117–118
    pneumopericardium in, 118
    pneumoperitoneum in, 118
    pneumothorax in, 117
    pulmonary interstitial emphysema in, 118
  definition of, 117
  incidence of, 117
  management of, 118–119
    pneumomediastinum in, 118
    pneumopericardium in, 118
    pneumoperitoneum in, 118–119
    pneumothorax in, 118
    pulmonary interstitial emphysema in, 119
  outcome of, 119
  pathophysiology of, 117
  pulmonary, 89
Airway, in neonatal resuscitation, 82
  opening of, 83–84
    mouth and nares suctioning in, 83–84
    positioning for, 83, *83*
Albuterol, in bronchopulmonary dysplasia,
    114
Albuterol/terbutaline, in ventilation therapy,
    157
Alcohol abuse, breast-feeding and, 534
Alkalosis, metabolic, 298
Aminophylline, in methylxanthine therapy, 132
  in ventilation therapy, 156
Amniocentesis, 447–448
Amniotic bands, 465
Analgesia, obstetrical. See *Obstetrical analgesia.*

Anemia, 328–333
  clinical assessment in, 331
  clinical presentation in, 331
  complications of, 332–333
  definition of, 328
  diagnostic studies in, 332, 332t
  differential diagnosis in, 332
  etiologic factors in, 329–331
    hemolysis in, 329–331
      ABO incompatibility in, 330, 330t
      blood group incompatibilities in, 329–331
      enzymatic defect in, 330
      intrauterine infection in, 331
      Rh incompatibility in, 329–330. See also
        Rh incompatibility.
    hemorrhage in, 329
    iatrogenic post-natal phlebotomy in, 331
    prematurity in, 331
  in sick newborn, 50
  outcome of, 333
  patient care management in, 333
  physical examination in, 332
Anencephaly, 88, 399–400
Anesthesia, obstetrical, 29–31. See also
    Obstetrical anesthesia.
Antepartum care, 6–7
  initial lab work in, 7
  initial visit in, 6–7
    medical history in, 6–7
    obstetrical history in, 6
  routine and diagnostic lab work in, 7
    glucose screen in, 7
    glucose tolerance test in, 7
Antepartum period, conditions related to,
      17–20. See also individual conditions.
  diabetes mellitus in, 19–20
  pregnancy-induced hypertension in, 17–19
Antepartum visits, 8–9
  frequency of, 8
  routine assessments in, 8–9
Antibiotics, 511–513
  definitions in, 511–512
  for bacterial infections, 356, 357t
  for meningitis, 421–422
  for pneumonia, 104
  for respiratory distress syndrome, 101
  for sick newborns, 53
  for urinary tract infections, 354
  newborn considerations in, 512–513
  principles of use in, 512
Anus, imperforate, 242–243
    high, 242
    low, 242
Aorta, coarctation of, 213–214
Aortic stenosis, 214–215
Apgar scores, 40, 49, 81, 698
Apnea, 125–133
  causes of, 128–129
    cardiovascular disorders in, 128–129
    central nervous system disorders in, 129
    drugs in, 129
    environmental, 129
    hematopoietic, 129
    infection in, 129
    metabolic, 129
    reflex stimulation in, 129
    respiratory disorders in, 128
  central, 126
  definition of, 125–126
  evaluation of, 129–131
    documentation of episodes in, 130

Apnea (*Continued*)
    laboratory work-up in, 130
    neonatal risk factors in, 130
    perinatal risk factors in, 129–130
    physical examination in, 130
    pneumogram in, 131
  home monitoring of, 133
    effectiveness of, 133
    family support for, 133
    indications for, 133
  idiopathic, 126–127
  management of, 131–133
    assisted ventilation in, 133
    continuous positive airway pressure in, 131
    cutaneous stimulation in, 131
    neck roll in, 131
    pharmacological therapy in, 131–133. See
        also individual agents.
    prone position and, 131
    reflexes triggering in, 131
  mixed, 126
  obstructive, 126
  of prematurity, 126–127
  pathogenesis of, 127–128
    chemoreceptors in, 127
      hypercapnia and, 127
      hypoxemia and, 127
    immature central respiratory center in, 127
    mechanoreceptors, 127–128
    protective reflexes and, 128
    sleep state and, 128
    thermal afferents and, 127
  periodic breathing and, 125
  primary, 126
  secondary, 126
  types of, 126–127
Arnold-Chiari malformation, common features
      of, 404
  myelomeningocele and, 404–405
  patient care management in, 404
Arthrogryposis multiplex congenita, 468
Artifact, 613
Ascites, 634, *634*
Asphyxia, case study of, 602–605
    hypoxic-ischemic encephalopathy in,
        604–605
    management in, 602–603
    presenting problem in, 602
  neonatal resuscitation and, 78
    meconium in, 78
    tissue hypoxia in, 78
Assessment of newborn, 40–47, 57–74
  activity in, 65
  auscultation/palpation in, 66–68
    abdomen/trunk in, 68
      anal area and, 68
      bladder and, 68
      kidneys and, 68
      liver and, 68
      organ enlargement and, 68
      spine and, 68
      umbilical cord in, 68
    chest/lungs in, 67–68
      breasts and nipples in, 67
      bronchial breath sounds in, 67
      respiratory rate and pattern in, 67
    heart in, 66–67. See also *Heart.*
  body part examination in, 69–74. See also
      individual parts.
  body temperature in, 42
  clinical behavior sequence in, 40, *41*

Assessment of newborn (*Continued*)
  color in, 66
  general condition in, 65–66
  genitalia in, 69. See also *Genitalia*.
  gestational age in, 58–65. See also *Gestational age assessment*.
  head in, 41
  heart sounds in, 41
  intestines in, 41–42
  morphology in, 66
  neurologic examination in, 74
  nutrition in, 66
  perinatal history review in, 57–58
    labor and delivery history in, 58
    prenatal history in, 58
    resuscitation required in, 58
  physical examination in, 40–42, 65
  posture in, 65
  respirations/breath sounds in, 41, 65–66
  skin in, 40–41, 65
  state in, 65
Atrial septal defect, 211, *211*
Autosome, 444

B
Bacterial infections. See *Infections, bacterial*.
Bacteroides fragilis, 421–422
Bag and mask ventilation, 84
Bag to endotracheal tube ventilation, 84–85
Ballard method, for gestational age assessment, 59, *59*
Beckwith's syndrome, 64
Beckwith-Wiedemann syndrome, 452–453
Behavioral organization, 427–430
  assessment of, 428
  definition of, 427
  infant's capacity for, 427, 427–428
  intervention strategies in, 428–430
    attention-interactional system in, 429
    autonomic system in, 428
    awake states in, 429
    motor system in, 428
    self-regulatory system in, 429–430
    sleep states in, 428
    transitional states in, 429
Bilirubin, metabolism of, 246
  origin of, 246
Biophysical profile, 10
  management after, 10
  scoring in, 10
Birth asphyxia, 48–49
Birth defect, March of Dimes' definition of, 443
Birth trauma, 62
Birthweight, blood pressure by, 67, *67*
  very low, case study of, 599–602
    fluid and electrolyte management in, 601–602
    initial management in, 599–600
Bladder. See *Urinary bladder*.
Blisters, sucking, 74
Blood cells, development of, 322–327
  blood volume in, 326–327
  erythropoiesis in, 323–324
  hematocrit in, 324, 324t
  hematopoiesis in, 322–323, *323*
  hemoglobin in, 324
  platelets in, 326
  red, count in, during pregnancy, 5
    in newborn, 324t, 325
    development of, *323*, 324–325

Blood cells (*Continued*)
    function of, 324–325
    indices in, 324t, 325
      mean corpuscular hemoglobin concentration in, 325
      mean corpuscular hemoglobin in, 325
      mean corpuscular volume in, 325
    packed, 339
  white, count in, during pregnancy, 5
    evaluation of, 341
    in newborn, 326, 326t
    development of, *323*, 325–326
    function of, 325
    granulocytes in, 325–326
    lymphocytes in, 326
    monocytes in, 326
Blood count, complete, evaluation of, 341–342
    neutrophil counts in, 341–342, *342*
    response to infection in, 341
    white blood cells in, 341
Blood flow, cerebral, 397–398
    autoregulation of, 397–398
    factors affecting, 397
  concepts of, 199
  uteroplacental, 17
Blood gas interpretation, 164–167
  acceptable values in, 164, 164t
  compensation/correction of acidosis-alkalosis in, 165–166, 166t
  process of, 167
  respiratory/metabolic acidosis and alkalosis in, 164–165
Blood pressure, by birthweight, 67, *67*
  during pregnancy, 5
  in congenital heart disease diagnosis, 204–205
Blood products, 339–341
  albumin in, 340
  components in, 339
  fresh frozen plasma in, 339
  granulocytes, 339–340
  packed red blood cells in, 339
  platelets in, 340
  whole blood, 339
Body substance isolation, 362
Bonding, family-infant, 542–545
  assessment in, 542–543
  definitions in, 542
  evaluation of, 544–545
  interventions for encouragement of, 543–544
Bowel atresia and stenosis, 630–631
Boyle's law, in assisted ventilation, 149
Brachial nerve plexus injury, 409–410
  Duchenne-Erb palsy and, 409
  Klumpke's paralysis and, 409
Bradycardia, 66
Brain, anatomy of, 396–397
  brainstem in, 397
  cerebellum in, 396
  cerebrum in, 396–397
Brain injury, 407–410. See also specific conditions.
Brainstem, 397
Breast-feeding, infant in crisis and, 544
  pre-term infant and, 437
    improving chances for success in, 437
    indicators for, 437
  substance abuse and, 534
    AIDS in, 534
    alcohol in, 534
    cocaine and methamphetamines in, 534

Breast-feeding (*Continued*)
  heroin in, 534
  marijuana in, 534
  nicotine in, 534
Breast milk, 269–271
  advantages of, 269
  disadvantages of, 270–271
  establishing and maintaining adequate supply
    of, 271
  full-term infants and, 269
  pre-term infants and, 269
Breasts, during puerperium, 12
  in gestational age assessment, 60
  in newborn assessment, 67
  physiologic changes in, 5
Breathing, See also *Respiration; Respiratory* entries.
  in neonatal resuscitation, 82
Breech delivery, 26–28
  assessment and management of, 27–28
    cesarean delivery and, 28
    newborn in, 28
    vaginal delivery and, 27–28
  clinical presentation of, 27
  complications of, 27
    fetal/newborn, 27
    maternal, 27
  etiology/predisposing factors in, 26–27
    maternal, 26–27
    placental/fetal, 27
  incidence of, 26
Bronchodilators, 156–157
Bronchogenic cyst, 121
Bronchopulmonary dysplasia, 111–116
  clinical presentation of, 113
  complications of, 113–114
  definition of, 111–112
  diagnosis of, 113
  etiology of, 112–113
    assisted ventilation in, 112
    early fluid intake in, 112
    gestational age in, 112–113
    nutritional deficiencies in, 112
    oxygen toxicity in, 112
    shunting in, 112
  incidence of, 112
  management of, 114–115
    bronchodilators in, 114
    cardiac evaluation in, 114–115
    diuretics in, 114
    fluid restriction in, 114
    nutrition in, 115
    respiratory support in, 114
    steroids in, 115
    team approach in, 115
    tracheostomy in, 115
  outcome of, 115–116
  pathophysiology of, 113
  radiologic evaluation of, 617, *618*
Bullous impetigo, 481
Bunnell Life Pulse, 173

C
Café au lait spots, 477, *478*
Caffeine, in methylxanthine therapy, 132
  theophylline vs., 132
Calcium, 293–295
  disorders of, 293–295
  fetal metabolism and, 293
  homeostasis in, 293

Calcium (*Continued*)
  in pre-term infant nutrition, 262–263
  in total parenteral nutrition, 267, 268t
  neonatal metabolism and, 293
Calories, in pre-term infant nutrition, 259, 259t
  in total parenteral nutrition, 265
Candidiasis, acute disseminated, 358
  cutaneous, 358
  oral, 72
Capillary blood sampling, *639*, 639–640
Caput succedaneum, 69, 408
Carbohydrates, in pre-term infant nutrition, 260
  in total parenteral nutrition, 266t, 266–267
    complications associated with, 268
Cardiac output, 197, 199
  calculation of, 197
  definition of, 197
  stroke volume in, 197, 199
    contractility and, 199
    pre-load and, 197, 199
Cardinal movements, during labor, 10
Cardiothoracic ratio, 613
Cardiovascular disorders, 193–229. See also
    individual disorders.
Cardiovascular system, adaptation at birth of,
    38, *39*
  ductus arteriosus and, 38
  ductus venosus and, 38
  foramen ovale and, 38
  postnatal circulation and, 38
  umbilical cord and, 38
  disorders of, apnea and, 128–129
  embryology of, 194–197
    cardiac development in, 194–195, *194–196*
    circulatory development in, 196–197
    great vessel development in, 196, *196*
  lesions with congested vascularity in, 625–627
  lesions with decreased pulmonary vascularity
    in, 627
  of sick newborn, clinical findings and, 50
    congenital heart disease and, 50
    persistent fetal shunts and, 50
    physical assessment and, 47
  physiologic changes in, 5
  physiology of, 197–199
    cardiac depolarization in, 197
    cardiac output in, 197
    concepts of blood flow in, 199
    normal circulation in, 197, *198*
    stroke volume in, 197, 199
      contractility and, 199
      pre-load and, 197, 199
  radiologic evaluation of, 624–627. See also
    individual parts and conditions.
Case studies, 586–608
  asphyxia in, 602–605
    hypoxic-ischemic encephalopathy and,
      604–605
    management in, 602–603
    presenting problem in, 602
  congenital diaphragmatic hernia in, 596–597
  herpes simplex virus infection in, 592–595
    management in, 592–593
    presenting problem in, 592
  hyaline membrane disease in, 605–608
  hypoplastic left heart syndrome in, 597–599
  necrotizing enterocolitis in, 586–589
    management in, 587–588
    presenting problem in, 587
  substance abuse in, 589–592
    management in, 590

Case studies (*Continued*)
    presenting problem in, 590
    very low birthweight in, 599–602
        fluid and electrolyte management in,
            601–602
        initial management in, 599–600
Cataracts, 71, 491–492
Central nervous system, disorders of, apnea
        and, 129
    in pain management, 695–696
    neonatal resuscitation and, 77
    of sick newborn, 47
Cephalohematoma, 69, 407–408
Cerebellum, 396
Cerebral blood flow, autoregulation of, 397–398
    factors affecting, 397
Cerebrum, 396–397
Cesarean delivery, 31
Chemoreceptors, apnea and, 127
    hypercapnia and, 127
    hypoxemia and, 127
Chest, normal, x-ray appearance of, 616, *616*
Chest compressions, in neonatal resuscitation,
        85
Chest tubes, *621*, 637
Chlamydia trachomatis, 489–490
Chloasma, 4
Chloral hydrate, in persistent pulmonary
        hypertension of newborn, 109
    in ventilation therapy, 160
Chlorothiazide, in bronchopulmonary dysplasia,
        114
    in congestive heart failure management, 227
    in ventilation therapy, 158
Choanal atresia, 71, 88, 120
Chondrodystrophies, 121
Chorionic villus sampling, 448–449
    abdominal, 449
    vaginal, 449
Chromium, in total parenteral nutrition, 268t
Chromosomes, heterogeneous, 444
    homologous, 444
Circulation, extracorporeal, 182
    blood flow in, 182
    blood-surface interface in, 182
    gas exchange in, 182
    in neonatal resuscitation, 82
Circumcision, 389–390
Clavicle, fracture of, 469, *634*, *634*
    intervention in, 469
    physical examination in, 469
    radiologic evaluation of, *634*, *634*
    types of, 469
Cleft lip/palate, 453–454
Clubfoot. See *Talipes equinovarus.*
Coagulation, disseminated intravascular,
        334–336
    clinical assessment of, 335
    clinical presentation in, 334–335, *335*
    complications of, 335
    definition of, 334
    diagnostic studies in, 329t, 335
    differential diagnosis in, 335
    outcome of, 336
    patient care management in, 336
    physical examination in, 335
    precipitating factors in, 334
    hemostatic mechanisms in, 327
    newborn deficiencies in, 327
    process of, 327–328, *328*
    tests for, 328, 329t

Cocaine, 523–525, 534
    action of, 524
    in pregnancy, 524–525
        fetal and newborn effects of, 524–525
        maternal effects of, 524
    incidence of abuse of, 523–524
    pharmacology of, 524
Collodion baby, 482, *482*
Colorado Intrauterine Growth Charts, 61, *62*
Compliance, in assisted ventilation, 149
Congenital heart disease, 50, 199–207
    acyanotic lesions in, 50
    admixture lesions in, 50
    congestive heart failure and, 205
    diagnosis of, 200–207
        arterial blood gases in, 205–206
        cardiac catheterization in, 207
        chest x-ray in, 206
        clinical presentation in, 202–205
            blood pressure in, 204–205
            congestive heart failure in, 205, 205t–206t
            cyanosis in, 202
            ejection clicks in, 203
            heart sounds in, 202–204
            murmurs in, 203–204, 204t. See also
                Murmurs.
            peripheral pulses in, 204
            respiratory pattern in, 202
        echocardiography in, 207
        electrocardiography in, 206
        history in, 200–202
            associated cardiac anomalies in, 201
            delivery mode in, 201
            gestational age in, 200–201
            maternal disease in, 201, 201t
        laboratory data in, 207
        ultrasonography in, 202
    environmental factors in, 199–200
        alcohol and, 200
        amphetamine and, 200
        anticoagulants and, 200
        anticonvulsants and, 200
        antineoplastic medications and, 200
        lithium and, 200
        trimethadione and, 200
    environmental hazards and, 200
    genetic factors in, 199
    incidence of, 199–200
    maternal diseases and, 200, 201t
    obstructive lesions in, 50
    sex preferences associated with, 200
Congestive heart failure, 224–227
    causes of, in first week of life, 205t
        in second through fourth weeks of life,
            206t
    clinical features of, 225
    congenital heart disease and, 205
    definition of, 224
    etiology of, 205t–206t, 224
    management of, 225–227
        fluid and nutritional support in, 226
        oxygen consumption in, 226
        pharmacologic therapy in, 226–227, 227t
            chlorothiazide in, 227
            digoxin in, 226, 227t
            diuretics in, 226
            ethacrynic acid in, 226
            inotropic agents in, 227
        positioning in, 225
    manifestations of, 225, 225t
    severity assessment guidelines for, 225, 226t

Conjunctiva, 486
Conjunctivitis, 488–490. See also *Chlamydia trachomatis; Neisseria gonorrhoeae.*
Constipation, during pregnancy, 4
Contraction stress test, 9–10
Coombs' test, 332
Copper, in total parenteral nutrition, 268t
Cornelia de Lange syndrome, 454–455
Corticosteroids, 158
Cranial sutures, 69–70, 70
Craniosynostosis, 70, 405–407, 455
   care management in, 455
   clinical presentation of, 406, 455
   complications of, 455
   definition of, 405, 406
   diagnostic studies in, 406
   incidence of, 406, 455
   outcome in, 407, 455
   pathophysiology of, 405–406
   patient care management in, 407
Craniotabes, 70
Crisis manifestations, 556–558
   coping methods in, 558
   interpersonal behaviors in, 556–557
     family members in, 557
     infant in, 556–557
     NICU staff in, 557
     spouse or partner in, 556
   intrapersonal behaviors in, 557–558
Crisis origins, 550–556
   adolescence in, 551–552
   situational, 554–556
     low birthweight in, 555
     possible adverse outcomes in, 555–556
     prematurity in, 555
   sociocultural, 552–554
     family relationship disruption in, 553
     father's profile in, 553–554
     mother's profile in, 553
     peer group relationship disruption in, 552
     risks to infant in, 554
   transitional (adolescent), 550–551
     physical and physiologic development in, 550–551
       for both, 550
       for females, 550
       for males, 551
     psychosocial changes in, 551
Crisis resolution, 549, 549–550, 558–562
   events stimulating crisis occurrence and, 549–550
   intervention and, 549
   negative, 559–560
     neglect or abuse of infant in, 560
     role confusion in, 559
     self-isolation in, 560
   new resources and, 549
   origins and, 549
   positive, 558–559
     adult role attainment in, 558–559
     aid(s) to, 560–562
       facilitation of role adjustment as, 560
       resources use as, 561–562, 562
       support systems enhancement as, 560–561
     effective caretaking in, 559
     strong parent-infant bond in, 559, 559
   probability factors and, 549
Crouzon syndrome, 456
Cryotherapy, care during, 495

Cryptorchidism, 316, 388–389
Curare, 109
Cutis aplasia, 483, 483
Cutis marmorata, 474, 475
Cyanosis, central, 202
   in newborn assessment, 66
   peripheral, 202
Cyst, bronchogenic, 121
Cystic adenomatoid malformation, 121
Cystic fibrosis, 303
Cystic hygroma, 72, 120–121
Cytomegalovirus, 497–498
   in neonatal infections, 358–359

D
Dalton's law, in assisted ventilation, 150
Dehydration, 288–289
Dermatitis, *Candida* diaper, 480
Dermis, 472
Dexamethasone, 158
Diabetes mellitus, 19–20
   assessment and management of, 20
     gestational diabetes, 20
     newborn in, 20
     pre-existing diabetes in, 20
   infant of diabetic mother and, 284–285
   maternal, and large for gestational age infants, 62
     and small for gestational age infants, 64
   potential complications of, 19–20
     fetal/newborn, 19–20
     maternal, 19
Diaper dermatitis, *Candida*, 480
Diaphragm, eventration of, 621, 622
   paralysis of, 621, 622
Diaphragmatic hernia, 243–244
   congenital, case study of, 596–597
     radiologic evaluation of, 622–624, 623
   lung hypoplasia and, 243
Diffusion, augmented, 171
   coaxial, 171, 171
Digitalis, 227t, 229
Digoxin, 226, 227t
Diploid, 444
Discharge planning, 565–569
   challenges influencing, 566
   criteria for consideration of, 566
   goals and objectives of, 565
   nurse's role in, 566–569
     assessment in, 567
     assumptions in, 566–567
     plan development in, 567–568
       reimbursement resources in, 568
       specific provider requirements in, 567–568
     plan evaluation in, 568–569
     plan implementation in, 568
Disseminated intravascular coagulation. See *Coagulation, disseminated intravascular.*
Diuretics, 513–514
   in ventilation therapy, 157–158
   newborn considerations in, 513–514
   principles of use in, 513
Dobutamine, in persistent pulmonary hypertension of newborn, 109
   in shock management, 229
   in ventilation therapy, 159
Dopamine, in persistent pulmonary hypertension of newborn, 109
   in shock management, 229

Dopamine (*Continued*)
  in ventilation therapy, 158–159
Doxapram, 132–133
  action mechanism of, 132
  dosage of, 133
  pharmacokinetics of, 132
  side effects of, 133
Drugs. See also individual types.
  absorption of, 504–507
    administration sites in, 504–505
      gastrointestinal, 504–505
      inhalation, 505
      intramuscular, 505
      intravenous, 505
      subcutaneous, 505
      topical, 505
    definition of, 504
    in newborn, 505–507
      inhalation in, 506
      intramuscular/subcutaneous route in, 506–507
      intravenous route in, 507
      oral route in, 505–506
      rectal route in, 506
      topical route in, 506
  administration of, 517–518
  apnea and, 129, 131–133
  cardiovascular, 514–515
    antiarrhythmic, 515
    antihypertensive, 514
    definition of, 514
    inotropic, 514
    newborn considerations in, 515
    principles of use in, 515
    types of, 514–515
    vasodilator, 515
  definition of, 502
  distribution of, 507–509
    body compartments in, 507
    definition of, 507
    drug movement in, 508
    in newborn, 508–509
      body compartments in, 508
      drug movement in, 509
      protein binding in, 509
    protein-binding sites in, 507–508
  excretion of, 510–511
    definition of, 510
    in newborn, 511
  for central nervous system, 516–517
    definitions in, 516
    newborn considerations in, 516–517
    principles of use in, 516
  in neonatal resuscitation, 82, 85–87, 86
  in persistent pulmonary hypertension, 108–110
  metabolism of, 509–510
    definition of, 509
    in newborn, 510
Dubowitz method, for gestational age assessment, 59
Duchenne-Erb palsy, brachial nerve plexus injury and, 409
Ductus arteriosus, 38
  patent, 207–209
    anatomy of, 208, 208
    clinical features of, 208
    hemodynamics of, 208
    incidence of, 207–208
    management of, 208–209

Ductus venosus, 38
Duodenal atresia, 239–240
  stenosis and, 630, 630
Dwarfism, achondroplasia in, 635
  thanatophoric, 635, 636
Dysplastic kidney disease, multicystic, 378–379

E
Ear(s), in gestational age assessment, 60
  in newborn assessment, 71
    ear canals and, 71
    preauricular or auricular skin tags or pits and, 71
    shape and position of, 71
Ecchymoses, 74
Elastic recoil, in assisted ventilation, 149
Electrolytes, 260–261
Emphysema, congenital lobar, 121
  pulmonary interstitial, 617, 618
Encephalocele, 88, 405
Encephalopathy, hypoxic-ischemic, 417–419
  asphyxia and, case study of, 602–605
  mild, 417
  moderate, 417–418
  severe, 418
Endocardial cushion defect, 212, 212–213
Endocrine system, disorders of, 306–320. See also individual glands and disorders.
  glands of, 306
  hormones in, 306–307
    function of, 307
    production of, 306–307
    regulation of, 307
Endotracheal intubation, 635–636, 636, 644–646
Enteral feedings, 271–277. See also individual types.
  advantages of, 271–272
  facilitating tolerance of, 276–277
    non-nutritive sucking in, 276–277
    positioning in, 277
    stress reduction in, 277
  initiation of, 272
Enterocolitis, necrotizing. See *Necrotizing enterocolitis.*
Environment, apnea and, 129
  in neonatal resuscitation, 82
Epidermis, 472
Epidermolysis bullosa, 481–482
Epinephrine, in neonatal resuscitation, 82, 85–86
Epispadias, 69
Epstein's pearls, 71, 475–476, 476
Equinovarus, congenital. See *Talipes equinovarus.*
Erythema toxicum, 74, 474–475, 475
Erythropoiesis, 323–324
Escherichia coli, antibiotics for, 421
  in neonatal infections, 355
Esophageal atresia, 237–238. See also *Tracheoesophageal fistula.*
  radiologic evaluation of, 628, 629
  with tracheoesophageal fistula, radiologic evaluation of, 628, 629
Esophagus, 628
Ethacrynic acid, 226
Ethical issues, 665–671
  decision making in, 666–668
    conclusion in, 668
    decision maker qualifications in, 667
    information collection in, 667

Ethical issues (*Continued*)
recognition of dilemma in, 667
definitions in, 665–666
dilemma resolution resources in, 670
institutional policies in, 671
nurse's role in, 670
shared values in, 671
team communication style in, 670–671
dimensions in, 668
management of uncertainty in, 669
medical treatment of pregnant women in, 669–670
parental role in, 668–669
principles of, 666
Exosurf Neonatal, 139–142
administration guidelines for, 140t, 140–141
anticipated response to, 141–142
chest expansion and, 142
hypocapnia and, 142
mucous plugs and, 142
pulmonary hemorrhage and, 142
transcutaneous oxygen saturation and, 142
dosage administration and, 141
prophylactic treatment criteria for, 139
rescue treatment criteria for, 139
results of, vs. placebo, 139, 139t
special considerations for, 142
suspension preparation and, 141
ventilator settings and, 140–141
Extracorporeal membrane oxygenation, 177–188
blood gas monitoring device for, 181
cannulation in, 182
nursing responsibilities and interventions in, 183t–185t
circuit components of, 179–181, 180
activated clotting time machine in, 181
bladder box assembly in, 180–181
bubble-detector in, 181
cannulas in, 179–180
heat exchanger in, 181
membrane oxygenator in, 181
polyvinylchloride (PVC) tubing in, 180
roller head pump in, 181
circuit emergency procedures for, 188t
complications of, 186t–187t
contraindications to, 178
criteria for use of, 178, 179t
definition of, 177
extracorporeal circulation physiology and, 182
blood flow in, 182
blood-surface interface in, 182
gas exchange in, 182
follow-up evaluations and, 188
historical perspective of, 177–178
infant care and, 182–188
parental support and, 188
specialist responsibilities and interventions in, 186t
venoarterial perfusion and, 178–179
advantages of, 178–179
risks of, 179
technique for, 178
weaning/decannulation in, 185
Extraocular muscles, 487
Extremities, in newborn assessment, 72–73
Eye(s). See also individual disorders.
anatomy of, 485–487, 486
birth trauma and, 488
bony orbit of, 486
care of, 44

Eye(s) (*Continued*)
conjunctiva of, 486
extraocular muscles and, 487
globe of, 486–487
anterior cavity of, 487
inner layer of, 486–487
lens of, 487
middle layer (vascular tunic) of, 486
outer layer (fibrous tunic) of, 486
posterior cavity of, 487
retina of, 486–487
uveal tract of, 486
in gestational age assessment, 60, 61
in newborn assessment, 71
cataracts and, 71
iris and, 71
Mongolian slanting and, 71
pupil response and, 71
red reflex and, 71
subconjunctival hemorrhages and, 71
tears and, 71
lacrimal system of, 486
patient assessment and, 487–488
protective structures of, 485–486
Eyelids, 485

F
Face, in newborn assessment, 72
Family in crisis, 537–545
definition of, 538
family-infant bonding in, 542–545
assessment in, 542–543
definitions in, 542
evaluation of, 544–545
interventions for encouragement of, 543–544
grief and loss in, 540–541
assessment in, 540–541
definitions in, 540
interventions for facilitating grief in, 541
interventions in perinatal loss in, 541
identification of, 538–540
assessment in, 538–539
evaluation in, 539–540
intervention in, 539
parental needs in, 545
psychological tasks of, 538
Fat, in pre-term infant nutrition, 260
in total parenteral nutrition, 266, 266t
complications associated with, 267–268
Feeding abilities, 433–437
nutritive sucking in, 434–437
breast-feeding pre-term infant and, 437
improving chances for success in, 437
indicators for, 437
common problems in, 435–436
fatigue in, 435–436
initiation criteria in, 434
mechanical considerations in, 435
patterns of, 434
poor lip closure in, 436
poor suck-swallow-breathe coordination in, 435
preparation for, 434–435
state disorganization in, 436
"stop" signs in, 436–437
sustained closure of jaws in, 436
weak, arrhythmic suck in, 436
successful oral, 433–434

Feeding abilities (*Continued*)
goals of, 433–434
variables affecting, 434
sucking response in, 433
Fentanyl citrate, in infant pain management, 698–699
in persistent pulmonary hypertension of newborn, 110
in ventilation therapy, 160
Fetal alcohol syndrome, 526–528
birth order in, 526
characteristics in, 526
central nervous system abnormalities in, 526
facial dysmorphology in, 526
growth disturbances in, 526
diagnosis of, 526
dosage of alcohol in, 526
effects during pregnancy of, 526
gestational stage in, 526
history in, 526
incidence of, 526
newborn withdrawal from alcohol in, 528
nursing considerations for, 528
pharmacology of ethanol in, 526
Fetal anomalies, 443–460. See also individual disorders; *Genetics*.
evaluation in, 451–452
causation consideration in, 452
family history in, 451
physical examination in, 451–452
prenatal history in, 451
family care management in, 452
newborn care management in, 451
diagnosis in, 451
physical problems prevention in, 451
prenatal diagnosis of, 446–450
advantages of, 446
amniocentesis in, 447–448. See also *Amniocentesis*.
chorionic villus sampling in, 448–449. See also *Chorionic villus sampling*.
genetic counseling in, 449–450. See also *Genetic counseling*.
maternal serum alpha-fetoprotein in, 446–447
percutaneous umbilical blood sampling in, 449. See also *Umbilical blood sampling*.
ultrasound in, 447
Fetal surveillance, antepartum, 9–10
biophysical profile in, 10
contraction stress test in, 9–10
non-stress test in, 9
Fetus, circulation and, 36, 37
harlequin, 483
hematology and, 36, 38
lung characteristics of, 36
metabolism of, 36, 38
Film, expiratory, 613
exposure of, 613
inspiratory, 613
lordotic, 613
Fluid(s), in pre-term infant nutrition, 258–259
factors indicating decrease of, 259
factors indicating increase of, 258–259
requirements for, 258–259
in total parenteral nutrition, 265
Fluid overload, 289–290
Fluorescence polarization test, 8
Fontanelles, 70, *70*
Foramen ovale, 38

Fractures, long bone, 635
radiologic evaluation of, 634–635. See also individual types.
Functional residual capacity, 149
Furosemide, in bronchopulmonary dysplasia, 114
in congestive heart failure management, 226
in ventilation therapy, 157

G
Gag reflex, 72
Gamete, 444
Gas exchange mechanisms, 170–171
effectiveness of, 171
in high-frequency ventilation, 170–171
augmented diffusion and, 171
coaxial diffusion and, 171, *171*
entrainment and, 171, *171*
inter-regional gas mixing and, 171
in spontaneous and conventional mechanical ventilation, 170
Gastric perforation, 630
Gastrointestinal system, disorders of, 233–252. See also individual disorders.
abdominal wall defects in, 234–237
intestinal obstruction in, 237–245
embryonic development of, 233–234
functions of, 234
neonatal resuscitation and, 77
of pre-term infant, anatomic characteristics of, 255
feeding-induced hormones in, 255
function of, 255
nutrient store deficiencies in, 255–256
physiologic characteristics of, 255
physiologic changes in, 4
radiologic evaluation of, 627–634. See also individual parts and conditions.
Gastroschisis, *235*, 235–236
Gastrostomy feedings, 275
Gavage feedings, 273–274
advantages of, 274
continuous, indications for, 274
procedure for, 274
vs. intermittent, 274
disadvantages of, 274
indications for, 273
intermittent procedure in, 273–274
parenteral nutrition and, 273
Gene, definition of, 444
dominant, 444
recessive, 444
Genetic counseling, 449–450
definition of, 449
discussion of alternatives in, 450
indications for, 450
methods of, 450
principles of, 450
Genetics, 443–445
chromosomal defects in, 445–446
abnormal number in, 445
causes of, 445
mosaicism in, 445
polyploidy in, 445
abnormal structure in, 446
deletion in, 446
environmental influences in, 446
incidence of, 446
polygenic defects in, 446
translocation in, 446

Genetics (*Continued*)
  definitions in, 443–444
  dominance and recessiveness in, 444–445
    autosomal dominant characteristics in, 444–445
    autosomal recessive characteristics in, 445
    chromosome combinations in, 444
    dominant gene in, 444
    heterogeneous chromosomes in, 444
    homologous chromosomes in, 444
    phenotype in, 444
    recessive gene in, 444
    x-linked dominant disorder characteristics in, 445
    x-linked recessive disorder characteristics in, 445
Genitalia, female, labia majora, 69
    pseudohermaphroditism in, 69
  in gestational age assessment, 60
  in newborn assessment, 69
  male, epispadias in, 69
    hydrocele in, 69
    hypospadias in, 69
    scrotum in, 69
    testes in, 69
Genotype, 444
Gestation, divisions of, 3
  length of, 3
Gestational age assessment, 7–8, 58–65
  breast tissue and areola in, 60
  ears in, 60
  eyes in, 60, 61
  fetal heart tones in, 8
  fundal height in, 8
  genitalia in, 60
  hair in, 60
  infants at risk in, 62–65
    large for gestational age complications in, 62, 64, 64
      Beckwith's syndrome in, 64
      birth trauma in, 62
      maternal diabetes in, 62
      thermoregulation problems in, 64
    small for gestational age complications in, 64–65
      chromosomal defects in, 64
      hypoglycemia in, 64
      intrauterine growth retardation in, 64
      maternal diabetes in, 64
      meconium aspiration in, 64
      polycythemia in, 65
      thermoregulation problems in, 64
  laboratory assessments in, 8
  lanugo in, 60
  last menstrual period in, 7–8
  neurologic signs in, 60–61
    flexion angles and joint mobility in, 61
    posture in, 60–61
  newborn classification in, 61–62
    appropriate for gestational age in, 61–62
    clinical estimate of gestation in, 61
    growth charts in, 61, 62
    large for gestational age in, 62
    neonatal mortality risk in, 62, 63
    small for gestational age in, 61
  obstetrical methods for, 58
  pediatric methods for, 59
  pelvic examination in, 8
  physical signs in, 60
  purpose of, 58
  quickening in, 8

Gestational age assessment (*Continued*)
  skin in, 60
  sole creases in, 60
  sonography in, 8
  tool(s) for, 59
    Ballard method as, 59, 59
    Dubowitz method as, 59
Glomerular filtration rate, 5
Glucocorticoids, lung development and, 96–97
Glucose-6-phosphate dehydrogenase deficiency, 302–303
Glucose tolerance test, 7
Graves' disease, 310
Grief, 540–541
  anticipatory, 540
  assessment of, 540–541
  chronic, 540
  definition of, 540
  interventions for facilitating, 541
Growth, adequate, standards for, 256

H
Haemophilus influenzae, 355
Hair growth, during pregnancy, 4
  in gestational age assessment, 60
Hands, in newborn assessment, 72
Haploid, 444
Harlequin fetus, 483
Head, in newborn assessment, 69–71
    caput succedaneum and, 69
    cephalohematoma and, 69
    fontanelles and, 70, 70
    macrocephaly and, 69
    microcephaly and, 69
    scalp and, 70–71
    sutures and, 69–70, 70
Hearing loss, 437–439
  central auditory dysfunction and, 438
  conductive, 438
  follow-up in, 439
  identification of high risk infants in, 439, 440
  implications for caregivers in, 439
  incidence of, 437
  mixed, 438
  ototoxic, 439
  screening tools in, 438–439
    auditory brain stem response in, 439
    behavioral observation audiometry in, 438
    Crib-O-Gram in, 438–439
    high-risk register in, 438
  sensorineural, 438
  types of, 438
Heart, congenital disease of. See *Congenital heart disease.*
  failure of. See *Congestive heart failure.*
  in newborn auscultation/palpation, 66–67
    blood pressure and, 67, 67
    bounding pulses and, 66–67
    bradycardia and, 66
    femoral pulses and, 66
    muffled or shifted heart sounds and, 66
    murmurs and, 66
    point of maximal intensity and, 66
    precordial activity and, 66
    tachycardia and, 66
  output of. See *Cardiac output.*
  radiologic evaluation of, left-sided obstruction in, 626–627
    left-to-right shunt in, 625–626
    position in, 625, 625

Heart (*Continued*)
  pulmonary vascularity and, 625, *626*
  size in, *624*, 624–625
Hemangioma, cavernous, 479–480
  Kasabach-Merritt syndrome and, 480
  Klippel-Trenaunay-Weber syndrome and, 480
  strawberry, 478, *479*
Hematocrit, 324, 324t
Hematologic changes, during pregnancy, 5–6. See also under *Blood.*
Hematologic disorders, 322–342. See also individual disorders.
Hematopoiesis, 322–323, *323*
Hemorrhagic disease, 333–334
Henry's law, in assisted ventilation, 150
Hepatitis B, 359–360
  transmission of, 359
  treatment of, 359–360
  vaccine for, 694t
Heroin, 528–529, 534
  fetal effects of, 528–529
  maternal effects of, 528
  methadone vs., 529
  newborn effects of, 529
  pharmacology of, 528
Herpes simplex virus, 359, *480*, 480–481
  case study of, 592–595
    management in, 592–593
    presenting problem in, 592
Hip dislocation, congenital, 468
Hip dysplasia, congenital, 73, *73*
Hirschsprung's disease, 243
  meconium plug syndrome and, 242
  radiologic evaluation of, 632, *632*
Human immunodeficiency virus (HIV), 360–361
Hyaline membrane disease, 98–102. See also *Respiratory distress syndrome.*
  case study of, 605–608
  radiologic evaluation of, 616–617, *617*
  Survanta rescue treatment study and, 143
    administration procedure in, 143
    criteria for, 143
    exclusion criteria for, 143
Hydrocele, 69
Hydrocephalus, 69, 400–403
  congenital, 401–402
  definition of, 400
  myelomeningocele and, 404
  outcome in, 403
  pathophysiology of, 400–401
  post-hemorrhagic, 402–403
Hydrochlorothiazide, 158
Hydronephrosis, 379–381
  clinical assessment in, 379
  clinical presentation in, 379
  complications in, 380
  definition of, 379
  diagnostic studies in, 380
  differential diagnosis in, 380
  disease states in, 379
  incidence of, 379
  outcome in, 380–381
  patient care management in, 380
  physical examination in, 379
Hydrops fetalis, 251–252
  definition of, 251
  diagnosis of, 252
  etiology of, 251–252
    cardiovascular, 251
    chromosomal, 252

Hydrops fetalis (*Continued*)
    gastrointestinal, 252
    hematologic, 251
    infection, 251
    maternal conditions in, 252
    placenta/cord in, 251
    pulmonary, 251
    renal, 251
  immediate neonatal conditions in, 252
  management of, 252
Hyperammonemia, 301–302
Hyperbilirubinemia, 246–251
  ABO incompatibility and, 330
  bilirubin metabolism in, 246
  bilirubin origin in, 246
  conjugated, 250–251
    causes of, 248t, 250–251
    management of, 251
  exchange transfusion for, 249–250
    complications of, 250
    indications for, 250
    post-exchange care in, 250
    procedure for, 250
    serum bilirubin level and, 250t
  in newborn assessment, 66
  management of, 248–249
  natural history of, 246
  non-physiologic, 247
    breastfeeding and, 247
    indications of, 247
    labor and delivery history in, 247
    liver disease and, 247
    maternal drugs and, 247, 249t
    patient history in, 247
  phototherapy for, 249
  physiologic, 246–247
    causes of, 246–247, 248t
    definition of, 246
    treatment of, 247
Hypercalcemia, 294–295
Hyperglycemia, 285–286
Hyperkalemia, 292
Hypermagnesemia, 296
Hypernatremia, 291
Hypertelorism, 72
Hypertension, 373–375
  persistent pulmonary, of newborn, 105–110. See also *Persistent pulmonary hypertension.*
  pregnancy-induced, 17–19
    assessment and management of, 18–19
      eclampsia in, 18
      newborn assessment in, 19
      severe pre-eclampsia in, 18
    incidence of, 17
    potential complications of, 18
    predisposing factors for, 17
    signs and symptoms of, 9, 17
  states of, 373–374
    endocrine component in, 373
    renal component in, 373
    vascular component in, 373
Hyperthyroidism, 310–311
  Graves' disease in, 310
Hypocalcemia, 293–294
Hypoglycemia, 282–284
  in sick newborn, 50–51
  in small for gestational age infants, 64
Hypokalemia, 291–292
Hypomagnesemia, 295–296
Hyponatremia, 290–291

Hypoplastic left heart syndrome, 215–216
  anatomy of, 215, *215*
  case study of, 597–599
Hypoplastic right heart syndrome, 627
Hypospadias, 69, 316, *384*, 384–385
Hypothermia, 83
Hypothyroidism, 307–310
  acquired, 308
  clinical presentation of, 309
  complications of, 309
  congenital, 307
    biosynthesis defects in, 307
    maternal factors causing, 307
    morphogenesis defects in, 307
  diagnosis of, 308–309
    maternal prenatal history in, 308
    newborn screening for, 308
    thyroid function tests in, 308t, 308–309
  outcome of, 309–310
  patient care management in, 309
  transient, 308
Hypovolemic shock, acute, 50
Hypoxic-ischemic encephalopathy, 417–419
  asphyxia and, case study of, 602–605
  mild, 417
  moderate, 417–418
  severe, 418

I
Ichthyosis, 482–483
  bullous, 483
  definition of, 482
  lamellar, 483
  treatment of, 483
  vulgaris, 482
  x-linked, 482
Immune system, neonatal resuscitation and, 77
Immunology, 346–347
  cellular immunity in, *346*, 347
    non-specific, 347
    specific, 347
  humoral immunity in, 346–347
    immunoglobulin A in, 346
    immunoglobulin E in, 347
    immunoglobulin G in, 346
    immunoglobulin M in, 346
    immunoglobulins in, 346, *346*
  neonatal host defense limitations in, 347
Imperforate anus, See *Anus.*
Infant formula, 270t, 271
  elemental, 271
  milk-based, 271
  recommendations for, 271
  soy-based, 271
Infant of diabetic mother, 284–285
Infections, 345–362. See also individual
      conditions.
  bacterial, 353–354
    antibiotic therapy in, 356, 357t
    common sites of, 353–354
      meningitis in, 353
      neonatal ophthalmia in, 354
      pneumonia in, 353
      sepsis in, 353
      urinary tract in, 354
    epidemiologic history in, 353
    gram-negative organisms in, 355
    gram-positive organisms in, 354–355

Infections (*Continued*)
    organism transmission in, 348
    parasites in, 355–356
    pathogens in, 354–356
    transfusion therapy in, 356
      exchange, 356
      intravenous immune globulin in, 356
      neutrophil in, 356
  clinical assessment in, 348
  clinical manifestations in, 348–349
    cardiovascular, 348–349
    gastrointestinal, 348–349
    neurologic, 348–349
    respiratory, 348–349
    skin in, 348–349
  control of, 362
    body substance isolation in, 362
    universal precautions in, 362
  diagnostic evaluation in, 352
    cultures in, 352
      blood in, 352
      cerebrospinal fluid in, 352
    follow-up in, 352
  fungal, 357–358
  hematologic evaluation in, 349–352
    complete blood count in, 349–351
      differential in, 349–351, *350–351*
      white blood count in, 349
    diagnostic aids in, 351–352
  predisposing risk factors identification in, 348
  viral, 358–361
Informed consent, 678–679
  capacity and, 678
  court orders and, 679
  information giving in, 678
  parental role in, 678
  refusal of, 678–679
  risks or benefits of treatment in, 678
Inguinal hernia, 387–388
Insulin, 6
Intensive care unit, developmental support in,
      426–441
    auditory assessment and, 437–439. See
        also *Hearing loss.*
    behavioral organization in, 427–430. See
        also *Behavioral organization.*
    concepts of, 426–427
    feeding abilities assessment in, 433–437.
        See also *Feeding abilities.*
    fostering parent-infant interaction in, 440
      intervention strategies in, 440
      key to, 440
    neuromotor development in, 430
      maturation in, 430
      sequence of, 430
    plan for, 441
    positioning techniques in, 430–433. See
        also *Positioning techniques.*
    requirements for, 427
Interlobar fissure, 613
Intracerebellar hemorrhage, 411–412
Intracranial hemorrhage, 410–414. See also
      individual types.
  neonatal resuscitation and, 89
Intrapartum period, conditions related to,
      20–28. See also individual conditions.
    abruptio placentae in, 22–23
    breech delivery in, 26–28
    placenta previa in, 23–24
    pre-term labor in, 20–22, 21t

Intrapartum period (*Continued*)
 shoulder dystocia in, 25–26
 umbilical cord prolapse in, 24–25
Intravenous line placement, peripheral,
  641–643, 642
Iron, in pre-term infant nutrition, 263
 action of, 263
 supplementation in, 263
Isoproterenol, in persistent pulmonary
  hypertension of newborn, 109
 in shock management, 229
 in ventilation therapy, 157

J
Jaundice. See *Hyperbilirubinemia.*
Jejunal/ileal atresia, 240–241

K
Kasabach-Merritt syndrome, cavernous
  hemangioma and, 480
Kidney(s), embryology of, 366
 mesonephros in, 366
 metanephros in, 366
 pronephros in, 366
 failure of. See *Renal failure.*
 in newborn assessment, 68
 physiologic changes in, 5
Kleihauer-Betke test, 332
Klinefelter's syndrome, 316
Klippel-Feil syndrome, 466
Klippel-Trenaunay-Weber syndrome, cavernous
  hemangioma and, 480
Klumpke's paralysis, brachial nerve plexus
  injury and, 409

L
Labia majora, 69
Labor, normal, 10
 phases of, 10
 placenta and, 36
 pre-term. See *Pre-term labor.*
 seven cardinal movements in, 10
 stress hormones and, 36
Labor management, 10–11
 assessments in, 10–11
 low-risk patient in, 11
  auscultation and, 11
  fetal heart rate patterns and, 11
  fetal monitoring and, 11
Lacrimal system, 486
Lanugo, 60
Laplace's law, 150–151
Larynx, obstruction of, 121
Lecithin/sphingomyelin ratio test, 8
Legal issues, 673–682
 documentation in, 676–678
  errors in, 677–678
  objectivity in, 676
  patient's progress in, 676
  promptness of, 676–677
 informed consent in, 678–679. See also
   Informed consent.
  court orders and, 679
  information giving in, 678
  parental role in, 678
  refusal of, 678–679
  risks or benefits of treatment in, 678
 liability in, 674–676

Legal issues (*Continued*)
  costs of, 676
  negligence and, 675
  nurse's role in, 674–675
  quality assurance department and, 675–676
 malpractice in, 680–681. See also *Malpractice.*
  establishment of, 680
  national practitioner data bank and,
    680–681
  nurse's risk of suit for, 680
  prevention of, 681
   documentation in, 681
   nursing skills in, 681
   patient rights in, 681
 scope of practice in, 679–680
  professional organizations standards and,
    679–680
  state medical practice acts and, 679
 standard of care in, 673–674. See also
   Standard of care.
  expert witnesses testimony in, 674
  institutional policies and procedures in, 674
  professional literature in, 674
  professional organizations' standards in, 674
  reasonableness and prudence in, 674
  state and federal regulations in, 674
Listeria monocytogenes, antibiotics for, 421
 in neonatal infections, 355
Liver, in newborn assessment, 68
 neonatal resuscitation and, 77
 physiologic changes in, 4
Lobar emphysema, congenital, 624, 624
Lorazepam, 416
Lung(s), See also *Pulmonary* entries.
 development of, 95–97
  embryonic, 95–96
  glucocorticoids and, 96–97
  surface-active phospholipids in, 96
 hyperexpanded, 613
 hypoexpanded, 613
 neonatal resuscitation and, 77
Lung capacity, total, 149
Lung disease, chronic, 116

M
Macrocephaly, 69
Macrostomia, 72
Magnesium, 295–296
 disorders of, 295–296
 homeostasis of, 295
 in pre-term infant nutrition, 262–263
 in total parenteral nutrition, 268t
Malpractice, 680–681
 definition of, 680
 establishment of, 680
 national practitioner data bank and, 680–681
 nurse's risk of suit for, 680
 prevention of, 681
  documentation in, 681
  nursing skills in, 681
  patient rights in, 681
Malrotation, 239
Manganese, in total parenteral nutrition, 268t
Maple syrup urine disease, 301
Marijuana, 530–531, 534
 fetal effects of, 530–531
 newborn effects of, 531
 pharmacology of, 530

Mask of pregnancy, 4
Maternal risk factors, conditions and substances
    affecting pregnant woman and, 14
    fetus and, 14
    perinatal assessment of newborn and, 14,
        15t–16t
    placenta and, 14
    placental transport mechanisms and, 16–17
Mean airway pressure, 149, 154
Mechanoreceptors, apnea and, 127–128
Meconium, 110
Meconium aspiration syndrome, 110–111
    in small for gestational age infants, 64
    radiologic evaluation of, 618, *619*
Meconium ileus, 241
    radiologic evaluation of, *626*, 631
Meconium peritonitis, 633–634
Meconium plug syndrome, 242
    Hirschsprung's disease and, 242
    radiologic evaluation of, 632
Melasma, 4
Meningitis, 353, 420–422
    acquisition of, 353
    antibiotics for, 421–422
    clinical manifestations of, 353
    congenital presentation of, 420–421
    definition of, 420
    diagnostic studies in, 421
    incidence of, 420
    outcome of, 422
    pathophysiology of, 420
    patient care management in, 421–422
Mesonephros, 366
Metabolic acidosis. See *Acidosis, metabolic.*
Metabolic alkalosis. See *Alkalosis, metabolic.*
Metabolism, acid-base balance in, 296–298
    buffering system in, 296
    compensation in, 296–297
    disorders of, 297–298. See also *Acidosis;*
        Alkalosis.
    kidney regulation in, 296
    lung regulation in, 296
    pH in, 296
    physiology in, 296–297
    carbohydrate disorders of, 302
    disorders of, 281–303
    electrolyte balance in, 290–296. See also
        individual types.
    fluid balance in, 286–290
        assessment of, 288
        disorders of, 288–290. See also individual
            disorders.
        fluid requirements in, 287
        maintenance of, 287–288
        physiologic factors affecting, 286
        postnatal influences on, 287, 287t
        renal function in, 286
    glucose, 282–286
        disorders of, 282–286. See also individual
            disorders.
        homeostasis in, 282
            fetal, 282
            neonatal, 282
            physiology of, 282
    inborn errors of, 298–300, 300t. See also
        individual disorders.
    organic acid disorders of, 301
Metanephros, 366
Metatarsus adductus, 467, 467–468
    incidence of, 467

Metatarsus adductus (*Continued*)
    intervention in, 468
    physical examination in, 467
Methadone, 528–529
    fetal effects of, 528–529
    heroin vs., 529
    maternal effects of, 528
    newborn effects of, 529
    pharmacology of, 528
Methamphetamine, 525–526
    action of, 525
    newborn effects of, 525–526
    pharmacology of, 525
Methylxanthine therapy, 131–132
    action mechanism of, 131–132
    aminophylline in, 132
    caffeine in, 132
    caffeine vs. theophylline in, 132
    pharmacokinetics of, 132
    side effects of, 132
    theophylline in, 132
Metric conversion tables, 691t–693t
    for length, 692t
    for temperature, 691t
    for weight (mass), 693t
Microcephaly, 69, 400
Micrognathia, 72, 120
Microphallus, 316
Microstomia, 72
Midazolam hydrochloride, 160
Midgut volvulus, 631–632
Milia, 74, 475, *476*
Miliaria, 476, *476*
Müllerian aplasia, 316
Mongolian slanting, of eyes, 71
Mongolian spots, 74, 476–477, *477*
Moniliasis, 72, 358
Morphine sulfate, in infant pain management,
        698
    in persistent pulmonary hypertension of
        newborn, 109–110
    in ventilation therapy, 160
Mosaicism, 445
Mouth, in newborn assessment, 71–72
    Epstein's pearls and, 71
    macrostomia and, 71
    micrognathia and, 72
    microstomia and, 71
    natal teeth and, 72
    thrush and, 72
Murmurs, 203–204
    causes of, 203
    evaluation of, 203–204
    grading of, 203, 204t
    incidence of, 203
    location within cardiac cycle of, 204
    sound quality of, 204
Muscular system, 463
Myelomeningocele, 88, 403–405
    Arnold-Chiari malformation and, 404–405
    hydrocephalus and, 404

N

Naloxone hydrochloride, in neonatal
        resuscitation, 82, 87
Nasal cannula, in assisted ventilation, 152, 161
Nasolacrimal duct obstruction, 490–491
Natal teeth, 72
Neck, in newborn assessment, 72

Necrotizing enterocolitis, 244–246
   case study of, 586–589
   radiologic evaluation of, 632–633, *633*
Neisseria gonorrhoeae, 355, 488–489
Neonatal abstinence syndrome, 529–530
   autonomic system dysfunction in, 529–530
   definition of, 529
   duration of, 529
   gastrointestinal abnormalities of, 530
   incidence of, 529
   neurologic signs of, 529
   onset of, 529
   presentation of, 529
   respiratory signs of, 530
   scoring system for, 530
Neurologic system, assessment of, 398–399
   observation in, 398, 398t
   physical examination in, 398–399
     cranial nerve function in, 398–399, 399t
     muscle tone in, 399
     reflexes in, 399
   brain anatomy in, 396–397
    brainstem in, 397
    cerebellum in, 396
    cerebrum in, 396–397
   disorders of, 394–422. See also individual
     disorders.
   embryologic development in, 394–396, 395t
    dorsal induction in, 394–395
    myelination in, 396
    neuronal migration in, 395–396
    neuronal organization in, 396
    neuronal proliferation in, 395
    ventral induction in, 395
   physiology of, 397–398
    cerebral blood flow in, 397–398
     autoregulation of, 397–398
     factors affecting, 397
    glucose metabolism in, 397
Neuromotor development, 430
   maturation of, 430
   sequence of, 430
Neutral thermal environment, 42–44
   cold stress pathophysiology and, 43–44
   definition of, 42
   heat loss and, 43
   heat production and, 42–43
   hypothermia pathophysiology and, 43–44
   nursery temperature and, 44
   temperatures and, 42, 42t
Neutrophil, maturation stages of, 349, *350*
Nevus simplex, 477–478
Newborn, apnea and, 125–133. See also *Apnea.*
   assessment of. See *Assessment of newborn.*
   cardiovascular adaptation at birth of, 38, *39*
    ductus arteriosus and, 38
    ductus venosus and, 38
    foramen ovale and, 38
    postnatal circulation and, 38
    umbilical cord and, 38
   classification of. See *Gestational age assessment.*
   medications in transition nursery and, 44–47.
     See also *Transition nursery.*
   neutral thermal environment and, 42–44. See
     also *Neutral thermal environment.*
   perinatal assessment of, maternal risk factors
     and, 14, 15t–16t
   pulmonary adaptation at birth of, 38, 40
    lung compliance and, 40
    stimuli for initiating respiration and, 38

Newborn (*Continued*)
    surfactant and, 40
    thoracic squeeze and, 40
   sick, 47–53. See also individual problems.
    congenital anomalies and, 51
    diagnostic tools and, 48
     hematocrit in, 48
     orogastric tube passage in, 48
     pulse oximetry in, 48
     urine sample in, 48
    handling of, 52–53
     antibiotics in, 53
     glucose supply in, 52
     naloxone hydrochloride in, 53
     non-nutritive sucking in, 52
     oxygen supply in, 52–53
     volume expanders in, 53
    initial stabilization of, 51–53
    maternal medications/drug abuse and, 51
    observation of, 51–52
    perinatal history and, 47
    physical assessment of, 47–48
     cardiovascular system in, 47
     central nervous system in, 47
     morphology in, 47–48
     respiratory system in, 47
     skin in, 47
Nicotine, 531, 534
   dose-related response in, 531
   newborn effects of, 531
   reduced oxygen availability and, 531
Non-stress test, 9
Nose, 71
   choanal atresia and, 71
   nostril patency and, 71
Nursery, transition. See *Transition nursery.*
Nutrition, 254–277
   adequate growth standards and, 256
   assessment in, 275–276
    anthropometric measurements in, 275–276
    feeding tolerance in, 276
   breast milk in, 269–271. See also *Breast milk.*
   enteral feedings in, 271–277. See also
     individual types.
    advantages of, 271–272
    facilitating tolerance of, 276–277
     non-nutritive sucking in, 276–277
     positioning in, 277
     stress reduction in, 277
    initiation of, 272
   for full-term infants, 256–257
    caloric and fluid requirements in, 256
    protein, fat, and carbohydrate intake in, 256
     breast milk and, 256
     commercial formulas and, 256
     supplements and, 256
   for pre-term infants, 257–264
    calories in, 259, 259t
    carbohydrates in, 260
    electrolytes in, 260–261
    fat in, 260
    general considerations in, 257–258, 258t
    minerals in, 262t, 262–264
     calcium in, 262–263
     iron in, 263
     magnesium in, 262–263
     phosphorus in, 262–263
     zinc in, 263–264
    protein in, 259–260
    vitamins in, 261t, 261–262

Nutrition (*Continued*)
 vitamin A in, 261–262
 vitamin D in, 262
 vitamin E in, 262
 vitamin K in, 262
 water in, 258–259
  factors indicating decrease of, 259
  factors indicating increase of, 258–259
  requirements for, 258–259
 gastrointestinal system and, of pre-term
   infant, 255–256. See also
   Gastrointestinal system.
 in bronchopulmonary dysplasia, 112, 115
 in newborn assessment, 66
 oral. See *Oral feedings.*
 parenteral, 264–269. See also *Parenteral
   feedings.*

O
Obstetrical analgesia, 28–29
 assessment and management of, 28–29
 potential complications of, 28
Obstetrical anesthesia, 29–31
 general, assessment and management of, 29
  potential complications of, 29
 regional, assessment and management of,
   30–31
  allergic reaction in, 30–31
  high spinal in, 30
  hypotension in, 30
  toxic reaction in, 30
  potential complications of, 29–30
   epidural anesthesia in, 29–30
   fetal/newborn, 30
   maternal, 29–30
   pudendal block in, 30
   spinal and epidural anesthesia in, 29
Omphalocele, 234, 234–235
Operative delivery. See *Cesarean delivery.*
Ophthalmia, 354
Oral feedings, 272–273
 advantages of, 272
 disadvantages of, 272–273
 indications for, 272
 oxygenation and, 273
 pre-term infants breast feeding in, 273
 procedure for, 272
 test-weighing and, 273
Orbit, bony, 486
Orthopedic conditions, 462–469. See also
   individual conditions.
 clinical assessment in, 463–464
  anterior chest in, 463
  family history in, 463
  head and neck in, 463
  lower extremities in, 464
  medication history in, 463
  perinatal factors in, 463
  physical examination in, 463–464
  posterior chest in, 463–464
  trunk and spine in, 463–464
  upper extremities in, 464
 lower extremities in, 466–469
 neck abnormalities in, 465–466
 pathologic conditions in, 464–465
  etiology of, 464
  limb abnormalities in, 464
Osteogenesis imperfecta, 468–469
 etiology of, 468

Osteogenesis imperfecta (*Continued*)
 intervention in, 469
 outcome in, 469
 physical examination in, 468–469
 radiologic evaluation of, 469, 635
Oxygenation, extracorporeal membrane. See
   Extracorporeal membrane oxygenation.
Oxyhood, 152, 161

P
Pain management, 695–697
 attenuation of stress response in, 696
 infant pain responses in, 696
  behavioral, 696
  biochemical, 696
  physiologic, 696
 interventions in, 696–697
  nonpharmacologic, 696
  pharmacologic, 160, 696–697
   fentanyl in, 110, 160, 696–697
   morphine in, 109–110, 160, 696
Pain transmission, nervous system development
   and, 695–696
 cortical maturity in, 695–696
 interacting components in, 695
 nerve fiber myelination in, 695
 thalamocortical pain fibers/hypothalamus
   in, 695
Pallor, in newborn assessment, 66
Palmar erythema, 4
Pancreas, annular, 630
Pancuronium bromide, in persistent pulmonary
   hypertension of newborn, 109
 in ventilation therapy, 159–160
Parent education, 53–54
 at delivery, 53
 before delivery, 53
 during post-partum period, 54
 during transition, 53–54
 upon transfer to level II or III setting, 54
Parenteral feedings, 264–269
 administration of, 264
  central route in, 264
  general considerations in, 264
  monitoring schedule in, 264, 265t
  peripheral route in, 264
 calcium in, 267
 calories in, 267
 carbohydrates in, 266t, 266–267
 complications associated with, 267–269
  carbohydrates and, 268
  fat and, 267–268
  infection in, 268
  prevention of, 269
  protein and, 267
  vitamin imbalance in, 268
 fat in, 266, 266t
 guidelines in, 264–267
 indications for, 264
 minerals in, 267, 268t
 phosphorus in, 267
 protein in, 265–266, 266t
 vitamins in, 267, 267t
 water in, 265
Patent ductus arteriosus. See *Ductus arteriosus.*
Patent urachus, 383–384
Peak inspiratory pressure, 153
Pentobarbital, 160
Perihilar, 613

Periventricular-intraventricular hemorrhage, 412–414
  clinical presentation of, 412
  diagnostic studies in, 413
  grading system for, 412, *413*
  incidence of, 412
  outcome in, 413
  pathophysiology of, 412
  patient care management in, 413–414
Periventricular leukomalacia, 419–420
Persistent pulmonary hypertension, 105–110
  clinical presentation of, 106–107
    cardiovascular system in, 107
    history of hypoxia or asphyxia in, 106
    metabolic system in, 107
    respiratory system in, 106–107
  complications of, 107–108
  definition of, 105
  diagnosis of, 107
  differential diagnosis in, 107
  etiology of, 106
    pulmonary vascular bed in, 106
    pulmonary vasoconstriction in, 106
    pulmonary vessels in, 106
  management of, 108–110
    extracorporeal membrane oxygenation in, 110
    pharmacologic support in, 108–110. See also individual agents.
      analgesics/sedatives in, 109–110
      muscle relaxants in, 108–109
      pulmonary vasodilators in, 109
      vasopressors in, 109
    specialized monitoring in, 108
    stimulation in, 108
    supportive care in, 108
    ventilation in, 108
  outcome of, 110
  pathophysiology of, 106
  radiologic evaluation of, 627
Pharmacodynamics, 502–504
  definition of, 502
  drug action mechanisms in, 502–503
  drug dose and clinical response relationship in, 503
  effects of medications in, 503–504
  receptor concept in, 502
Pharmacokinetics, 502
Pharmacology, 501–518. See also under *Drugs.*
  definition of, 502
  pharmacodynamics in, 502–504
    drug action mechanisms in, 502–503
    drug dose and clinical response relationship in, 503
    effects of medications in, 503–504
    receptor concept in, 502
  pharmacokinetics in, *504,* 504–511
  principles of, 502–511
  terminology of, 502
Pharmacotherapy, 502
Phenobarbital, 416
Phenotype, 444
Phenylketonuria, 300–301
Phenytoin, 416
Phosphate, in total parenteral nutrition, 268t
Phosphatidylglycerol test, 8
Phospholipids, surface-active, 96
Phosphorus, in pre-term infant nutrition, 262–263
  in total parenteral nutrition, 267

Phrenic nerve paralysis, 410
Pigmented nevus, 477
Placenta, circulation and, 35–36
  labor and, 36
Placenta previa, 23–24
  assessment and management of, 24
    marginal placenta previa in, 24
    partial or total placenta previa in, 24
  clinical presentation of, 23–24
  definition of, 23
  incidence of, 23
  potential complications of, 24
  predisposing factors for, 23
Placental transport mechanisms, 16–17
  concentration gradient in, 16–17
  diffusing distance in, 17
  placental area in, 16
  uteroplacental blood flow in, 17
Plethora, in newborn assessment, 66
Pleural effusion, 613
Pneumomediastinum, 620, *621*
Pneumonia, 102–104, 353
  clinical presentation of, 103, 353
    physical examination in, 103
    prolonged labor in, 103
    signs and symptoms in, 103
  complications of, 104
  definition of, 102
  diagnosis of, 103–104, 353
  differential diagnosis of, 104
  etiology of, 102–103
    aspiration in, 103
    bacteria in, 102
    viruses in, 103
  incidence of, 102
  intrauterine, definition of, 102
    pathophysiology of, 103
  management of, 104
    antibiotic therapy in, 104
    blood pressure monitoring in, 104
  neonatal, definition of, 102
    pathophysiology of, 103
  outcome of, 104
  pathophysiology of, 103
  radiologic evaluation of, 619, *620*
  transmission of, 353
Pneumopericardium, 620–621, *621*
Pneumoperitoneum, *631,* 633
Pneumothorax, 619–620, *620*
Polycystic kidney disease, infantile, 376–378
  clinical assessment in, 377
  clinical presentation of, 376–377
  complications in, 377
  diagnostic studies in, 377
  differential diagnosis in, 377
  etiology of, 376
  incidence of, 376
  outcome of, 378
  patient care management in, 377
  physical examination in, 377
Polycythemia, 338–339
  in sick newborn, 50
  in small for gestational age infants, 65
Polydactyly, 72, 464
Polyploidy, 445
Port-wine stain, 478
  Sturge-Weber syndrome and, 478, *479*
Portal venous air, 633
Positioning techniques, 430–433
  areas of treatment in, 432

Positioning techniques (*Continued*)
  goals of, 430–431
  indications for, 432, *433*
  principles of, 431
  prone position in, 432
    benefits of, 432
    principles of, 432
  purpose of, 430
  side-lying position in, 432
    benefits of, 432
    principles of, 432
  strategies in, 431–432
  supine position in, 432
    flexor patterns and, 432
    principles of, 432
Positive airway pressure, continuous,
    endotracheal, 152
  in assisted ventilation, 152
  mask, 152
  nasal, 152
Positive end-expiratory pressure, in initiating
    assisted ventilation, 153–154
  inadvertent, 149
Posture, in gestational age assessment, 660
  in newborn assessment, 65
Potassium, 291–292
  disorders of, 291–292
  homeostasis of, 291
  in total parenteral nutrition, 268t
Potter's syndrome, *375*, 375–376
Pregnancy, diabetogenic effect of, 6
  endocrine changes during, 6
  metabolic changes during, 6
  physiologic anemia during, 5
  physiologic changes during, 4–6. See also
      individual systems and organs.
  post-term, 4
  pre-term, 4
  term, 4
Prematurity, signs and symptoms of, 9
Pre-term labor, 20–22
  assessment and management of, 21–22
    drug therapy in, 22
    education in, 21
    high-risk women in, 21–22
    screening in, 21
  clinical presentation of, 21
  definition of, 20
  incidence of, 20
  potential complications of, 21
  predisposing factors for, 21, 21t
Pronephros, 366
Protein, in pre-term infant nutrition, 259–260
  in total parenteral nutrition, 265–266, 266t
    complications associated with, 267
Prune-belly syndrome, 236–237
Pseudohermaphroditism, 69
  female, 316
  male, 316
Pseudomonas aeruginosa, antibiotics for, 421
  in neonatal infections, 355
Puerperium, 11–12
  breasts in, 12
  definition of, 11
  immunizations in, 12
  lochia in, 11
  placental site regeneration in, 11
  uterine involution in, 11
Pulmonary atresia, 220, 220–221
Pulmonary edema, *622*, *623*

Pulmonary hemorrhage, 119–120
Pulmonary hypertension, persistent. See
    Persistent pulmonary hypertension.
Pulmonary hypoplasia, 87, 119
Pulmonary interstitial emphysema, 617, *618*
Pulmonary stenosis, 219–220
  anatomy of, 219, *219*
  radiologic evaluation of, 627
Pulmonary surfactant system, 137
Pulmonary venous connection, total anomalous,
    223, 223–224
Pulse oximetry, in assisted ventilation, 155, *156*
  nursing care and, 162–163
Pustular melanosis, transient, 477
Pyloric stenosis, 238–239
  radiologic evaluation of, 630

Q

Quality assurance, 684–688
  assessment in, 685–686
    monitoring in, 686
      concurrent review in, 686
      prospective review in, 686
      retrospective review in, 686
    outcome components in, 685–686
    process components in, 685
    standards in, 685
    structure components in, 685
  definition of, 684–685
  evaluation in, 686–687
    data analysis in, 686
    plan of action in, 686–687
  interdisciplinary, 687
  plan for, 685
  trends in, 687
Quickening, 8

R

Rad, 613
Radial artery puncture, 640–641
Radiologic evaluation, 612–637. See also
    individual conditions and systems.
  basic concepts in, 612–613
  commonly used views in, 613–614, *614*
  radiographic densities in, 614
  terminology in, 613
  x-ray interpretation in, 614–615
    abdomen in, 615
    diaphragms in, 615
    heart in, 615
    respiratory system in, 615
    skeletal system in, 615
    thymus in, 615
    trachea in, 615
    tubes and catheters in, 615
Radiolucent, 613
Radiopaque, 613
Radius, absent, 465
Red reflex, 71
Reflex(es), gag, 72
  in newborn, 72
  protective, 128, 129, 131
  red, 71
  root, 72
  suck, 72
  swallow, 72

Renal failure, 369–373
  clinical assessment of, 371
  clinical presentation of, 370–371
  complications of, 372
  definition of, 369
  diagnostic studies in, 371
    blood in, 371
    ultrasound in, 371
    urinalysis in, 371
  differential diagnosis in, 371–372
  etiology of, 369–370
    post-renal in, 370
    pre-renal in, 369–370
    renal parenchymal in, 370
  incidence of, 370
  outcome in, 373
  patient care management in, 372–373
  states of, 370
Renal vein thrombosis, 381–382
Research, 653–663
  basic principles of, 653–655
  conceptual framework development in, 657
  data measurement planning in, 659
  definition of study purpose in, 656
  design selection in, 658
  dissemination of findings in, 660
  ethics in, 654–655
  hypothesis formation in, 658
  implications for nursing in, 661–663
    acceptance promotion in, 662
    participation prerogatives in, 661–662
    question provision in, 662
    study outcomes dissemination in, 662–663
  interpretation of findings in, 659–660
  literature review in, 656–657
  methods of, 654
  problem identification in, 656
  process of, 656–660
  purposes of, 653–654
  question identification in, 655–656
    clinical patient care experience in, 655
    nursing practice questions in, 655–656
    study feasibility in, 656
  role of, 660–661
    intellectual stimulation in, 661
    quality of care issues in, 660–661
  sample selection in, 658–659
  study limitations in, 657
  study terms in, 658
Resistance, in assisted ventilation, 149
Respiration, in newborn assessment, 65–66, 67
  physiology of, 97
    first breath and, 97
    in utero, 97
    pulmonary adaptation and, 97
    stimulation to breathe and, 97
  stimulation of, 83
Respiratory disorders, 98–122. See also
        individual disorders.
  apnea and, 128
  due to cardiovascular and hematologic
      disorders, 122
  due to central nervous system disorders,
      121–122
  due to diaphragmatic disorders, 122
  due to renal disorders, 122
  due to thoracic disorders, 121
  due to upper airway disorders, 120–121
Respiratory distress syndrome, 98–102
  clinical course of, 100

Respiratory distress syndrome (*Continued*)
  clinical presentation of, 99
    lung compliance in, 99
    prematurity in, 99
    respiratory difficulty in, 99
  complications of, 100–101
    cardiovascular, 100
    hematologic, 101
    metabolic, 101
    neurologic, 101
    oliguric, 101
    pulmonary, 100
    secondary infectious, 101
  definition of, 98
  diagnosis of, 99–100
  differential diagnosis in, 100
  etiology of, 98
    precipitating factors in, 98
    unlikely factors in, 98
  incidence of, 98
  management of, 101
    antibiotics in, 101
    blood pressure monitoring in, 101
    sodium bicarbonate in, 101
    supportive, 101
  outcome of, 101
  pathophysiology of, 98–99
    lack of surfactant in, 99
    pulmonary adaptation prerequisites in, 98
    pulmonary ischemia in, 99
    very immature infant and, 99
  prevention of, 101
  surfactant replacement therapy for, 136–137.
        See also *Exosurf Neonatal; Survanta.*
Respiratory system, adaptation at birth of, 38, 40
    lung compliance and, 40
    stimuli for initiating respiration and, 38
    surfactant and, 40
    thoracic squeeze and, 40
  of sick newborn, clinical presentations and,
      49–50
  physical assessment and, 47
  physiologic changes in, 4
  radiologic evaluation of, 616–622. See also
        individual parts and conditions.
Resuscitation, 76–90
  abdominal wall defects and, 87–88
  airway opening in, 82, 83–84
    mouth and nares suctioning in, 83–84
    positioning for, 83, *83*
  anatomy and physiology and, 77–78
  anteriorly situated glottis and, 77
  asphyxia physiology and, 78
    meconium in, 78
    tissue hypoxia in, 78
  bag and mask ventilation in, 84
  bag to endotracheal tube ventilation in, 84–85
  breathing and, 77, 82
  chemical, 85–87
    drugs and solutions used in, 85–87, 86t.
        See also individual types.
    indications for, 85
  chest compressions in, 85
  choanal atresia and, 88
  circulation in, 82
  complications of, 89
  decision making process in, 81, *82*
  decreased muscle mass and, 77
  decreased subcutaneous fat and, 77
  definition of, 76

Resuscitation (*Continued*)
  drugs/medication in, 82
  environment in, 82
  equipment for, 80–81
  evaluation in, 84
  extremely low birthweight infant and, 89
  head size to body size ratio and, 77
  hypothermia prevention in, 83
  immature systems and, 77
  initial steps in, 82–84
  neural tube defects and, 88
  oxygen in, 84
  positive-pressure ventilation in, 84–85
  post-resuscitation care in, 89–90
    arterial blood gases and, 89
    family support in, 90
    fluids/electrolytes in, 90
    glucose monitoring in, 89
    infection screening in, 90
    vital signs monitoring in, 90
    x-rays in, 89–90
  preparation for, 79–89
    delivery room in, 80
    general, 80
    non-delivery room, 80
    personnel in, 80
  pulmonary hypoplasia and, 87
  respiration stimulation in, 83
  risk factors in, 78–79
    intrapartum, 79
    post-partum, 79
    pre-partum (maternal), 79
  short neck and, 77
  surface area to body size ratio and, 77
  undiagnosed multiple gestation and, 88
  venous access and, 77, 78
Retained lung fluid syndrome, 104–105
Retinopathy of prematurity, 492–495
  complications of, 494
  etiology of, 493
  incidence of, 493
  outcome in, 495
  pathophysiology of, 493
  patient care in, 494–495
    cryotherapy in, 495
    parent education in, 495
    precautions in, 494
    results in, 494
    sensory stimulation in, 494
  physical examination in, 494
Retrolental fibroplasia. See *Retinopathy of prematurity.*
Rh incompatibility, 329–330
  definition of, 329
  infant presentation in, 330
  predisposing factors in, 329–330
  prophylactic therapy for, 330
Rib, fracture of, 635, *635*
Roentgen, 613
Root reflex, 72
Rotation, 613
Rubella syndrome, congenital, 481, *481*, 495–497
  clinical presentation in, 496
  complications of, 496
  etiology of, 496
  incidence of, 496
  outcome in, 497
  pathophysiology of, 495–496
  patient care in, 496
 in neonatal infections, 358

S
Scalp, 70–71
Screw Principle of Woods, for shoulder dystocia, 26
Scrotum, 69
Seizures, 414–416
  clinical presentations of, 415
  definition of, 414
  diagnostic studies in, 415
  focal clonic, 415
  genetic, 414–415
  intracerebral meningitis in, 414
  lorazepam for, 416
  metabolic encephalopathies in, 414
  multifocal clonic, 415
  myoclonic, 415
  outcome in, 416, 416t
  pathophysiology of, 414–415
  patient care management in, 416
  phenobarbital for, 416
  phenytoin for, 416
  structural, 414
  subtle, 415
  tonic, 415
  withdrawal from maternal drugs in, 414
Selenium, 268t
Sepsis, 353
  in sick newborn, 51
  incidence of, 353
  presentation of, 353
Sex chromosome, 444
Sexual development, disorders of, 314–320
  clinical assessment of, 317
    findings in, 317, *317–318*
    genitalia examination in, 317
  clinical presentation of, 316–317
  diagnosis of, 318
  patient care management in, 318–320
    care of parents in, 319
    gender assignment in, 318–319
    outcome of, 319–320
    treatment in, 319
 in embryo/fetus, 314–315
    genital duct differentiation in, *315*, 315–316
    gonad development in, 315
    gonadal differentiation in, 315
Shock, 227–229
  cardiogenic, 227
  clinical indications of, 228
    blood volume indicators in, 228
    cardiac function indicators in, 228
    cardiopulmonary status changes in, 228
    coagulation defects in, 228
    metabolic disturbances in, 228
    septic shock indicators in, 228
    urinary output in, 228
  definition of, 227
  distributive, 228
  hypovolemic, 227
  management of, 228–229
    acidosis in, 228
    blood volume and red cell mass in, 229
    cardiac output in, 229
    digitalis in, 227t, 229
    dobutamine in, 229
    dopamine in, 229
    inotropic agents in, 229
    isoproterenol in, 229
   fluid and electrolyte balance in, 228
   infectious process and, 229

Shock (*Continued*)
    oxygenation and ventilation in, 228
Shoulder dystocia, 25–26
Simian crease, 72
Skeletal system, 462
    appendicular skeleton in, 462
    axial skeleton in, 462
    changes during pregnancy to, 5
    joints in, 462
    radiologic evaluation of, 634–635. See also
        individual parts and conditions.
Skin, 471–483
    anatomy of, 471–472, 472
    appearance of, factors affecting, 474
    assessment of, 474
    benign lesions of, 74
    care of, 473–474
        pre-term infant in, 473
        term infant in, 473
        umbilical cord in, 474
    dermis in, 472
    differences in, 473
    epidermis in, 472
    functions of, 472
    in gestational age assessment, 60
    in newborn assessment, 65, 73–74
    lesions of, 474–483. See also individual
        conditions.
        definitions in, 474
        hereditary, 481–483
        infectious, 480–481
        pigmented, 476–477
        vascular, 477–480
    normal variations in, 474–476
    of sick newborn, physical assessment and, 47
    physiologic changes in, 4
    subcutaneous layer, 472
Skinfold, 613
Skull fractures, 408–409
    radiologic evaluation of, 635
Sleep state, apnea and, 128
Sodium, 290–291
    disorders of, 290–291
    homeostasis of, 290
    in total parenteral nutrition, 268t
Sodium bicarbonate, in neonatal resuscitation,
        82, 86–87
    in respiratory distress syndrome, 101
Sole creases, 60
Spider angiomata, 4
Spine, 68
Spironolactone, 157–158
Standard of care, 673–674
    definition of, 673–674
    expert witnesses testimony in, 674
    institutional policies and procedures in, 674
    professional literature in, 674
    professional organizations standards in, 674
    reasonableness and prudence in, 674
    state and federal regulations in, 674
Staphylococcus aureus, antibiotics for, 421
    in neonatal infections, 354
Staphylococcus epidermidis, antibiotics for, 421
    in neonatal infections, 355
Stomach. See also under *Gastro*.
    radiologic evaluation of, 629–630
Streptococcus, group B, antibiotics for, 421
    in neonatal infections, 354
Striae gravidarum (stretch marks), 4
Sturge-Weber syndrome, port-wine stain and,
        478, 479

Subarachnoid hemorrhage, 411
Subdural hemorrhage, 410–411
Subgaleal hemorrhage, 408
Substance abuse, case study of, 589–592
    management in, 590
    presenting problem in, 590
    perinatal, 523–535. See also individual
        substances.
        breast-feeding and, 534
            AIDS in, 534
            alcohol in, 534
            cocaine and methamphetamines in, 534
            heroin in, 534
            marijuana in, 534
            nicotine in, 534
        ethical considerations and, 534–535
        legal issues and, 534
        management recommendations in, 532–533
        maternal-infant relationship in, 532
        nursing intervention in, 533
        problems associated with, 531–532
        psychological profile in, 532
Suck reflex, 72
Sucking blisters, 74
Supine hypotension, 5
Surfactant, adaptation at birth and, 40
    clinical use of, 138–145. See also *Exosurf
        Neonatal; Survanta*.
    definition of, 96
    functional characteristics of, 137
    historical overview of, 137
    pulmonary surfactant system and, 137
    replacement, artificial lung-expanding
        compound as, 138
        Exosurf Neonatal as, 138
        modified natural surfactants as, 138
        natural human surfactant as, 138
        synthetic surfactants as, 138
        types of, 138
        whole surfactant as, 138
Surfactant replacement therapy, 136–146
    respiratory distress syndrome and, 136–137.
        See also *Exosurf Neonatal; Survanta*.
Survanta, 142–145
    acute clinical effects of, 145
    administration guidelines for, 144–145
    dosage administration for, 144–145
    patient positioning and, 145
    prevention protocol for, 142–143
    prevention treatment criteria for, 144
    recommendations for use of, 144
    rescue treatment criteria for, 144
    rescue treatment study of, 143
        criteria for, 143
        hyaline membrane disease and, 143
            administration procedure in, 143
            criteria for, 143
            exclusion criteria for, 143
    solution preparation for, 144
    ventilator settings and, 145
Swallow reflex, 72
Syndactyly, 72, 464–465
Syphilis, 361–362

T
Tachycardia, 66
Tachypnea, transient, 618, *619*
Talipes equinovarus, 73, 467

Technical procedures, 638–649. *See also individual procedures, e.g. Capillary blood sampling.*
Teenage. *See Adolescence.*
Testes, 69
Tetralogy of Fallot, 218–219
    anatomy of, 218, *218*
    radiologic evaluation of, 627
Theophylline, in bronchopulmonary dysplasia, 114
    in methylxanthine therapy, 132
        caffeine vs., 132
Thoracentesis, 643–644
Thrombocytopenia, 336–338
    clinical assessment of, 337
    clinical presentation of, 337
    complications of, 338
    definition of, 336
    diagnostic studies in, 337
    differential diagnosis in, 337
    etiologic factors in, 336–337
        impaired platelet production in, 337
        platelet destruction in, 336–337
        platelet interference in, 337
    outcome of, 338
    patient care management in, 338
    physical examination in, 337
Thromboembolism, during pregnancy, 6
Thrush, 72, 357–358, 480
Thymus, 616
Thyroid gland, anatomy of, 307
    changes during pregnancy in, 6
    fetal development of, 307
    functions of, 307
    hormones of, 307
    physiology of, at birth, 307
Tidal volume, 149
Tolazoline, in persistent pulmonary hypertension of newborn, 109
    in ventilation therapy, 159
Torticollis, 465–466
    definition of, 465, *466*
    intervention in, 466
    muscular defect in, 465
    physical examination in, 466
    radiologic examination in, 466
    skeletal defect in, 465–466
Toxoplasmosis, 361, 498–499
    in neonatal infections, 361
Trachea, obstruction of, 121
    radiologic evaluation of, 616
Tracheoesophageal fistula, *237*, 237–238
    esophageal atresia with, 628, *629*
    radiologic evaluation of, 628–629
Transfusion therapy, 340
    erythropoietin, 340
    exchange, 340, 356
    for neonatal infections, 356
    intravenous immune globulin in, 356
    neutrophil, 356
    partial exchange, 340
    reactions to, 340–341
    replacement, 340
Transition nursery, eye care and, 44
    glucose needs and, 45–46
        feeding and, 46
            evaluation prior to, 46
            guidelines for, 46
            sterile water test feeding in, 46

Transition nursery (*Continued*)
    screening blood glucose determination and, 45–46
    hepatitis vaccine and, 45, 694t
    medications in, 44–47
    ongoing family education in, 46–47
    transfer from, 47
    vitamin K and, 44–45
        dosage of, 44–45
        function of, 45
        maternal risk factors and, 45
Translocation, 445
Transport, 573–583
    back/return, 574–575
    documentation in, 581
        logistic, 581
        patient care, 581
    environment in, 581
        altitude in, 581
        dysbarism in, 581
        effects of motion in, 581
        noise and vibration in, 581
    equipment in, 577–579
        intravenous therapy, 577t–578t
        medications in, 578t–579t
        recommended, 577
        respiratory, 577t
        thermoregulation and monitoring, 578t
    ethical issues in, 582
    historical, 573–574
    legal issues in, 582, *582*
    maternal, neonatal outcomes and, 574
    one-way, 574
    peer review in, 583
    personnel in, 576–577
        EMT/paramedics in, 576
        physicians in, 576
        registered nurses in, 576
        requirements for, 577
        respiratory therapists in, 576
        roles for, 576
        selection of, 576
        team composition in, 576
    philosophy of, 574–575
    process for, 579–580
        en route to receiving hospital in, 580
        en route to referral hospital in, 580
        referral call in, 579
        stabilization at referral hospital in, 580
    quality control in, 582–583
    quality improvement in, 583
    two-way, 574
    vehicle selection in, 575–576
        ambulance in, 575
        fixed-wing aircraft in, 575–576
        general considerations in, 575
        helicopters in, 575
Transposition of great vessels, 216–217, *217*
Transpyloric feedings, 274–275
    advantages of, 275
    disadvantages of, 275
    indications for, 274
    procedure for, 275
Trauma, birth, 62
    neonatal resuscitation and, 89
Traumatic nerve palsy, 410
Tricuspid atresia, *221*, 221–222
Trisomy 13, 458
Trisomy 18, 457–458
Trisomy 21, 456–457

Truncus arteriosus, 222, 222–223
Turner's syndrome, 316, 459

U
Ultrasound, in fetal anomalies diagnosis, 447
Umbilical artery catheterization, 646–649
    complications of, 648–649
    equipment for, 646
    indications for, 646
    precautions in, 646
    procedure for, 647–648, 647–648
    radiologic evaluation of, 636–637, 637
Umbilical blood sampling, percutaneous, 449
Umbilical cord, cardiovascular adaptation at
        birth and, 38
    catheters for, dangers of, 89
    in newborn assessment, 68
Umbilical cord prolapse, 24–25
Umbilical vessel catheters, neonatal resuscitation
        and, 89
Universal precautions, 362
Urachus, patent, 383–384
Ureters, physiological changes in, 5
Urinary bladder, 68
    exstrophy of, 385–387
        clinical assessment in, 386
        clinical presentation of, 385–386
        complications in, 386–387
        definition of, 385, 386
        differential diagnosis in, 386
        disease states in, 385
        etiology of, 385
        incidence of, 385
        outcome in, 387
        patient care management in, 387
        physical assessment in, 386
Urinary system, anatomy of, gross, 366
        microscopic, 366–367
    blood flow in, 367
    disorders of, 365–390. See also individual
            disorders.
    embryology of, 365–366
        kidney in, 366
        urinary tract in, 366
        vascular supply in, 366
    hemodynamics of, 367
    neonatal resuscitation and, 77
    physiologic changes in, 5
        glomerular filtration rate and, 5
        kidney enlargement and, 5
    physiology of, 368–369
        acid-base balance in, 369
        concentration and dilution mechanism in,
            369
        glomerular filtration in, 368
        post-natal changes in, 368
        tubular function in, 368–369
Urinary tract infections, 354, 382–383
    antibiotics in, 354
    clinical manifestations of, 354, 382–383
    common pathogens in, 354
    complications in, 383
    diagnostic studies in, 383
    differential diagnosis in, 383
    disease states in, 382
    etiology of, 382
    outcome in, 383
    patient care management in, 383

V
Vascular nevi, 74
Vater association, 459–460
Venipuncture, 640
Venoarterial perfusion, 178–179
Ventilation, 148–167
    airway management in, 161
    assisted, initiating, 153–154
        types of, 153
    bag and mask, 84
    bag to endotracheal tube, 84–85
    blood gas interpretation in, 164–167
        acceptable values in, 164, 164t
        compensation/correction of acidosis-
            alkalosis in, 165–166, 166t
        process of, 167
        respiratory/metabolic acidosis and alkalosis
            in, 164–165
    blood gas measurement in, 156
    Boyle's law and, 149
    compliance in, 149
    control of breathing and, 151, 151t
    Dalton's law and, 150
    elastic recoil in, 149
    equipment function in, 161–162
    functional residual capacity in, 149
    gas trapping in, 149
    Henry's law and, 150
    high-frequency, 170–176
        bronchopulmonary dysplasia prevention
            and, 175
        definition of, 170
        diaphragmatic hernia treatment and, 175
        flow-interrupted, 172
        gas exchange mechanisms and, 170–171,
            171
        hypoplastic lungs treatment and, 175
        indications for, 172
        jet, complications of, 175
            definition of, 172
            entrainment during, 171, 171
            parameters for, 173–174
            patient care and, 174, 174–175
            ventilator design for, 173
        oscillatory, complications of, 173
            definition of, 172
            parameters for, 173
            patient care and, 173
            ventilator design for, 172–173
        persistent pulmonary hypertension
            treatment and, 175
        physiology of, 170–171
        positive-pressure, 172
        respiratory distress syndrome treatment
            and, 175
    inadvertent positive end-expiratory pressure
        in, 149
    Laplace's law and, 150–151
    mean airway pressure in, 149
    monitoring and, 162–163
    negative-pressure, intermittent, 153
    nursing care and, 161–163
    oxygen therapy and, 152–153
        assisted ventilation and, 152–153
        continuous positive airway pressure in,
            152
        nasal cannula in, 152
        oxyhood in, 152
    patient care in, 153–154
    physical assessment in, 154

Ventilation (*Continued*)
    auscultation in, 154
    observation in, 154, *155*
    physiology in, 149–151
    positive-pressure, 84–85
      intermittent, 153
    pulse oximetry in, 155, *156*
    resistance in, 149
    tidal volume in, 149
    total lung capacity in, 149
    transcutaneous monitoring in, 155–156
    ventilation-perfusion ratio in, 149, *150*
    vital capacity in, 149
    weaning from ventilator in, 163–164
      extubating in, 163–164
      indications for, 163
      nursing care and, 164
      techniques for, 163
    work of breathing in, 149
Ventilation-perfusion ratio, 149, *150*
Ventilation therapy, medications used during,
    156–161. See also individual drugs.
Ventricular septal defect, 209–210, *210*
Viral infections. See *Infections, viral.*
Vital capacity, 149
Vitamin A, in pre-term infant nutrition, 261–262
    deficiency of, 261–262
    excess of, 262
    function of, 261

Vitamin A (*Continued*)
  in total parenteral nutrition, 267t
    complications associated with, 268
Vitamin B, 267t
Vitamin C, 267t
Vitamin D, in pre-term infant nutrition, 262
  in total parenteral nutrition, 267t
Vitamin E, in pre-term infant nutrition, 262
  in total parenteral nutrition, 267t
Vitamin K, for newborn, 44–45
    dosage of, 44–45
    function of, 45
    maternal risk factors and, 45
  in pre-term infant nutrition, 262
  in total parenteral nutrition, 267t
Volume expanders, in neonatal resuscitation, 82,
    86

W
Work of breathing, in assisted ventilation, 149

Z
Zinc, in pre-term infant nutrition, 263–264
  in total parenteral nutrition, 268t